PATHOLOGY ANNUAL

PART 1

1982

SERIES EDITORS

SHELDON C. SOMMERS, M.D.

Consultant Pathologist, Lenox Hill Hospital, New York, New York; Clinical Professor of Pathology, Columbia University College of Physicians and Surgeons, New York, New York; Clinical Professor of Pathology, University of Southern California School of Medicine, Los Angeles, California

PAUL PETER ROSEN, M.D.

Attending Pathologist, Memorial Hospital for Cancer and Allied Diseases, Memorial Sloan-Kettering Cancer Center, New York, New York; Associate Member, Sloan-Kettering Institute, New York, New York; Associate Professor of Pathology, Cornell University Medical College, New York, New York

PATHOLOGY ANNUAL

PART 1

VOLUME 17

1982

ACC APPLETON-CENTURY-CROFTS/Norwalk, Connecticut

82 83 84 85 86/10 9 8 7 6 5 4 3 2 1

Library of Congress Catalog Card Number: 66–20355

Prentice-Hall International, Inc., London
Prentice-Hall of Australia, Pty. Ltd., Sydney
Prentice-Hall of India Private Limited, New Delhi
Prentice-Hall of Japan, Inc., Tokyo
Prentice-Hall of Southeast Asia (Pte.) Ltd., Singapore
Whitehall Books Ltd., Wellington, New Zealand

PRINTED IN THE UNITED STATES OF AMERICA
0–8385–7765–2

CONTRIBUTORS

Kenneth W. Barwick, M.D.
Assistant Professor of Pathology, Yale University Hospital, New Haven, Connecticut

Robert R. Belliveau, M.D.
Chairman, Department of Pathology, Southern Nevada Memorial Hospital, Las Vegas, Nevada

Bruce L. Bender, M.D.
Pathologist, Forbes Health System, East Suburban Health Center, Monroeville, Pennsylvania (Formerly Assistant Professor of Pathology, Department of Pathology, University of Pittsburgh School of Medicine; Pathologist, Department of Pathology, Presbyterian-University Hospital, Pittsburgh, Pennsylvania)

John W. Bolen, M.D.
Assistant Professor of Pathology, University of Washington, Seattle, Washington

Joel N. Buxbaum, M.D.
Professor of Medicine, Department of Medicine, New York University School of Medicine; General Medical Research, New York Veterans Administration Medical Center, New York, New York

Maria M. Dabska, M.D.
Professor and Chief, Department of Pathology, Maria Sklodowska-Curie Memorial Institute of Oncology, Warsaw, Poland

Ivan Damjanov, M.D.
Professor of Pathology, Department of Pathology and Laboratory Medicine, Hahnemann Medical College, Philadelphia, Pennsylvania

Frederick R. Eilber, M.D.
Professor of Surgery, Division of Oncology, Department of Surgery, UCLA School of Medicine, Los Angeles, California; Surgical Service, Veterans Administration Hospital, Sepulveda, California

Diane C. Farhi, M.D.
Instructor, Department of Pathology, University of Colorado Health Sciences Center, Denver, Colorado

Helen D. Feiner, M.D.
Assistant Professor of Pathology, Department of Pathology, New York University School of Medicine, New York, New York

Arnold J. Felsenfeld, M.D.
Assistant Professor of Medicine, University of Oklahoma Health Sciences Center and Veterans Administration Medical Center, Oklahoma City, Oklahoma

Gerald Fine, M.D.
Chief, Division of Anatomic Pathology, Department of Pathology, Henry Ford Hospital, Detroit, Michigan; Clinical Professor of Pathology, Medical School, University of Michigan, Ann Arbor, Michigan

William J. Frable, M.D.
Professor of Surgical Pathology, Virginia Commonwealth University, Health Sciences Division, Medical College of Virginia, Richmond, Virginia

Gloria R. Gallo, M.D., M.S.
Associate Professor of Pathology, Department of Pathology, New York University School of Medicine, New York, New York

Steven I. Hajdu, M.D.
Attending Pathologist, Chief of the Cytology Service, Memorial Sloan-Kettering Cancer Center; Associate Professor of Pathology, Cornell University Medical College, New York, New York

Michael Kashgarian, M.D.
Professor of Pathology, Yale University Hospital, New Haven, Connecticut

Tadeusz Koszarowski, M.D.
Professor of Surgery, Director of the Maria Sklodowska-Curie Memorial Institute of Oncology, Warsaw, Poland

Francisco Llach, M.D.
Professor of Medicine, University of Oklahoma Health Sciences Center and Veterans Administration Medical Center, Oklahoma City, Oklahoma

Gregor Mikuz, M.D.
Assistant Professor of Pathology, Department of Pathology, University School of Medicine, University of Innsbruck, Innsbruck, Austria

Donald L. Morton, M.D.
Professor and Chief, Division of Oncology, Department of Surgery, UCLA School of Medicine, Los Angeles, California; Surgical Service, Veterans Administration Hospital, Sepulveda, California

William M. Murphy, M.D.
Associate Professor of Pathology and Urology, Baptist Memorial Hospital, Memphis, Tennessee

George K. Nagy, M.D.
Pathologist, St. Vincent Hospital; Associate Professor of Pathology, University of Massachusetts Medical School, Worcester, Massachusetts

Derrick J. Pounder, MB, ChB, FRCPA
Specialist Pathologist, Division of Tissue Pathology, Institute of Medical and Veterinary Science, Adelaide, South Australia

Ali H. Qizilbash, M.B., B.S., F.R.C.P.(C)
Head, Cytopathology, Department of Pathology, St. Joseph's Hospital; Professor of Pathology, McMaster University, Hamilton, Ontario

Paul Peter Rosen, M.D.
Attending Pathologist, Memorial Hospital for Cancer and Allied Diseases, Memorial Sloan-Kettering Cancer Center, New York, New York; Associate Professor of Pathology, Cornell University Medical College, New York, New York

Robert Rowland, BSc(Hons), MB, BS, MRCPath, FRCPA
Deputy Head of Division of Tissue Pathology, Institute of Medical and Veterinary Science, Adelaide, South Australia

Gurdip S. Sidhu, M.D.
Pathologist and Director, Electron Microscopy Laboratory, New York Veterans Administration Medical Center; Assistant Professor of Pathology, New York University School of Medicine, New York, New York

Steven G. Silverberg, M.D.
Professor of Pathology and Chief of Anatomic Pathology, The George Washington University Medical Center, Washington, D.C.

Mark S. Soloway, M.D.
Professor of Urology, University of Tennessee Center for the Health Sciences, Memphis, Tennessee

Herman D. Suit, M.D.
Chief, Department of Radiation Medicine, Massachusetts General Hospital; Professor of Radiation Therapy, Harvard Medical School, Boston, Massachusetts

David Thorning, M.D.
Associate Professor of Pathology, University of Washington; Chief, Electron Microscopy, Veteran's Administration Medical Center, Seattle, Washington

Sharon W. Weiss, M.D.
Assistant Chairman, Department of Soft Tissue Pathology, Armed Forces Institute of Pathology, Washington, D.C.

Eduardo J. Yunis, M.D.
Professor of Pathology, Department of Pathology, University of Pittsburgh School of Medicine; Chief, Department of Pathology, Children's Hospital of Pittsburgh, Pittsburgh, Pennsylvania

CONTENTS

PATHOLOGY ANNUAL

PART 1

1982

PATHOLOGIC STUDIES IN COLORECTAL CANCER

A Guide to the Surgical Pathology Examination of Colorectal Specimens and Review of Features of Prognostic Significance

ALI H. QIZILBASH

Cancer of the colon and rectum is becoming the most important malignancy in North America today. It is second in mortality to cancer of the lung in men and of the breast in women.[1] In 1981, approximately 120,000 new cases of colorectal cancer will be diagnosed in the United States.[1]

There are approximately 500,000 living persons in the United States who have cancer of the colorectum.[2] Mortality figures show that there has been little change since 1950[1] in the survival rate for such cancer; the 5-year survival rates for the period 1950 to 1959 were 42 percent for males and 46 percent for females. For the period 1965 to 1969 the rates were 43 and 46 percent, respectively.

Surgical specimens from patients with tumors of the colorectum continue to be among the tissue specimens most frequently examined by pathologists. The way in which this examination is done, and the final reporting of the results, play an important role in assessing the prognosis. The clinical staging of colorectal cancer is not accurate because of the difficulty encountered in clinically assessing the extent of the disease. However, the careful and systematic examination of surgical specimens gives the clinician valuable information regarding the configuration and grade of a lesion, the extent of spread, and the extent of vascular and lymphatic invasion if any—factors which have an important bearing on the patient's ultimate survival. Additionally, with increasing interest in more individualized methods of treatment for cancer of the large bowel, accurately compiled pathologic data assist in delineating patients suitable for local treatment or adjuvant chemotherapy.

Analysis of surgical pathology reports show that no uniform standard for reporting exists, and some workers have compiled essential information for pathology reports.[3] The American Joint Committee for Cancer Staging and End Result Reporting[4] has developed a system of clinical and pathologic staging—the

TNM system—for the purpose of standardizing the classification of cancer in various sites. The TNM system provides a basis for categorizing the extent of disease; essential site-specific information is recorded on standard data forms. The method of reporting used is not crucial as long as the factors important in making the prognosis are accurately recorded.

The surgical pathologist has an important role to play in the emerging multidisciplinary setting in the treatment of patients with cancer in various organs. The time-honored triad of pathologist, radiologist, and surgeon must now be expanded to include the radiotherapist and the oncologist or chemotherapist. It is not only enough to be able to make a diagnosis—prior knowledge of the patient and the results of previous investigations and biopsy are important in the subsequent handling of surgical specimens.

GENERAL CONSIDERATIONS

The surgical pathologist is responsible for the pathology specimen once it is removed from the patient. It is his responsibility to make sure that the specimen is properly handled and promptly delivered to the processing laboratory. All large specimens should be sent in the fresh state to prevent distortion by fixatives. The bowel undergoes considerable shrinkage on fixation, with the result that the adequacy of the resected margins may be underestimated if measurements are taken following fixation. Bowel specimens should be examined right away and not left to be handled at the end of the day, after the other, smaller specimens have been examined.

An accurate and detailed gross examination of the specimen is important and cannot be overemphasized. This should be supplemented by photographs of the specimen in the fresh state where possible. In addition, we have found line drawings depicting the lesions and relationships to important landmarks and margins to be very useful. Fixation of the specimen is necessary before blocks are taken for sections, and care should be taken in handling specimens in preparation for fixation. If any washing is required—such as the flushing of feces out of the bowel—it should be done with a weak solution of formalin or isotonic saline, and not with tap water. The choice of fixative is a personal matter, but we have found a 10 percent dilution of 40 percent formaldehyde in normal saline, buffered to neutrality, to be a satisfactory fixative. Although formalin penetrates slowly, the tissues do not harden unduly even after prolonged fixation, and the results are good if prior specimen preparation is adequate. It takes from 24 to 48 hours before a specimen of bowel is fixed satisfactorily, enabling adequate blocks to be taken. In my experience, frozen sections are rarely employed unless the resection margin is very close to the tumor, or when they are necessitated by some unexpected finding at surgery.

METHOD OF EXAMINATION OF THE LARGE-BOWEL SPECIMEN

The unopened specimen received from the operating room should be carefully examined, with note taken of the external features. The segment of the bowel should be identified—as for example, whether it is from a right hemicolectomy, a sigmoid resection, or an abdominoperineal excision. The length of the bowel and its diameter both above and below the lesion are recorded. Note is made if the appendix or a segment of terminal ileum are present, and their measurements and characteristics are recorded. The amount and features of the mesentery are next recorded. Note is made of the appearance of the serosa of the bowel. Any other lesions noted grossly, such as diverticula, perforations, or tumor deposits, are recorded.

Once the initial gross examination described above is completed, the specimen should be prepared for fixation. Some workers[5] advocate inflating the specimens with formalin. Although this is a good method for preserving specimens for museum purposes, I personally favor, for routine purposes, the alternate method described below. Following gross examination, the specimen is opened lengthwise along the antimesenteric border. In case of the rectum and anus, it is cut open with scissors along the midline anteriorly. A slight deviation may be necessary to avoid cutting through the tumor. The mucosa is then gently rinsed to get rid of the feces. The size of the tumor (in three dimensions) and the site are next recorded. Multiple cancers should be described and labeled separately (Fig. 1). The relationship of the lesion to the pectinate line, ileocecal valve, or other landmarks is noted. The color, consistency, and configuration of the tumor should be recorded. It is important to accurately record if the tumor is polypoid and involving, for instance, only one-fourth of the circumference of the bowel, or whether it is a constrictive, napkin-ring type of lesion causing complete obstruction.

The tumor should next be sliced through the region of deepest penetration to note the extent of local spread (Fig. 2). In the majority of cases, gross examination will give a fairly good idea of the extent of local spread. However, this should always be confirmed histologically. The distance of the tumor from the resected margins should be recorded. Any other lesions—for example, polyps—and their size, number, location, etc., should be noted. The length of the stalks should be recorded. The presence of diverticula and changes of inflammatory bowel disease, such as ischemia or ulcerative colitis, should be documented.

The presence or absence of lymphatic spread is next studied. The best way to examine the lymph nodes is to turn the specimen over and cut a series of thin slices through the extrarectal and colonic tissues from the outside in, hinging these slices on the uncut wall of the bowel. The lymph nodes can easily be felt and seen, and can be removed for microscopic study. Another way of looking for lymph nodes is to remove the glands in groups, for example, fatty tissue containing lymph nodes is removed separately from the immediate vicinity of the cancer, as well as fatty tissue distal or proximal to the tumor. The topmost glands located at the point of ligation of the vascular pedicle should always be identified. Following separation of the fat containing the various groups of lymph nodes, the search for the lymph nodes is undertaken. The lymph nodes are separated from the fat and put in a fixative overnight. The nodes are identified as to location.

No difficulty is usually encountered in finding large lymph nodes involved by cancer. However, finding normal-sized lymph nodes may pose a problem for the inexperienced. I have found that sampling lymph nodes is easier before fixation, when lymph nodes appear light pink to gray in color in contrast to the yellow color of the surrounding fatty tissue. After fixation in formalin, the nodes appear pale

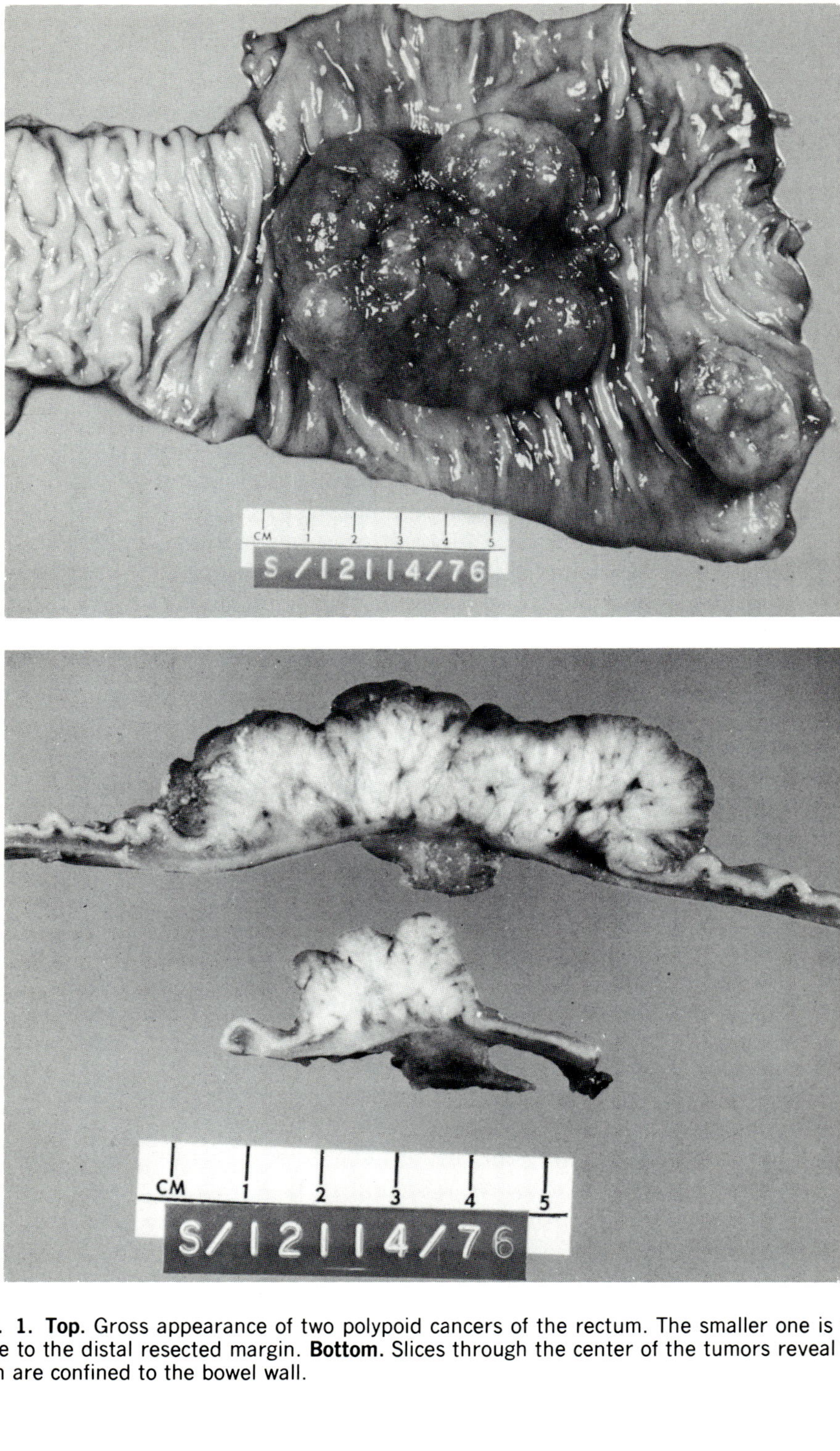

FIG. 1. Top. Gross appearance of two polypoid cancers of the rectum. The smaller one is very close to the distal resected margin. **Bottom.** Slices through the center of the tumors reveal that both are confined to the bowel wall.

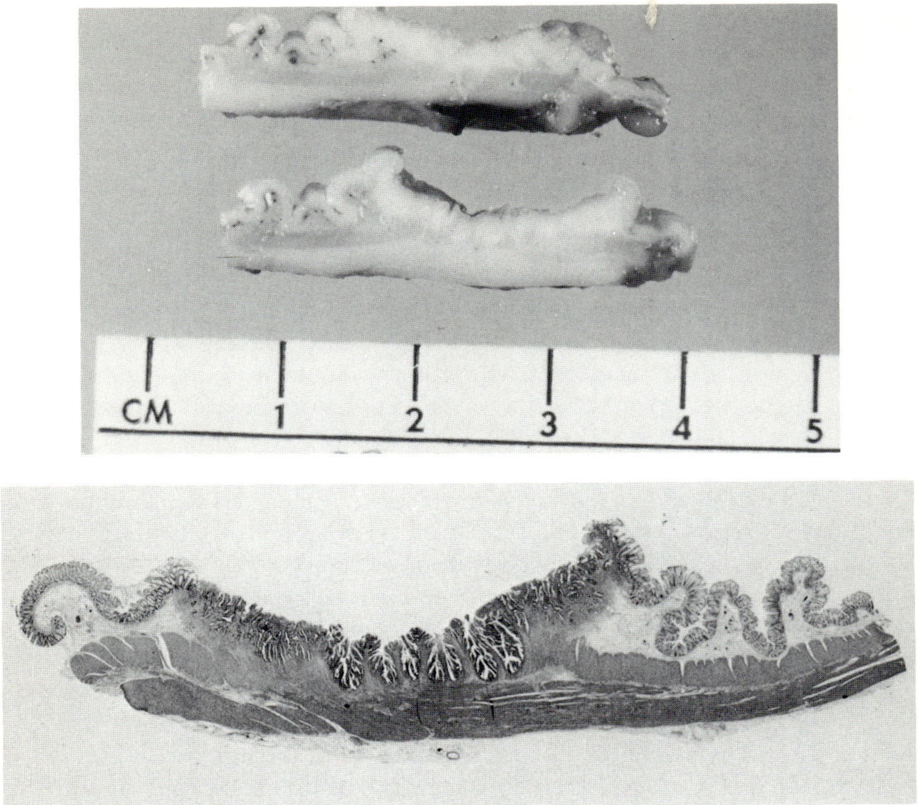

FIG. 2. Top. Slices of an ulcerated adenocarcinoma from the area of deepest penetration show that the lesion is confined to the bowel wall. **Bottom.** The large section confirms the gross impression. H&E. ×3.

gray, and separation from the surrounding fatty tissue becomes more difficult. Clearing techniques have been used to identify lymph nodes; the mesentery is immersed in graded alcohols followed by xylene to remove fat. This, however, is time-consuming, expensive, and not recommended for routine work. Following the search for lymph nodes, the veins should be carefully examined for the presence of tumor.

With the gross examination completed, the specimen is then pinned on a corkboard and fixed for 24 hours in formalin. After overnight fixation, I usually remove the specimen from the corkboard and let it lie flat in formalin until the late afternoon, when blocks are taken. The numbers of blocks one takes depend on the size of the cancer. Small lesions may require taking only two blocks, whereas larger ones may necessitate examining 6 to 12 sections, especially if the tumor is necrotic. On the average, I find four sections of the tumor quite adequate. The blocks taken should include the junction of the tumor and the adjacent bowel mucosa, and at least one block should be routinely taken from the region of deepest penetration, consisting of about equal parts of tumor and apparently normal tissue. Sections should be taken of the proximal and distal margins. If the tumor is situated in close proximity to the resected margin, I usually take a longitudinal section, to include the tumor and the margin. Otherwise, transverse sections, which would comprise most of the circumference, are taken. The use of India ink to determine surgical margins is to be recommended; however, fixed tissues do not take the ink as successfully as fresh tissue, so that margins should be inked prior to fixation.

If more than one tumor is present, the blocks from each tumor must be separately labeled. Polyps and other mucosal lesions should be sectioned. With rare exceptions, sections should be taken from all polyps. Small polyps can easily be embedded whole; however, large ones may require trimming. The polyps should be blocked in such a way so as to include the head and the stalk. In patients with familial polyposis it may be necessary to examine dozens of polyps. Large villous adenomas are notorious for harboring small foci of carcinoma; therefore, multiple sections of these should be taken. Random sections of the colon away from the tumor should be routinely taken. All lymph nodes identified and removed previously should be blocked and appropriately labeled. The highest lymph nodes at the point of vessel ligation should be separately blocked. Sections from the extracolonic tissues should be included, for the study of mesenteric vessels. Sections from right hemicolectomy specimens should include the appendix and the terminal ileum. In abdominoperineal resections, blocks from the anus should be taken for histologic study.

The size of the tissue blocks taken for histologic study varies in different laboratories, and thus one cannot arbitrarily recommend the optimum number of blocks. I personally take a minimum of four blocks, including one through the center, to include the area of deepest penetration of the tumor, and multiple sections from the periphery of the tumor and the adjacent nonneoplastic tissues. In addition, I usually take, in selected cases for a large section, a longitudinal block of tissue of the entire tumor and surrounding fatty tissue.

STUDY OF COLORECTAL CANCER BY LARGE SECTIONS

For the past 10 years I have been using large sections cut on a Leitz sledge microtome for the study of tumors of the gastrointestinal tract. After 24 hours fixation in formalin, longitudinal or cross-sections of bowel, including the entire tumor and surrounding tissues, are cut. A thin slice of tissue from the center of the lesion, of approximately 0.75 cm thickness, is selected. Care should be taken not to make the blocks very thin since a fair amount of rough cutting is necessary before a satisfactory slide is obtained. The size of the blocks varies, depending on the lesion; however, blocks of up to approximately 9.0 cm by 7.0 cm can be cut. These are mounted on large glass slides 10.0 cm by 8.0 cm in size, and are studied both grossly and microscopically.

The total time involved from the time that a slice of tissue is selected to the time that the stained slide is made is approximately a week; however, this largely depends on the size of the block. I routinely fix a large slice of tissue for an additional 12 hours before beginning processing. The volume of the fixative should be at least 10 times that of the specimen. The processing is done manually by a technologist who transfers the specimen daily through graded changes in alcohol. The specimen is then cleared using two changes of chloroform. Impregnation is accomplished by transfer of the specimen through two changes of paraffin. The slice of tissue is then ready for embedding. The cutting of sections on a sledge microtome has not been a major problem. The method described above provides uniformly thin sections of about 6 μ thickness. Not all tumors are so studied, but one can select those that can best be examined by this method. I have found the method very useful in the study of large polyps of the gastrointestinal tract (Figs. 3 to 5). The large sections that are used have the advantage of preservation of the anatomic relationships of the tissues. In the case of polyps, a section along the long axis of the entire lesion is very effective in demonstrating malignant change and the extent of invasion in the stalk. (Figs. 6 and 7). In the case of a carcinoma, the configuration, extent, and pattern of spread through the bowel wall and into the adjacent tissues

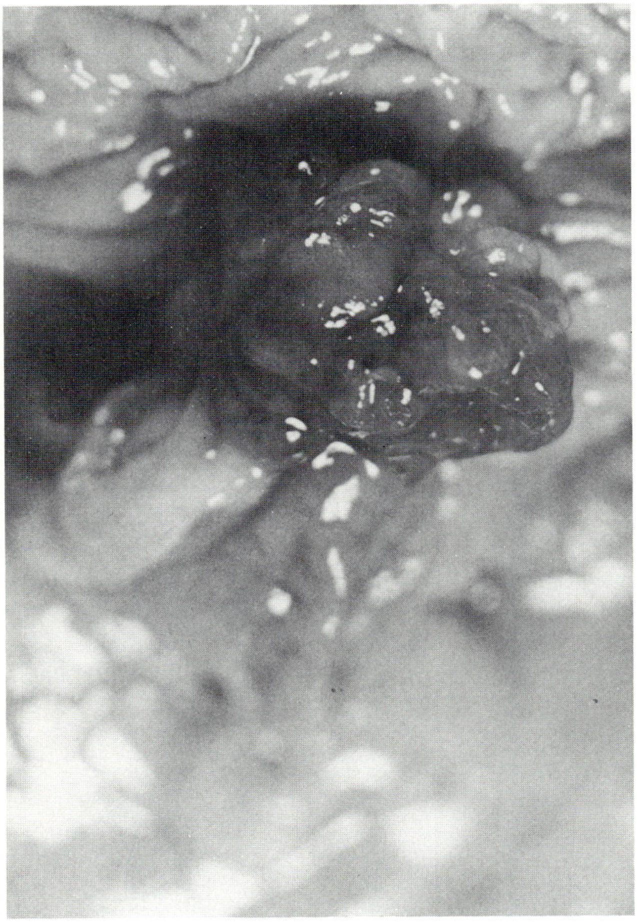

FIG. 3. Gross specimen of colon with a 2.5 cm adenoma on a long stalk. (Continued)

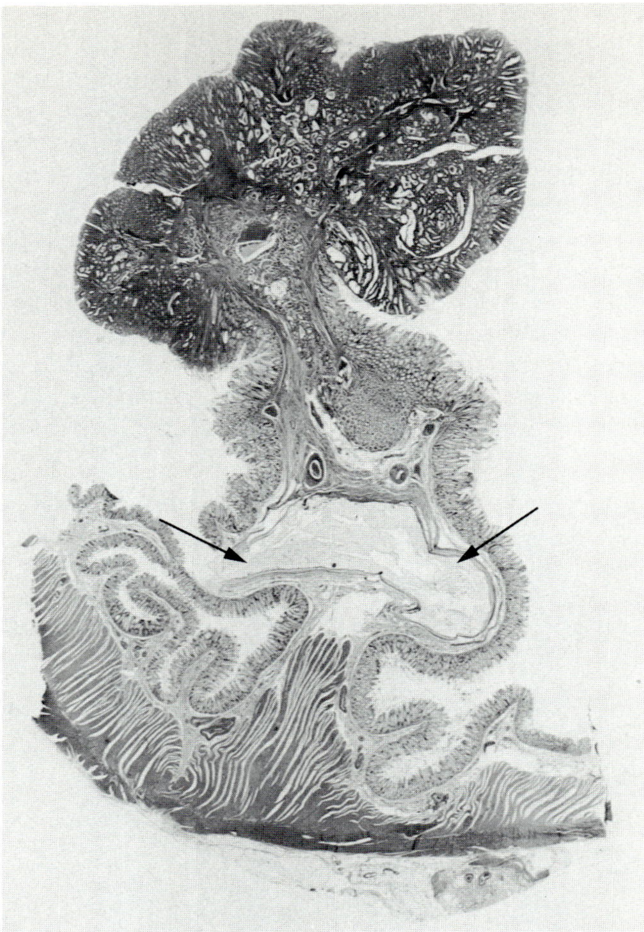

FIG. 3 (cont.). Large section of the adenoma, stalk, and colon. This is an unusual adenoma with misplaced epithelium and lakes of mucus within the stalk (arrows). H&E. ×3.

are best studied by this method (Figs. 8 to 13). Similarly, variation in tumor morphology from one area to another is also best appreciated in the large sections that are used (Fig. 14). The relationships of cancer to lesions situated in the immediate vicinity are also best demonstrated by large sections (Figs. 15 and 16).

MICROSCOPIC EXAMINATION OF SPECIMENS

The microscopic study forms an important part of the examination of colorectal specimens. The pathology report should contain information on the following features of the tumors: histologic type, grade, tumor margins, degree of inflammatory reaction, extent of direct spread, lymph node involvement, and perineural involvement. Synchronous tumors, such as a second cancer or a polyp, should also

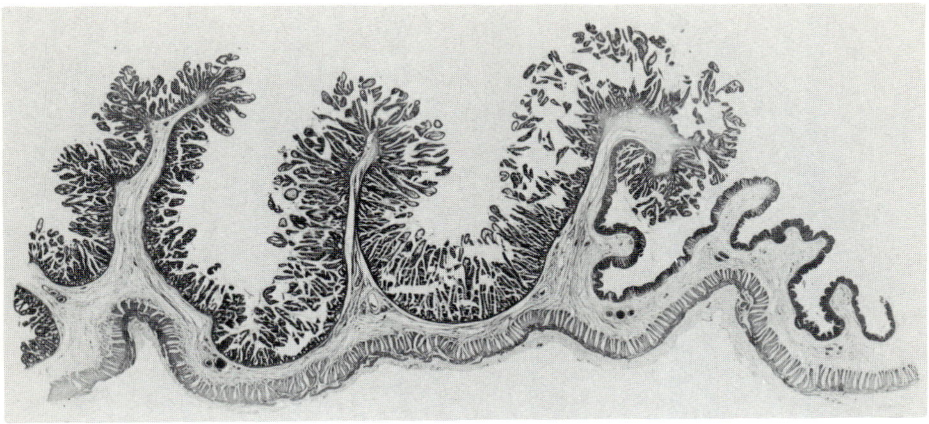

FIG. 4. Large section of sessile villous adenoma colon. This was an 8 cm flat tumor arising in the cecum of a 72-year-old woman. H&E. ×2.25.

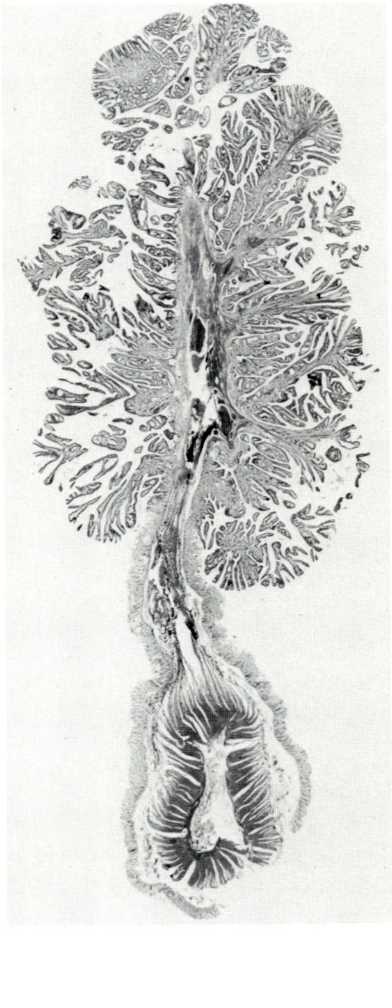

FIG. 5. Large section of a 5 cm pedunculated villous adenoma. The majority of villous tumors are sessile but some may acquire a stalk as seen here. H&E. ×2.25.

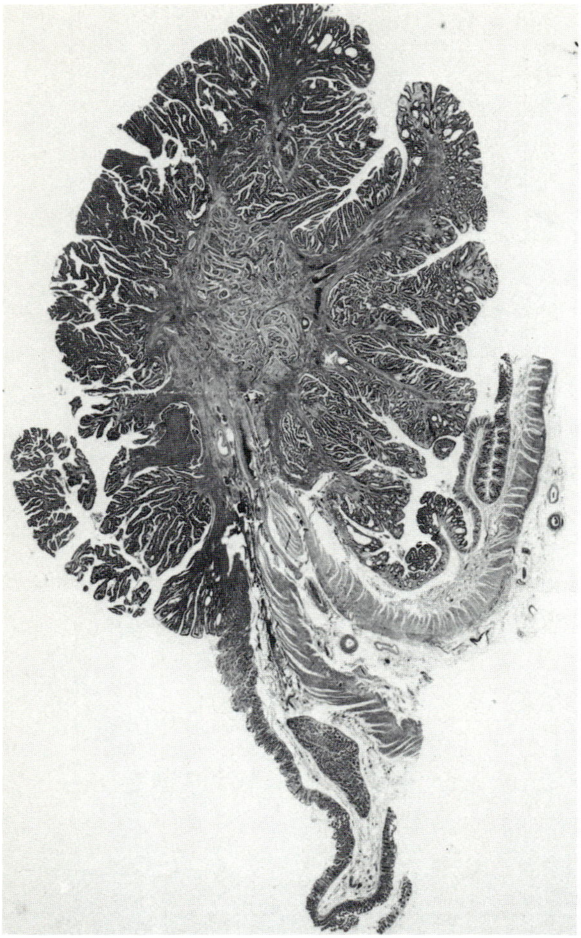

FIG. 6. Large section of a villotubular adenoma showing invasive cancer in the stalk. H&E. ×2.25.

be described in the above terms. The type of polyp—whether hyperplastic, tubular, or a villous adenoma—should be recorded.

Histologic Type

Most malignant tumors of the large bowel are adenocarcinomas forming tubules or glands. However, mucinous (Fig. 17), signet ring (Fig. 18), undifferentiated (Fig. 19) and other types of tumor—such as squamous carcinoma and carcinoid (Fig. 20)—may also be found and should be so classified.

Histologic Grade

The degree of differentiation of a tumor should be recorded. I favor a three- rather than a four-grade system. Only adenocarcinomas should be graded. Grade 1 carcinomas resemble adenomas, with well-formed tubules and the least degree of

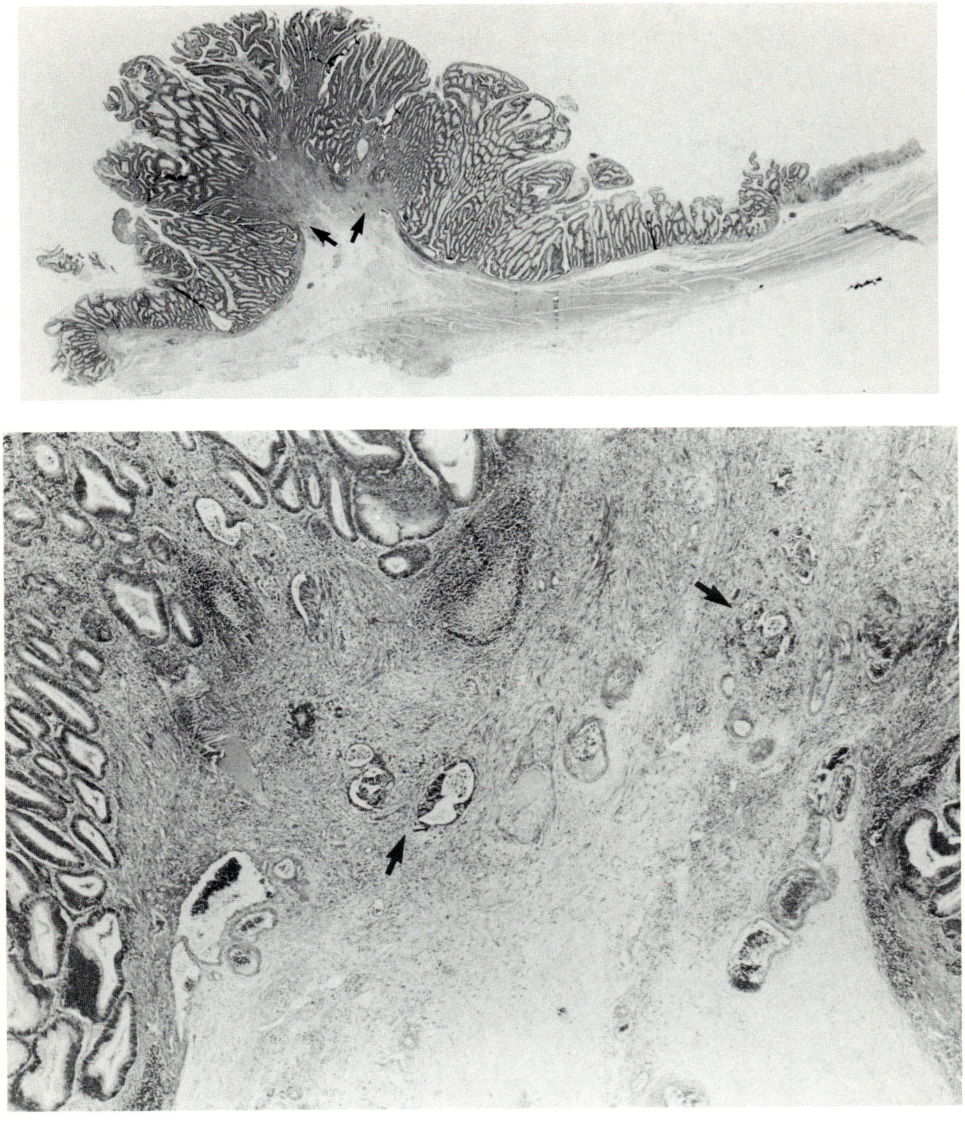

FIG. 7. Top. Large section of a sessile villous adenoma with early cancer (arrows). H&E.×3. **Bottom.** Carcinomatous foci in the stalk (arrows). H&E.×50.

pleomorphism and mitotic rate (Fig. 21). Grade 3 cancers are the least differentiated (Fig. 22), with occasional recognizable glandular structures. The lining cells are pleomorphic with a high mitotic count. Grade 2 lesions are intermediate between grade 1 and grade 3 lesions (Fig. 23). Mucoid and diffusely infiltrating signet-ring cancers should be classified separately and are not included in this grading scheme. The prognosis of such a tumor depends on other histologic features, such as extent of disease, as well as vascular and lymphatic involvement.

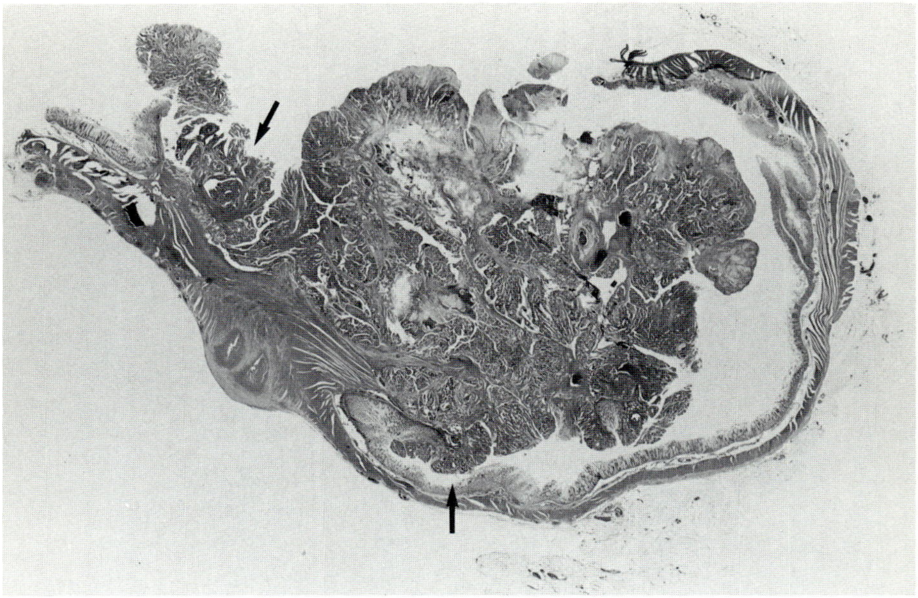

FIG. 8. A cross-section from a large polypoid cancer filling the lumen of the bowel. Remnants of villous adenoma are still identifiable at the edges of the tumor (arrows). H&E. ×1.5.

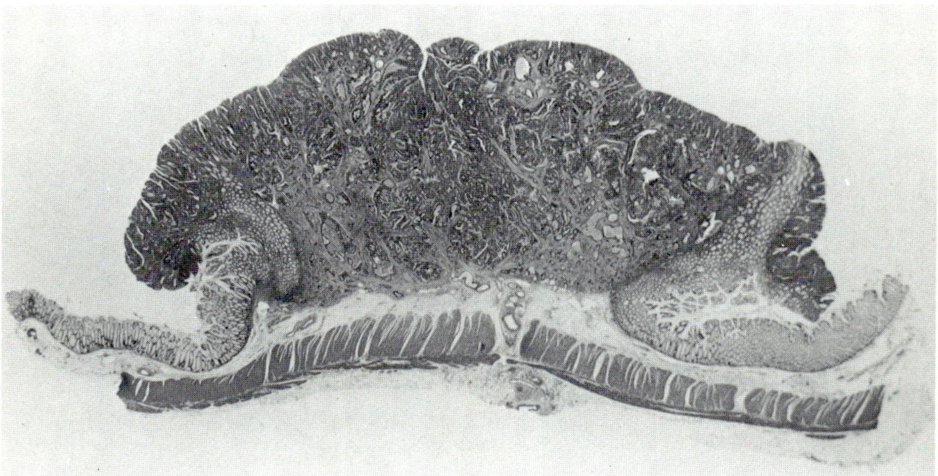

FIG. 9. A large polypoid, so-called early cancer infiltrating only the submucosa. H&E. ×2.25.

Tumor Margins

The borders of the tumor, whether pushing—i.e., with sharp demarcation between the tumor and host tissue (Fig. 24)—or infiltrative, i.e., poorly defined, with intermixture between tumor elements and host tissue (Fig. 25) should be recorded.

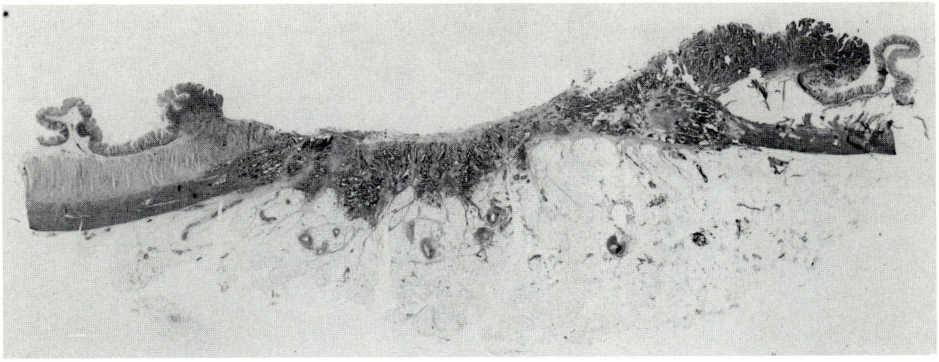

FIG. 10. Large section of an ulcerated adenocarcinoma growing through the full thickness of the bowel wall and infiltrating the mesenteric fat. H&E. ×2.25.

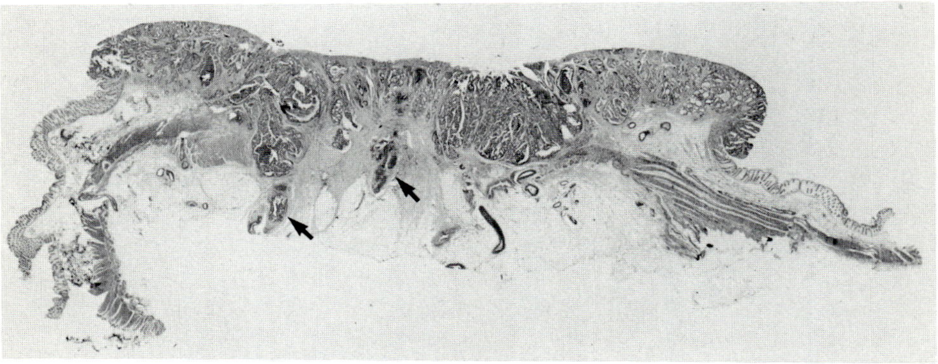

FIG. 11. Large section showing direct infiltration into the mesenteric fat with venous involvement (arrows). H&E. ×2.25.

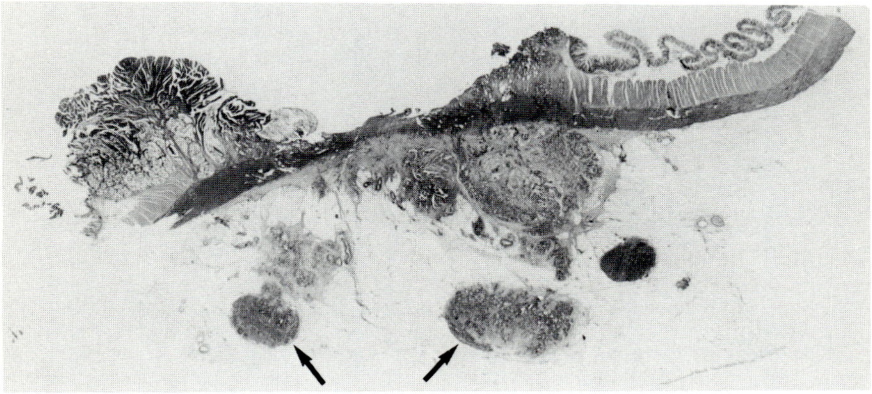

FIG. 12. Ulcerated adenocarcinoma arising in a villous adenoma. The tumor has spread into the surrounding fatty tissue and involves the mesenteric lymph nodes (arrows). H&E. ×2.25.

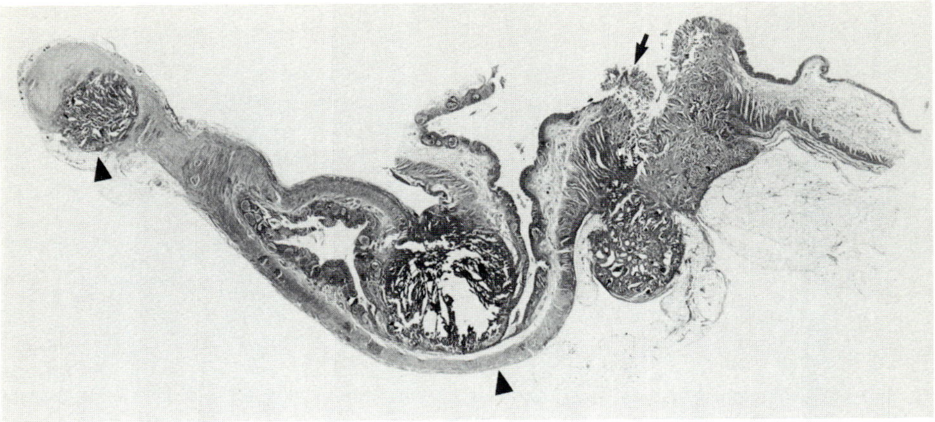

FIG. 13. Right hemicolectomy specimen showing a small ulcerated adenocarcinoma of the cecum (arrow) which has spread into surrounding mesenteric fat. Tumor metastases are also noted in the base and the tip of the appendix (arrowheads). H&E. ×1.5.

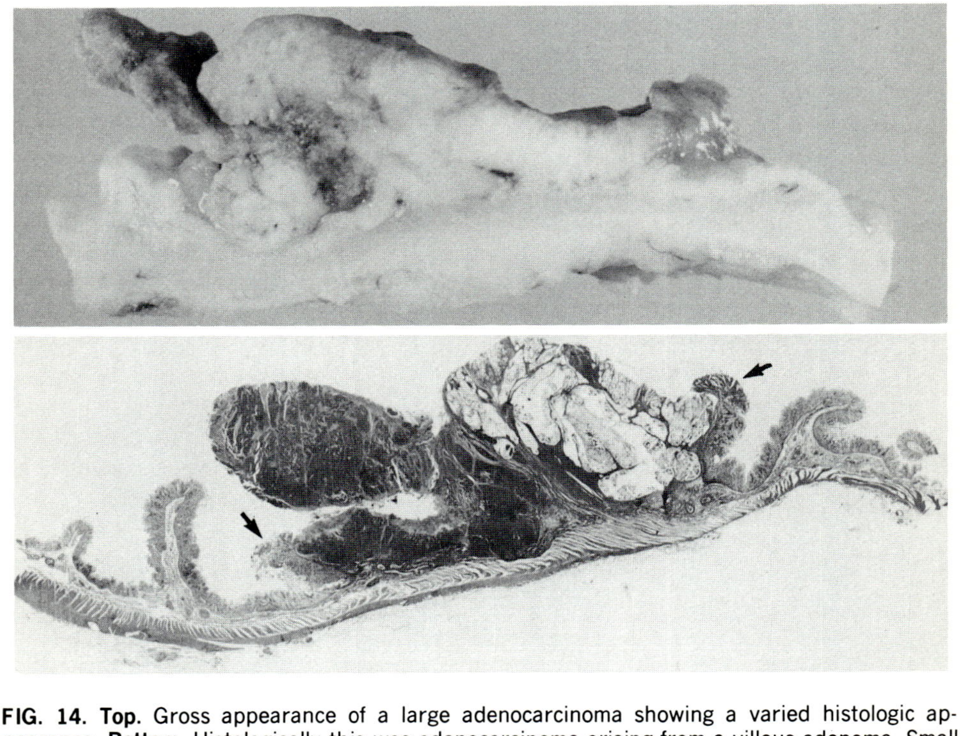

FIG. 14. Top. Gross appearance of a large adenocarcinoma showing a varied histologic appearance. **Bottom.** Histologically this was adenocarcinoma arising from a villous adenoma. Small remnants of villous adenoma are seen at the two edges of the tumor (arrows). Half of the invasive carcinoma is mucinous or colloid and the other half undifferentiated. The tumor was still confined to the bowel wall and no lymph nodes were involved. H&E. ×1.5.

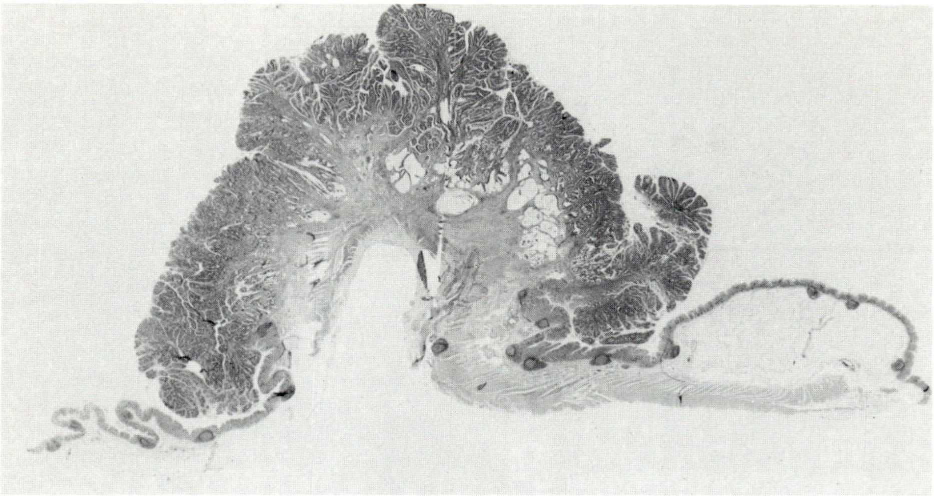

FIG. 15. Mucinous adenocarcinoma arising in a villous adenoma. Note the adjacent benign lipoma separate from the cancer. H&E. ×2.25.

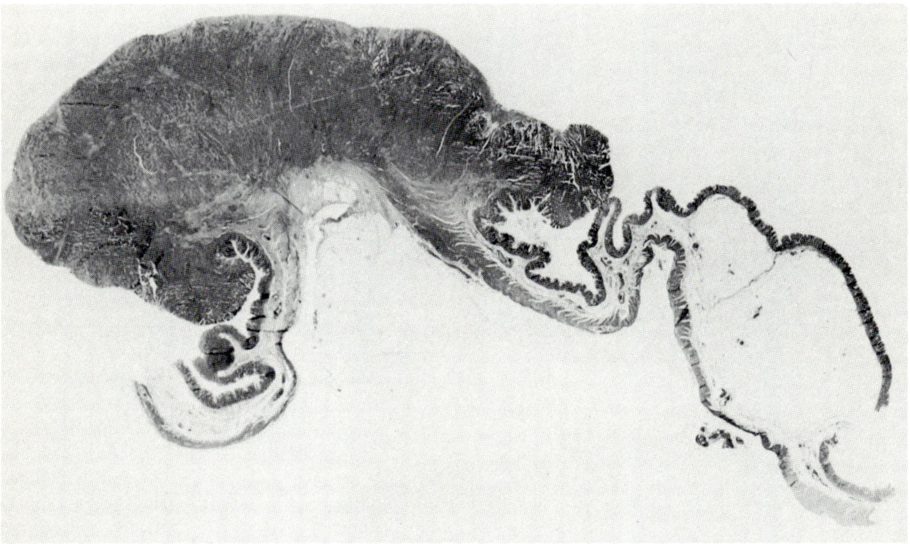

FIG. 16. An undifferentiated carcinoma and submucosal lipoma adjacent to each other. H&E. ×2.25.

Inflammatory Reaction

The presence or absence of lymphocytes, plasma cells, and macrophages at the margins of the tumor should be noted. I personally grade the inflammatory reaction, when present, into mild and severe (Fig. 26).

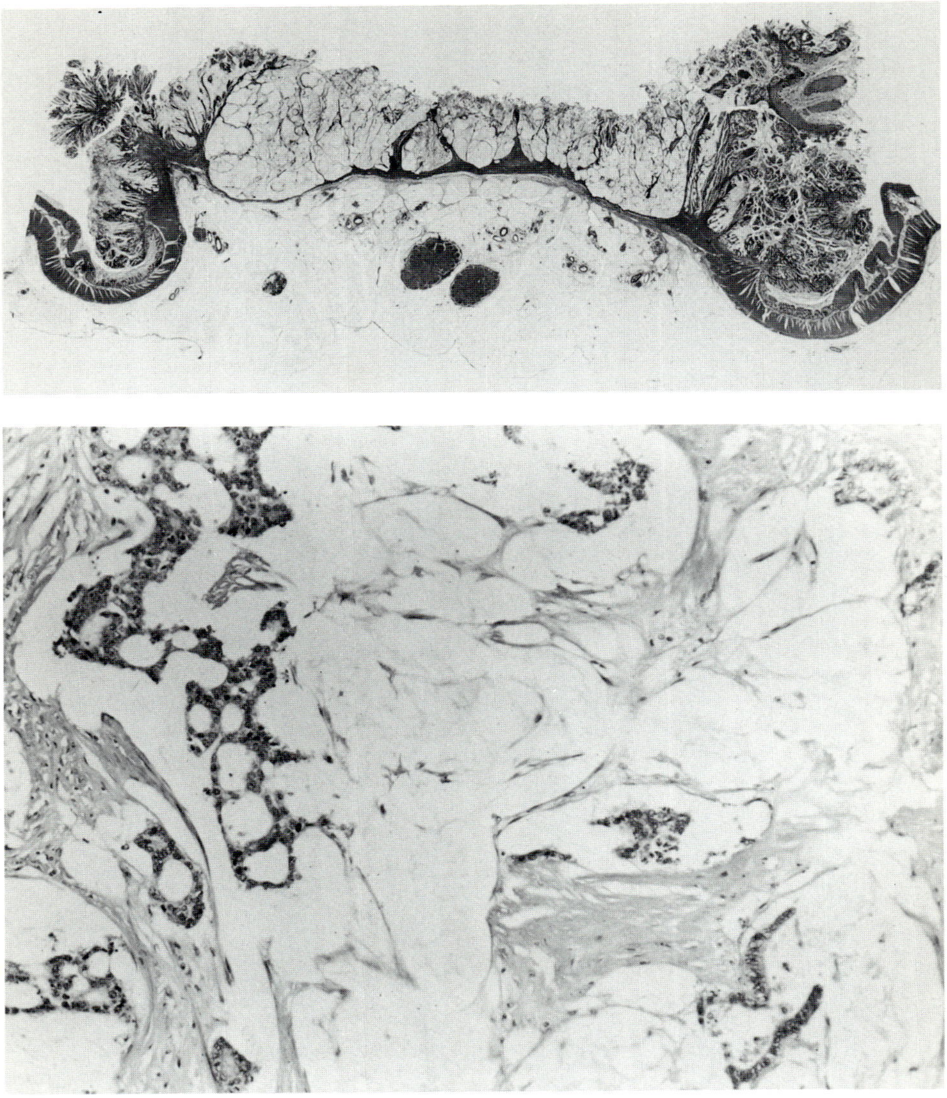

FIG. 17. Top. Large section of a mucinous carcinoma. The tumor is confined to the bowel wall. Two lymph nodes in the mesenteric fat are uninvolved by the tumor. H&E. ×1.5. **Bottom.** Lakes of mucous-containing nests of malignant tumor cells. H&E. ×200.

Extent of Spread

The gross impression of the extent of spread of a tumor through the bowel wall should always be confirmed histologically. I use Dukes'[6] original classification (Fig. 27) in describing the extent of spread, though others find the Astler and Coller[7] modification more meaningful (Fig. 28). According to Dukes' original classification, a lesion is labeled as "A" when the cancer is confined to the bowel wall; that

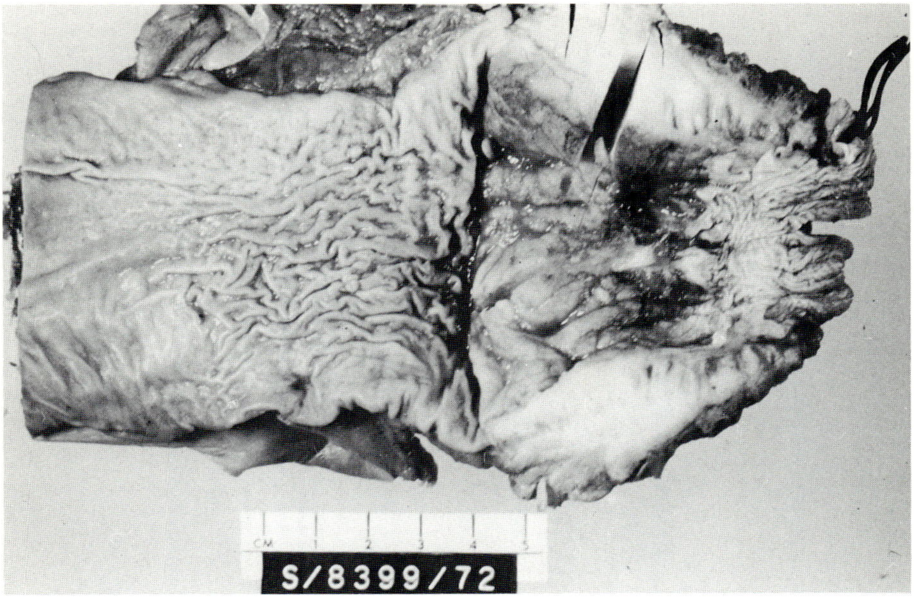

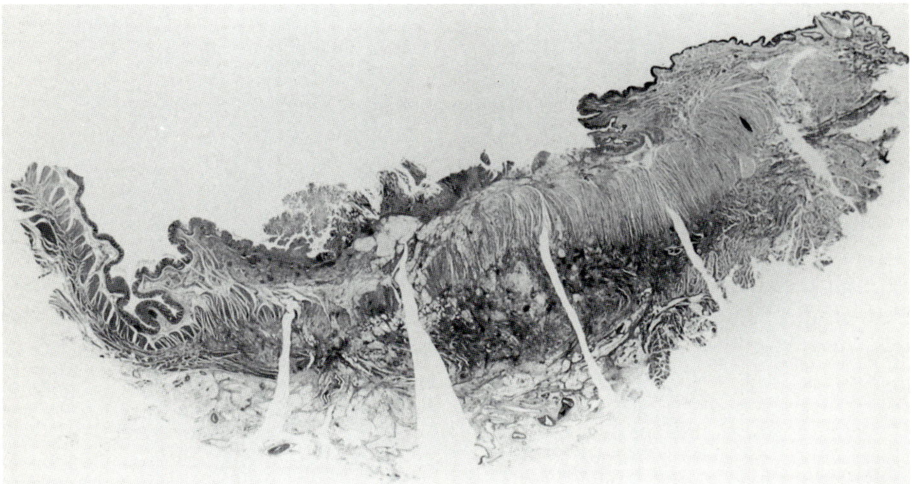

FIG. 18. Top. Linitis plastica—signet ring cancer of the rectum. Note the distal half of the rectum is infiltrated by cancer. From Dis Colon Rectum 17:540, 1974. **Bottom.** Large section showing infiltration of the entire wall and surrounding fibro-fatty and muscular tissue by cancer cells. Compare the thickness of the rectum in the involved and non-involved areas. H&E. ×1.5. From Dis Colon Rectum 17:540, 1974. (Continued)

is, it has not yet penetrated through the muscularis propria. Dukes' "B" lesions are those in which the cancer has spread by direct extension into the serosa and beyond, but in which the lymph nodes are not involved. Dukes' "C" lesions are those associated with lymph node metastases. The extent of spread into the adjoining tissues and the completeness of excision should be recorded.

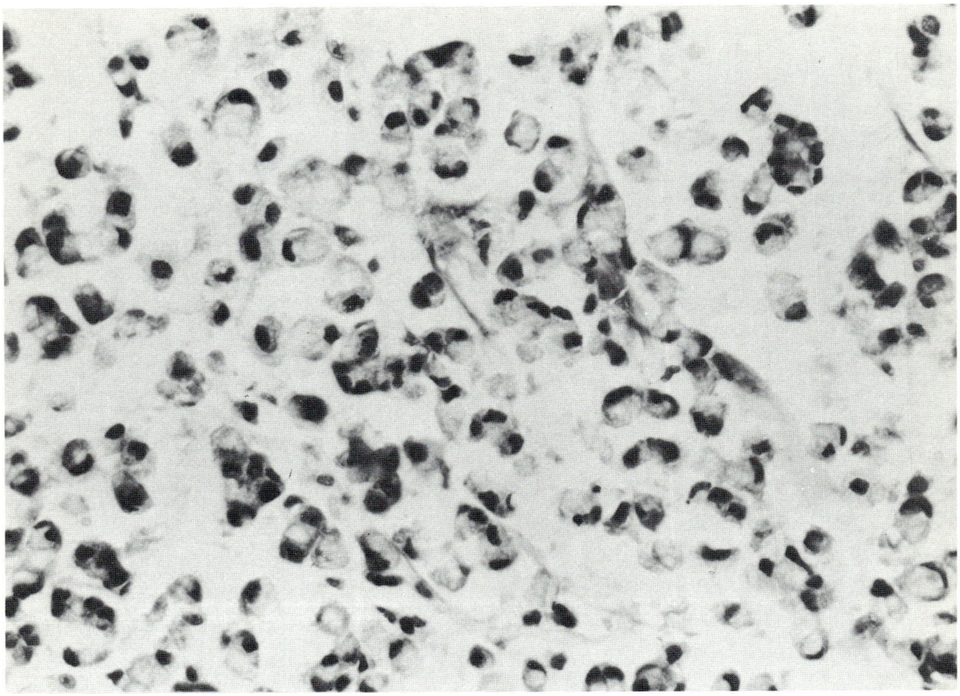

FIG. 18 (cont.). Signet ring carcinoma cells infiltrating the wall of the rectum. H&E. ×480.

Lymph Node Involvement

The total number of lymph nodes found and the number involved by metastatic tumor should be noted. The location of the involved nodes, whether adjacent to the tumor or at the high point of vessel ligation, should be documented (Figs. 29 and 30).

Perineural and Vascular Involvement

This should be sought for and recorded (Figs. 31 and 32). Venous invasion is readily apparent in the majority of cases; however, when difficulty is encountered in identifying a vein, special stains, for example, Weigert's or Verhoeff's hematoxylin and VanGieson elastic stains, may be used. I do not routinely use elastic stains. In many cases venous invasion can be diagnosed by the presence of tumor tissue in an endothelial-lined space containing red blood cells or associated with a small thrombus and surrounded by a rim of muscle. The presence of an adjacent artery is also helpful in the identification of the vein. In cases in which the diagnosis is doubtful, I do resort to the use of elastic stains.

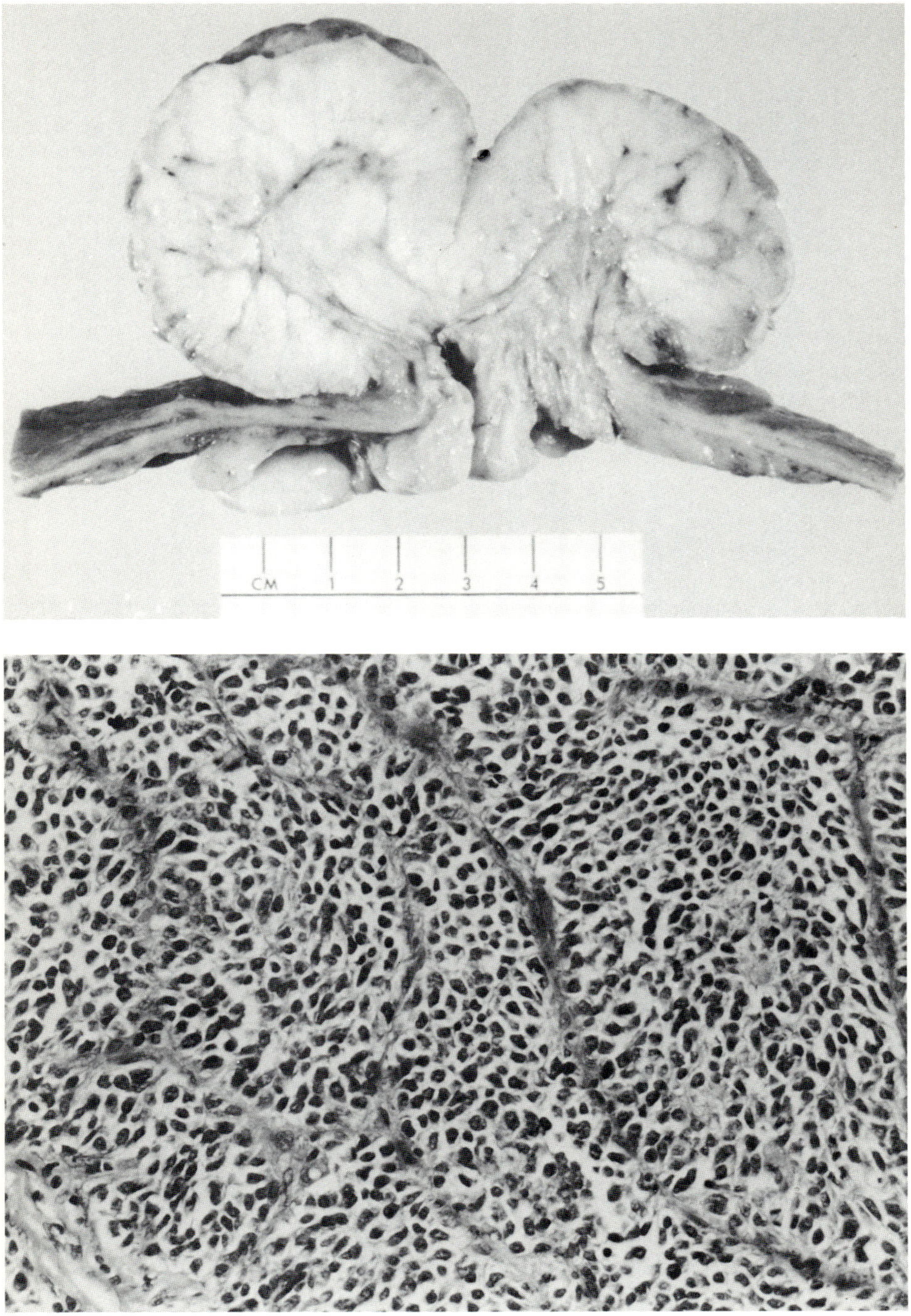

FIG. 19. Top. Gross appearance of large, polypoid, undifferentiated carcinoma of the cecum. **Bottom.** Histologically the tumor exhibited extensive necrosis. Viable portions of the tumor were undifferentiated and composed of small oval-to-round tumor cells. H&E. ×200.

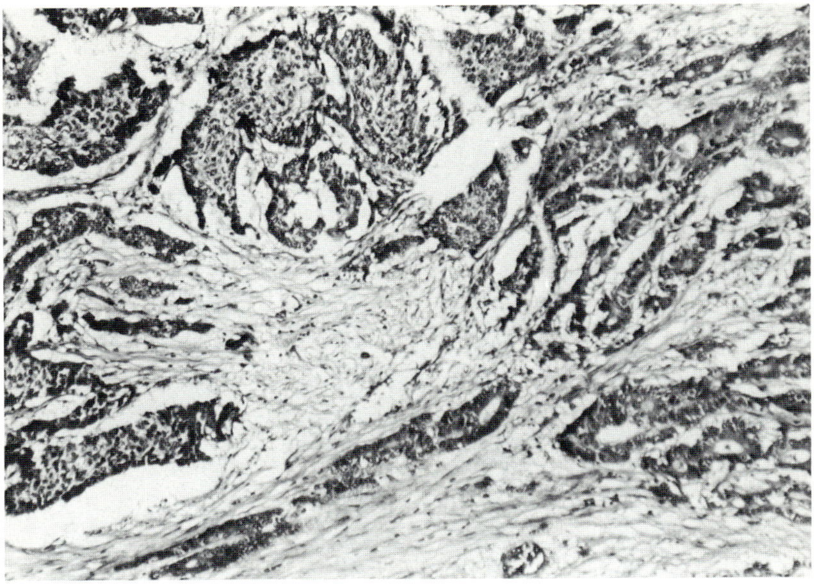

FIG. 20. Mixed carcinoid and adenocarcinoma. Both patterns are seen. Solid islands of carcinoid tumor are seen merging into areas showing glandular differentiation. In other portions of the tumor colloid areas were present. H&E. ×170.

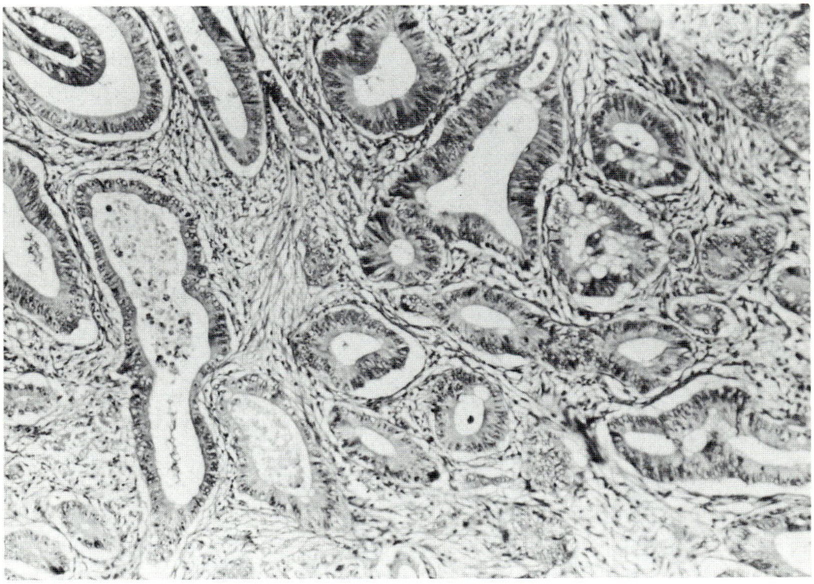

FIG. 21. Grade 1 adenocarcinoma. H&E. ×170.

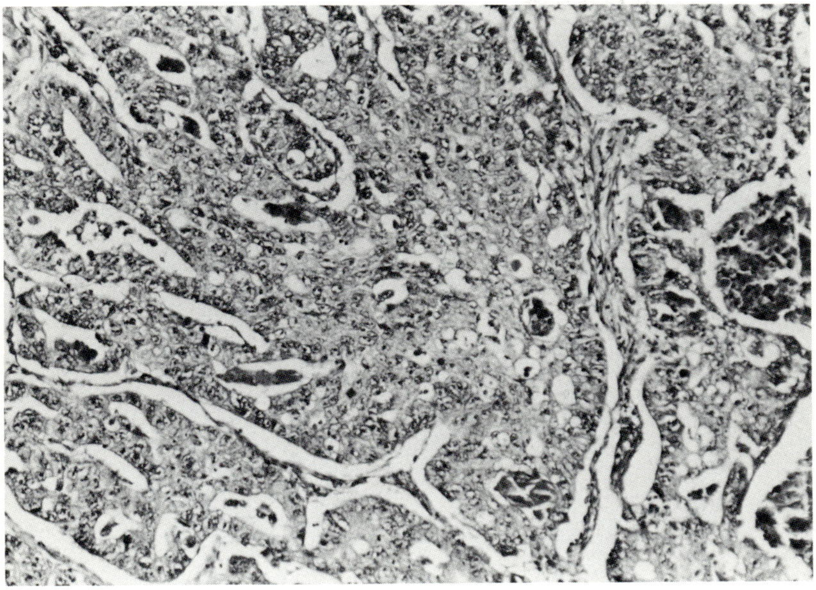

FIG. 22. Grade 3 adenocarcinoma. H&E. ×170.

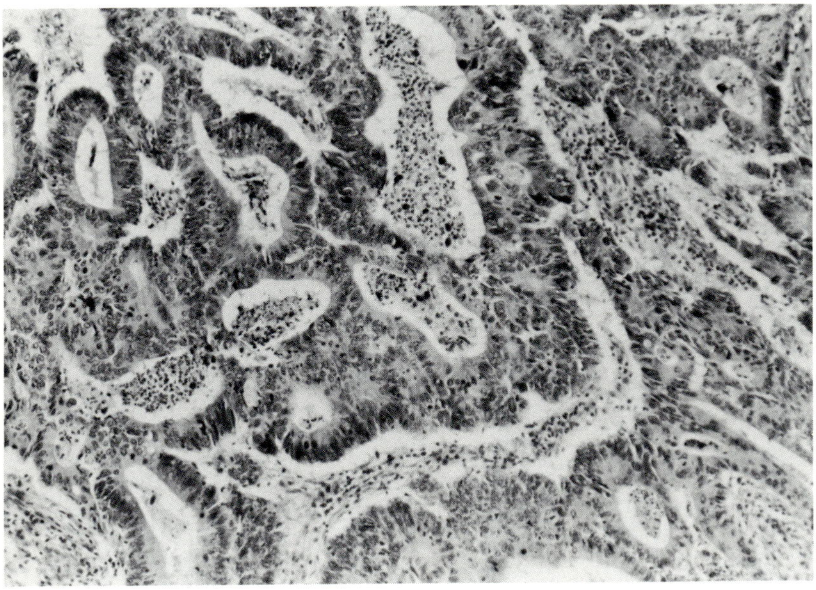

FIG. 23. Grade 2 adenocarcinoma. H&E. ×170.

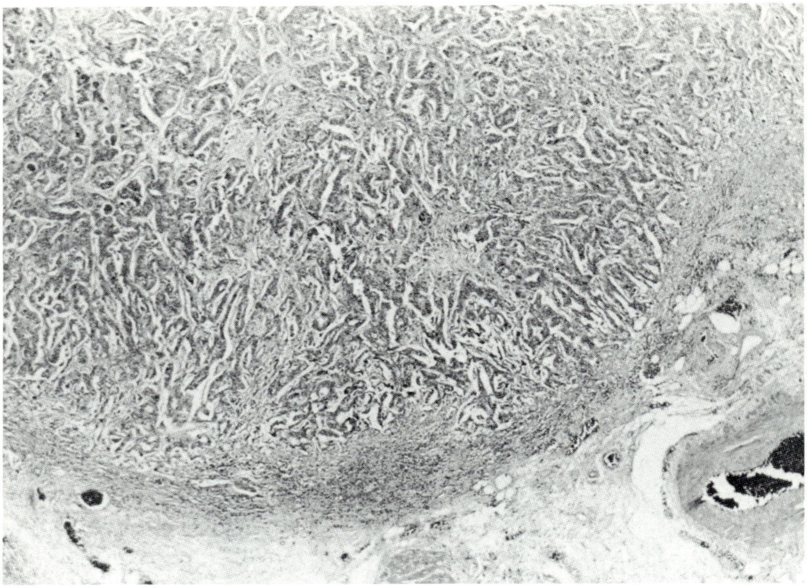

FIG. 24. Pushing tumor margin with sharp demarcation between the tumor and host tissue. H&E. ×43.

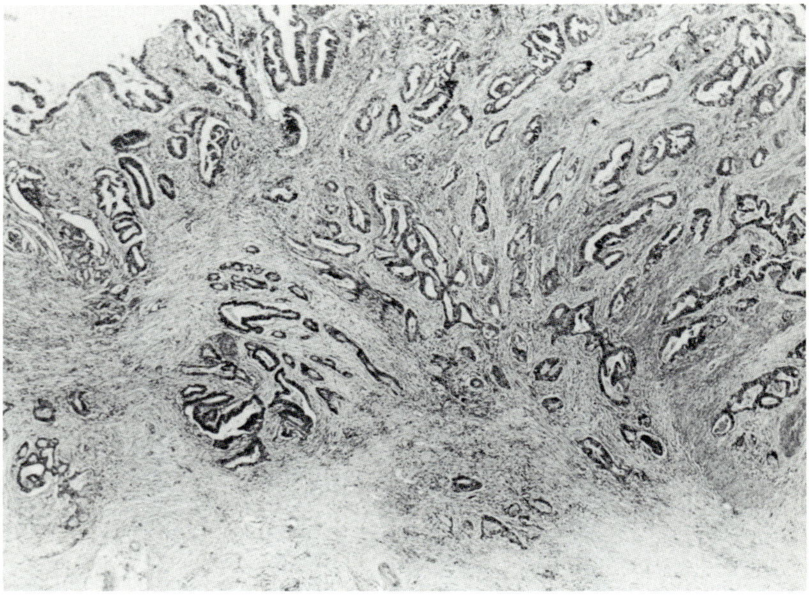

FIG. 25. Infiltrative tumor margin with intermixture between tumor elements and host tissue. H&E. ×43.

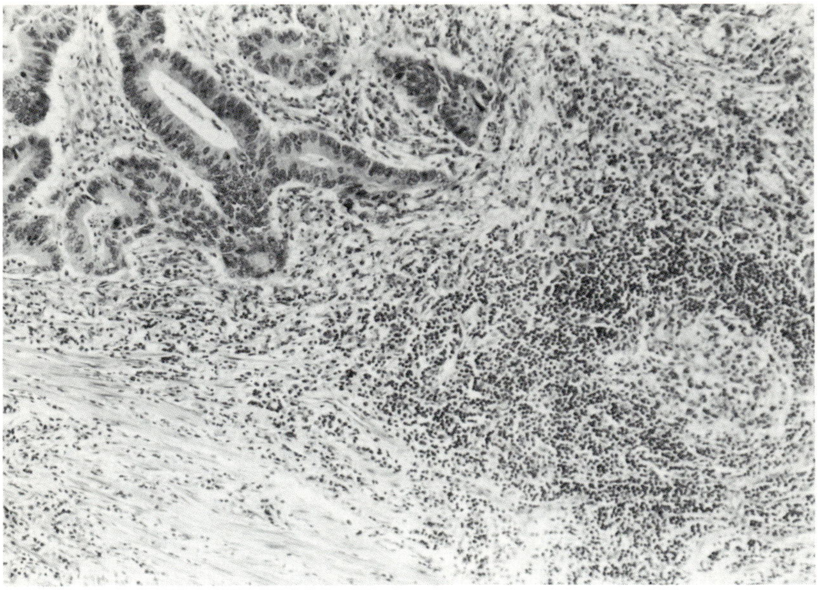

FIG. 26. A well-developed inflammatory reaction at the advancing margin of a cancer. H&E. ×170.

Other Synchronous Tumors

A second cancer or polyp should be described in the terms stated above, and the type of polyp, whether hyperplastic, tubular, or a villous adenoma, should be documented.

The final diagnosis should summarize the information on the location, extent of spread (Dukes' stage), and degree of differentiation of the lesion or lesions. The number and location of the involved lymph nodes should be stated. Such a systematically organized pathology report has many advantages and is important both in patient-care and research. Although such a report may contain some items which others may find nonessential, it reflects the thoroughness of pathologic examination and data collection.

VALUE OF A STANDARDIZED REPORTING SYSTEM

Buckwalter and Kent[3] believe that surgical pathology reports on specimens from patients with cancer of the colon and rectum can be standardized to facilitate the compiling of data and the evaluation of patient prognosis. Furthermore, they suggest that such standardized reporting can be used as a method of quality control in establishing minimum standards for data collection.

Examination of surgical pathology reports on patients with colorectal cancer from the five McMaster University Teaching Hospitals in Hamilton, Ontario, disclosed that though generally satisfactory, some were incomplete, with the

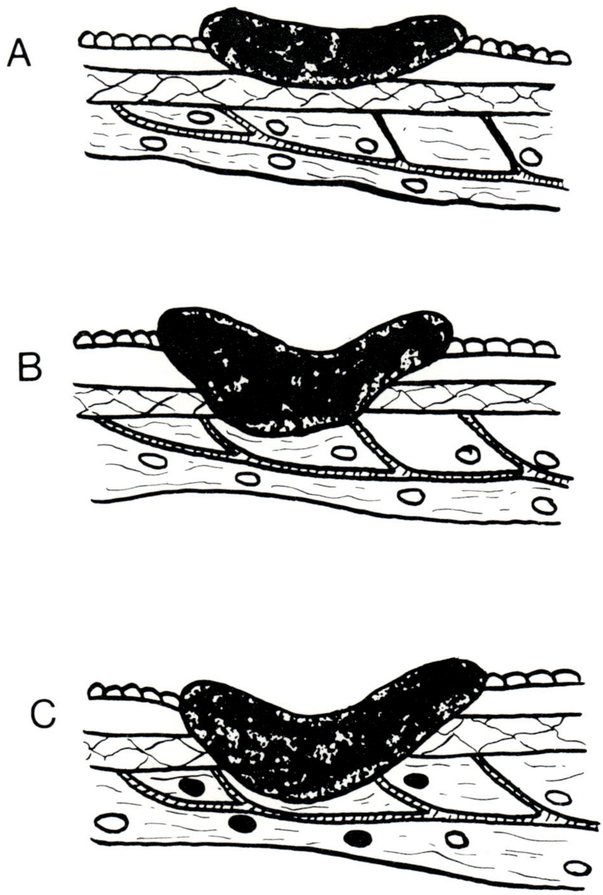

FIG. 27. Dukes' classification of spread of colorectal carcinoma. **A.** Cancer confined to wall of bowel. **B.** Direct spread of cancer through the muscle layers into serosa or surrounding fatty tissue. Lymph nodes not involved. **C.** Metastases in regional lymph nodes.

absence of essential or desirable pathologic data. This led us to develop a standard pathology report form for data collection on all patients with cancer of the colorectum admitted to the five McMaster University Teaching Hospitals. In 1977 a gastrointestinal oncology panel was formed with representation from all the hospitals. The panel members consisted of surgeons, gastroenterologists, radiotherapists, a diagnostic radiologist, a medical oncologist, and a pathologist. We agreed on the need for a standardized pathology reporting system. This led to the development of such a form, which was circulated to all pathology departments in the five hospitals and approved by the pathologists in the system.

The necessary data on the standardized form were arranged in a check-list fashion (Table 1). A guide to the examination of the large bowel, to Dukes' staging, and to the grading of tumors was also prepared and was sent with the standardized report form to all pathology departments in the city. It was requested that the various surgical pathology laboratories in the five hospitals send a descriptive pathology report with essential data to the physician or to the patient's chart in the usual manner, but in addition, fill in the standardized form and return it to a designated person at the local cancer clinic. The forms were reviewed by me, and

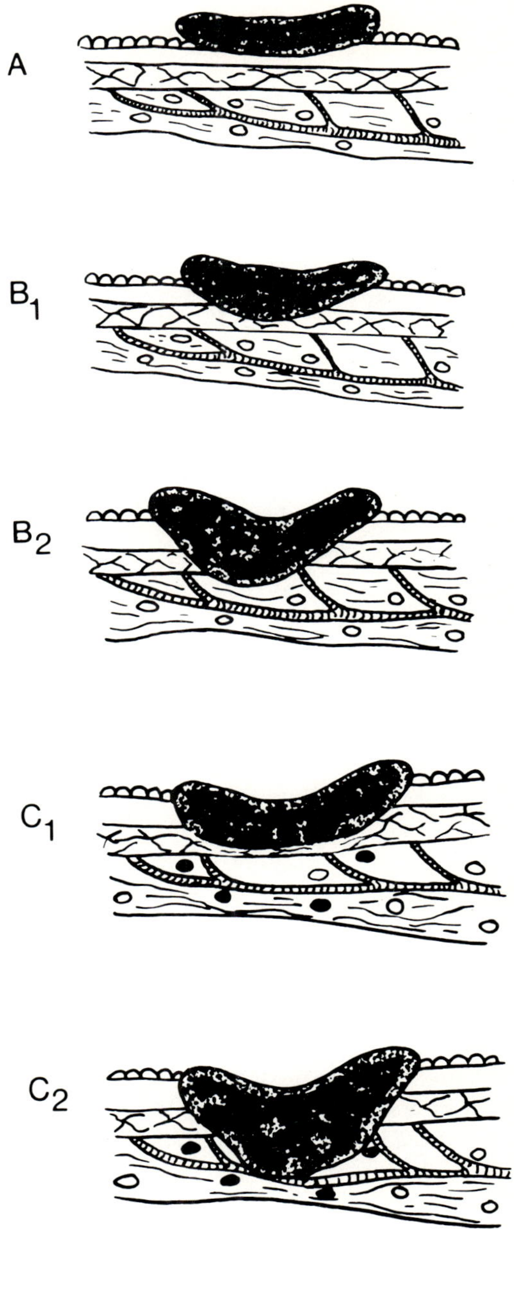

FIG. 28. Astler and Coller's modification of Dukes' classification. **A.** Carcinoma limited to mucosa. **B_1.** Extending into muscularis propria but not penetrating it. Negative lymph nodes. **B_2.** Penetrating the muscularis propria. Negative lymph nodes. **C_1.** Limited to wall with positive lymph nodes. **C_2.** Penetrating the wall with positive lymph nodes.

the data were presented to the oncology committee and pathologists for information and discussion. The form we prepared consists of three pages, including information we felt it was essential to collect. It was the responsibility of the pathologist or the resident, and not the histology technologist or the clerical staff, to fill in the form.

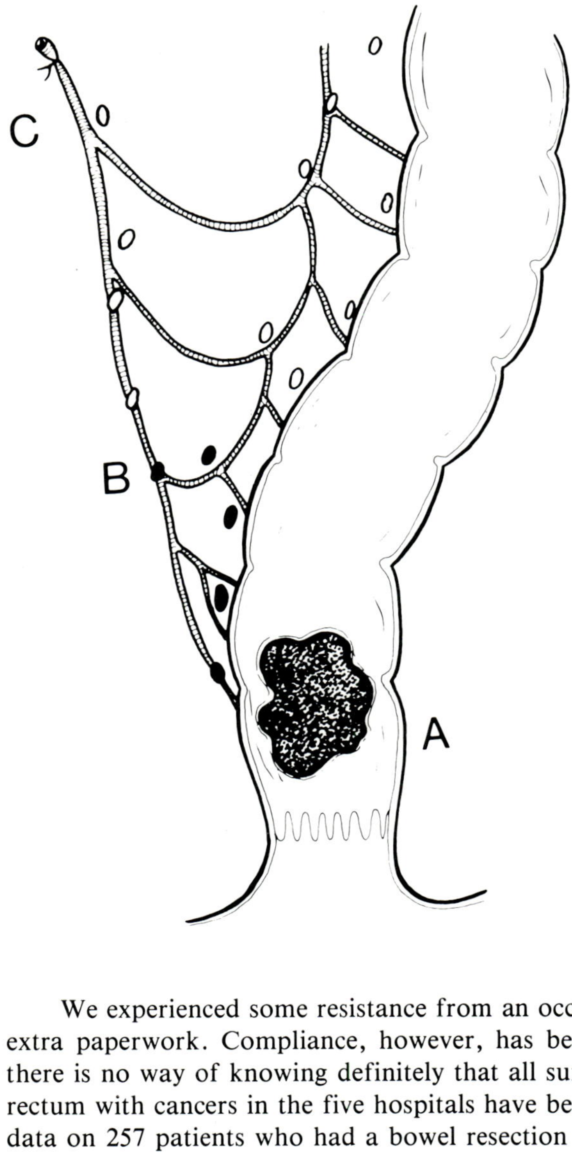

FIG. 29. Lymph nodes at point of vessel ligation, free of tumor. **A.** Carcinoma of rectum. **B.** Lymph nodes adjacent to tumor involved by metastases. **C.** Lymph nodes at point of vessel ligation negative for tumor.

We experienced some resistance from an occasional pathologist regarding this extra paperwork. Compliance, however, has been generally good, and although there is no way of knowing definitely that all surgical specimens of the colon and rectum with cancers in the five hospitals have been so recorded, we have reviewed data on 257 patients who had a bowel resection for cancer from January 1978 to December 1979. Over 100 cases collected during 1980 still await review.

The results of the study are summarized below. During 1978 and 1979, 257 patients underwent a bowel resection for cancer of the colorectum. There were 138 women and 119 men with an age range from 21 to 97 years. There were 266 cancers confirmed histologically in these 257 patients. Nine patients had a second synchronous cancer in the resected bowel. The distribution of these 266 carcinomas is shown in Figure 33. The location of the cancer was not documented in five patients. The majority (70 percent) of cancers were left-sided in location. Of the 62 patients with rectal cancer, 38 underwent abdominoperineal resection.

The tumor configuration was as follows: 143 (54 percent) were of the ulcerative

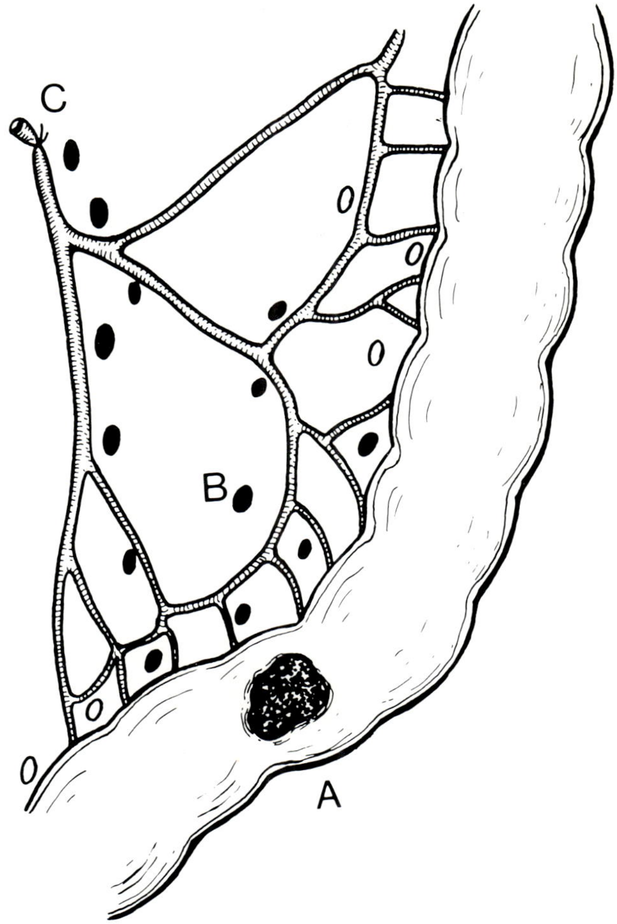

FIG. 30. Lymph nodes at point of vessel ligation contain deposits of tumor. **A.** Carcinoma of colon. Lymph nodes adjacent to tumor **(B)** and at highest point of vessel ligation **(C)** are involved by metastatic tumor.

type with heaped ulcer margins; 73 (28 percent) were polypoid in type; 38 (14 percent) were constrictive and had a napkin-ring-like appearance; 3 (1 percent) showed a segmental narrowing; and in 9 (3 percent) the exact type was not recorded. Histologically, the majority were tubular adenocarcinomas with 244 (91 percent) representing this subtype: 14 (5 percent) were mucinous carcinoma; 4 (2 percent) were signet-ring-type cancers; and 2 (1 percent) were examples of adenosquamous and undifferentiated carcinoma, respectively.

The histologic grades of the 244 adenocarcinomas in the study were as follows: 68 (28 percent) were well-differentiated (grade 1) lesions; 145 (59 percent) were moderately differentiated (grade 2); and 31 (13 percent) were poorly differentiated (grade 3). According to Dukes' staging, 44 (16 percent) were stage "A"; 116 (44 percent) were stage "B"; and 106 (40 percent) were stage "C."

Local inflammatory reaction was present in approximately 75 percent of cases. This was graded as mild in 65 percent and marked in 10 percent of the cases. Ten or less lymph nodes were found in 74 percent of the specimens, and 11 to 20 nodes

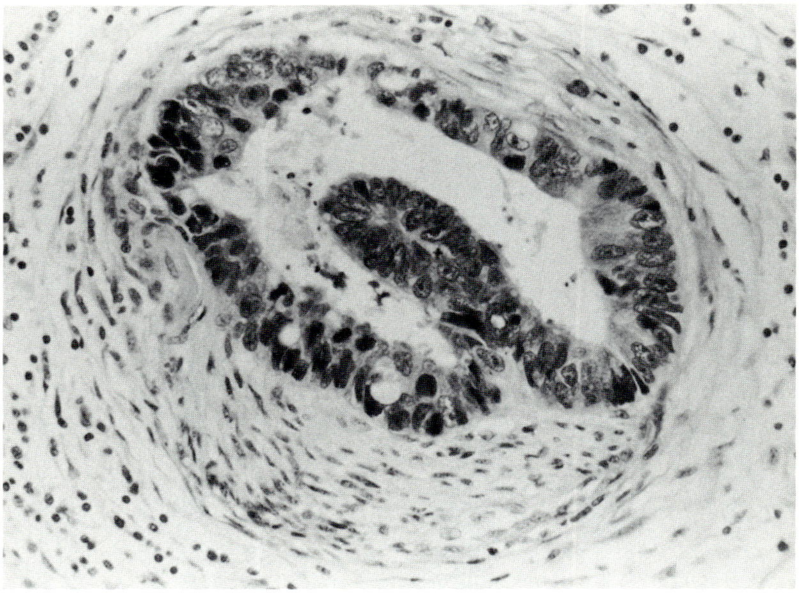

FIG. 31. Perineural involvement. H&E. ×408.

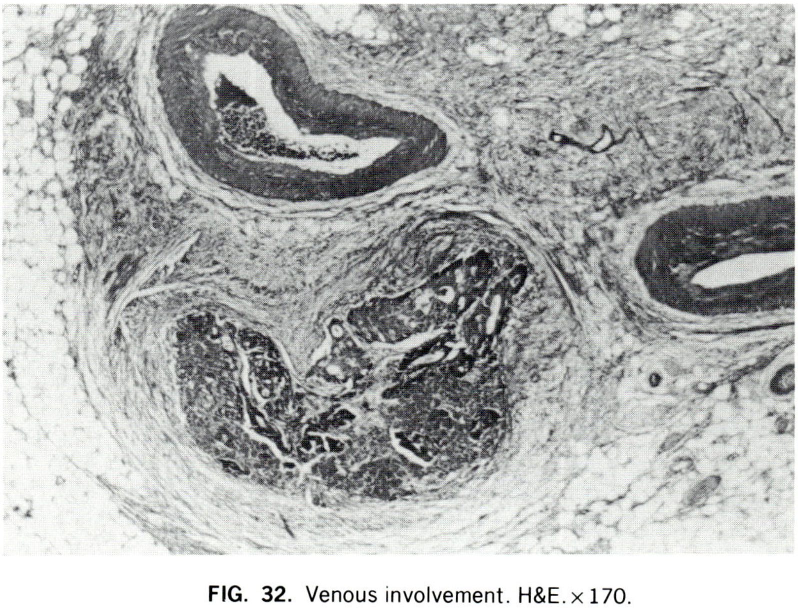

FIG. 32. Venous involvement. H&E. ×170.

were identified in 8 percent. In 18 percent of the reports, the exact number of nodes was not stated. Lymph nodes were involved with metastatic carcinoma in 40 percent of the specimens. In 80 percent of these the number of lymph nodes involved was four or less.

Venous involvement was present in 23 patients. The relationship of venous involvement to the histologic grade and Dukes' stage of cancers is seen in Table 2. When present, venous involvement was commonly found in Dukes' "C" lesions and in tumors with grade 2 or 3 histology.

Benign adenomatous epithelium was recognized in 30 (11 percent) of the 266 cancers in the study, suggesting origin in an adenoma. In 24 (9 percent) the adenomas were villous in type, and in 6 (2 percent) they were tubular.

In 87 patients, multiple synchronous tumors were found in the bowel at the time of surgery. In 78 (30 percent) of the patients these were adenomas. Forty-six were tubular in type and 22 were villous or had a mixed villo-tubular pattern. In 29 patients multiple adenomas were present, varying from 2 to 30 in number. Nine patients (3.5 percent) had a second cancer elsewhere in the bowel. The combined incidence of a synchronous tumor, either benign or malignant, in our series, was therefore 33.5 percent.

Five percent of the patients also had had a previous carcinoma removed from elsewhere in the bowel. The true metachronous rate in our series of 257 patients can only be arrived at by proper investigation and follow-up in future years.

Other associated lesions documented in these 257 patients included hyperplastic polyps in 10 percent of cases. This is one-third the incidence of adenomas in the study and probably shows that these common hyperplastic lesions are not accurately documented. In addition, three cecal lipomas, eight ileocecal lipomatoses, and one neurofibroma were also found. Diverticulosis was present in 16 patients. One patient had chronic idiopathic ulcerative colitis prior to developing carcinoma.

DISCUSSION

A careful and sytematic pathologic examination of the colorectum in patients with cancer is important in providing the clinician with valuable information for staging and prognosis. It has been suggested that the use of a standardized pathology report form may play an important role in accumulating data on patients with cancer from multiple institutions and in evaluating patient prognosis.[3] Our experience with such a standardized pathology report system demonstrates that this is feasible on a multiple-institution basis.

A number of features present in resected specimens from patients with colorectal cancer are important in predicting prognosis. Since clinical staging is difficult to apply in cancers of the colorectum, accurate recording of the pathologic data becomes increasingly important. Review of the literature reveals that tumor size,[8-11] tumor configuration,[12-14] circumference of intestinal wall involvement,[11,13,14] obstruction,[15,16] distance of the resected margin from the tumor,[17,18] depth of infiltration,[7,10,19,20] tumor grade,[13,21] tumor margin,[22,23] local inflammatory infiltrate,[19,25]

TABLE 1. Carcinoma of the Large Bowel Pathology Report

Name____________________ Age________ Sex________

Surgical No.____________________ Hospital________________

Patients's Physician____________________ Pathologist________________

Gross Examination

1. Primary Tumor
   (A) Location:
   - ☐ Cecum
   - ☐ Ascending colon
   - ☐ Hepatic flexure
   - ☐ Transverse colon
   - ☐ Splenic flexure
   - ☐ Descending colon
   - ☐ Sigmoid colon
   - ☐ Rectum above peritoneal reflection
   - ☐ Rectum below peritoneal reflection
     Distance from pectinate line________cm
     Length of resected bowel________cm
     Distance of tumor from distal resected margin________cm

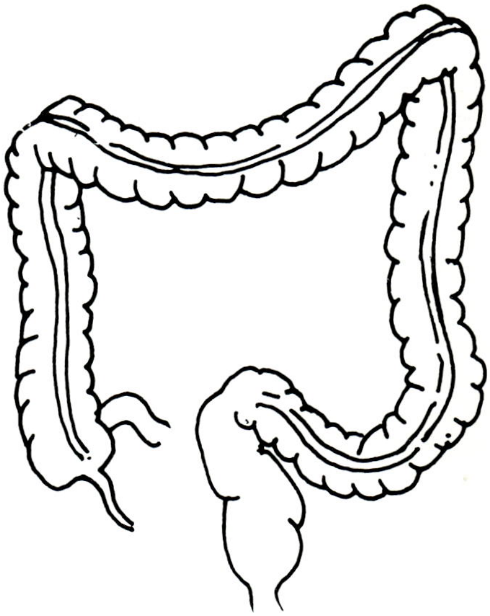

   (B) Size: Width________ cm

   Length________ cm

   Elevation________ cm

   Thickness________ cm

   (C) Configuration:
   - ☐ Polypoid
   - ☐ Ulcerated
   - ☐ Constrictive, i.e., napkin-ring type
   - ☐ Segmental
   - ☐ Diffuse, infiltration linitis plastica type

2. Lymph nodes
   (A) Adjacent to tumor. No. examined________________

   (B) At point of ligation of mesenteric vessels. No. examined________________

3. Peritoneum and attached mesocolon
   - ☐ Tumor implants present
   - ☐ Local ☐ Distant ☐ Omental

TABLE 1. (continued)

4. Perforation

☐ Present ☐ With abscess ☐ With fistula

Histologic Examination

5. Extent of spread

Dukes' classification

☐ A

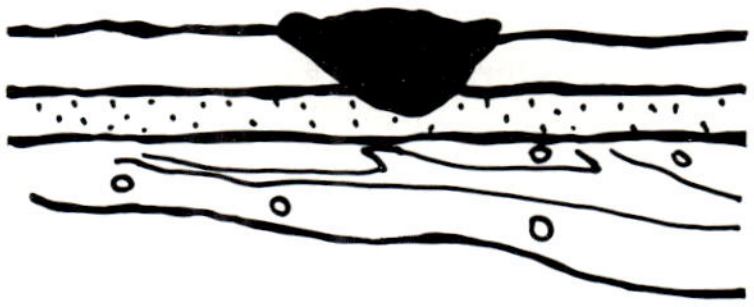

☐ B

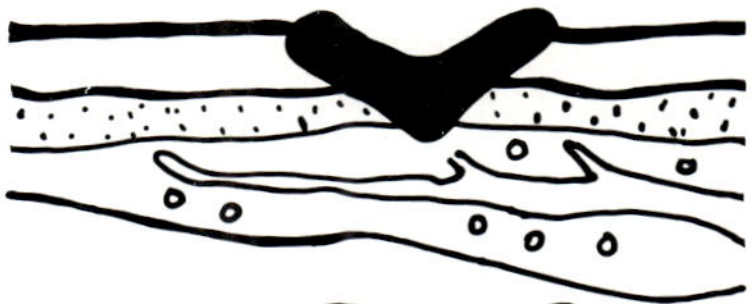

☐ C

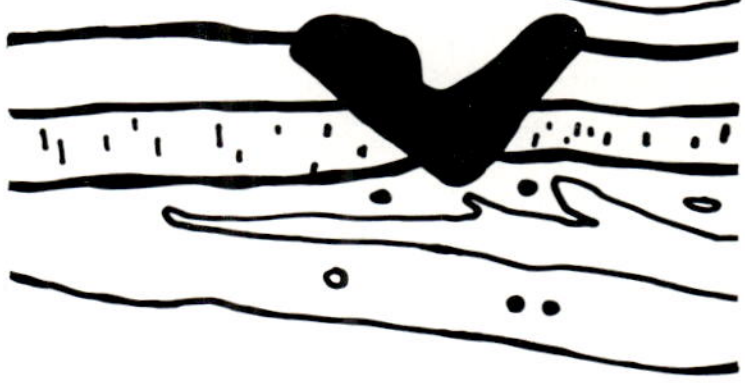

6. Histologic Type

☐ Adenocarcinoma

☐ Signet-ring carcinoma

☐ Mucinous carcinoma

☐ Undifferentiated carcinoma

☐ Other

Specify ____

____

7. Histologic Grade

☐ Well-differentiated (1)

☐ Moderately differentiated (2)

☐ Poorly differentiated (3)

8. Other Histologic Features

(A) Cellular reaction (lymphocytic, plasmacytic, and histiocytic)

☐ None ☐ Present ☐ Mild ☐ Marked

(B) Desmoplastic reaction

☐ None ☐ Present ☐ Mild ☐ Marked

9. Lymph node involvement

(A) Adjacent to tumor. No. examined_________ No. involved_________________

TABLE 1. (continued)

(B) At point of ligation of mesenteric vessels. No. examined________________
No. involved________________

10. Lymph vessel involvement
☐ Present Location: ☐ (A) Bowel wall ☐ (B) Outside bowel

11. Perineural involvement
☐ Present Location: ☐ (A) Bowel wall ☐ (B) Outside bowel

12. Blood vessel examination
☐ Venous involvement present Location: ☐ Bowel wall ☐ Outside bowel
☐ Thrombosis ☐ Ischemic changes bowel

13. Other simultaneous lesions
(Illustrate in Figure 1 and please specify below, e.g., size, location, number, and type of lesion)

Tumors.

Second carcinoma________________
____

Polyps________________
____

Other conditions (e.g., diverticula, ulcerative colitis, etc.) ________________
____
____

14. Final Diagnosis

15. Previous biopsy ☐ Yes ☐ No Surgical No. ________________
Diagnosis________________

and venous and perineural involvement,[17,19,20,22,27,28] are important in estimating prognosis.

Goodwin and Brown[8] showed a relationship between tumor size and depth of infiltration. Osnes,[9] on the other hand, found higher survival after resection of large tumors as compared with small tumors. Recently, Cohen and associates found that 42 percent of ulcerative adenocarcinomas greater than 4 cm in size[10] penetrated grossly through the rectal wall, compared to 12 percent of tumors less than 4 cm. However, Grinnell[11] did not find any relationship between size and frequency of metastases in tumors of the rectum. Our studies show no definite correlation between tumor size, extent of spread, and lymph node metastases. Although 21 percent of tumors less than 4 cm in size were in Dukes' stage "A" as compared to 12

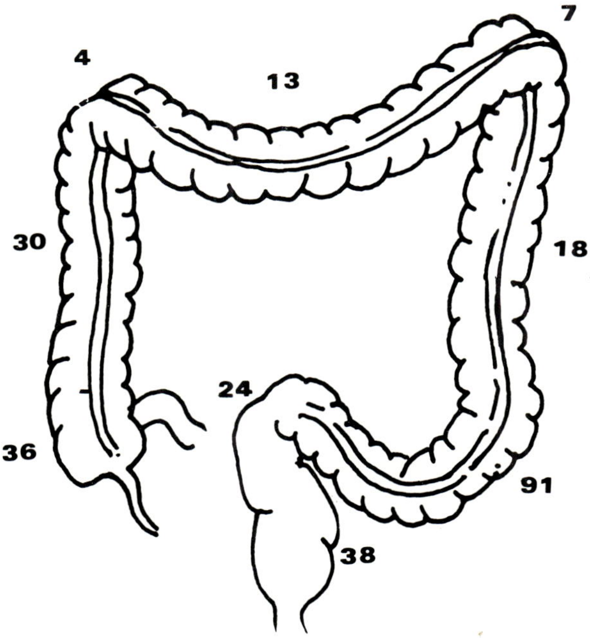

FIG. 33. Location of tumors. A total of 266 cancers were present in 257 patients; location not documented in 5.

percent of tumors greater than 4 cm, 44 percent of tumors less than 4 cm in size were in Dukes' stage "C" as compared with 40 percent greater than 4 cm in size.

Tumor shape also appears to have some prognostic significance. Polypoid tumors tend to grow slowly and to metastasize late in disease as compared to sessile tumors, which rapidly infiltrate the wall and metastasize to lymph nodes.[12-14] In our series of 266 cancers, 28 percent were polypoid whereas 54 percent were of the ulcerative type. Of the polypoid tumors, 32 percent were confined to the bowel wall (Dukes' "A"), whereas this was true in only 6 percent of the ulcerated cancers. Twenty-one percent of the polypoid tumors had lymph node metastases (Dukes' "C") compared to 47 percent of the ulcerated cancers.

TABLE 2. Relationship of Venous Involvement to Histologic Grade and Dukes' Stage

Dukes' Stage	No. with Venous Involvement	Histologic Grade		
		1	2	3
A	0	0	0	0
B	4	0	2	2
C	19	2	8	9
Total	23	2	10	11

The proportion of the circumference of the colon involved by cancer also influences prognosis. Grinnell[11,13] found a higher frequency of lymph node metastases and venous involvement, and poorer 5-year survival, in annular tumors involving the entire circumference of the bowel. Similarly, Coller et al.[14] found a greater frequency of lymph node metastases with tumors involving a large circumference of the bowel wall. Obstruction of the lumen is also associated with poor prognosis. The 5-year survival with tumors producing complete obstruction of the bowel is about one-half that in cases of nonobstructing carcinomas.[15,16] Tumors producing obstruction tend to be annular lesions with involvement of the entire circumference of the bowel wall, and therefore tend to be advanced cancers associated with a poor prognosis. Fourteen percent of our tumors were annular lesions with a napkin-ring configuration. All had spread beyond the wall of the bowel, with lymph node metastases in half of the cases.

There is evidence to suggest that 5 cm is an adequate margin of resection for tumors of the colorectum. Copeland[17] found suture line recurrence in 18 percent of cases if one or both of the resected margins was less that 5 cm. The recurrence rate for the whole group, however, was 10 percent. Furthermore, they found a 51 percent 5-year survival in the group of patients with more than 5 cm of normal intestine proximal and distal to the tumor, compared to a 38 percent 5-year survival in patients in whom less than a 5 cm margin of normal intestine was resected. Grinnell[18] found that the maximal distal permeation of lymphatics in the wall of the colon by carcinoma was of the order of 4 cm, and that a 5 cm margin of resection appeared adequate. From personal experience, I regard a 2 cm margin as quite adequate.

The depth of infiltration through the bowel wall is inversely related to survival, whether or not lymph nodes are involved.[7,19] The depth of infiltration correlates well with the frequency of venous invasion and lymph node metastases.[19] There are data suggesting that the most dramatic decrease in survival occurs when the muscle layers are penetrated by cancer. Seefeld and Bargen[20] showed that the incidence of venous invasion was dependent on the extent of mural penetration. Only 3 of the 20 cases in which there was venous invasion were of the Dukes' "B" type, compared to 17 cases which were Dukes' "C." There were no Dukes' "A" cases with venous involvement. Lymph node metastases also increased with deeper penetration of the rectal or colonic wall by cancer. Astler and Coller[7] showed that tumors infiltrating the muscle but not through it (B1) had a 3.9 percent lymph nodal involvement whereas those lesions which penetrated the muscle completely (B2) had 35 percent lymph nodal involvement. This suggests that a muscle coat of the bowel acts as an important barrier to metastases. Astler and Coller[7] also showed that the 5-year survival diminished by about 12 percent with tumor extension through the muscle coat of the bowel (B2), in contrast to cases in which tumor penetration was limited to the muscularis propria (B1). Transmural growth is also associated with a higher incidence of pelvic recurrence of cancer. In one recent study the pelvic recurrence rate with gross transmural invasion was twice that with microscopic transmural invasion only.[10]

The degree of differentiation of a tumor, or its histologic grade, has prognostic significance. Poorly differentiated tumors are associated with greater local spread, venous involvement, metastases to lymph nodes, and distant spread. Dukes[21] graded adenocarcinomas into four categories and found that this gave a fairly accurate index of the degree of malignancy. The 5-year survival with grade 1 lesions was 60 percent, whereas none of the patients with grade 4 lesions survived. Grinnell[13] used the architectural pattern of tumor cells—for example, glandular differentiation, polarity of the cells, and invasive tendency—as a degree of differentiation and found these features useful in predicting prognosis. With a three-grade system, 28 percent of the cancers in our study were well differentiated, 59 percent moderately differentiated, and 13 percent poorly differentiated. There was good correlation between the grade of the tumor and the Dukes' stage. Twenty-seven percent of our well-differentiated tumors were in Dukes' stage "A" as compared with 10 percent that showed moderate differentiation. None of the poorly differentiated cancers were in Dukes' stage A. Sixty percent of poorly differentiated carcinomas were in Dukes' stage "C" compared with 40 percent of moderate and 19 percent of well-differentiated lesions. Similarly, 54 percent of our mucinous carcinomas were in Dukes' "C" stage at the time of diagnosis.

Spratt and Spjut[22] showed that the study of advancing margins of the tumor provides information regarding prognosis. They showed that patients with tumors exhibiting infiltrating margins did poorly in contrast to those with tumors having circumscribed borders. Ackerman and Rosai[23] also noted that tumors with infiltrating borders had a higher incidence of lymphatic spread and distant metastases. Moreover, they showed that carcinomas with pushing borders and surrounded by an inflammatory infiltrate of lymphocytes and plasma cells did not metastasize as frequently as carcinomas devoid of an inflammatory reaction. Spratt and Spjut[22] also graded the inflammatory reaction around the cancer from none to severe, and demonstrated doubling of the 5-year survival rate in lesions associated with severe reaction. Similarly, Murray et al.[24] found a 46 percent 5-year survival in patients with Dukes' "B" carcinoma without local inflammatory reaction, and an 89 percent 5-year survival in those cases associated with such a reaction. In our study, local inflammatory reaction was present in 75 percent of the cases. This is similar to the incidence recorded by Wartman,[25] although Murray et al.[24] found this feature in 52 percent of their cases.

Recently, Pihl et al.[26] have shown that perivascular lymphocytic cuffing (Fig. 34) occupying more than 5 percent of a section through the muscular layers and pericolic subserosal fat adjacent to a carcinoma is associated with a longer disease-free interval, as compared with those lesions where this reaction is absent. Moreover they found that paracortical lymph node hyperplasia—i.e., T-lymphocytic hyperplasia—occupying an area of more than 15 percent of the lymph node section indicated a favorable association with survival. The combined paracortical hyperplasia in regional lymph nodes and perivascular lymphocytic cuffing in the primary tumors were associated with significantly fewer recurrences and deaths among those patients who showed this combination. However, sinus histiocytosis and cortical lymph node hyperplasia did not significantly affect the disease-free interval or overall survival.

Pihl et al. hypothesized that paracortical lymph node hyperplasia and perivascular lymphocytic cuffing in the primary tumor were expressions of a chain

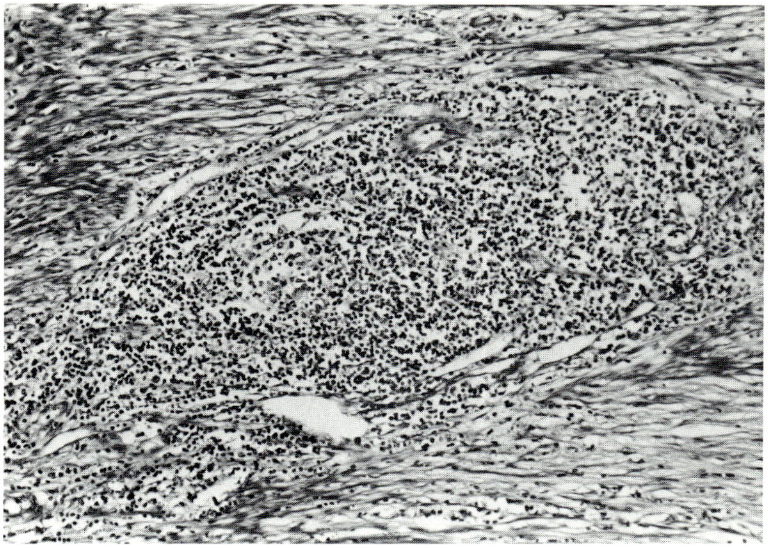

FIG. 34. Perivascular lymphocytic cuffing in the wall of the rectum in a patient with carcinoma. H&E. ×170.

of events initiated by the recognition of tumor antigen in the regional lymph nodes and followed by the proliferation by cytotoxic lymphoid cells in the paracortex. Some of these cytotoxic lymphoid cells, on leaving the lymph nodes via postnodal lymphatics, would reach the tumor site via the blood supply and appear in sections as perivascular lymphocytic cuffing. Pihl et al.[26] suggest that the absence of these immunomorphologic features can be used as a guide for identifying a subgroup of Dukes' "B" patients associated with poor prognosis in whom adjuvant chemotherapy may be justified. Tsakraklides and associates[27] did not find the morphologic changes in the regional lymph nodes to be important in predicting prognosis although patients with germinal center predominance—i.e., B-lymphocytic hyperplasia—did have a higher 5-year survival; however, the difference was not significant. Sinus histiocytosis was not frequently seen and was observed only in three patients in the study of Tsakraklides et al. However, Murray et al.[24] found sinus histiocytosis in 33 percent of patients with carcinoma of the colon. Furthermore, this was associated with an increased 5-year survival. For both stage "B" and "C" cancers the 5-year survival in the presence of sinus histiocytosis in regional lymph nodes was 76 percent, and in its absence the survival rate was 58 percent.

It is well recognized that the presence of metastases in regional lymph nodes adversely affects prognosis. Survival rates are reduced by one-half if regional lymph nodes contain metastases.[7,9,12,13,17,21] It is therefore important that node dissection be done carefully, and that all lymph nodes found be examined histologically for evidence of metastases, since gross determination of lymph node involvement is unreliable. There also appears to be a good correlation between the number of lymph nodes involved and survival. An increase in the number of involved lymph nodes is associated with a decrease in survival. Dukes,[28] Spratt and Spjut,[22] and

Copeland et al.[17] have shown that patients with colorectal cancer having more than five involved lymph nodes have a 5-year survival of less than 19 percent. The location of the lymph nodes involved by metastases also has prognostic implications. Involvement of lymph nodes farthest from the tumor, i.e., at the point of transection of the main vascular pedicle, is associated with a poorer prognosis than, for example, the involvement only of the lymph nodes adjacent to the tumor.[19] Grinnell[29] showed that when lymph nodes nearest to the point of transection of the main vessels were involved, the 5-year survival rate for cancers of the colorectum was 18 percent, but that if the nodes were uninvolved the survival rate was 53 percent. A retrograde pattern of metastases, although uncommon, is associated with a very poor prognosis.[30]

Venous involvement in cancer of the colon and rectum implies a poor prognosis.[17,19,20,22,29] Visceral metastases are more frequent when venous invasion is present. Venous invasion is rarely found before nodal involvement, but may occur in approximately 15 percent of cases without lymph node metastases.[20] The incidence of venous invasion in cancer of the colorectum varies from a little over 10 percent[31] to 61 percent.[32] Dukes[28,33] found gross invasion of veins in 17 percent of patients with rectal cancer, in 12 percent of cases of carcinoma of the left colon, and in 6 percent of growths in the right colon. Brown and Warren[32] reported an incidence of 61 percent in an autopsy study of 165 cases of cancer of the rectum. The high incidence can be explained on the basis of advanced disease with a greater chance of venous invasion. Seefeld and Bargen[20] found venous invasion in 20 percent of patients with cancer of the rectum. Grinnell[29] studied both cancer of the rectum and colon and found very little difference in the incidence of venous involvement. Thirty-three percent of tumors of the colon and 36 percent of those in the rectum had evidence of vascular invasion. In Grinnell's[29] series, 3 percent of Dukes' "A," 25 percent of Dukes' "B," and 49 percent of Dukes' "C" lesions demonstrated venous invasion. In our series venous involvement was demonstrated in 23 cases. There was a direct relationship between Dukes' stage, histologic grade, and venous invasion (Table 2). Nineteen of the cancers with venous invasion were Dukes' "C" cases and 21 of the 23 cancers were of histologic grade 2 and 3. Only four Dukes' "B" tumors had venous involvement and none of the cancers showing venous involvement were stage "A" lesions. Thus, in 17 percent of our cases venous involvement was present in the absence of lymph nodal involvement. It is apparent that stage of the disease influences venous involvement.

The method of examining the specimen also plays an important part in detecting venous involvement. Careful examination of the specimen with study of multiple sections and the use of elastic stains greatly increases detection of the incidence of venous involvement. Khankhanian et al.[34] have shown that vascular invasion confined within the bowel wall is not necessarily associated with poor prognosis. They studied 143 Dukes' "B" cancers, 27 with vascular involvement, and found no difference in either the tumor-free interval or the overall survival period in the groups with or without involvement. Grinnell,[29] however, showed a poorer prognosis in patients with Dukes' "B" cancer and venous invasion (5-year survival rate 60 percent) than in those with Dukes' "B" lesions that did not show venous invasion (5-year survival rate 88 percent).

Perineural invasion also is associated with a poor prognosis in colorectal cancer.[20,22] Seefeld and Bargen[20] showed that the frequency of perineural involvement increased with the poorer grade of a lesion, and was related to the Dukes' stage. Perineural involvement increased from about 14 percent in grade 1 to 37.5 percent in grade 4 tumors. The incidence of perineural involvement increased from 33 percent in Dukes' stage "B" to 66 percent in Dukes' "C" cases. No perineural involvement was found in Dukes' "A" cases. They further demonstrated a definite increase in the incidence of local recurrences. Eighty-one percent of the patients with perineural involvement developed local recurrences, compared with 30 percent in whom no perineural involvement could be demonstrated.

Muto et al.[35] have demonstrated contiguous benign tumor, either villous or tubular adenoma, in approximately 14 percent of cancers of the colorectum. Heald and Bussey[36] have shown the incidence of contiguous benign adenoma in relation to multiple synchronous invasive adenocarcinomas to be of the order of 27 percent. These studies suggest that adenocarcinomas of the colorectum evolve through a polyp–cancer sequence. In our series of 266 cancers, benign adenomatous epithelium was present in 30, or 11 percent, of the cancers. In 24 (9 percent) the adenomatous epithelium was villous in type, and in 6 (2 percent) it was tubular. Our studies confirm that the villous type of growth pattern has a higher malignant potential. Although tubular adenomas are more common, the villous adenomas show a much higher incidence of malignant transformation.

In 87 of our cases multiple synchronous tumors, either benign or malignant, were found in the bowel at the time of surgery. In 78 patients, these synchronous lesions were benign adenomas; in 9 patients, a second carcinoma was present elsewhere in the bowel. This combined incidence of benign and malignant synchronous tumors in our series was 33.5 percent. In the St. Marks Hospital experience with 3,002 patients, the incidence of multiple synchronous tumors, both benign and malignant, was 20 percent.[35] In a separate study from St. Marks Hospital of 157 multiple synchronous cancers, there were 78, or 50 percent of cases, with separate benign adenomas.[36] Additionally, 5 percent of our patients developed a second or metachronous cancer. Muto et al.[35] found a 7 percent metachronous rate in a 25-year follow-up of patients with tumors of the colorectum. Of the other associated lesions found in the surgical specimens of colorectum in our study, the one that deserves some comment is the so-called hyperplastic polyp. Hyperplastic polyps were recorded in only 10 percent of the cases in the study reported here, whereas adenomas were found in 30 percent. Hyperplastic polyps are common lesions and are found in the majority of colorectal specimens resected for cancer. Arthur,[36] for example, found metaplastic (hyperplastic) polyps in over 80 percent of rectums resected for cancer. It would appear that these small nodules are not being recorded accurately.

EXAMINATION OF POLYPECTOMY SPECIMENS

Biopsies from cancers of the colorectum obtained at the time of proctosigmoidoscopy or at colonoscopy are very helpful in establishing or confirming the diagnosis of malignancy and determining its histologic type. Orientation is not very crucial. On the other hand, diagnosing invasive cancer in polyps by biopsies is difficult. With the increasing use of colonoscopy, polypectomy is now being done in a majority of patients with polyps without resorting to laparotomy. Most polyps visualized during colonoscopy can be completely removed by cautery snare. The procedure is safe, with a low complication rate.

It is now widely accepted that adenomas of the large bowel are premalignant, although only a very small minority develop into cancer.[35] This risk varies with the size and type of adenoma. Polyps of less than 1 cm in size are rarely malignant. The incidence of invasive carcinoma in adenomas less than 1 cm is 0.3 percent, reaching 46 percent in lesions over 2 cm in size.[35] However, adenomas over 2 cm are relatively uncommon, representing less than 20 percent of all polyps.[35] In a recent study of 160 adenomas removed at colonoscopy, we found only 18, or 11 percent, to be over 2 cm.[37] The incidence of invasive cancer in these large adenomas was 22 percent (4 of 18), whereas none of the 82 adenomas under 1 cm in size showed histologic evidence of invasive cancer. Moreover, 2 of the 60—or 3 percent—adenomas between 1.0 and 1.9 cm contained invasive cancer.

Current evidence indicates that tubular adenomas have a low risk of malignant transformation in comparison with villous adenomas. Muto et al.[35] found a 4.8 percent incidence of invasive cancer in tubular adenomas compared with a 40.7 percent incidence in villous adenomas. However, Gillespie et al.,[38] in a polypectomy study, found invasive carcinoma in 2.2 percent of tubular adenomas, 5.8 percent of mixed villo-tubular, and 18 percent of villous adenomas. In a recent study,[37] we found 6 invasive cancers in 160 adenomas. None of the 108 tubular adenomas showed evidence of cancer, but three of the 36 or 8 percent of villo-tubular adenomas, and 3 of the 16 or 19 percent of villous adenomas harbored invasive cancers.

Malignant change—i.e., invasive carcinoma—in adenomas will be overlooked if one only examines small biopsies from these tumors. Therefore, histologic examination should be based on a thorough, complete examination of the excised polyp. This is best achieved by examining entire polyps (Fig. 35). Proper orientation is important. The majority of adenomas are small, being under 2 cm in size, so that it is possible to examine the entire lesion embedded in one block. Larger lesions may require some trimming. Sections should be cut along the long axis and include both the head and the stalk. The lines of resection must be included in the sections. I do not slice off the base of the stalk for histologic study. I embed the entire polyp and have it sectioned along the axis so that the head and the entire stalk are present on one slide and the relationship of the tumor to the stalk and line of resection is preserved. In the case of sessile polyps, the margins can be inked for easier identification.

Multiple sections are usually studied to exclude invasive cancer. A diagnosis of invasive carcinoma is made only when carcinomatous elements are found in the connective tissue stroma, below the level of the muscularis mucosa (Fig. 36). Cancer superficial to the muscularis mucosa, the so-called intramucosal cancer, very rarely metastasizes to regional lymph nodes,[39] and if completely excised needs no further treatment.

The management of patients with invasive cancer arising in pedunculated

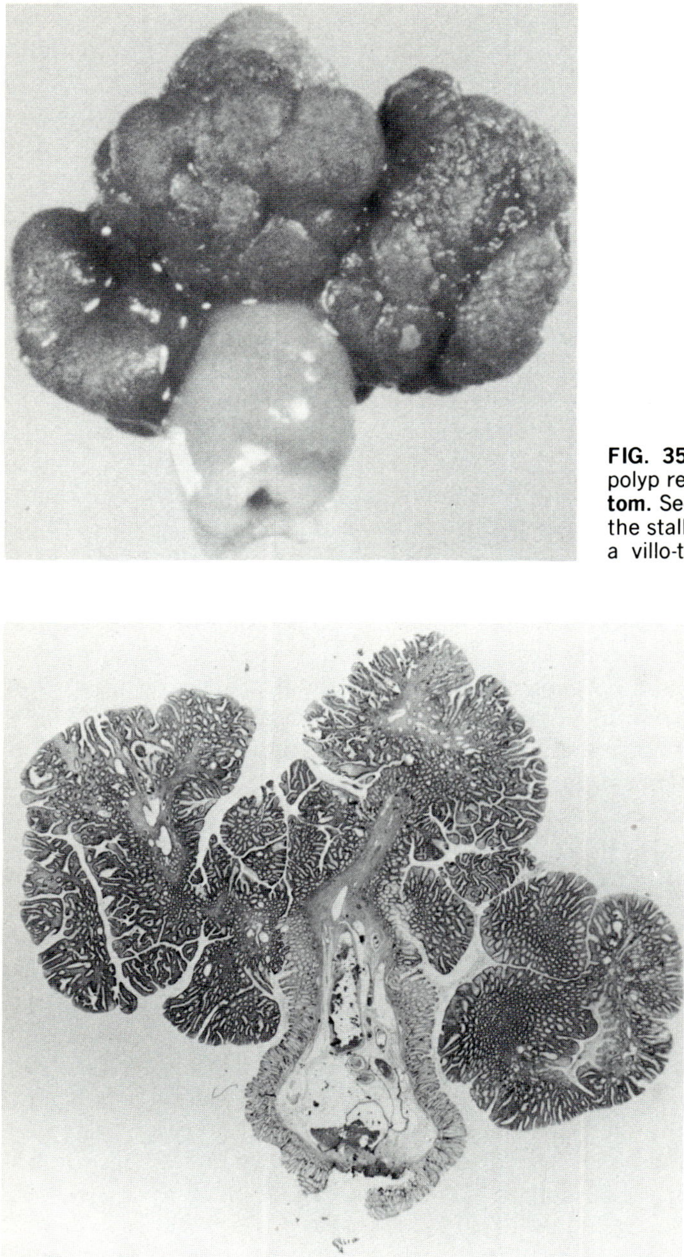

FIG. 35. Top. A 3 cm pedunculated polyp removed at polypectomy. **Bottom.** Section showing the head and the stalk. Histologically the lesion is a villo-tubular adenoma. H&E. ×3.

adenomas is controversial. Some workers recommend that local colonoscopic excision alone is sufficient treatment if the lesion is adequately resected and the malignant focus is moderately to well differentiated on histologic examination.[38] Polyps with poorly differentiated cancers and/or vascular and lymphatic invasion justify further surgical treatment. Most surgeons advocate further surgical resection in pa-

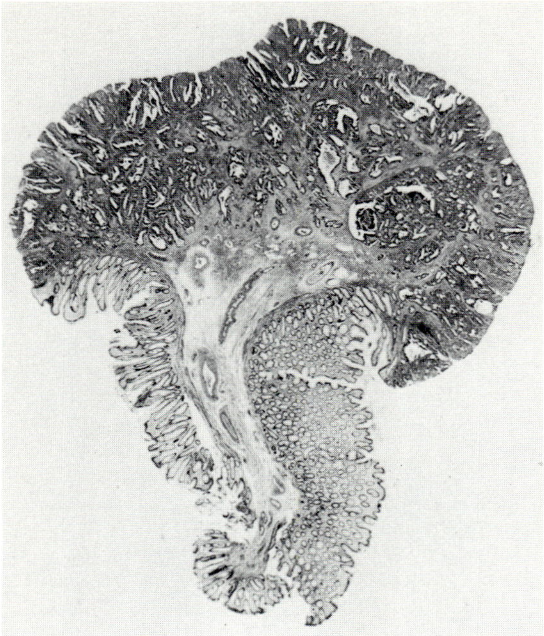

FIG. 36. Malignant polyp. Carcinomatous elements are present in the connective tissue of this polyp, below the level of muscularis mucosa. Resection margin is free of tumor. H&E. ×5.25. From Dis Colon Rectum 23:529, 1980.

tients with sessile adenomas exhibiting invasive cancer.[40] However, colonoscopic excision may have to suffice in poor-risk cases.

Pedunculated adenomas with misplaced epithelium in the stalk[37] must be distinguished from adenomas with invasive cancer. The former lesions show adenomatous epithelium and lamina propria above and below the muscularis mucosae (Figs. 37 and 38). The branching muscularis mucosa is usually thickened and surrounds islands of benign adenomatous epithelium. Recent hemorrhage and hemosiderin pigment is nearly always present, which is a clue to the diagnosis. Cystic change is not uncommon, with lakes of mucus in the stalk (Fig. 38), and separation from mucinous carcinoma may pose a problem for the inexperienced.

Another type of polyp which deserves brief mention is polypoid carcinoma. These lesions are protuberant carcinomas in which no evidence of benign epithelium is found at the time of diagnosis (Fig. 39). One percent of tumors removed at colonoscopy in one recent study were examples of polypoid carcinomas.[38] We found 4, or 2.2 percent, of 182 polyps removed from 100 patients during colonoscopy to represent polypoid carcinoma.[37] Three of these tumors were between 1.0 and 1.9 cm in size and one was over 2 cm. All four patients underwent subsequent bowel resection. The three cancers under 2.0 cm in size were initially adequately excised and were moderate to well-differentiated. No evidence of residual disease was found in the resected colons in these three cases. However, residual cancer was present in the fourth case, with metastases to the regional lymph nodes.

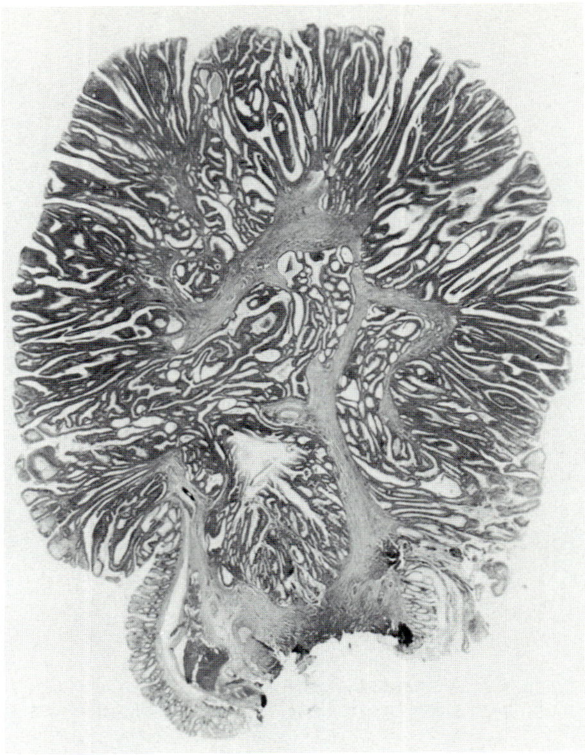

FIG. 37. Villo-tubular adenoma with misplaced epithelium in the stalk. Note the admixture of adenomatous epithelium and branching muscularis mucosa in the connective tissue stroma of the stalk. H&E. ×3.75. From Dis Colon Rectum 23:529, 1980.

This was incompletely excised initially and moreover was poorly differentiated. It would appear that well- and moderately differentiated cancers, either arising in adenomas or presenting as polyps, may be adequately treated by local excision as long as the excision is complete and the lesion is well- to moderately differentiated. Gillespie et al.[38] also advocate a similar line of treatment for these early large-bowel cancers.

SUMMARY

The results of a careful and systematic examination of surgical specimens from patients with tumors of the colorectum play an important role in patient care and the assessment of prognosis. An accurate and detailed gross examination of the specimen is important. Photographs and line drawings are very useful. Proper handling of the specimen and fixation for 24 to 48 hours are essential before satisfactory blocks can be taken for sectioning. Lymph nodes adjacent to the lesion and at the point of ligation of the vascular pedicle should be removed for section-

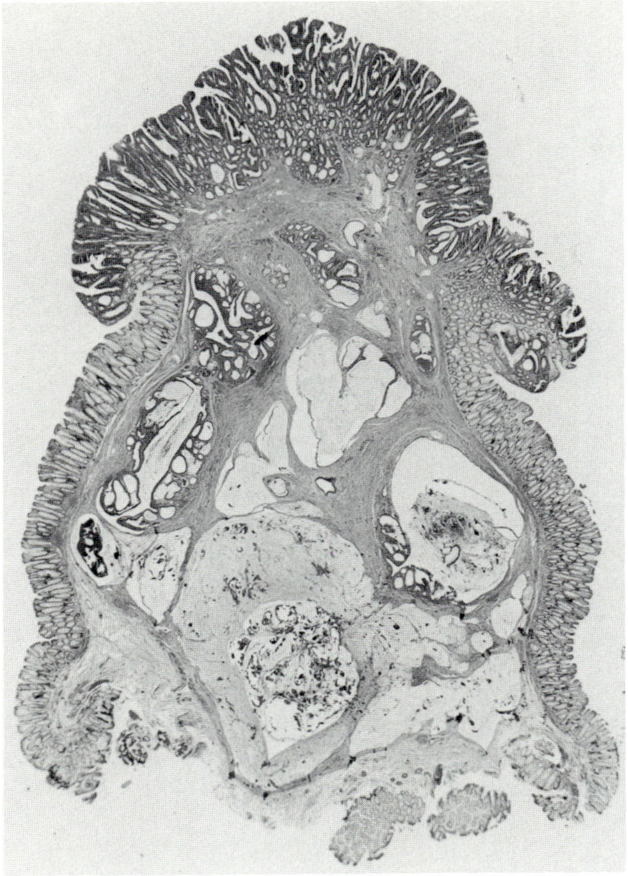

FIG. 38. Villo-tubular adenoma with misplaced epithelium in the stalk with large lakes of mucus. H&E. ×3. From Dis Colon Rectum 23:529, 1980.

ing. Multiple blocks of the tumor and adjacent tissues should be taken for histologic study. All blocks should be appropriately labeled and properly identified. I have found the use of large sections of the entire lesion a very satisfactory method of studying cancers and polyps; in such preparations the anatomic relationships remain undisturbed. The pathology report should include information on the site or sites of tumor, the size, configuration, and circumference of the bowel wall involved, obstruction, distance of the resected margin from the tumor, depth of infiltration, tumor grade, tumor margin, local inflammatory reaction, lymph node involvement and location, and venous and perineural invasion. There is evidence in the literature to suggest that all of the above pathologic features are either essential or desirable for pathology reports and have varying degrees of prognostic value. The literature on the prognostic value of immunomorphologic features in non-tumorous regional lymph nodes is contradictory. Cortical, paracortical, and sinus hyperplasia have been reported to be both associated with or to have no relation to

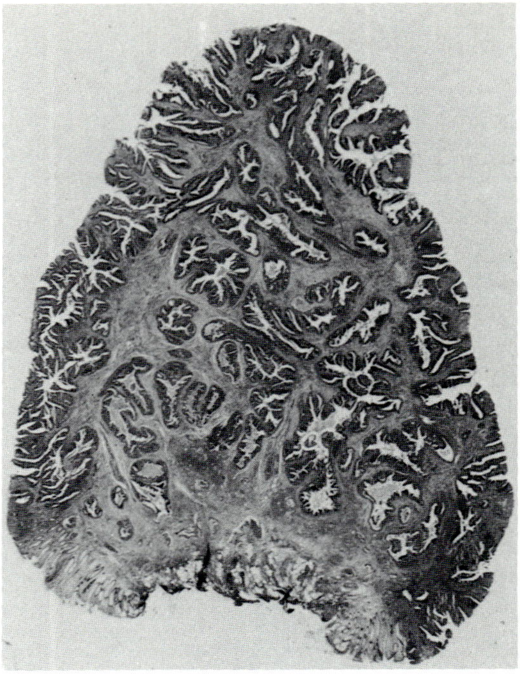

FIG. 39. Polypoid carcinoma. The entire lesion is malignant. The lesion was apparently completely resected. However, since the cancer elements were close to the resection margin, a segmental resection of the colon and lymph node dissection was done. No residual tumor was present in the colon and the lymph nodes were free of tumor. H&E. ×5.25. From Dis Colon Rectum 23:529, 1980.

prognosis. However, careful documentation of the changes in lymph nodes may in time shed light on their value, if any, with regard to survival.

We have found a standardized pathology reporting system very useful in compiling data and evaluating patient prognosis. Moreover, this system of reporting can be used as a method of quality control in establishing minimum standards for data collection, as originally suggested by Buckwalter and Kent.[3] In a regional multiinstitutional study such as ours, differences attributable to subjective variations among different observers are likely to occur, and may have some bearing when different pathologic features are eventually correlated with survival.

ACKNOWLEDGMENTS

The author gratefully acknowledges the collaboration of the numerous pathologists and pathology residents in the McMaster University Teaching Hospitals, Hamilton, and the members of the regional G.I. Oncology group, for without their support and cooperation this study could not have been possible.

I am specially grateful to the histology staff of Henderson General Hospital, Hamilton, and in particular to Mrs. R. Staat for her dedication and technical expertise in the preparation of the large microscopic sections. Thanks are due also to Miss Christine Marshall-Smith for the reproductions of the gross and microscopic photographs and to Mrs. R. Quinn for the typing of this manuscript.

REFERENCES

1. Silverberg E: Cancer Statistics. CA 31:13, 1981
2. Levin DL, Devesa SS, Godwin JD, Silverman DT: Cancer Rates and Risks, ed 2. Bethesda, Md, DHEW Publication No. (NIH) 75–691, 1974
3. Buckwalter JA, Kent TH: Colonic cancer. Essential information for a pathologic report. Arch Pathol 95:366, 1973
4. Manual for Staging of Cancer. American Joint Committee for Cancer Staging and End Results Reporting. Chicago, Whiting Press, 1978, pp 77–83
5. Dukes CE, Bussey HJR, Lamb GW: The examination and classification of operation specimens of intestinal cancer. Bull Int Assoc Med Mus 28:55, 1948
6. Dukes CE: The classification of cancer of the rectum. J Pathol Bacteriol 35:323, 1932
7. Astler VB, Coller FA: Prognostic significance of direct extension of carcinoma of the colon & rectum. Ann Surg 139:846, 1954
8. Goodwin JD, Brown CC: Some prognostic factors in survival of patients with cancer of the colon & rectum. J Chron Dis 28:441, 1975
9. Osnes S: Carcinoma of the colon and rectum. A study of 353 cases with special reference to prognosis. Acta Chir Scand 110:378, 1955
10. Cohen AM, Wood WC, Gunderson LL, Shinnar M: Pathological studies in rectal cancer. Cancer 45:2965, 1980
11. Grinnell RS: The lymphatic and venous spread of carcinoma of rectum. Ann Surg 116:200, 1942
12. Rankin FW, Olsen PF: The hopeful prognosis in cases of carcinoma of the colon. Surg Gynecol Obstet 56:366, 1933
13. Grinnell RS: The grading and prognosis of carcinoma of the colon and rectum. Ann Surg 109:500, 1939
14. Coller FA, Kay EB, MacIntyre RS: Regional lymphatic metastases of carcinoma of the rectum. Surgery 8:294, 1940
15. Wilder TC, Dockerty MB, Waugh JM: A clinicopathologic study of obstructing carcinomas of the right portion of colon. Surg Gynecol Obstet 113:353, 1961
16. Minister JJ: Comparison of obstructing and non-obstructing carcinoma of the colon. Cancer 17:242, 1964
17. Copeland EM, Miller LD, Jones RS: Prognostic factors in carcinoma of the colon and rectum. Am J Surg 116:875, 1968
18. Grinnell RS: Distal intramural spread of carcinoma of the rectum and rectosigmoid. Surg Gynecol Obstet 99:421, 1954
19. Dukes CE, Bussey HJR: The spread of rectal cancer and its effect on prognosis. Br J Cancer 12:309, 1958
20. Seefeld PH, Bargen JA: The spread of carcinoma of the rectum. Invasion of lymphatics, veins and nerves. Ann Surg 118:76, 1943
21. Dukes CE: Histological grading of rectal cancer. Proc R Soc Med 30:371, 1936
22. Spratt JS, Spjut HJ: Prevalence and prognosis of individual clinical and pathologic variables associated with colorectal carcinomas. Cancer 20:1976, 1967
23. Ackerman LV, Rosai J: Surgical Pathology, ed 5. St. Louis, Mosby, 1974, p 471
24. Murray D, Hreno A, Dutton J, Hampson LG: Prognosis in colon cancer. A pathologic reassessment. Arch Surg 110:908, 1975
25. Wartman WB: Sinus cell hyperplasia of lymph nodes regional to adenocarcinoma of the breast and colon. Br J Cancer 13:389, 1959

26. Pihl E, Malahy MA, Khankhanian N, et al.: Immunomorphological features of prognostic significance in Dukes' class B colorectal carcinoma. Cancer Res 37:4145, 1977
27. Tsakraklides V, Wanebo HJ, Sternberg SS, et al.: Prognostic evaluation of regional lymph node morphology in colorectal cancer. Am J Surg 129:174, 1975
28. Dukes CE: The surgical pathology of rectal cancer. The President's address. Proc R Soc Med 37:131, 1944
29. Grinnell RS: The spread of carcinoma of the colon and rectum. Cancer 3:641, 1950
30. Grinnell RS: Lymphatic block with atypical and retrograde lymphatic metastases and spread in carcinoma of the colon and rectum. Ann Surg 163:272, 1966
31. Dionne L: The pattern of blood borne metastases from carcinoma of rectum. Cancer 18:775, 1965
32. Brown CE, Warren S: Visceral metastases from rectal carcinoma. Surg Gynecol Obstet 66:611, 1938
33. Dukes CE: Discussion on the pathology and treatment of carcinoma of the colon. Proc R Soc Med 38:381, 1944–1945
34. Khankhanian N, Mavligit GM, Russell WO, Schimek M: Prognostic significance of vascular invasion in colorectal cancer of Dukes B class. Cancer 39:1195, 1977
35. Muto T, Bussey HJR, Morson BC: The evolution of cancer of the colon and rectum. Cancer 36:2251, 1975
36. Heald RJ, Bussey HJR: Clinical experience at St. Marks Hospital with multiple synchronous cancers of the colon and rectum. Dis Col Rectum 18:6, 1975
37. Qizilbash AH, Meghji M, Castelli M: Pseudocarcinomatous invasion in adenomas of the colon and rectum. Dis Colon Rectum 23:529, 1980
38. Gillespie PE, Chambers TJ, Chan KW, et al.: Colonic adenomas, a colonoscopic survey. Gut 20:240, 1979
39. Strauss RA, Pascal RR: Invasive and metastasizing carcinoma in a small adenomatous polyp of the colon: Report of a case with demonstration of tumor associated antigen. Hum Pathol 6:256, 1975
40. Welch JP, Welch CE: Villous adenoma of the colorectum. Am J Surg 131:185, 1976

PSEUDOMETASTASES IN FEMALE GENITAL CANCER

DIANE C. FARHI AND STEVEN G. SILVERBERG

Within the past few years, staging laparotomy, including abdominal and pelvic lymphadenectomy with inspection of the peritoneal surface, multiple biopsies and fluid cytologies, and the removal of suspicious lesions, has become a widely used procedure in the treatment of a variety of female genital malignancies.[9,15,68] In the course of abdominal and pelvic surgery for either benign or suspected malignant disease, a number of lesions may be excised which present diagnostic challenges. The purpose of this review is to call the attention of the practicing pathologist to various lesions resembling metastatic carcinoma, with particular emphasis on female genital tract malignancies. Each of these lesions has, in fact, been mistakenly diagnosed as malignant, sometimes leading to exhaustive investigations for occult carcinoma, to unduly radical surgery, or to unnecessary radiation or chemotherapy. Examples of most of these lesions have been seen recently at our institution in consultation or on the surgical pathology service. Some are common and others are rare, but all have occasionally presented diagnostic challenges to experienced pathologists.

Since the surgical evaluation of metastatic disease includes biopsies of lymph nodes and peritonealized surfaces, the following discussion has been divided into those two broad categories. Pitfalls in the differential diagnosis of carcinoma in the lymph nodes can occur with a wide range of metaplastic Mullerian inclusions: decidual change, endometriosis, and endosalpingiosis. We suspect that some of these inclusions may also have an independent malignant potential, which will be discussed below. Nevus cells in lymph nodes, although not yet described in abdominal or pelvic nodes, are included as an additional pitfall source in the diagnosis of metastatic disease.

Peritoneal lesions requiring distinction from metastases include leiomyomatosis peritonealis disseminata, the same range of paramesonephric (Mullerian) metaplasia described in lymph nodes, and reactive and papillary mesothelial pro-

Supported in part by grant CA-15823 from the National Institutes of Health, and by a gift to the Department of Pathology from the R. J. Reynolds Industries, Inc.

liferations. Other lesions, such as granulomata,[69] are more readily diagnosed correctly and will not be discussed further.

LESIONS IN NODES

Mullerian Inclusions

Small glands and epithelial-lined cysts have been noted in abdominal and pelvic lymph nodes in women since the nineteenth century, when they were first reported by Ries[17] in a study of uterine carcinoma, and by Wertheim[18] in a case of cervical carcinoma. Then, as now, they were mistaken for metastatic tumor, and therein lies their significance.

Over the next several decades, a small but steadily growing body of literature appeared concerning these lymph node inclusions, summarized by Russell in 1945.[1] By that time, the main theories regarding the pathogenesis of such inclusions had been established. Various authors supported a derivation from Wolffian (mesonephric) duct remnants, alterations in lymph node endothelium, metaplasia of the peritoneum to form Mullerian-type (paramesonephric) structures, the lymphatic or venous migration of endometrium, and retrograde menstrual flow into the peritoneum.[1] Russell himself was noncommittal as to which theory he favored. He added to the literature one example of endometriosis, with a well-developed decidual reaction in a pelvic lymph node; this was found in a woman who died of a ruptured ectopic pregnancy.

In 1960, the problem of benign glandular inclusions in female pelvic lymph nodes was taken up by Lange, who exhaustively reviewed the largely German literature from 1900 to the 1950s.[19] He recognized that the inclusions did not fulfill the criteria for endometriosis, but was at a loss to account for them, and invoked "inflammatory" influences. He found that 34.3 percent of 178 lymph node dissections for cervical carcinoma had lymph node inclusions.

The second large-scale attempt to establish the incidence of glandular inclusions in pelvic nodes was published in 1962 by Huhn.[2] He found, with meticulous examination, that 41 percent of radical dissections for cervical carcinoma had benign glandular inclusions in at least one node. This figure has not been approached since his report. The histologic features of these inclusions are not well defined, although they are said to resemble "the glands of the endometrium."

Confusion persists concerning the histologic range of these glandular lymph node inclusions. Weir and Janovski drew attention to this in a single case of an inclusion not fulfilling the histologic criteria for endometriosis.[3] They termed this a paramesonephric (Mullerian) inclusion, or endosalpingiosis, pointing out its strong resemblance to tubal epithelium. Koss reported a single case of carcinoma arising in such an inclusion, yet considered the inclusion a form of endometriosis.[4]

By 1969, the concept of endosalpingiosis as distinct from endometriosis was established;[5-7] the former was characterized by glands lined by tubal-type epithelium, often ciliated, without accompanying stroma other than a fibrous capsule. A unifying concept of the pathogenesis of endosalpingiosis emerged: metaplasia of coelomic epithelium, which embryologically gives rise to the Mullerian or paramesonephric ducts,[16] was favored as the origin of endosalpingiosis.[5-7] Reports of the incidence of endosalpingiosis of the pelvic and paraaortic nodes in autopsy and surgical material have given it a range of from about 5 percent to 14 percent.[5,9,11,20]

In recent years, there have appeared several additional case reports drawing the attention of clinicians and pathologists to endosalpingiosis, or benign Mullerian inclusions, and their differential diagnosis,[8-11,13,14] including glands of uncertain origin in extraabdominal locations.[12] Despite careful search, Mullerian inclusions have been found only in women.[3]

At present, endosalpingiosis remains defined as the ectopic location of epithelium resembling that of the normal fallopian tube.[7,21] The inclusions may be single or multiple and are consistently located in capsular or cortical areas. They range in size from microscopic tubules to cysts 1 to 2 cm in diameter. Although they have been reported, rarely, as causing ureteral obstruction,[3] they usually appear to be of no clinical significance unless mistaken for carcinoma.

Histologically, endosalpingiosis is characterized by small to cystically dilated glands containing a single, well-oriented layer of cuboidal to columnar epithelium, surrounded by a thin rim of fibrous tissue (Fig. 1). No endometrial stroma (or evidence of recent or remote hemorrhage) is present, distinguishing endosalpingiosis from endometriosis. The cells are cytologically bland, showing regular round to oval nuclei (Fig. 2). Mucin-containing goblet cells are often present, as

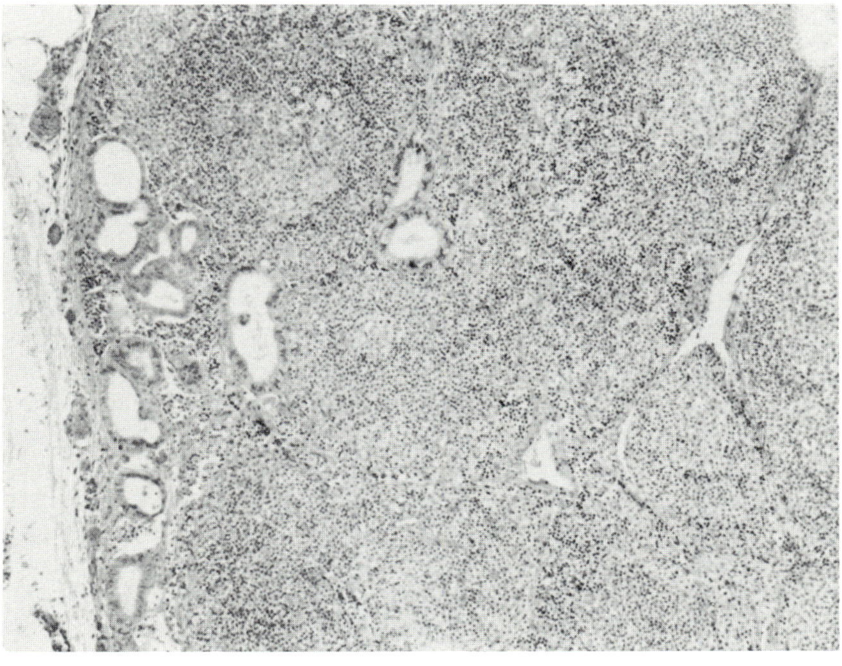

FIG. 1. Endosalpingiosis of an abdominal lymph node, showing small and cystically dilated glands in a subcapsular and cortical location. H&E. ×200.

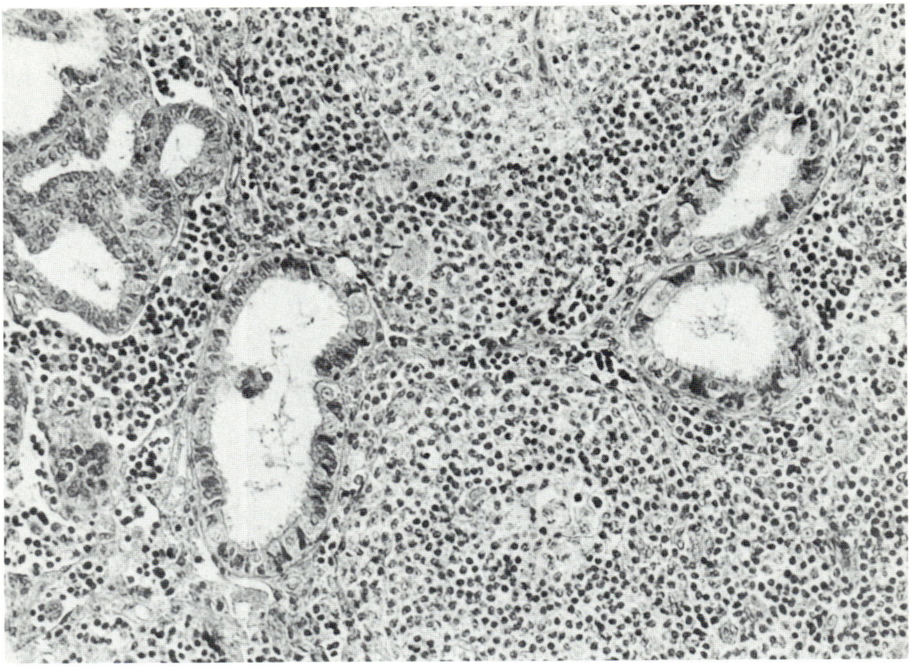

FIG. 2. Endosalpingiosis of an abdominal lymph node, showing detail of glands surrounded by a thin rim of fibrous tissue. A single layer of cuboidal to columnar cells is present. Many of the cells are ciliated, and a few are secretory. H&E. ×500.

well as variable numbers of tall columnar, pseudostratified ciliated cells, reinforcing the resemblance to endocervical and/or tubal epithelium. Foci of endometrial-type epithelium may also be encountered. Mitotic activity is extremely rare and usually absent. Significantly, intraluminal papillary projections and psammoma bodies[3,5,7,14,20,21] are common in endosalpingiosis, and thus are not helpful in distinguishing these inclusions from metastatic carcinoma.

In summary, a wide range of Mullerian-type inclusions may appear in the pelvic and abdominal lymph nodes in women. These represent a spectrum from decidualized stroma alone,[8] to a combination of stroma (decidualized or not) and endometrial-type glands, recognized as "endometriosis," to glands devoid of stroma, resembling endocervical and/or tubal mucosa and termed "endosalpingiosis." All of these mucosal types are derived embryologically from the paramesonephric (Mullerian) ducts, which are longitudinal invaginations of the coelomic epithelium. Metaplasia of coelomic epithelium trapped in lymph nodes and in abdominal or pelvic organs (see below) is the best available explanation for the occurrence of such inclusions. It seems best to simply term them paramesonephric or Mullerian inclusions. Their significance, beyond a rare case of obstructive uropathy or other mass effect, lies in their confusion with metastatic carcinoma, from which they may be distinguished by their typically capsular or septal location, lack of involvement of node sinuses, and the single layer of quite bland cells. The distinction from carcinoma constitutes a greater problem in a case of endosalpingiosis, where the readily recognized stroma of endometriosis is not present. At times it may be impossible to distinguish paramesonephric inclusions from metastases of a borderline ovarian carcinoma, in which case at least one author recommends that it may be best not to treat for metastatic disease.[14]

Finally, it is evident that a single node may contain more than one type of inclusion, as well as containing an inclusion and a true metastasis (Figs. 3 and 4).[5,11,13] Another important possibility is the development of a primary carcinoma in a paramesonephric inclusion. This has been reported in endometriosis of a pelvic lymph node[4] (although this was probably a case of endosalpingiosis), and we have seen two similar cases associated with borderline ovarian tumors (Figs. 5 and 6). There is no reason why malignant transformation may not occur in endosalpingiosis. In fact, it would seem likely that any systemic (e.g., hormonal) factors important in the induction of carcinoma in female Mullerian-derived mucosa would act on metaplastic Mullerian epithelium as well. This may account for the frequent association of endometrial carcinoma with endometrioid carcinoma of the ovary, for example. Although this combination is often considered to represent a primary and its metastasis, it has been noted that the survival rate in stage III endometrial carcinoma based on ovarian "metastasis" alone is much better than that seen with other types of pelvic dissemination. Thus, these lesions are more consistent with synchronous stage I primary tumors.[70] In some cases, the origin of the ovarian lesion in a focus of endometriosis can be demonstrated, effectively ruling out a metastasis from the endometrial tumor (Fig. 7). We have similar separate primary

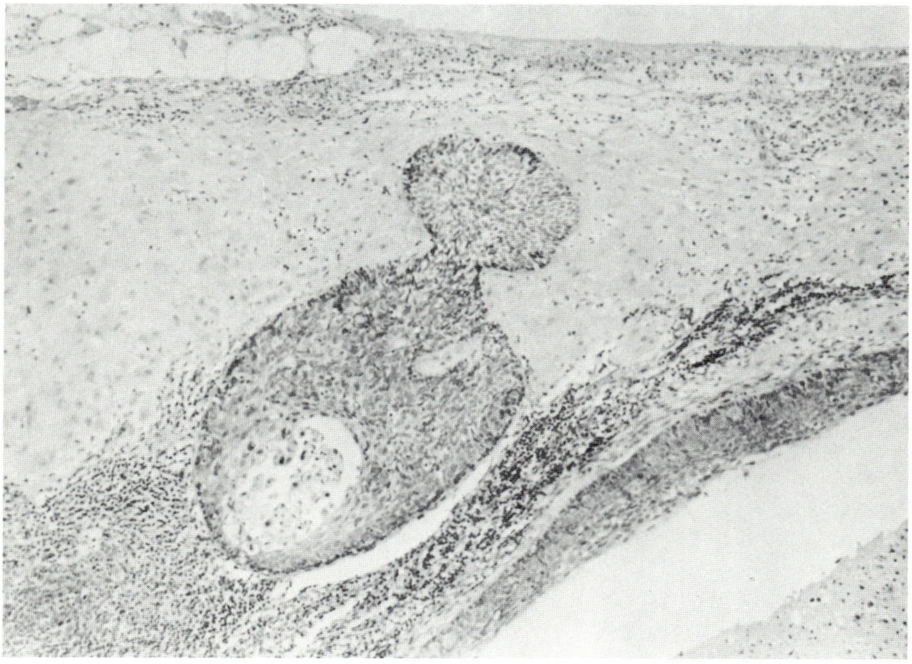

FIG. 3. Abdominal lymph node showing both metastatic cervical squamous cell carcinoma and a decidual reaction (evidence of paramesonephric metaplasia). H&E. ×200.

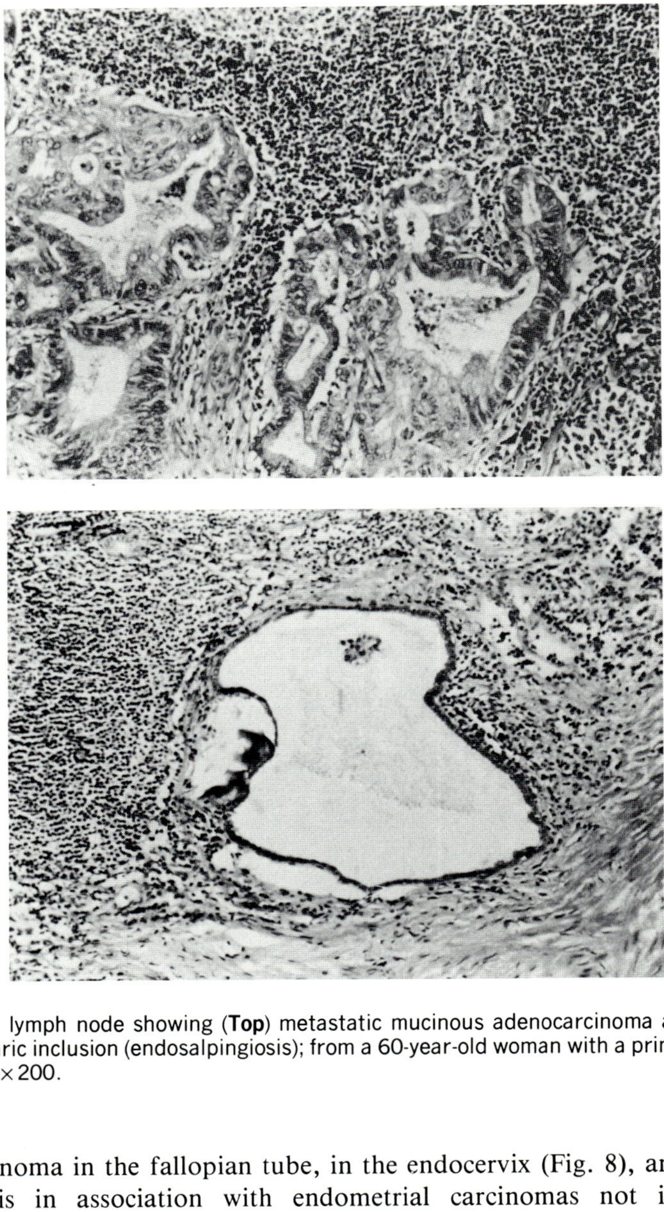

FIG. 4. Pelvic lymph node showing (**Top**) metastatic mucinous adenocarcinoma and (**Bottom**) a paramesonephric inclusion (endosalpingiosis); from a 60-year-old woman with a primary pelvic carcinoma. H&E. ×200.

foci of carcinoma in the fallopian tube, in the endocervix (Fig. 8), and in vaginal endometriosis in association with endometrial carcinomas not invading the myometrium, which are extremely unlikely to metastasize. Thus, there is ample evidence of a "field effect" or syndrome of upper female genital tract neoplasia,[71,72] which may involve nodal Mullerian epithelial inclusions as well.

Benign Nevus Cell Aggregates

Benign nests of nevus cells associated with lymph nodes are a second finding which may, like paramesonephric inclusions, be mistaken for metastatic tumor. Unlike

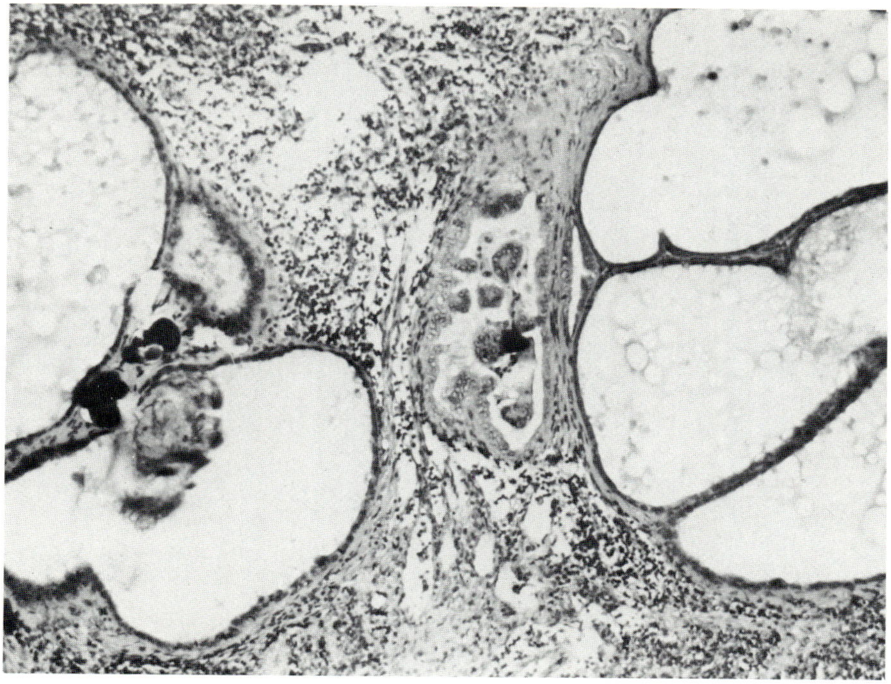

FIG. 5. Development of a borderline tumor in an otherwise typical focus of endosalpingiosis (right side of figure) in a pelvic lymph node. A borderline tumor was also present in the ovary. H&E. ×200.

Mullerian inclusions, they are not likely to be found in the course of pelvic or abdominal lymphadenectomies. The literature contains numerous examples of nevus cell aggregates with axillary nodes (36 cases),[22,24,27,28] groin nodes (9 cases),[24,25,31] and lymph nodes of the cervical region (5 cases),[22-24,27,28] but no examples in the thorax, abdomen, or pelvis. Nonetheless, these nevus cell aggregates are included here by virtue of their possible confusion with metastatic cancer, and in the context of female genital tract tumors can be encountered in groin dissections for vulvar carcinoma.

The occurrence of these cells in lymph nodes has been known for years, but observed only rarely. Stewart, in 1931, was the first to describe such a lesion in an axillary node, in the course of a discussion on neurogenic sarcoma.[32] The characteristic feature of the lesion is the presence of small, typically uniform, cytologically bland cells in the capsular connective tissue of the node. Many years later Stewart commented on having seen three such cases,[33] and in 1969 Johnson and Helwig published the first substantial series of nevus cell aggregates.[22] They reported six cases occurring in cervical and axillary nodes of patients with a wide variety of benign and malignant lesions. Two possible pathogenetic mechanisms were proposed: aberrant migration of melanocytes from the neural crest, and "benign metastasis" from a nevus in the skin drained by the involved node. Advocates of both the former[23,25,28] and the latter[24] theory have offered their opinions, but neither etiology has been proven.

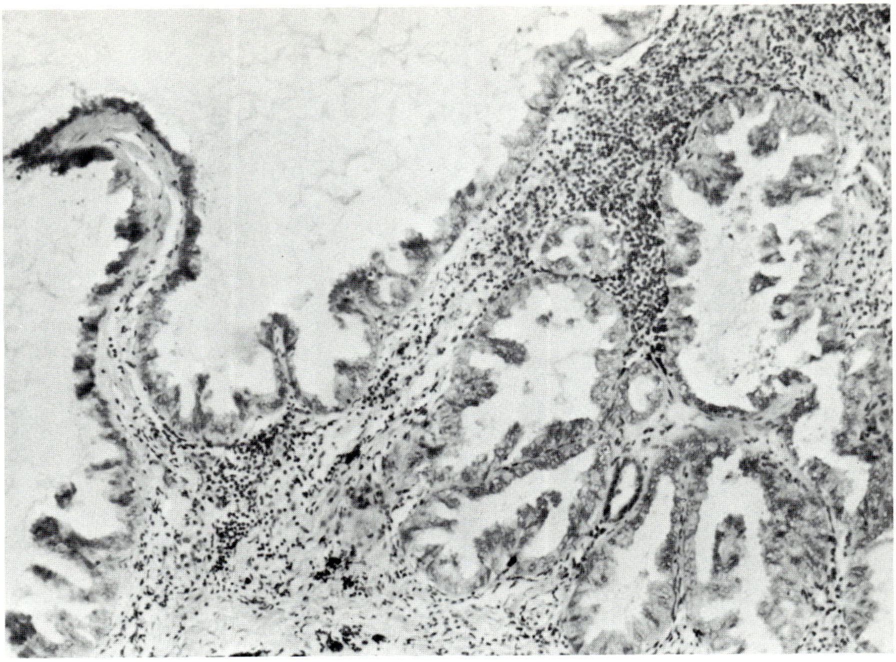

FIG. 6. Borderline tumor in a pelvic lymph node, developing in endosalpingiosis. A borderline tumor was also present in the ovary in this specimen which is a different case than Figure 5. H&E. ×200.

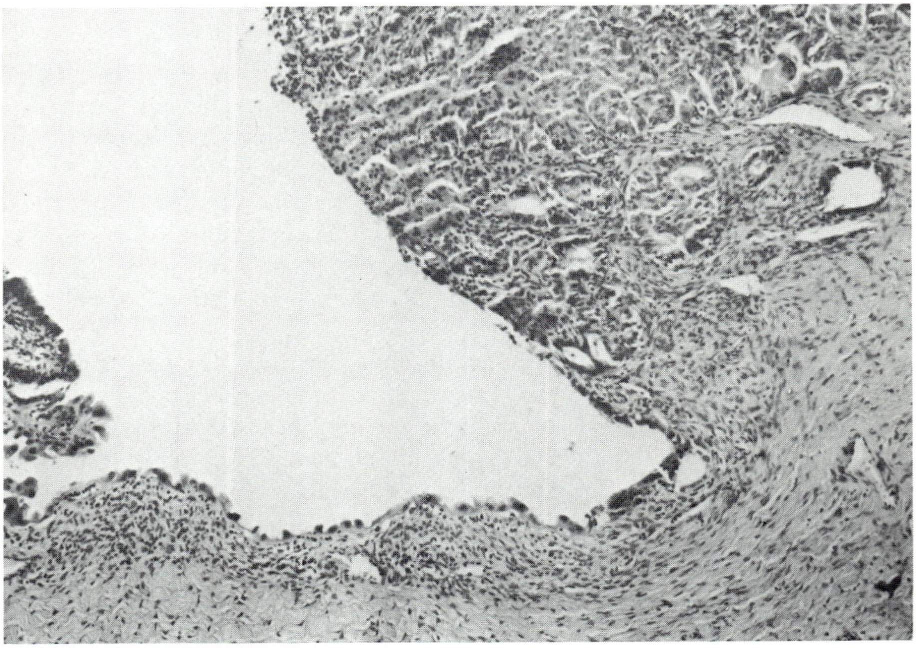

FIG. 7. Ovarian endometriosis with development of an endometrioid carcinoma, in a woman with carcinoma of the endometrium. H&E. ×200.

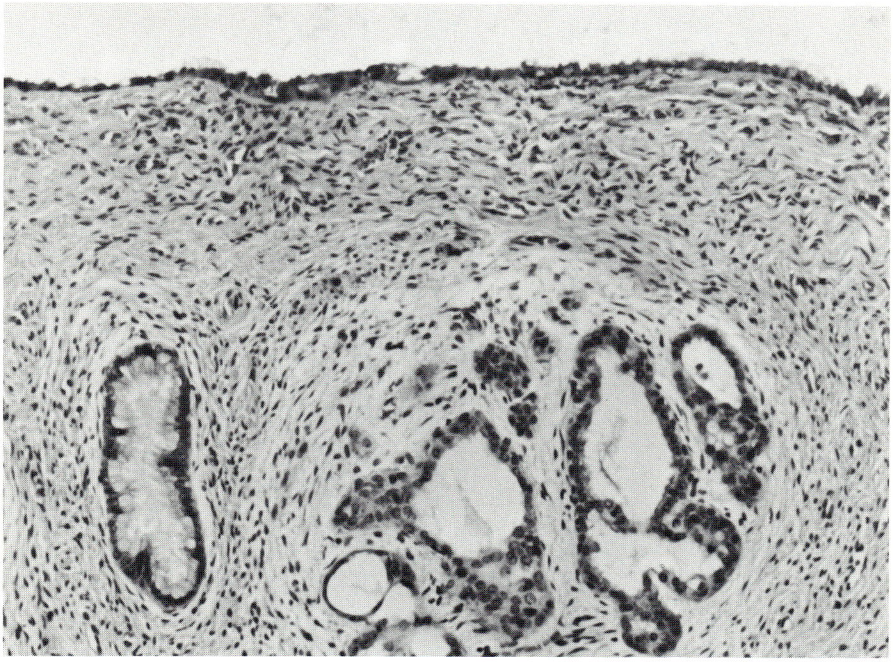

FIG. 8. Primary carcinoma of the endocervix in a patient with endometrial carcinoma, an example of the "field effect" of upper female genital tract neoplasia. H&E. ×200.

After Johnson and Helwig drew attention to these inclusions, case reports and series of cases steadily appeared in the literature.[23-31] With one exception, the inclusions were recognized as exact counterparts of nevi in the skin. Van der Berg[26] preferred to consider them "glomus cell clusters," recalling a resemblance that had been noted earlier.[22] In all, about 60 cases had been reported by 1980.

Incidence figures for these nevus cell inclusions have been derived from reviews of axillary, cervical, and inguinal node dissections. McCarthy et al. found that 6.2 percent of axillary dissections and 4.0 percent of inguinal dissections performed for malignant melanoma contained nevus cells, usually in just one node, but occasionally in two or even three. Ridolfi et al. reported an incidence of 0.33 percent in axillary dissections for breast carcinoma, and an incidence of 3.0 percent in node dissections from several sites for malignant melanoma.

The significance of nevus cells in lymph nodes, as with paramesonephric inclusions, lies in their recognition and distinction from metastatic carcinoma. This is particularly important when nodes are removed in the course of staging for breast carcinoma or melanoma; an unexpected clump of cells in a node may be mistaken for a metastasis, especially on frozen section examination.

The vast majority of nevus cells in nodes resemble their counterparts in the skin. Occasionally, blue nevi in nodes have been reported, with[28,30] and without[28] blue nevi in the associated skin. The typical lymph node nevus cell inclusion consists of a bandlike aggregate or "cap" of nevus cells in the node capsule (Fig. 9). This may extend along the delicate fibrous framework of the node into the hilum or into

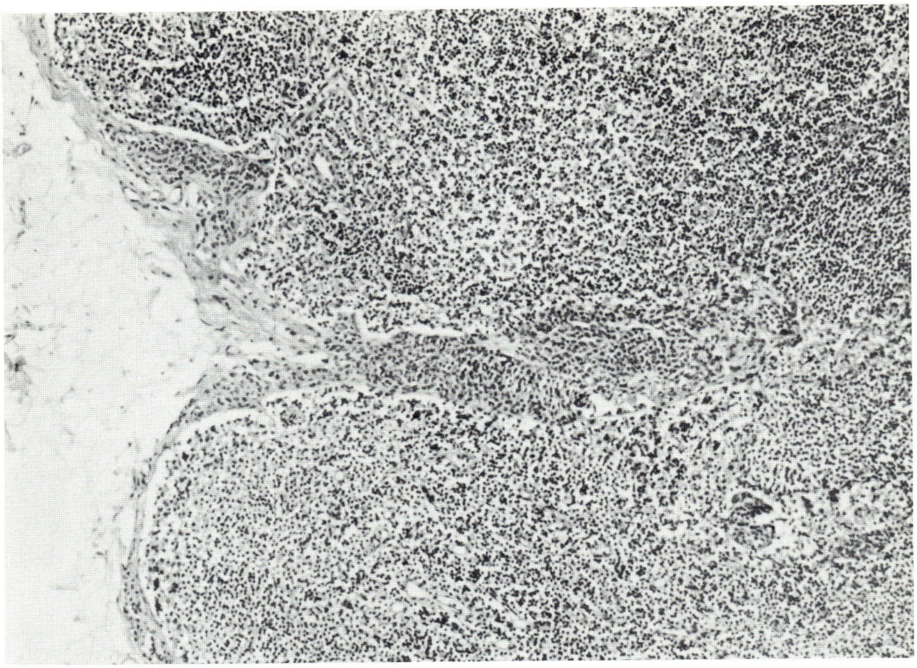

FIG. 9. Nevus cell aggregate in a lymph node, showing the characteristic capsular and septal distribution. H&E. ×200.

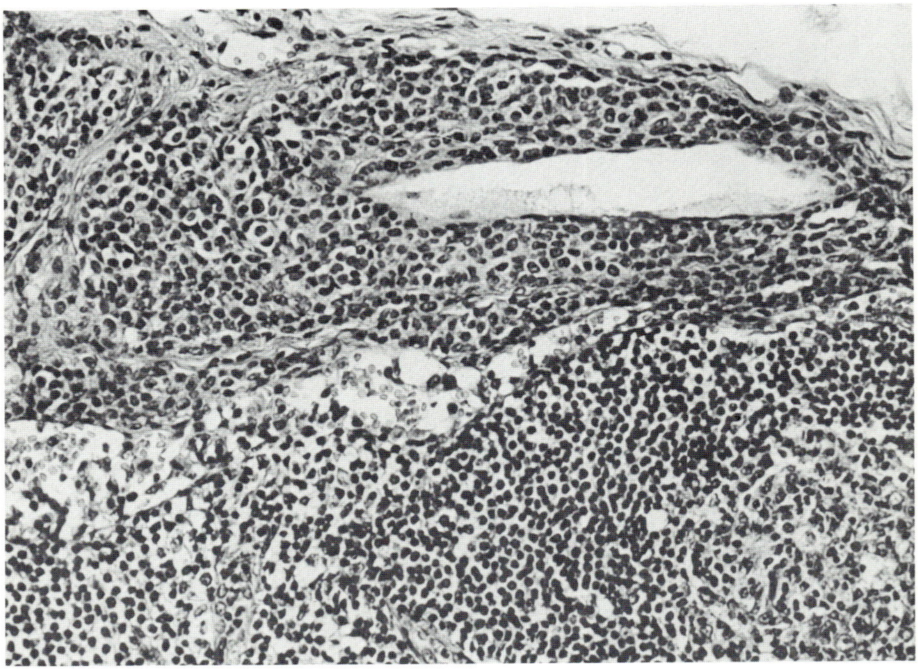

FIG. 10. Capsular nevus cell aggregate in a lymph node, showing bland cytology and sparing of capsular sinus. H&E. ×200.

the cortical parenchyma,[24,27] but does not encroach upon germinal centers or invade sinusoids. In this respect the inclusions resemble paramesonephric inclusions in lymph nodes. In two reports,[30,31] the nevus cells were described as lying within lymph node sinuses; McCarthy[24] has questioned this, suggesting that the nests may actually have been enmeshed in delicate fibrous strands. The cells may or may not be pigmented; when they are, special stains indicate that the pigment is melanin[22-24,27] and this has been confirmed recently by electron microscopy.[34]

The nevus cell aggregates often show clefts or spaces. The cells themselves are bland, round to ovoid, and show regular nuclei and scanty cytoplasm (Fig. 10). Cellular atypia and mitotic activity are virtually absent.

Nodal nevus cells may occur in conjunction with a malignant lesion. Cases with a single node harboring both nevus cells and Hodgkin's disease,[28] metastatic carcinoma,[27] and malignant melanoma[27] have been reported. In the latter two cases the nevus cell aggregate was "readily distinguished" from the metastasis by virtue of its characteristic location and bland cytologic appearance. Malignant transformation of a nodal nevus to a melanoma is a theoretical possibility, and has been invoked as an explanation for metastatic melanoma without an identifiable primary lesion.[23,24,27] However, no example of this transformation has yet been adequately documented.

LESIONS OF THE PERITONEUM

Leiomyomatosis Peritonealis Disseminata

While paramesonephric inclusions and nevi in nodes are most easily mistaken for malignant disease microscopically, leiomyomatosis peritonealis disseminata (LPD) is most worrisome on gross examination. The unexpected finding of an abdomen and pelvis studded with innumerable nodules in the course of a routine cesarean section or laparotomy can be disconcerting to the clinician and the pathologist. Several authors have pointed out the strong gross resemblance of LPD to widespread metastatic disease[35-50] of the female genital tract, and a few cases of LPD have been diagnosed as malignant tumors.[36,45]

The first report of LPD, though not yet named as such, was probably that of Willson and Peale in 1952.[35] Interestingly, they described the characteristic gross and microscopic features of LPD in a woman with a granulosa cell tumor of the ovary, a combination not reported since. This combination of lesions suggested that a hormonal effect might be important in the alteration or metaplasia of connective tissue cells, an effect documented in experimental animals.[35]

Sporadic reports of similar cases appeared during the next 25 years. In 1965, Taubert et al. described three cases and coined the term "leiomyomatosis peritonealis disseminata."[36] Two of these patients were pregnant and had an associated decidual reaction in the nodules, supporting Willson's impression of a hormonal influence. Taubert also favored a metaplastic origin of the nodules, likening them to endometriotis. (Subsequently, LPD was found in conjunction with endometriosis.[47,48]) Crosland, in 1973, reported a single case of LPD in a pregnant woman.[37] Parmley et al. in 1975 added two more cases of LPD in pregnant women, and questioned the previously held view that the nodules were composed of smooth muscle, preferring to consider them fibrotic remnants of decidual cells.[52] These two cases were studied by electron microscopy[37]; the conclusion was that the nodules were composed of fibroblasts, despite fixation so poor as to preclude evaluation for pinocytotic vesicles. A continuing debate was thus launched over the true nature of the cells within the nodules, overshadowing the question of their etiology.

In 1977, Goldberg[39] published a single case of LPD occurring in a woman receiving oral contraceptives; ultrastructural examination revealed the typical features of smooth muscle cells, including pinocytotic vesicles, a sparse endoplasmic reticulum, myofibrils, and cell junctions. He reviewed the possible etiology; metastases from a smooth muscle tumor of the uterus or gastrointestinal tract (uniformly rejected due to the subperitoneal location of the nodules), metaplasia of subcoelomic connective tissue, proliferation of smooth muscle in vessel walls, and fibrosis of a decidual reaction.

In the late 1970s and 1980, a flurry of case reports appeared,[40–42,44–51] several including electron microscopic examination.[41,44,46,47,50,51] Every ultrastructural study confirmed that the cells in LPD had characteristics of smooth muscle, though Nogales and Piesler also found evidence to suggest that they may be "myofibroblasts.[41,44]

In summary, by 1980, 20 cases of LPD had been reported, including 11 in pregnant women, 5 in women on oral contraceptives, and 1 in combination with an ovarian granulosa cell tumor. Cases occurring in pregnant women often showed an admixed decidual reaction, whereas others did not. The bulk of the light- and electron microscopic evidence favors a smooth muscle differentiation of the cells, with the occasional features of fibroblasts suggesting a spectrum of cell types from the fibroblast to the myofibroblast to the smooth muscle cell. The presence of decidual cells, when seen by light microscopy, has been confirmed ultrastructurally.[44] We have recently seen one case of LPD in a nonpregnant 37-year-old woman undergoing exploratory laparotomy for stage IB squamous cell carcinoma of the cervix; the nodules had ultrastructural characteristics of smooth muscle cells but no decidual cells (Figs. 11 and 12). It seems reasonable to accept a spectrum of cellular differentiation within LPD, with the smooth muscle cell as the predominant cell and an admixture of decidual or fibroblast-like cells in some cases. The latter cells appear to occur more frequently in the pregnant patient.

Despite the rare observation of nodules intimately associated with blood vessels,[39] the current favored mode of origin of LPD is metaplasia of subcoelomic connective tissue. Unlike paramesonephric metaplasia, the process appears to be limited to stroma rather than involving epithelium or mesothelium. It may even represent a metaplastic recapitulation of myometrium and endometrial stroma, without the endometrial epithelium characteristic of endometriosis. In this sense, it may be considered part of the spectrum of paramesonephric metaplasia in women.[36,43]

A hormonal influence is undoubtedly important in LPD, since 85 percent of cases are associated with pregnancy, oral contraceptive use, or a hormonally-active tumor. In one case, the nodules of LPD were shown to have a much higher affinity

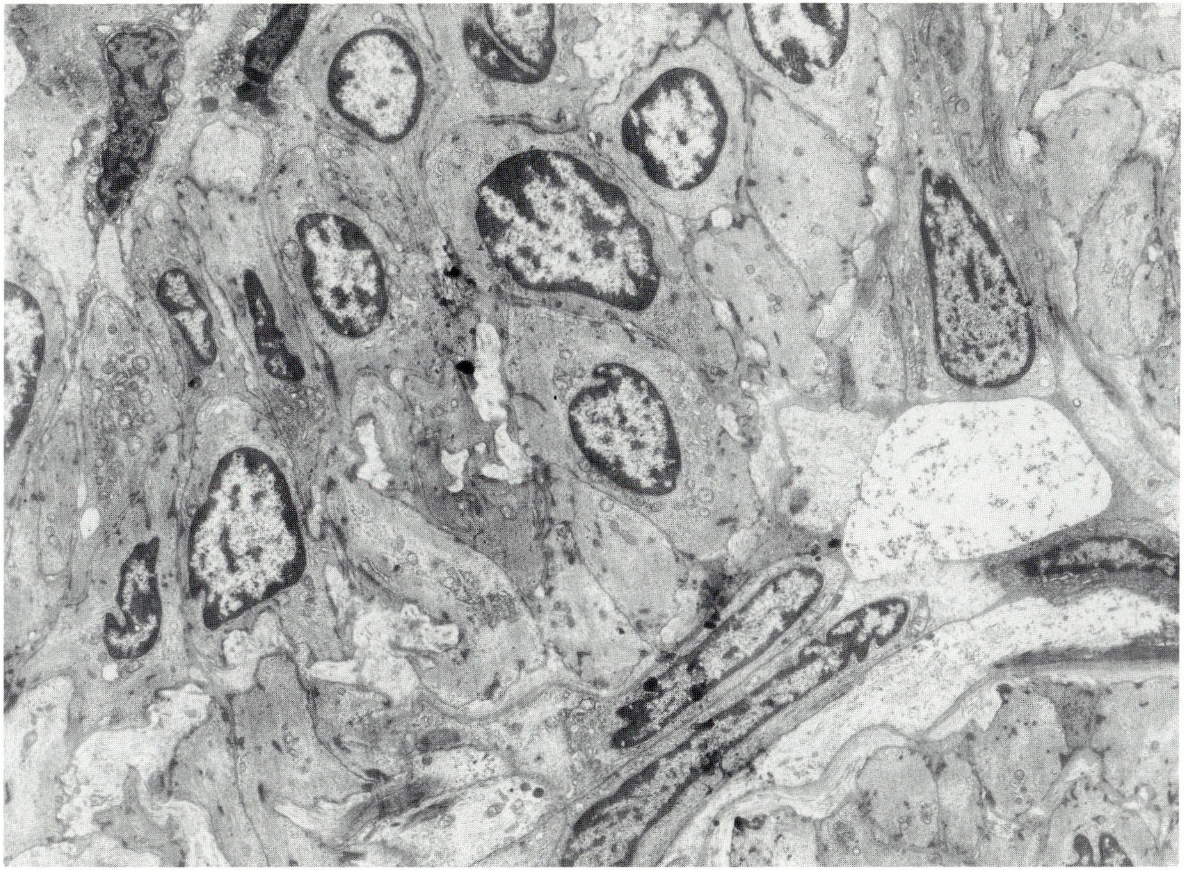

FIG. 11. Leiomyomatosis peritonealis disseminata; peritoneal nodule in a 37-year-old woman. Note abundance of plump, well-developed smooth muscle cells with numerous dense bodies. Scanty intercellular collagen is present. ×5,250.

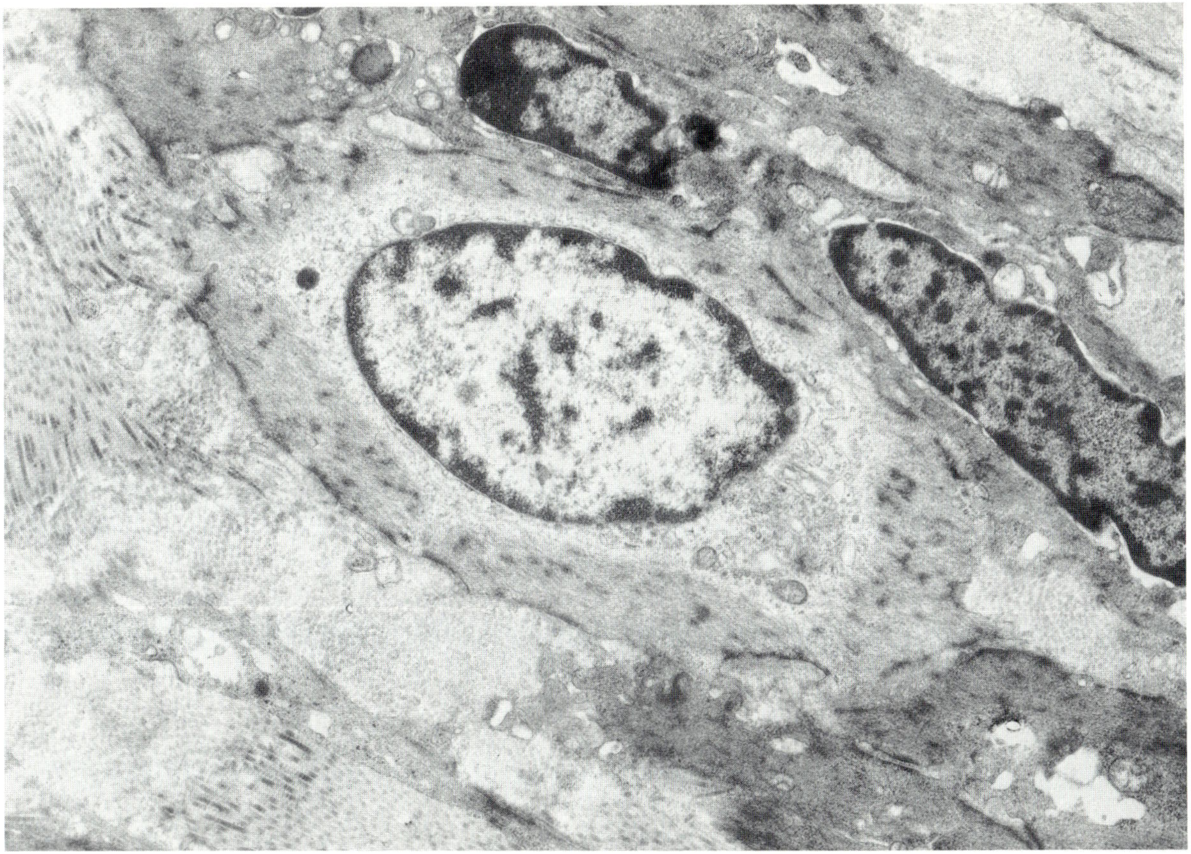

FIG. 12. Detail of leiomyomatosis peritonealis disseminata, showing an unusual cell characterized by a perinuclear "halo" containing an aggregate of organelles. More typical features of smooth muscle cells are also seen, including pinocytotic vesicles, dense bodies, myofibrils, and cell junctions. Possibly this represents a "myofibroblast." Note intercellular collagen. ×12,250.

for estrogen and progesterone binding than did myometrium from the same patient.[46]

Clinically and morphologically, the cases in the literature are quite similar. LPD is commonly discovered unexpectedly in the course of a cesarean section or laparotomy for pelvic pain. Our case is unusual in that exploration was done as a staging procedure for cervical carcinoma. The gross findings are striking, consisting of numerous firm, pale gray nodules ranging from a few millimeters to several centimeters in diameter. The nodules individually resemble benign leiomyomata, but create the impression of disseminated cancer. The entire peritoneum, including the surface of the pelvic organs, bowel, mesentery, and liver capsule, may be involved. Intramural leiomyomata of the uterus may be present or absent. Frozen-section examination is often requested, and on occasion a diagnosis of cancer has been rendered, followed by complete resection of the pelvic organs and mesentery. In our case, touch preparations were suspicious for metastatic carcinoma (Fig. 13), but a frozen section clearly demonstrated benign smooth muscle in omental fat.

Histologically, the nodules of LPD are submesothelial whorls of rather bland spindled cells resembling smooth muscle (Figs. 14 and 15). They may show a smooth, regular border or extend irregularly into the surrounding fat and connective tissue, suggesting metaplastic ''recruitment'' of adjacent cells.[40,47] The nodules may show areas of increased cellularity or hyalinization,[36] and usually contain collagen fibers. Cellular atypia is generally minimal, and mitoses are absent or rare. In a few cases, increased atypia[39] and mitotic activity[38] have been noted, with a rate of 1 to 3 mitoses per 10 high-power fields (HPF).[39,41,48,51]

The treatment of LPD is debatable. Many patients have undergone total abdominal hysterectomy and bilateral salpingo-oophorectomy; others have simply been delivered of their infants or have stopped taking oral contraceptives, with the resection of clinically significant leiomyomata being done. In every case for which follow-up data are available, either through physical examination or reexploration, the stabilization or regression of nodules has been observed.[35-37,39,40,45-51] This implies that termination of pregnancy or some other extraordinary hormonal stimulus may

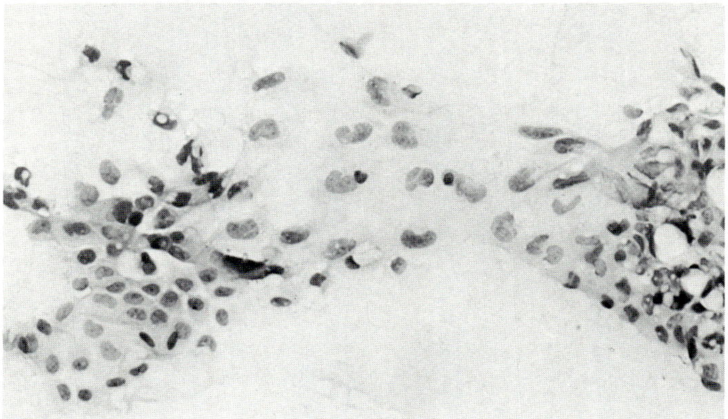

FIG. 13. Touch preparation of leiomyomatosis peritonealis disseminata, suggestive of metastatic carcinoma. Papanicolaou stain. ×200.

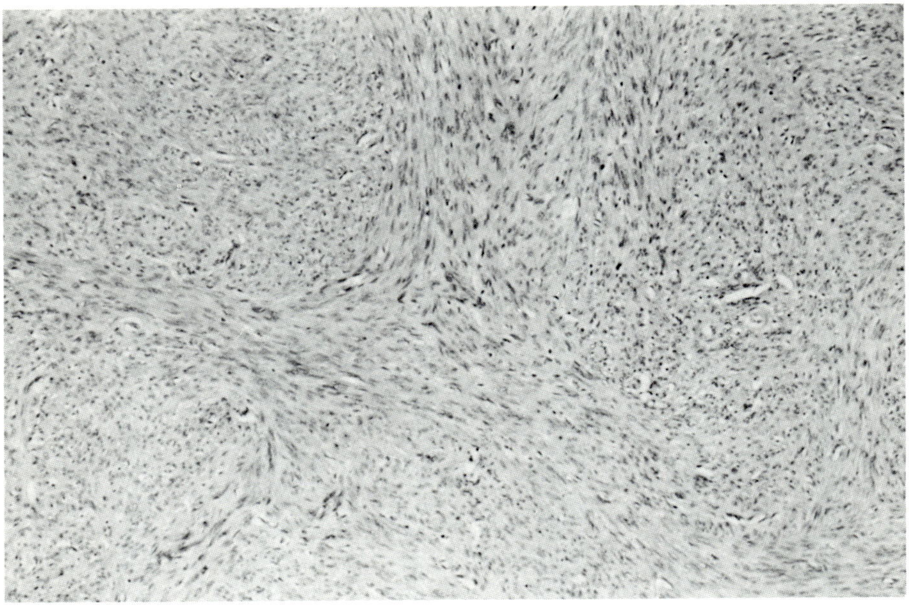

FIG. 14. Leiomyomatosis peritonealis disseminata, omental nodule in a 37-year-old woman undergoing staging laparotomy for cervical carcinoma. Note whorls of bland spindled cells resembling a uterine leiomyoma. H&E. ×200.

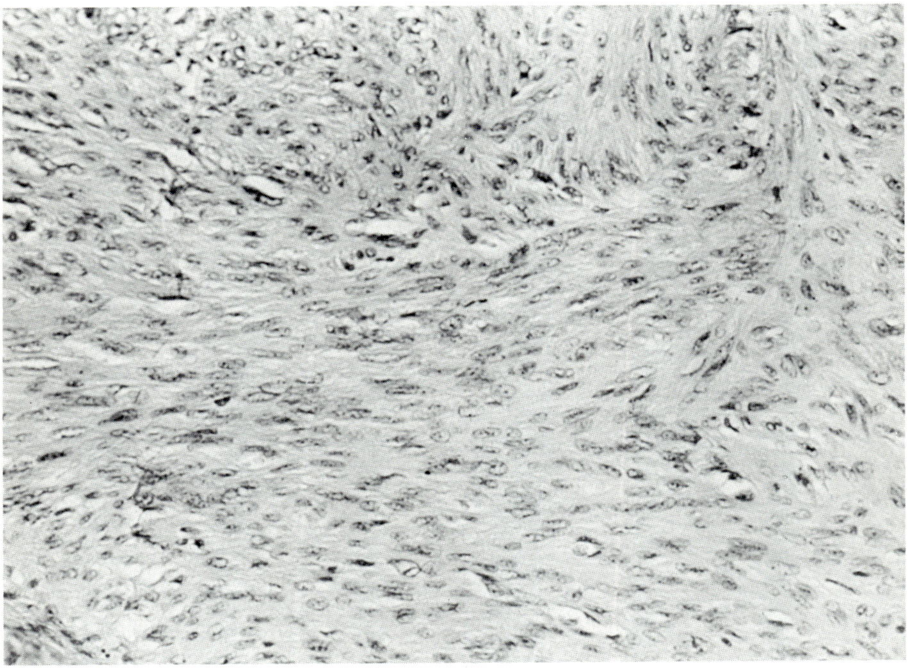

FIG. 15. Leiomyomatosis peritonealis disseminata, showing cytologic detail of an omental nodule. Note lack of cellular atypia and mitotic activity. H&E. ×500.

constitute sufficient treatment, and that castration is not necessarily the treatment of choice, a view shared by several other authors.[38,42,46,50]

Paramesonephric Inclusions of the Peritoneum

As discussed above with reference to lymph nodes, Mullerian or paramesonephric metaplasia of the peritoneum may occur to produce decidual reactions, endometriosis, or endosalpingiosis. Even leiomyomatosis peritonealis disseminata may be part of this spectrum, in light of its frequent association with decidua and occasional presentation with endometriosis. Such metaplasia is well recognized in lymph nodes, where it is believed to derive from the investing serosa. Metaplasia of the peritoneum lining the abdominal cavity and overlying the abdominal and pelvic organs is less well described. Clearly, such lesions need to be evaluated accurately to avoid a mistaken diagnosis of carcinoma, since current practice includes inspection and sampling of the peritoneum for metastatic female genital tract cancer.

Only a few reports specifically dealing with peritoneal lesions have appeared. Burmeister, in 1969, described two cases of peritoneal endosalpingiosis, one in a woman with endometriosis and one in a woman with bilateral ovarian cystadenocarcinomas.[7] He called attention to the presence of papillary configurations and psammoma bodies in endosalpingiosis. Irani, in 1976, cited a case of endometriosis of the peritoneum and pleura in a woman with hemorrhagic ascites and pleural effusions[53]; again, the differential diagnosis included metastatic ovarian cancer.

Twelve cases of paramesonephric metaplasia, or endosalpingiosis, of the peritoneum have been seen at the University of Colorado School of Medicine and in consultation by one of us (S.G.S.) in the past 3 years, indicating that despite the paucity of reports in the literature this is not a rare condition. The patients ranged from 21 to 64 years of age, and were explored for a variety of reasons, including pelvic inflammatory disease, endometriosis, and pelvic tumors. The latter consisted largely of ovarian tumors: four benign, three borderline, and one carcinoma. All of the ovarian tumors were serous except for one Brenner tumor, and in this case the endosalpingiosis (if this be the correct term here) resembled Walthard cell rests on the bowel serosa. The ovaries in the other 4 of our 12 cases contained no tumor, but always showed germinal inclusion cysts and/or surface papillations similar histologically to extraovarian endosalpingiosis. In each case one or more peritoneal "implants" were biopsied and suspected of comprising metastatic tumor. The "implants" occurred on the omentum, bowel, fallopian tubes, ovaries, and uterine serosa (Figs. 16 to 19). Papillary excrescences and psammoma bodies were often present, and in general the lesions resembled those described above in abdominal and pelvic lymph nodes. At times, if major degrees of proliferation and atypia are present, an accurate diagnosis may be nearly impossible, requiring total abdominal hysterectomy and bilateral salpingo-oophorectomy to rule out a true genital neoplasm. However, in the majority of cases a diagnosis of endosalpingiosis can be made with certainty, sparing the patient unnecessary surgery.

As with the similar inclusions in lymph nodes, and with endometriosis,[73] it is reasonable to suppose that foci of peritoneal endosalpingiosis may occasionally give

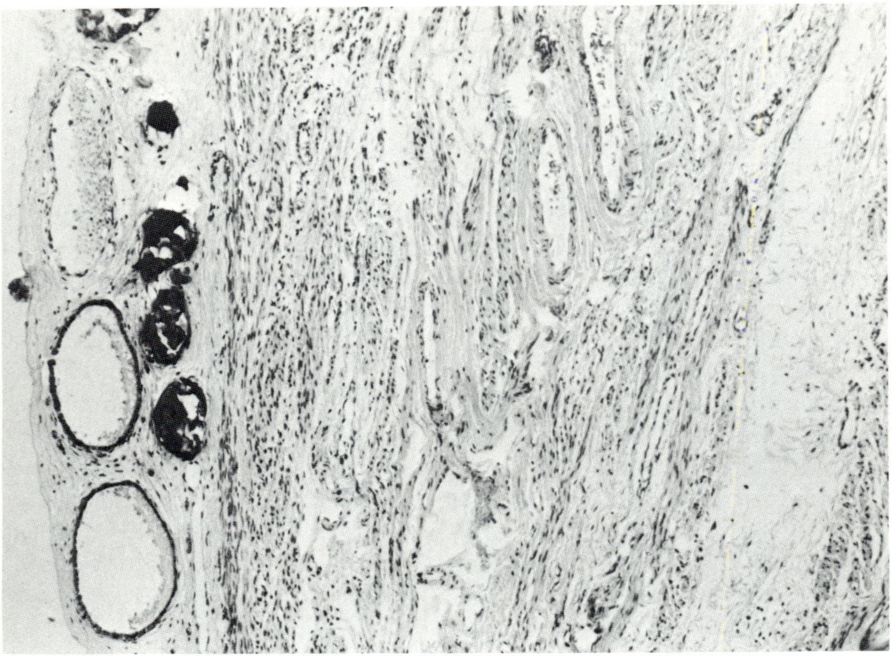

FIG. 16. Endosalpingiosis of the uterine serosa, showing small, dilated glands and microcalcifications. H&E. ×200.

rise to primary benign, borderline, or malignant tumors resembling those of the ovary which are derived from the coelomic surface mesothelium (serous, mucinous, endometrioid, clear cell, Brenner, etc.). Indeed, we have recently encountered a large mucinous tumor of the retroperitoneum, unattached to the pancreas or any other organ, the histology of which spanned the spectrum from benign through borderline to low-grade malignant ovarian carcinoma (Figs. 20 and 21). The ovaries in this case were reported as normal to inspection and palpation, but have not been excised for histologic examination. A few similar cases have been described in the literature.[74–77,79]

Mesothelial Proliferations

The nature of mesothelial proliferations of the peritoneum has been the subject of recent controversy. On the one hand, endometriosis, endosalpingiosis, and the ovarian epithelial neoplasms may be considered "mesothelial" disorders, since they presumably arise from Mullerian metaplasia of the peritoneum.[55] On the other hand, nonmetaplastic mesothelial proliferations can be clinically and pathologically recognized as bearing a strong resemblance to normal mesothelium. A gray zone, which is difficult to classify, probably exists between the two. Kannerstein[60] prefers

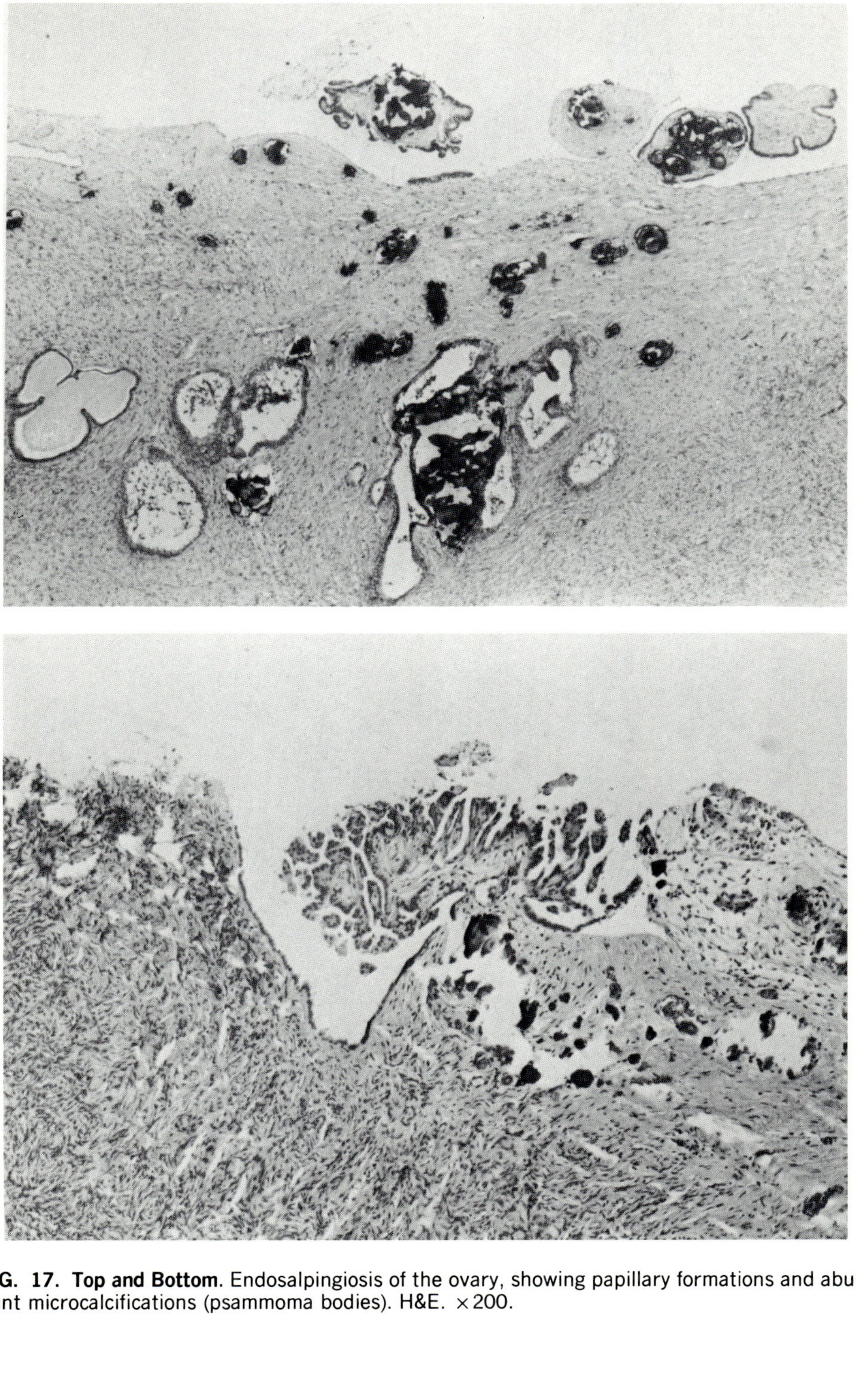

FIG. 17. Top and Bottom. Endosalpingiosis of the ovary, showing papillary formations and abundant microcalcifications (psammoma bodies). H&E. ×200.

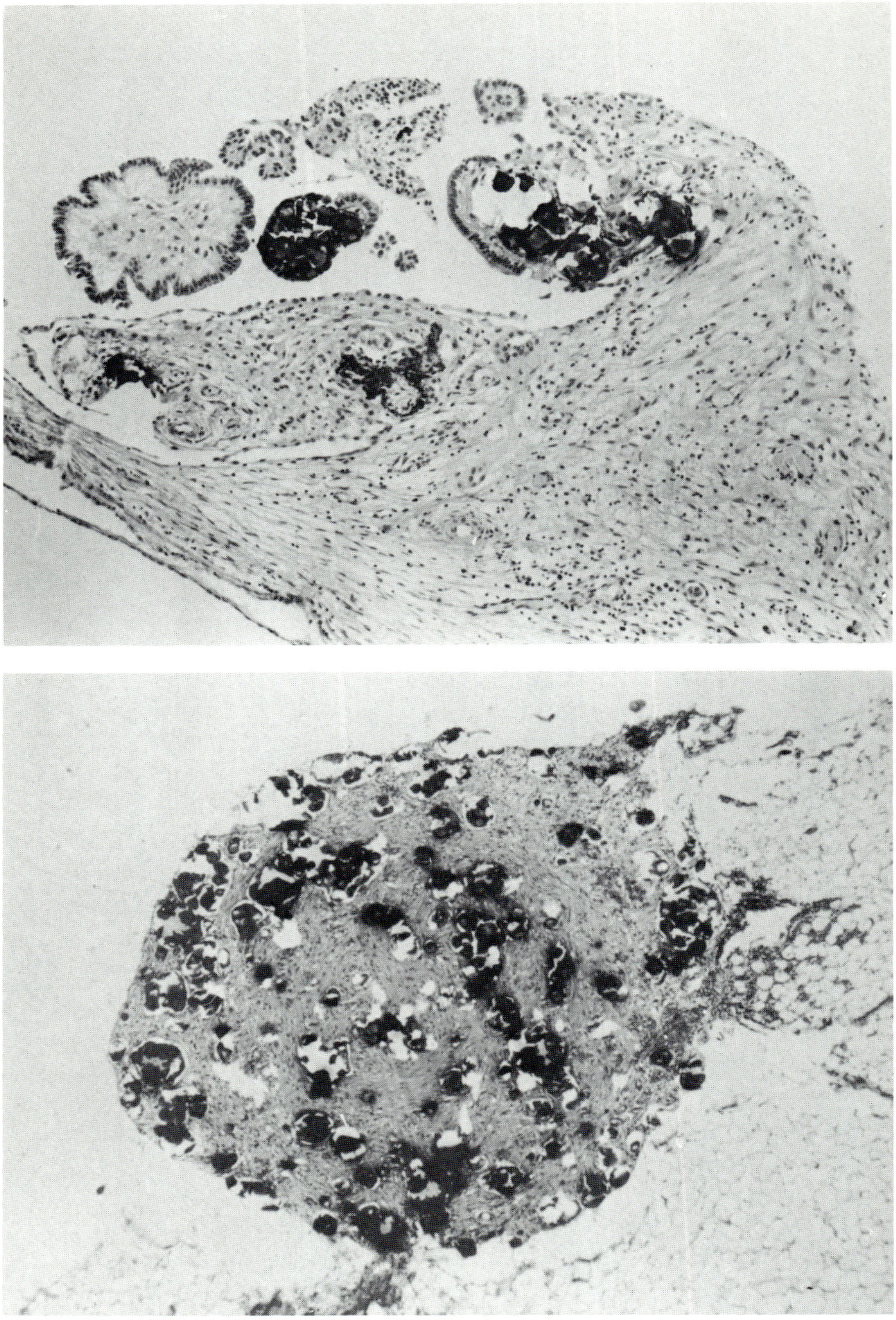

FIG. 18. Top and Bottom. Endosalpingiosis of the omentum. Note the papillary formations and the psammoma bodies, which may nearly replace the epithelial elements. H&E. ×200.

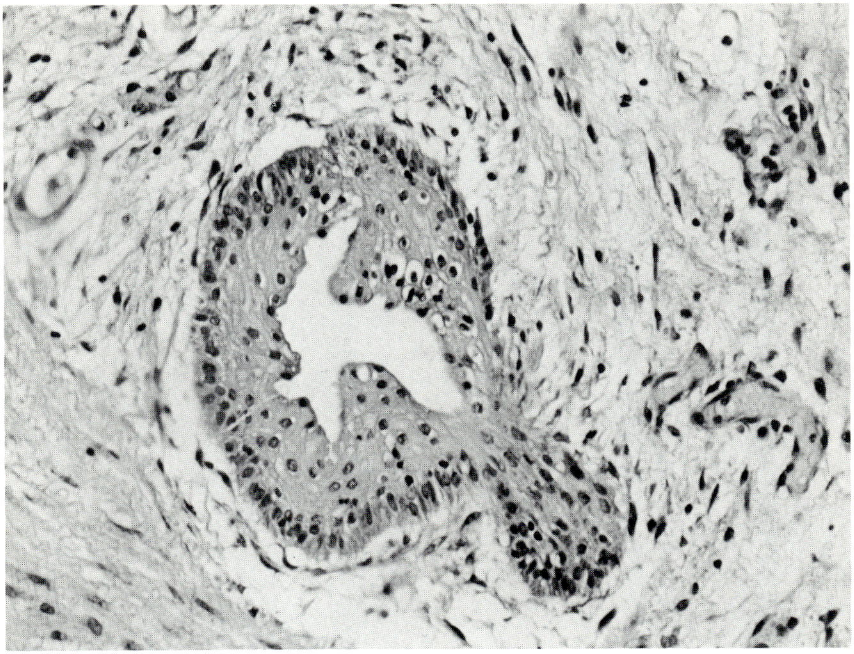

FIG. 19. Inclusion in bowel serosa showing Brenner-type epithelium; from a woman with an ovarian Brenner tumor. H&E. ×500.

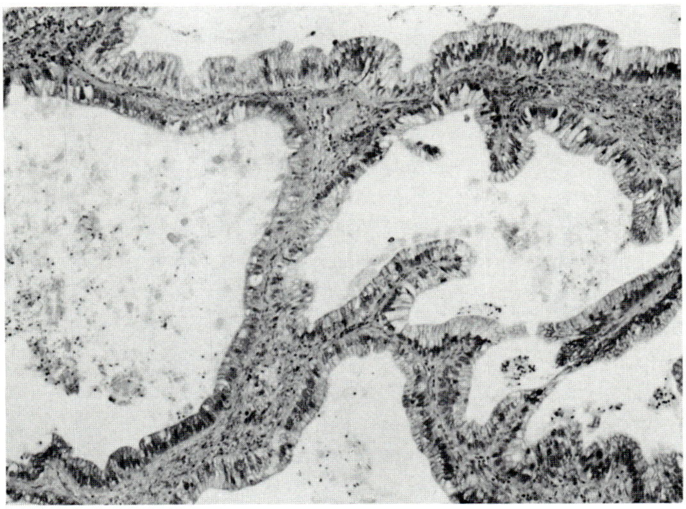

FIG. 20. Retroperitoneal mucinous tumor, showing transition between benign epithelium and borderline tumor. The ovaries were grossly normal. H&E. ×200.

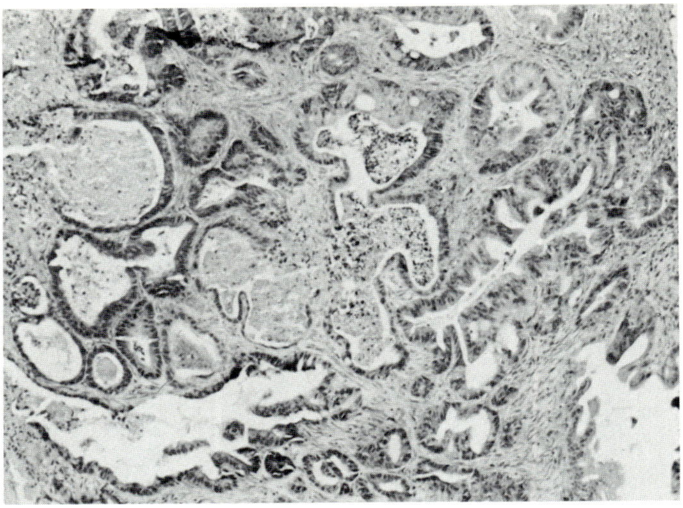

FIG. 21. Retroperitoneal mucinous tumor, showing areas of low-grade malignancy. H&E. ×200.

to consider all papillary lesions of the peritoneum in women as "papillary carcinoma arising from extraovarian tissue of Mullerian potentiality." However, there is histochemical and electron microscopic evidence to suggest that some of these proliferations are better considered mesothelial rather than epithelial.

The range of mesothelial lesions, excluding metaplasia, is broad. It includes nodular, reactive processes; papillary and cystic lesions (either reactive or neoplastic); and frankly malignant mesotheliomas, which may contain papillary areas. Any of these may present a diagnostic problem, but the following discussion will focus on those benign and reactive disorders most likely to be confused with metastatic carcinoma.

Until 1963, papillary mesotheliomas and adenomatoid tumors were not generally recognized as occurring outside the genital tract, and thus were not usually considered in the differential diagnosis of metastatic disease of the peritoneum. Hanrahan published the first case of such a tumor, a large, papillary, and solid omental mass in a 41-year-old woman, diagnosed on frozen section[54] as mucinous adenocarcinoma. The final diagnosis, however, was papillary mesothelioma, and a 5-year follow-up revealed no recurrence.

A second case was reported by Komorowski and Bobert: a cystic and papillary mass of the cul-de-sac and numerous smaller peritoneal masses in a 31-year-old woman.[56] These were diagnosed as peritoneal mesotheliomas, and the distinction from carcinoma was discussed. Differentiation of papillary mesotheliomas and adenomatoid tumors from papillary cystadenocarcinoma, even in males, may sometimes be quite difficult.[57,59]

A slightly different, though related, lesion was emphasized by Rosai and Dehner in 1975.[58] Nodular, reactive proliferations of mesothelium are often encountered in hernia sacs and other locations, where they may be mistaken for carcinoma. Rarely, they contain papillary areas and even psammoma bodies, rendering these features of little value in the distinction of these proliferations from carcinoma. Such cases have been seen at this institution in consultation (Figs. 22 and 23), specifically to rule out metastatic carcinoma.

Additional case reports of papillary mesothelial lesions have been sporadic.[63,64] Cystic mesotheliomas have been recently reviewed[65,76]; these are more often mistaken for lymphangiomas than for metastatic carcinoma (Figs. 24 and 25). We recognize 15 well-documented cases in the literature, including 5 of our own.[78] Although no case has yet proven lethal, recurrences have occurred in half of the patients followed for 2 years or more. Occasionally, mesotheliomas may also mimic leiomyomas.[61,62]

Clinically, reactive or neoplastic papillary mesotheliomas may be asymptomatic or may present as an abdominal or pelvic mass. They have been discovered incidentally during herniorrhaphy,[58] hysterectomy,[61,62] exploration for trauma,[63] or laparotomy for ovarian masses.[64] Cases in both males[58,63] and females[54,58,60,64] have been reported.

Grossly, the lesions range from a few millimeters to several centimeters in diameter, and are composed of varying amounts of solid, cystic, and papillary areas. Cystic areas contain clear, serous to gelatinous material.[65,67]

Microscopically, a similar range of patterns exists. Papillary fronds and cystic spaces are typically lined by a single layer of flattened to cuboidal or, less often, columnar cells, held together by a delicate fibrous framework. Cell stratification is not

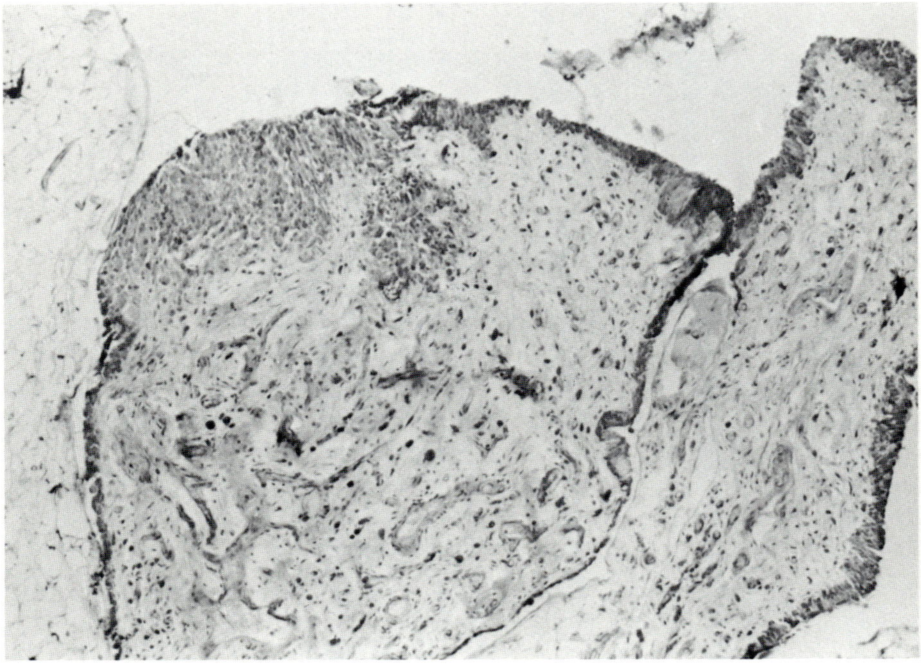

FIG. 22. Reactive mesothelial proliferation with a nodular aggregate of mesothelial cells from the peritoneum. H&E. ×200.

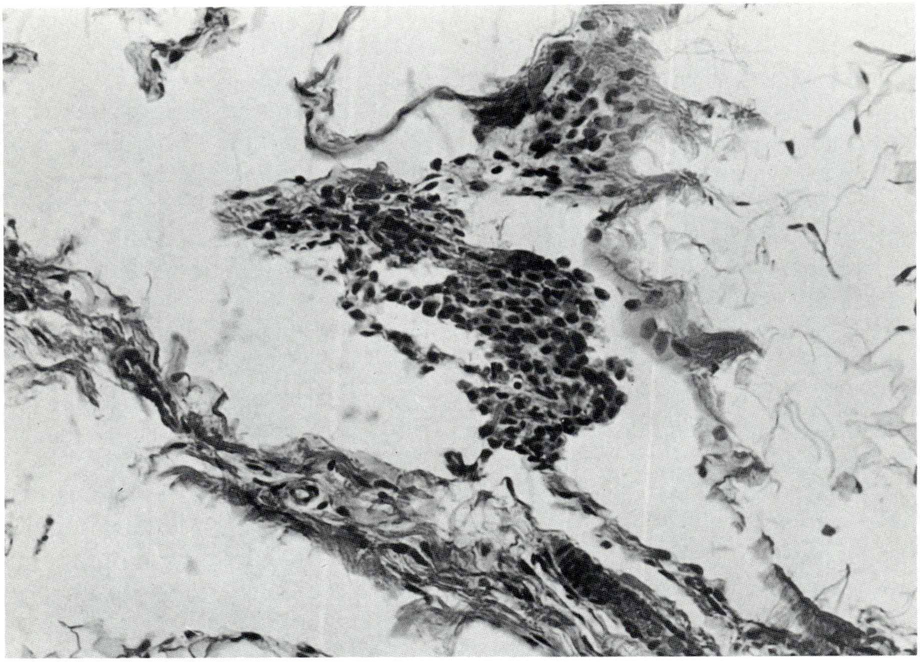

FIG. 23. Detail of an aggregate of reactive mesothelial cells, resembling metastatic carcinoma. Note the benign cytologic appearance. H&E. ×500.

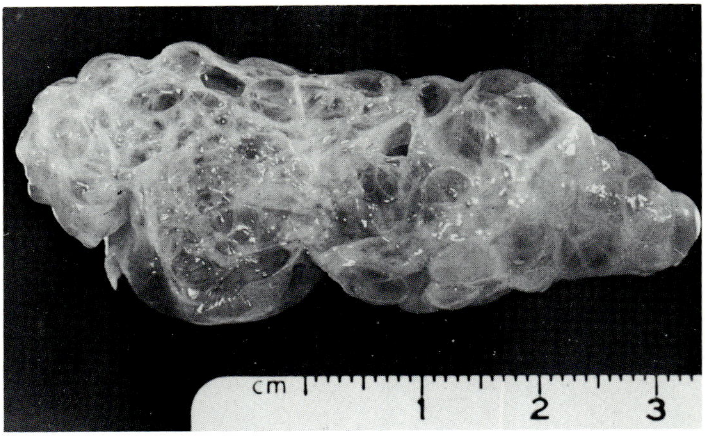

FIG. 24. Cystic mesothelioma of the adnexa in a 35-year-old woman; gross appearance.

seen. The columnar secretory and ciliated cells of endosalpingiosis and the stromal cells and hemorrhage of endometriosis are not present. Most lesions include dilated channels, gland-like areas, and solid nests characteristic of genital adenomatoid tumors, but unexpected in an extragenital setting. Foci of mesothelial hyperplasia may consist entirely of nodules of cuboidal cells. Whether flattened or rounded, the

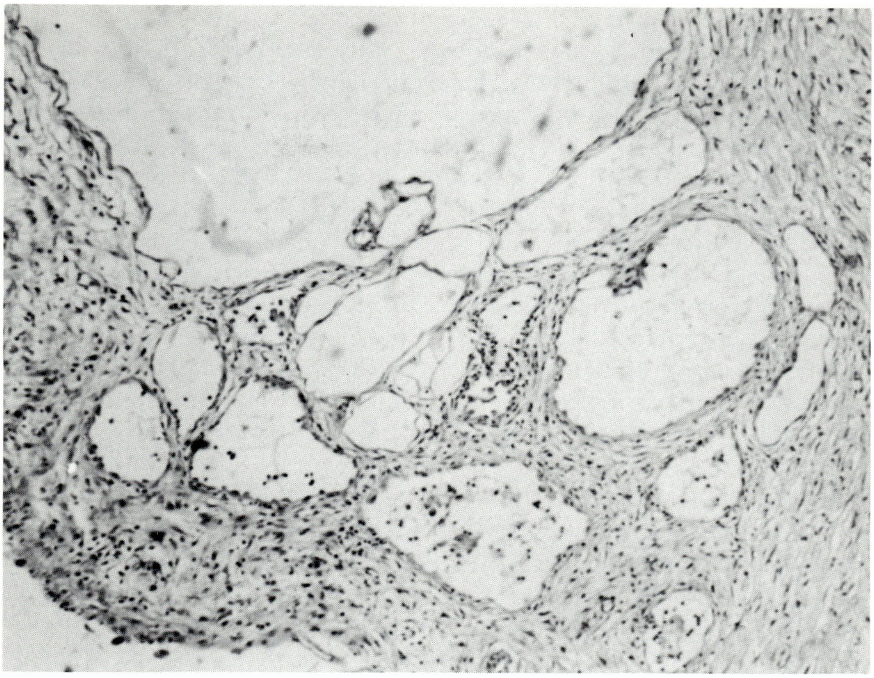

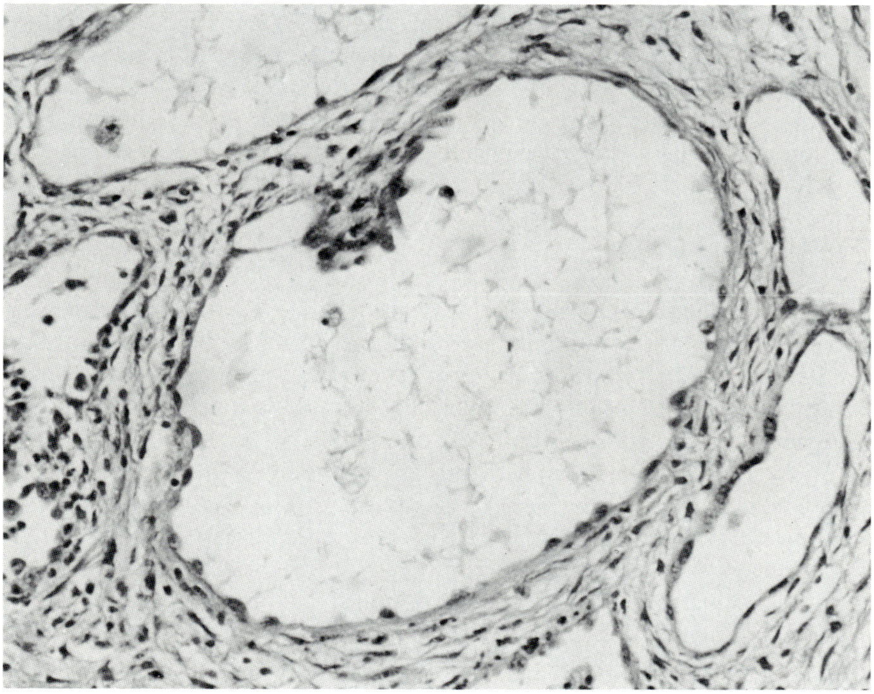

FIG. 25. Top. Cystic mesothelioma, composed of multiple dilated channels with occasional papillations. H&E. ×200. **Bottom.** Detail of cystic mesothelioma, illustrating single layer of flattened to cuboidal mesothelial cells. H&E. ×500.

cells are cytologically bland, showing uniform round to oval nuclei and moderate amounts of eosinophilic to slightly foamy cytoplasm. Cellular atypia and mitotic activity are usually absent, although numerous mitoses have been described in reactive hyperplasias.[58] Special stains reveal characteristics of mesothelial rather than epithelial cells, including negative mucicarmine[54,56,58,64] and a weak or negative periodic acid-Schiff (PAS) reaction after digestion with diastase.[54,58,63,64] Cytoplasmic vacuoles are sudanophilic.[54,56] The colloidal iron stain is positive and digestible with hyaluronidase,[63] and the alcian blue stain is negative.[58] Taken together, these findings indicate the presence of glycogen and neutral fat, the absence of neutral mucin, and the variable presence of acid mucopolysaccharides in the cells of papillary mesotheliomas. These may help distinguish a mesothelial proliferation from an epithelial neoplasm. Psammoma bodies (and, of course, papillations) are not helpful as indicators of carcinoma, since they have been described in reactive[58] and malignant mesothelial processes,[66] as well as in endosalpingiosis (see above).

Ultrastructural studies specifically directed to papillary mesotheliomas have not appeared in the literature. However, electron microscopy of the closely related cystic mesotheliomas has yielded evidence of their mesothelial origin, including numerous microvilli, desmosomes, and intracytoplasmic microfilaments.[65,67,78]

The biologic behavior of mesothelial tumors is notoriously difficult to predict. The hyperplastic lesions described by Rosai and Dehner clearly need no further treatment, although they may be mistaken for carcinoma.[58] Larger, cystic and papillary tumors may be multiple and recurrent.[56,65,67] Three- and 5-year follow-ups have shown no evidence of recurrent or disseminated tumor after the excision of a single papillary lesion.[54,63] Lack of invasion of the underlying omentum or other structures has been noted in some lesions.[56,58] At present, no definite recommendation beyond surgical excision of clinically significant masses seems indicated.

CONCLUSION

The differential diagnosis of metastatic cancer of the female genital tract can include a number of confusing imitative conditions. A variety of nonneoplastic and benign lesions of lymph nodes and the peritoneum has been reviewed, including the spectrum of paramesonephric (Mullerian) metaplasia, nevus cells in nodes, leiomyomatosis peritonealis disseminata, and papillary mesothelial proliferations. Most of these lesions can be distinguished from metastatic disease by careful histologic examination. Occasionally, the true nature of the lesion cannot be accurately determined, requiring surgery to delineate the disease. Features helpful in distinguishing each of these diagnostic look-alikes from carcinoma have been summarized and illustrated. The problem of multifocal primary tumors arising in separate female genital organs or in the genital tract and in a metaplastic inclusion has also been discussed. Here, the presence of benign elements, such as endometriosis or endosalpingiosis, or of foci of in situ carcinoma, may provide the only clue that a carcinoma is a separate primary rather than a metastatic lesion. In some cases, the histologic distinction between two primary tumors and a primary tumor with metastasis will be impossible, and the clinical setting then assumes paramount importance.

By calling attention to some of these lesions masquerading as metastatic cancer, we hope that some patients may be spared unnecessary diagnostic procedures and radical surgical and other therapies.

ACKNOWLEDGMENTS

The authors wish to thank Paul Peter Rosen, M.D., and Margaret Conley, M.D., for permission to use case material from their files.

REFERENCES

1. Russell HB: Decidual reaction of endometrium ectopic in an abdominal lymph node. Surg Gynecol Obstet 81:218–220, 1945
2. Huhn FO: Druseneinschlusse in Beckenlymphknoten der Frau. Virchows Arch [Pathol Anat] 335:84–100, 1962
3. Weir JH, Janovski NA: Paramesonepheric lymph node inclusions—A cause for obstructive uropathy. Obstet Gynecol 21(3):363–367, 1963
4. Koss LG: Miniature adenoacanthoma arising in an endometriotic cyst in an obturator lymph node. Cancer 15:1369–1372, 1963
5. Karp LA, Czernobilsky B: Glandular inclusions in pelvic and abdominal para-aortic lymph nodes. Am J Clin Pathol 52:212–218, 1969
6. Ferguson BR, Bennington JL, Haber SL: Histochemistry of mucosubstances and histology of mixed Mullerian pelvic lymph node glandular inclusions. Obstet Gynecol 33:617–625, 1969
7. Burmeister RE, Fechner RE, Franklin RR: Endosalpingiosis of the peritoneum. Obstet Gynecol 34:310–318, 1969
8. Covell LM, Discivllo AJ, Knapp RC: Decidual change in pelvic lymph nodes in the presence of cervical squamous cell carcinoma during pregnancy. Am J Obstet Gynecol 127:674–676, 1977
9. Delgado G, Chun B, Caglar H, Bapko F: Paraaortic lymphadenectomy in gynecologic malignancies confined to the pelvis. Obstet Gynecol 50:418–423, 1977
10. Kempson RL: Benign glandular inclusions in iliac lymph nodes. Am J Surg Pathol 2:321–325, 1978
11. Schnurr RC, Delgado G, Chun B: Benign glandular inclusions in para-aortic lymph nodes in women undergoing lymphadenectomies. Am J Obstet Gynecol 130:813–816, 1978
12. Silton RM: Letter to the editor. Am J Surg Pathol 3:285–286, 1979
13. Russell P, Laverty CR: Benign "Mullerian" nests in pelvic lymph node. Pathology 12:31, 129–130, 1980
14. Ehrmann RL, Federschneider JM, Knapp RC: Distinguishing lymph node metastases from benign glandular inclusions in low-grade ovarian carcinoma. Am J Obstet Gynecol 136:737–746, 1980
15. Langley II, Moore DW, Tarnasky JW, Roberts PHR: Radical hysterectomy and pelvic lymph node dissection. Gynecol Oncol 9:37–42, 1980
16. Moore KL: The Developing Human. Philadelphia, WB Saunders, 1973, pp 212–213
17. Ries E: Eine neue Operationsmethode des Uteruscarcinoms. Z Geburtsh Gynak 37:518, 1897
18. Wertheim E: Uber Lymphdrusenmetastasen bei Uteruscarcinomen. Z Geburtsh Gynak 48:545, 1903

19. Lange P: Clinical and histological studies on cervical carcinoma. Acta Pathol Microbiol Scand (Suppl 143) 50:123–137, 1960
20. Hsu YK, Parmley TH, Rosenshein NB, et al.: Neoplastic and non-neoplastic mesothelial proliferations in pelvic lymph nodes. Obstet Gynecol 55:83–88, 1980
21. Tutschka B, Lauchlan S: Endosalpingiosis. Obstet Gynecol 55 (Suppl): 575–605, 1980
22. Johnson WT, Helwig EB: Benign nevus cells in the capsule of lymph nodes. Cancer 23:747–753, 1969
23. Hart WR: Primary nevus of a lymph node. Am J Clin Pathol 55:88–92, 1971
24. McCarthy SW, Palmer AA, Bale PM, Hirst E: Naevus cells in lymph nodes. Pathology 6:351–358, 1974
25. Gray GE Jr, Dineen P: Benign nevus in lymph node. NY State J Med 76:754, 1976
26. Van den Berg FWT, Kaiserling E, Lennert K: Glomus-Zellnesten des Lymphknotens. Virchows Arch [Pathol Anat] 371:27–34, 1976
27. Ridolfi RL, Rosen PP, Thaler H: Nevus cell aggregates associated with lymph nodes: Estimated frequency and clinical significance. Cancer 39:164–171, 1977
28. Azzopardi JG, Ross CMD, Frizzera G: Blue naevi of lymph node capsule. Histopathology 1:451–461, 1977
29. Bertrand G, Rabreau M, George P: Présence de cellules naeviques dans les ganglions lymphatiques. A propos d'une observation. Arch Anat Cytol Pathol 28:58–62, 1980
30. Rodriguez HA, Ackerman LV: Cellular blue nevus. Cancer 21:393–405, 1968
31. Lerman RI, Murray D, O'Hara JM, et al.: Malignant melanoma of childhood. Cancer 25:436–449, 1970
32. Stewart FW, Copeland MM: Neurogenic sarcoma. Am J Cancer 15:1235–1320, 1931
33. Stewart FW: Early Cancer, Thayer Lecture, Johns Hopkins University, 1960. In Wood S Jr, Holyoke ED, Yarkley JH (eds): Mechanisms of Metastasis Production by Blood-Borne Cancer Cells. Canadian Cancer Conference 4. New York, Academic Press, 1961 p 172
34. Erlandson RA, Rosen PP: Electron microscopy of a nevus cell aggregate associated with an axillary lymph node. Cancer 49:269–272, 1982
35. Willson JR, Peale AR: Multiple peritoneal leiomyomas associated with a granulosa-cell tumor of the ovary. Am J Obstet Gynecol 64:204–208, 1952
36. Taubert H-D, Wissner SE, Haskins AL: Leiomyomatosis peritonealis disseminata: An unusual complication of genital leiomyomata. Obstet Gynecol 25:561–574, 1965
37. Crosland DB: Leiomyomatosis peritonealis disseminata: A case report. Am J Obstet Gynecol 117:179–181, 1973
38. Winn KJ, Woodruff JD, Parmley TH: Electronmicroscopic studies of leiomyomatosis peritonealis disseminata. Obstet Gynecol 48:225–227, 1976
39. Goldberg MF, Hurt WG, Frable WJ: Leiomyomatosis peritonealis disseminata: Report of a case and review of the literature. Obstet Gynecol 49(Suppl):465–525, 1977
40. Aterman K, Fraser GM, Lea RH: Disseminated peritoneal leiomyomatosis. Virchows Arch [Pathol Anat] 374:13–26, 1977
41. Nogales FF Jr, Matilla A, Carrascal E: Leiomyomatosis peritonealis disseminata: An ultrastructural study. Am J Clin Pathol 69:452–457, 1978
42. O'Sullivan BT: Leiomyomatosis peritonealis disseminata. Aust NZ J Obstet Gynecol 18:94–95, 1978
43. Herr JC, Platz CE, Heidger PM Jr, Curet LB: Smooth muscle within ovarian decidual nodules: A link to leiomyomatosis peritonealis disseminata? Obstet Gynecol 53:451–456, 1979
44. Pieslor PC, Orenstein JM, Hogan DL, Breslow A: Ultrastructure of myofibroblasts and decidualized cells in leiomyomatosis peritonealis disseminata. Am J Clin Pathol 72:875–882, 1979
45. Lim OW, Segal A, Ziel HK: Leiomyomatosis peritonealis disseminata associated with pregnancy. Obstet Gynecol 55:122–125, 1980
46. Sutherland JA, Wilson EA, Edger DE, Powell D: Ultrastructure and steroid-binding

studies in leiomyomatosis peritonealis disseminata. Am J Obstet Gynecol 136:992–996, 1980
47. Kuo T-T, London SN, Dinh TV: Endometriosis occurring in leiomyomatosis peritonealis disseminata. Am J Surg Pathol 4:197–204, 1980
48. Kaplan C, Benirschke K, Johnson KC: Leiomyomatosis peritonealis disseminata with endometrium. Obstet Gynecol 55:119–121, 1980
49. Del Castillo H, Rubio PA, Farrell EM: Leiomyomatosis peritonealis disseminata in the nonpregnant female: A case report. Int J Gynaecol Obstet 17:428–430, 1980
50. Williams LJ Jr, Pavlick FJ: Leiomyomatosis peritonealis disseminata: Two case reports and a review of the medical literature. Cancer 45:1726–1733, 1980
51. Fujii S, Okamura H, Nakashima N, et al.: Leiomyomatosis peritonealis disseminata. Obstet Gynecol 55(Suppl):795–835, 1980
52. Parmley TH, Woodruff JD, Winn K, et al.: The histogenesis of leiomyomatosis peritonealis disseminata (disseminated fibrosing deciduosis). Obstet Gynecol 46:511–516, 1975
53. Irani S, Atkinson L, Cabaniss C, Danovitch SH: Pleuroperitoneal endometriosis. Obstet Gynecol 47(Suppl):725–745, 1976
54. Hanrahan JB: A combined papillary mesothelioma and adenomatoid tumor of the omentum: Report of a case. Cancer 16:1497–1500, 1963
55. Parmley TH, Woodruff JD: The ovarian mesothelioma. Am J Obstet Gynecol 120:234–241, 1974
56. Komorowski RA, Bobert DH: Peritoneal mesothelioma presenting as an adnexal mass. South Med J 68:83–85, 1975
57. deKlerk DP, Nime F: Adenomatoid tumors (mesothelioma) of testicular and paratesticular tissue. Urology 6:635–641, 1975
58. Rosai J, Dehner LP: Nodular mesothelial hyperplasia in hernia sacs. Cancer 35:165–175, 1975
59. Kannerstein M, Churg J: Peritoneal mesothelioma. Hum Pathol 8:83–94, 1977
60. Kannerstein M, Churg J, McCaughey WTE, Hill DP: Papillary tumors of the peritoneum in women: Mesothelioma or papillary carcinoma. Am J Obstet Gynecol 127:306–314, 1977
61. Wood C, Bouchelle WH: Benign mesothelioma simulating a uterine leiomyoma. Am J Obstet Gynecol 132:225–226, 1978
62. Honoré LH: Uterine mesothelioma. Letter to the editor. Am J Obstet Gynecol 135:162, 1979
63. Craig JR, Hart WR: Extragenital adenomatoid tumor: Evidence for the mesothelial theory of origin. Cancer 43:1678–1681, 1979
64. Russell P, Laverty CR: Benign papillary mesothelioma of peritoneum. Pathology 10:316, 382–383, 1978
65. Mennemeyer R, Smith M: Multicystic, peritoneal mesothelioma: A report with electron microscopy of a case mimicking intra-abdominal cystic hygroma (lymphangioma). Cancer 44:692–698, 1979
66. Donaldson JC, Kaminsky DB, Elliott RC, et al.: Psammoma bodies in pleural fluid associated with a mesothelioma: Case report. Milit Med 144:476–479, 1979
67. Moore JH Jr, Crum CP, Chandler JG, Feldman PS: Benign cystic mesothelioma. Cancer 45:2395–2399, 1980
68. Abdulhayoglu G, Rich WM, Reynolds J, Disais PJ: Selective radiation therapy in Stage IB uterine cervical carcinoma following radical pelvic surgery. Gynecol Oncol 10:84–92, 1980
69. Chen KTK, Kostich ND, Rosai J: Peritoneal foreign body granulomas to keratin in uterine adenocanthoma. Arch Pathol Lab Med 102:174–177, 1978
70. Bruckman JE, Bloomer WD, Mack A, et al.: Stage III adenocarcinoma of the endometrium: Two prognostic groups. Gynecol Oncol 9:12–17, 1980
71. Dubravsky V, Schwab J: Das Problem des Carcinoma in situ der Endozervix, des Endometrium und der Endosalpinx. Ann Chir Gynaecol Fenn (Suppl 172) 59:4, 1970

72. Woodruff JD, Julian CG: Multiple malignancy in the upper genital canal. Am J Obstet Gynecol 103:810–822, 1969
73. Mostoufizadeh GH M, Scully RE: Malignant tumors arising in endometriosis. Clin Obstet Gynecol 23(3):951–963, 1980
74. Brooks JJ, Wheeler JE: Malignancy arising in extragonadal endometriosis. Cancer 40:3065–3073, 1977
75. Palladino VS, Troudell M: Extra-uterine Mullerian tumors: A review of the literature and the report of a case. Cancer 23:1413–1422, 1969
76. Labay GR, Feiner F: Malignant pleural endometriosis. Am J Obstet Gynecol 110:478–480, 1971
77. Hyman M: Extraovarian endometrioid carcinoma: Review of the literature and report of two cases with unusual features. Am J Clin Pathol 68:522–527, 1977
78. Katsube Y, Mukai K, Silverberg SG: Cystic mesothelioma of the peritoneum: A report of five cases with clinicopathologic considerations and ultrastructural findings. Cancer (in press)
79. Foyle A, Al-Jabi M, McCaughey WTE: Papillary peritoneal tumors in women. Am J Surg Pathol 5:241–250, 1981

HISTOGENETIC CLASSIFICATION OF PULMONARY CARCINOMAS

Peripheral Adenocarcinomas Studied by Light Microscopy, Histochemistry, and Electron Microscopy

JOHN W. BOLEN AND DAVID THORNING

Carcinomas of the lung have a variety of histologic growth patterns. The most widely recognized and accepted classification of these neoplasms, that proposed in 1967 by the World Health Organization (WHO), is based on these light-microscopically detected growth patterns and generally ignores neoplastic cell histogenesis. The WHO classification has been clinically useful, especially during the years when therapeutic regimens for carcinoma of the lung were limited; however, with the present availability of a larger variety of potentially useful therapeutic measures for this malignancy, a precise pretreatment identification of the neoplastic process is imperative for assessment of the effect of any one measure against that of another. Methods of observation other than by light microscopy have shown that histologic growth patterns are not always reliable indicators of the origin of a neoplastic cell type or of the degree of differentiation of neoplastic cells; these discrepancies are most notable in the WHO categories of small- and large-cell carcinomas.

As part of an ongoing study of pulmonary carcinomas, most biopsied neoplasms and all surgically resected neoplasms at this institution, as well as numerous others from local community hospitals, have been examined by both light and electron microscopy. An attempt was made to classify these neoplasms as originating from one or a combination of the cells found in the normal, uninjured epithelium, or in the injured, reactive, hyperplastic but nonneoplastic epithelium. A total of 243 neoplasms have been examined by these methods. Of this total, there were 57 peripheral adenocarcinomas; 42 of these 57 were histogenetically subclassified as outlined in Table 1, and 15 were either too poorly preserved or too poorly differentiated to be subclassified. From the group of 42, seven neoplasms were selected to illustrate the spectrum of histologic growth patterns and the variety of differentiated lung cell types. The histochemical and ultrastructural features useful in the process of cell-type identification will be detailed.

CASE MATERIAL

Clinical and anatomic data from the seven cases selected as illustrative are summarized in Table 2. The patients ranged in age from 59 to 77 years; four were men. All but one were treated by lobectomy; the exception, Case 3, had metastases to an excised supraclavicular node. All of the neoplasms were located in subpleural parenchymal sites away from major bronchi. They ranged in maximum diameter from 1.5 to 4.0 cm. The light-microscopic diagnoses were based on World Health Organization criteria.

The ultrastructural criteria for cellular differentiation generally parallel those of McDowell et al.[21] A secretory cell is one involved with the production of materials for extracellular transport. Such cells generally have a well-developed endoplasmic reticulum and Golgi apparatus, and often contain secretory granules. Adenocarcinomas are composed of secretory cells which may or may not form acini. It should be recognized that a tumor may show a poorly differentiated histologic growth pattern, i.e., few or no acini, but may still be composed of individually well-differentiated secretory cells. A structural cell features a prominent cytoskeletal system with an abundance of microfilaments in the form of tonofilaments, and a relatively poorly developed endoplasmic reticulum and Golgi apparatus. Desmosomes are generally frequent and well developed in structural cells, and there may or may not be evidence of keratin formation. Epidermoid car-

TABLE 1. Histogenetic Classification of Peripheral Adenocarcinomas

EM Cell Type	Light-Microscopic Diagnosis	No. Peripheral Adeno-carcinomas
Clara cell	Bronchioloalveolar carcinoma	9
	Poorly differentiated adenocarcinoma	10
	Large-cell undifferentiated carcinoma	4
		23
Goblet/small mucus granule	Bronchioloalveolar carcinoma	4
	Poorly differentiated adenocarcinoma	8
	Large-cell undifferentiated carcinoma	5
		17
Type II alveolar cell	Poorly differentiated adenocarcinoma	*2*
Indeterminate cell type	Poorly differentiated adenocarcinoma	8
	Large-cell undifferentiated carcinoma	7
		15
	Total peripheral adenocarcinomas	*57*

TABLE 2. Summary of Clinical and Anatomic Data

	Age	Sex	Specimen	Size/Location/Comment	Follow-up
Case 1	59	F	Right lower lobe	3.5 cm subpleural in posterior segment, metastatic to 2/7 bronchopulmonary nodes	No evidence of disease at 41 months
Case 2	57	M	Right upper lobe	3.6 cm subpleural	Dead, 7 months, active TB but no evidence of malignancy
Case 3	67	M	Supraclavicular lymph node	4.0 cm (by x-ray) subpleural nodule in right upper lobe	Dead, 4 months, disseminated carcinoma
Case 4	77	F	Right lower lobe	2.5 cm, subpleural	Lost to follow-up
Case 5	60	F	Right lower lobe	2.0 cm, subpleural	Dead, 1 month, extensive bilateral pulmonary carcinoma
Case 6	70	M	Left lower lobe	1.5 cm, subpleural	Alive, 24 months, no evidence of disease
Case 7	61	M	Right upper lobe	4.5 cm, subpleural, between posterior and apical segments	Dead, 6 months, disseminated carcinoma

TABLE 3. Summary of Pathologic Findings

	Light-Microscopic Diagnosis	PAS	Alcian Blue	Muci-carmine	EM Cell Type
Case 1	Bronchioloalveolar carcinoma	+	–	–	Clara cell
Case 2	Poorly differentiated adenocarcinoma	+	–	–	Clara cell
Case 3	Large cell undifferentiated carcinoma	+	Focally+	Focally+	Clara cell
Case 4	Bronchioloalveolar carcinoma	+	+	+	Goblet/small mucus granule
Case 5	Bronchioloalveolar carcinoma	+	+	+	Goblet/small mucus granule
Case 6	Poorly differentiated adenocarcinoma	–	–	–	Type II alveolar cell
Case 7	Poorly differentiated adenocarcinoma	–	–	–	Type II alveolar cell

cinomas are composed of such structural cells. The histochemical results and cell-type identification in the seven selected cases are summarized in Table 3.

METHODS

All specimens were fixed primarily in Millonig's phosphate-buffered formalin. For light microscopy, a portion of each specimen was processed by routine methods, cut into 3-μ-thick sections, and stained with H & E, periodic acid-Schiff (PAS) with and without diastase digestion, alcian blue with hyaluronidase treatment, and mucicarmine. For electron microscopy, another portion was postfixed in osmium tetroxide (OsO_4), processed by routine methods, cut into 60 to 90 nm-thick sections, and stained with uranyl acetate and lead citrate.

RESULTS

On the basis of histochemical staining and ultrastructural findings, the lesions in the seven selected cases were histogenetically classified as being derived from one of three secretory cell types: the Clara cell, the mucus secretory cell, or the type II alveolar cell.

Adenocarcinomas Derived from the Clara Cell

Cases 1, 2, and 3 demonstrated the histologic growth patterns of well-differentiated bronchioloalveolar adenocarcinoma, poorly differentiated adenocarcinoma, and large-cell undifferentiated carcinoma, respectively (Figs. 1, 2, and 3). The

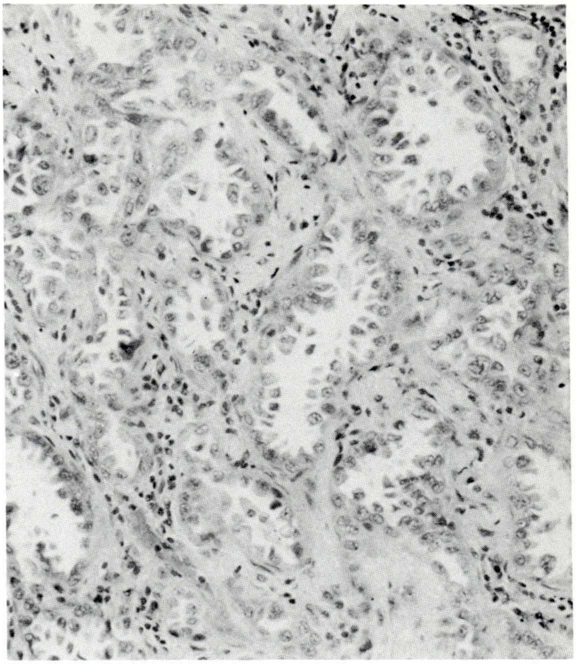

FIG. 1. Case 1. Neoplastic cells with bronchioloalveolar growth pattern.

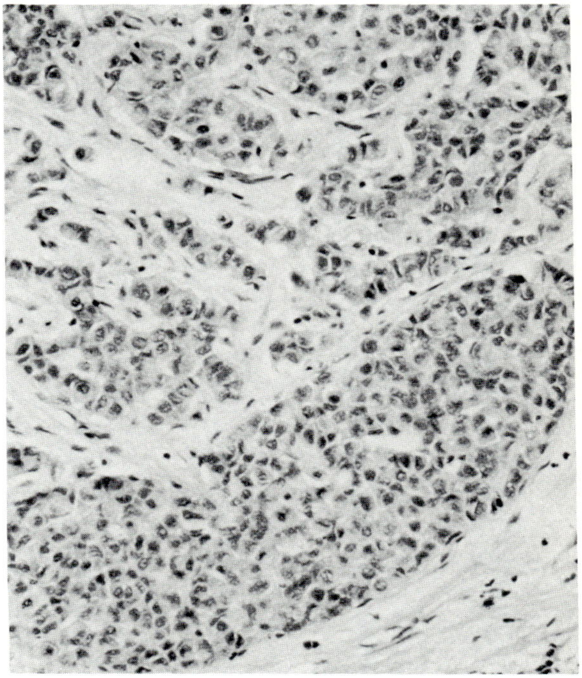

FIG. 2. Case 2. Neoplastic cells with poorly differentiated adenocarcinoma growth pattern.

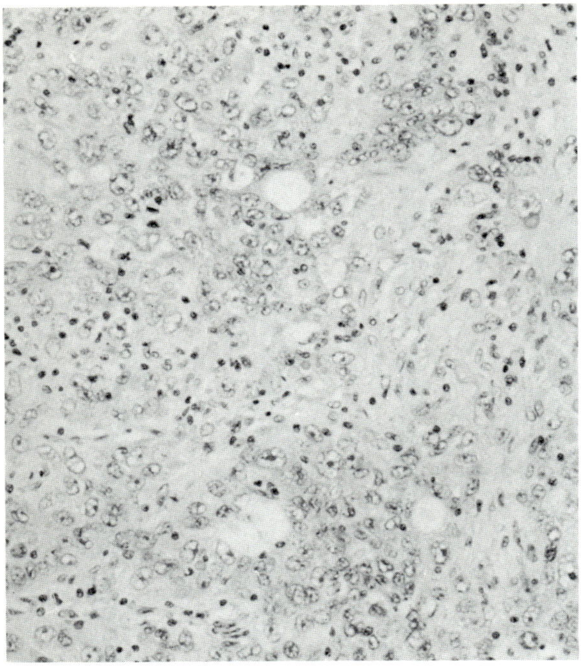

FIG. 3. Case 3. Neoplastic cells with large-cell undifferentiated carcinoma growth pattern.

specimens from all three cases contained readily identified PAS positive, diastase-resistant cytoplasmic substances. Mucicarmine and alcian blue stains were negative in Cases 1 and 2 and only focally positive in Case 3.

The ultrastructural features in the specimens examined were those of variably differentiated adenocarcinomas (Figs. 4, 5, 6, and 7). The numbers of observable intra- or intercellular acini were proportional to the level of differentiation predicted by light microscopy. Acini were lined by surface microvilli which were associated with an inconspicuous glycocalyx and terminal rootlets. Basal lamina separated nests of tumor cells from the alveolar connective tissue space in Case 1, but were absent in Cases 2 and 3. Despite the numerical variation in acini, individual neoplastic cells from all three cases exhibited the features of well-differentiated secretory cells. Their cytoplasm contained an abundance of rough endoplasmic reticulum (RER), prominent Golgi complexes, and numerous secretory granules. The granules generally ranged from 0.5 to 1.5μ in maximum diameter, and were round, irregularly ovoid, or crescentic in shape, with a uniformly condensed secretory product. Case 3 had, in addition to the predominant type of secretory cell, small numbers of cells which contained similar sized granules whose content was either an uncondensed flocculent material consistent with mucin, or a mixture of condensed and uncondensed materials (Fig. 8). These cells corresponded in number to the mucin-positive cells noted by light microscopy. In addition to secretory products, a few of the cells had bundles of perinuclear tonofilaments. The Case 2 specimen contained rare cells with an abundance of endoplasmic reticulum which focally formed so-called ribosomal-lamellar complexes composed of concentric membranes and interposed rows of ribosomes (Fig. 9).

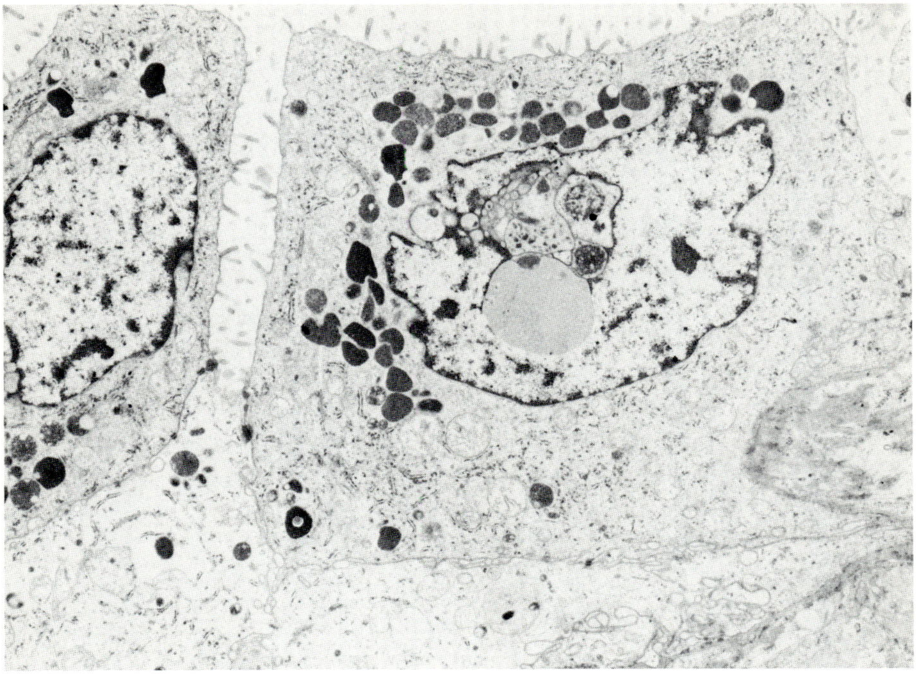

FIG. 4. Case 1. Neoplastic cell having characteristic Clara cell secretory granules which are electron dense and vary in shape. ×4,960.

Adenocarcinomas Derived from the Goblet/Small Mucus Granule Cell

Cases 4 and 5 demonstrated the histologic growth patterns of well-differentiated bronchioloalveolar adenocarcinomas (Figs. 10 and 11). Specimens from both cases contained an abundance of cytoplasmic PAS-positive, diastase-resistant, and alcian blue- and mucicarmine-positive material.

The ultrastructural features of the specimens from Cases 4 and 5 were those of well-differentiated adenocarcinomas. Both tumors contained numerous intercellular acini lined by short microvilli, and with a variably developed glycocalyx and terminal rootlets. The neoplastic cells in Case 4 were separated from the alveolar septal connective tissue by an intact basal lamina, while in Case 5 the basal lamina was only segmental. The specimen from Case 4 was uniformly composed of well-differentiated secretory cells with abundant interconnected segments of rough endoplasmic reticulum (RER), prominent Golgi zones, and numerous apically oriented secretory granules (Figs. 12 and 13). The majority of these granules were from 0.5 to 2.0μ in diameter, and contained an uncondensed granular-to-flocculent product; small numbers of granules were from 0.3 to 0.5μ in diameter and contained a condensed product. The larger granules often appeared to have coalesced with one another and to have fused with the apical cell membrane. The Case 5 specimen was composed of both moderately differentiated secretory cells and moderately differentiated structural cells with numerous transitional forms. The

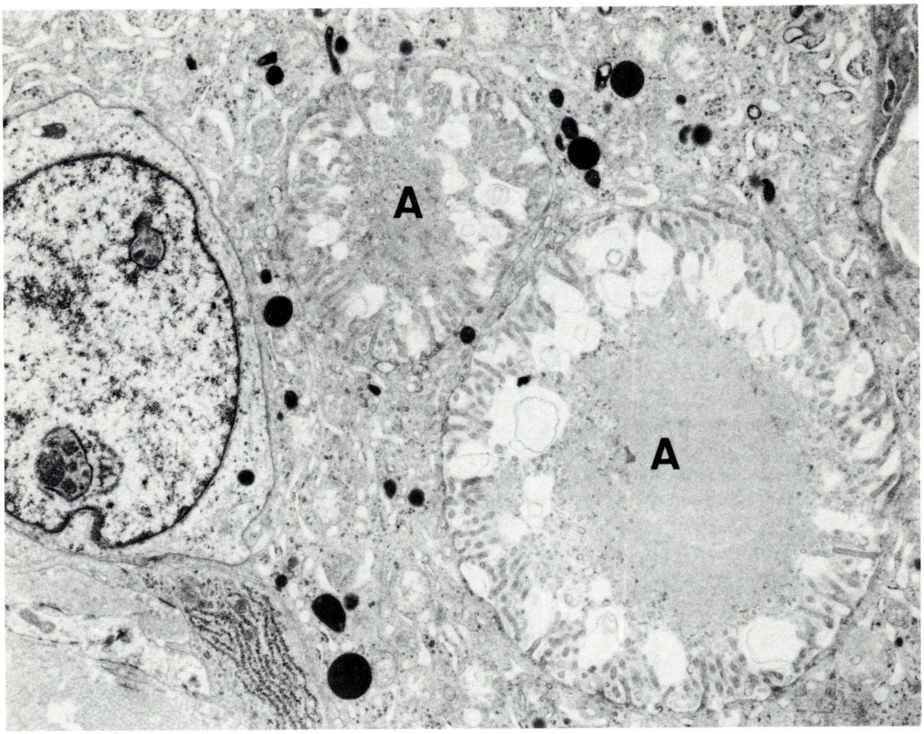

FIG. 5. Case 2. Neoplastic cell has intracellular acini (A) and Clara cell granules. ×7,200.

better-differentiated secretory cells had abundant rough endoplasmic reticulum, prominent Golgi zones, and apically oriented, 0.6 to 1.0μ secretory granules containing an uncondensed product. The structural cells were generally larger and contained an abundance of 6 to 8 nm microfilaments and a paucity of other common organelles; the microfilaments were both diffusely distributed throughout the cytoplasm and focally aggregated around the nucleus as tonofilaments (Fig. 14). Many other cells combined the secretory and cytoskeletal elements in various proportions. Rare neoplastic cells were joined by desmosomes to nonneoplastic, normally appearing, type II alveolar epithelial cells (Fig. 15).

Adenocarcinomas Derived From the Type II Alveolar Epithelial Cell

Cases 6 and 7 demonstrated the histologic growth patterns of poorly differentiated adenocarcinoma (Figs. 16 and 17). The Case 6 specimen contained small quantities of PAS-positive, diastase-sensitive material; however, PAS-positive, diastase-resistant, and mucicarmine- or alcian blue-positive materials were absent in both cases.

Despite the poorly differentiated histologic growth patterns, the lesions in both Cases 6 and 7 were composed of moderately differentiated secretory cells (Figs. 18,

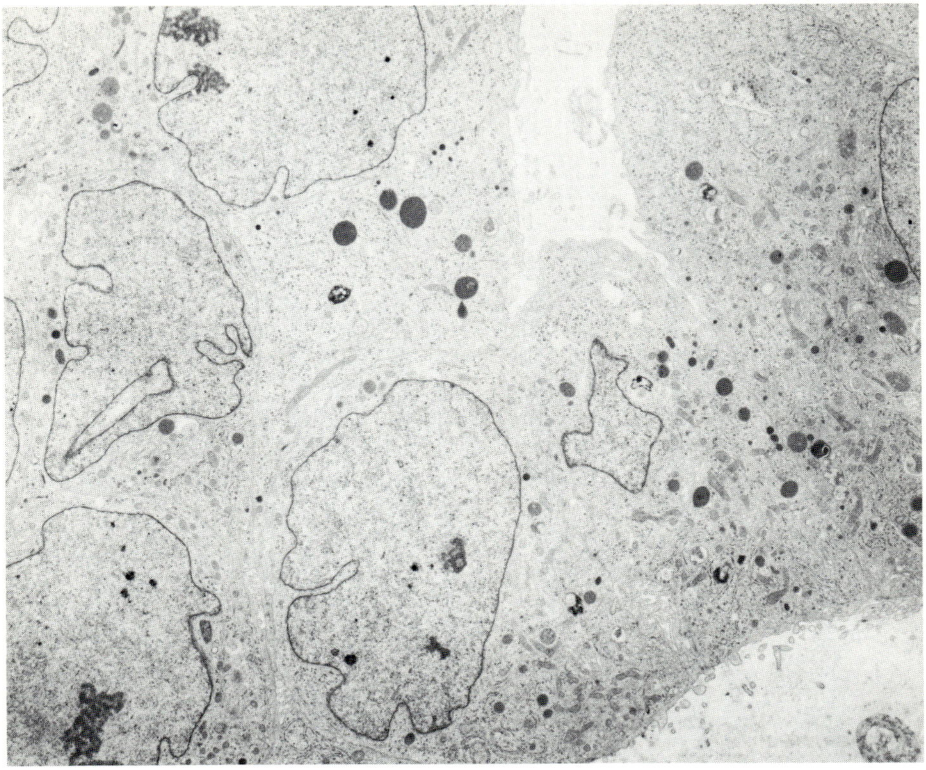

FIG. 6. Case 3. Aggregate of moderately differentiated secretory cells with characteristic Clara cell granules. ×4,200.

19, and 20). The cells formed infrequent intra- and intercellular acini, with surface microvilli having a distinct glycocalyx and inconspicuous terminal rootlets. Neoplastic cells were separated from the connective tissue space by an intact basal lamina in Case 6; however, they directly infiltrated the connective tissue space without intervening basal lamina in Case 7. Cytoplasmic organelles in the cells in both cases included multiple segments of rough endoplasmic reticulum, Golgi zones, and varying numbers of secretory granules. The secretory granules ranged from 0.5 to 2.2μ in diameter and contained a lamellated phospholipid membranous product. In addition, the Case 7 specimen contained similar-sized, clear, membrane-bound structures, suggesting previous extraction of a storage product. The Case 6 specimen had scattered multivesicular bodies containing varying quantities of lamellated phospholipid material, suggesting transitional forms to the mature phospholipid secretory product.

DISCUSSION

The most widely recognized and used system for classifying pulmonary neoplasms is that published by the World Health Organization in 1967.[15] This system divides lung neoplasms into 13 main types, most of which have several subtypes. The

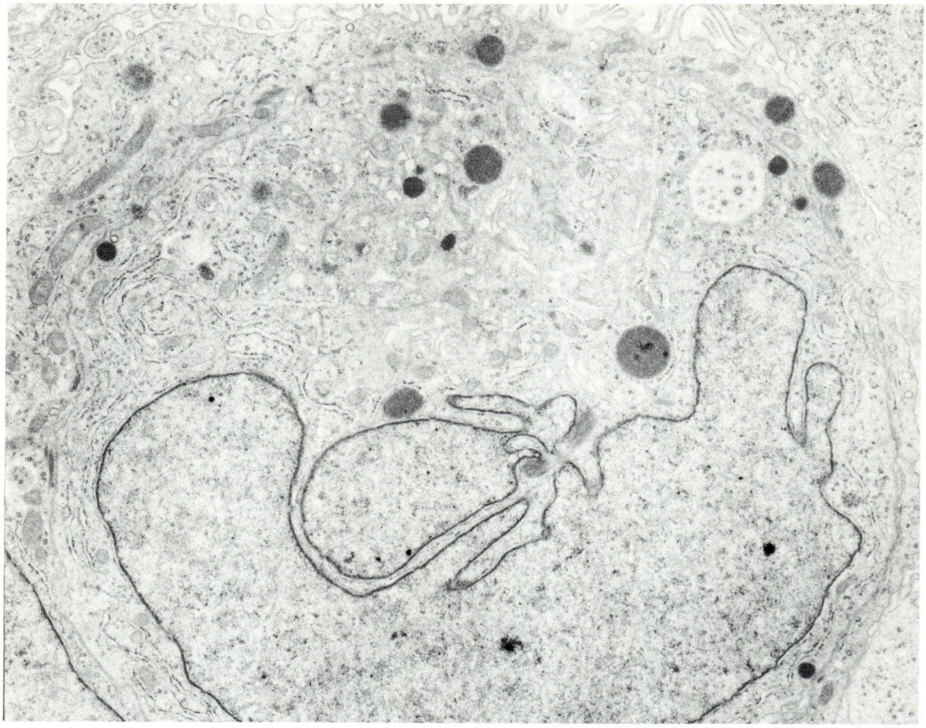

FIG. 7. Case 3. Neoplastic cell with an abundance of rough endoplasmic reticulum and electron-dense secretory granules. ×7,360.

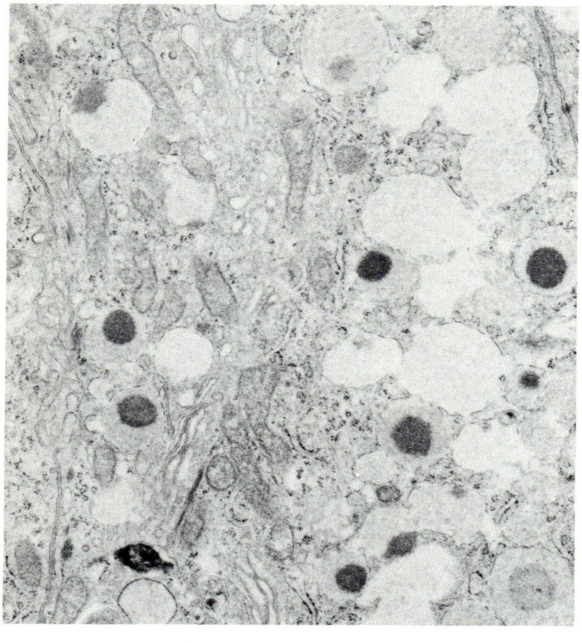

FIG. 8. Case 3. Another neoplastic cell has both a flocculent and electron-dense secretory product. ×12,600.

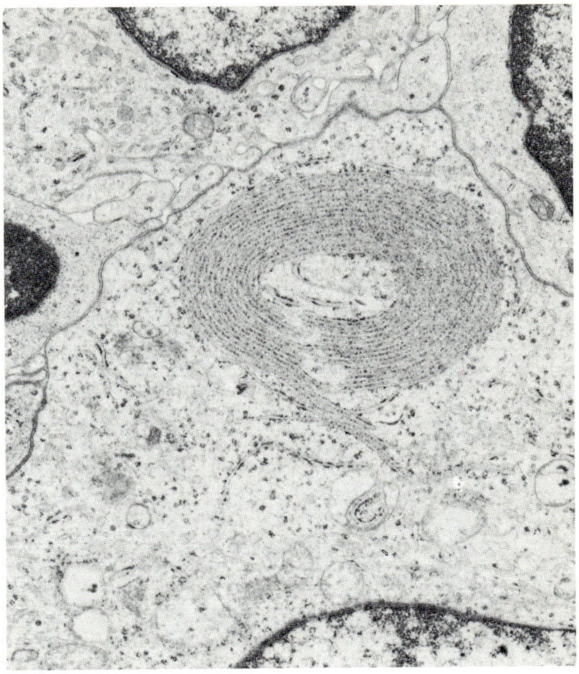

FIG. 9. Case 2. Neoplastic cell with ribosomal-lamellar complex. ×10,000.

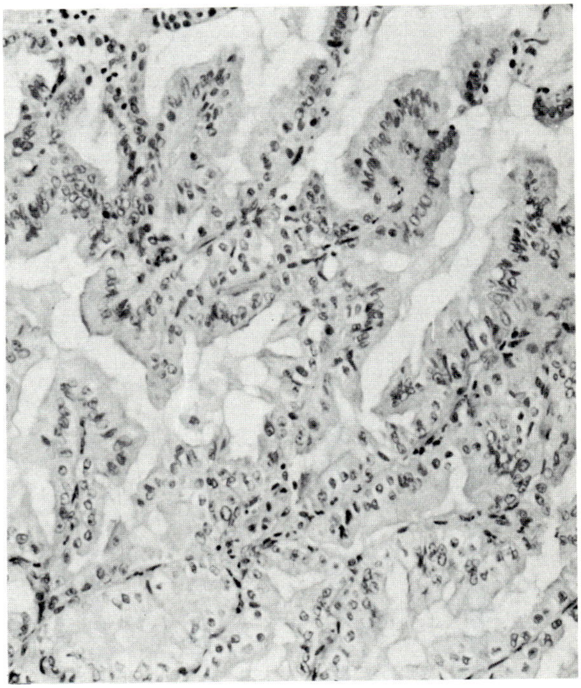

FIG. 10. Case 4. Neoplastic cells with bronchioloalveolar growth pattern.

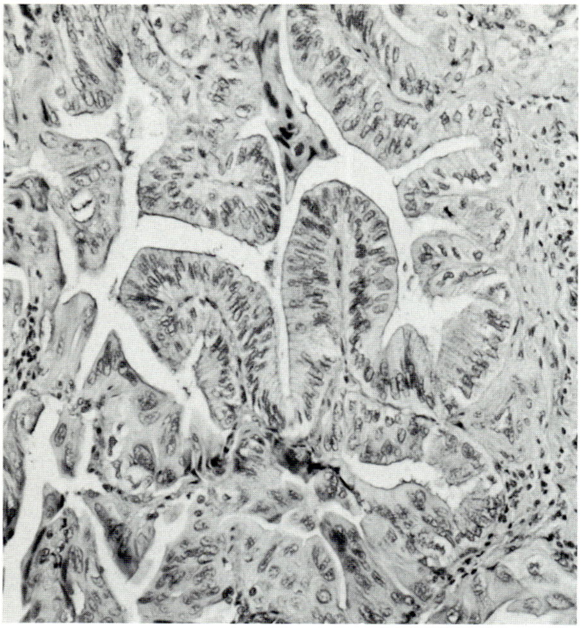

FIG. 11. Case 5. Neoplastic cells with bronchioloalveolar growth pattern.

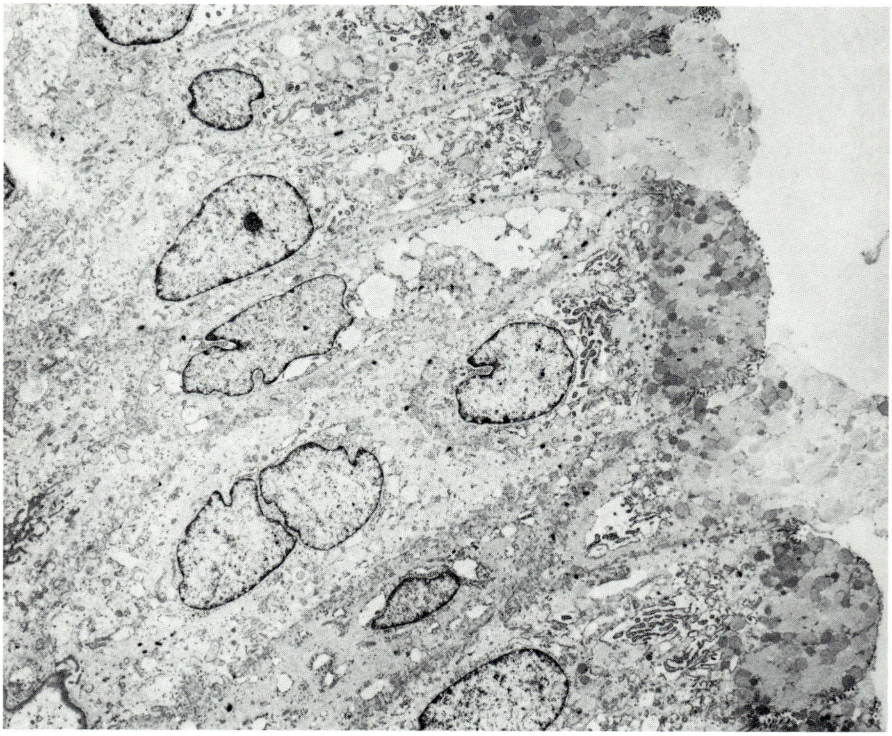

FIG. 12. Case 4. Neoplastic cells have apically concentrated secretory products. ×2,560.

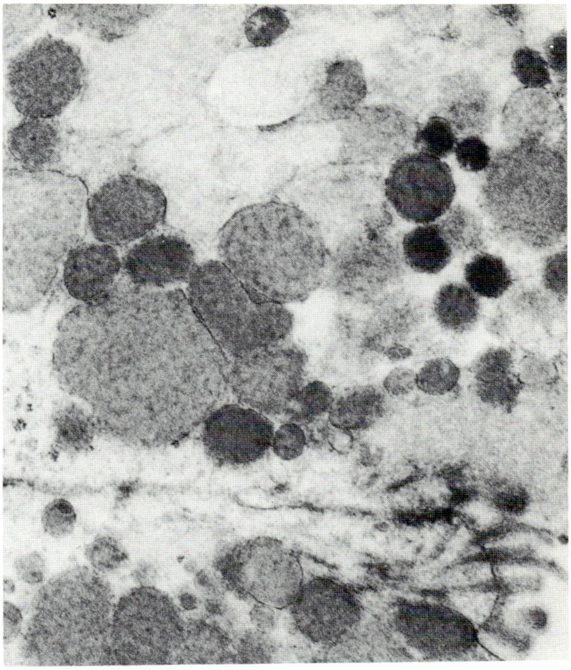

FIG. 13. Case 4. The secretory product is present in both flocculent and condensed forms. ×18,500.

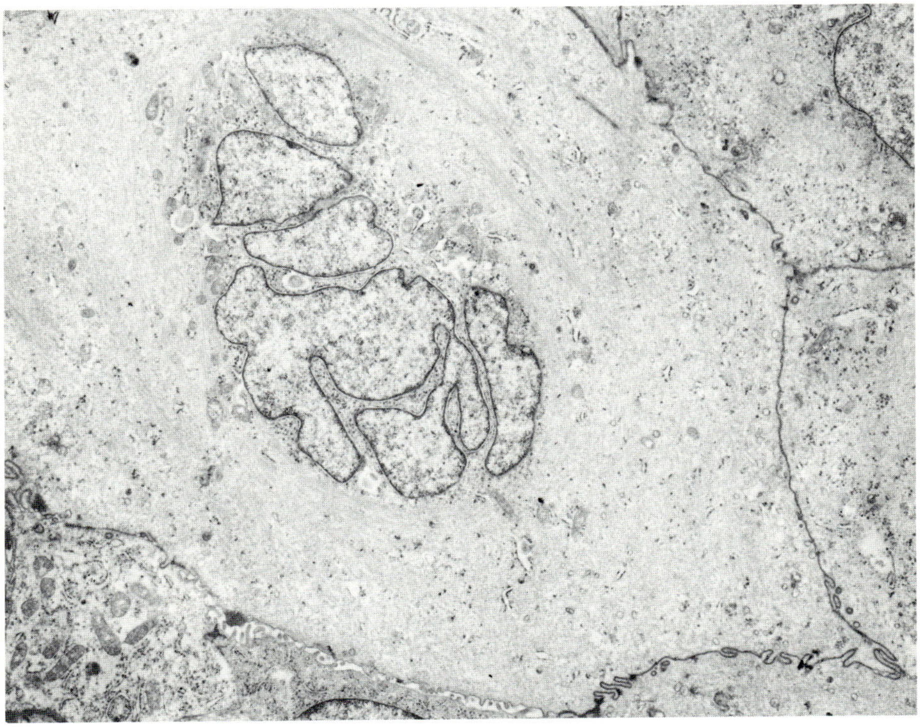

FIG. 14. Case 5. Neoplastic cell with an abundance of cytoskeletal microfilaments. ×4,400.

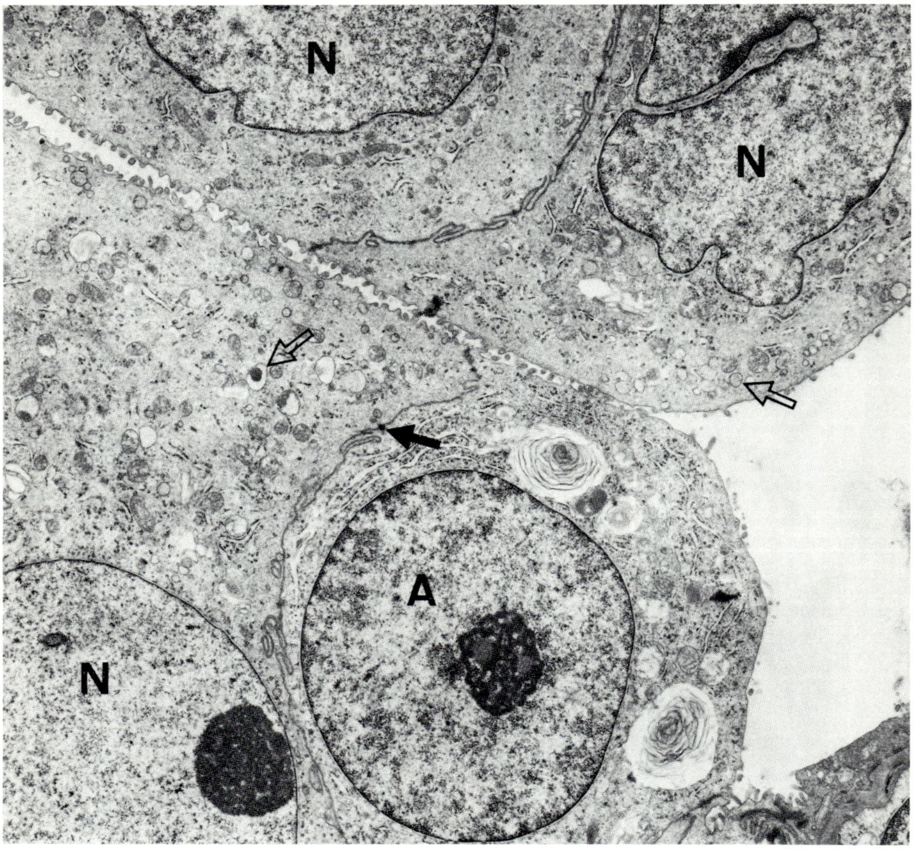

FIG. 15. Case 5. Neoplastic cells (N) adjacent to nonneoplastic type II alveolar epithelial cell (A). Note small junctional complex (solid arrow) and small mucous granules (open arrows) within neoplastic cells. ×6,400.

system is dependent upon the light-microscopic identification of various neoplastic growth patterns, with little consideration of histogenesis. In many instances, particularly in neoplasms exhibiting poorly developed growth patterns, it is difficult to apply the WHO diagnostic criteria with precision. Our experience over the past 5 years, using a combination of light and electron microscopy, indicates that the degree of neoplastic cell differentiation does not necessarily correlate with histologic growth patterns, cell sizes, and cell shapes. Furthermore, tissue fixation and/or section preparation often significantly interfere with the histologic evaluation. Using light and electron microscopy plus histochemical methods, we have tried to apply a histogenetic classification to epithelial neoplasms of the lung, and to assess the relative degree of neoplastic cell differentiation within the various classes. We feel this approach will provide a more accurate initial assessment of the neoplastic cell type and level of differentiation in a given case. If this proves cor-

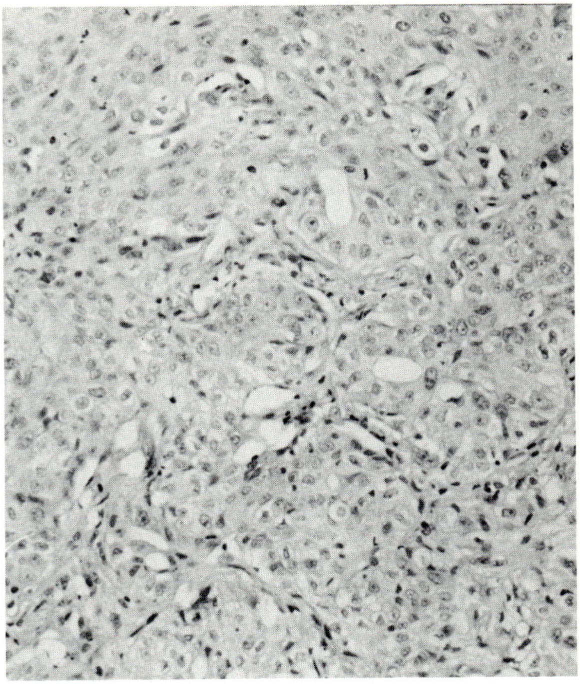

FIG. 16. Case 6. Neoplastic cells with poorly differentiated adenocarcinoma growth pattern.

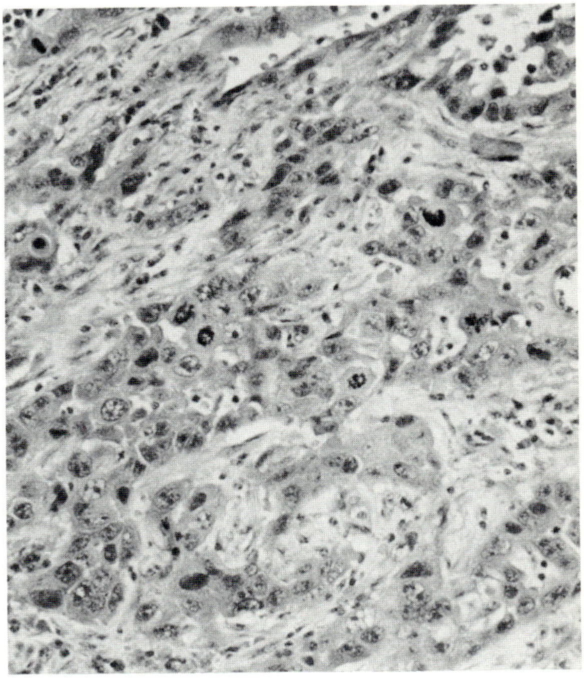

FIG. 17. Case 7. Neoplastic cells with poorly differentiated adenocarcinoma growth pattern.

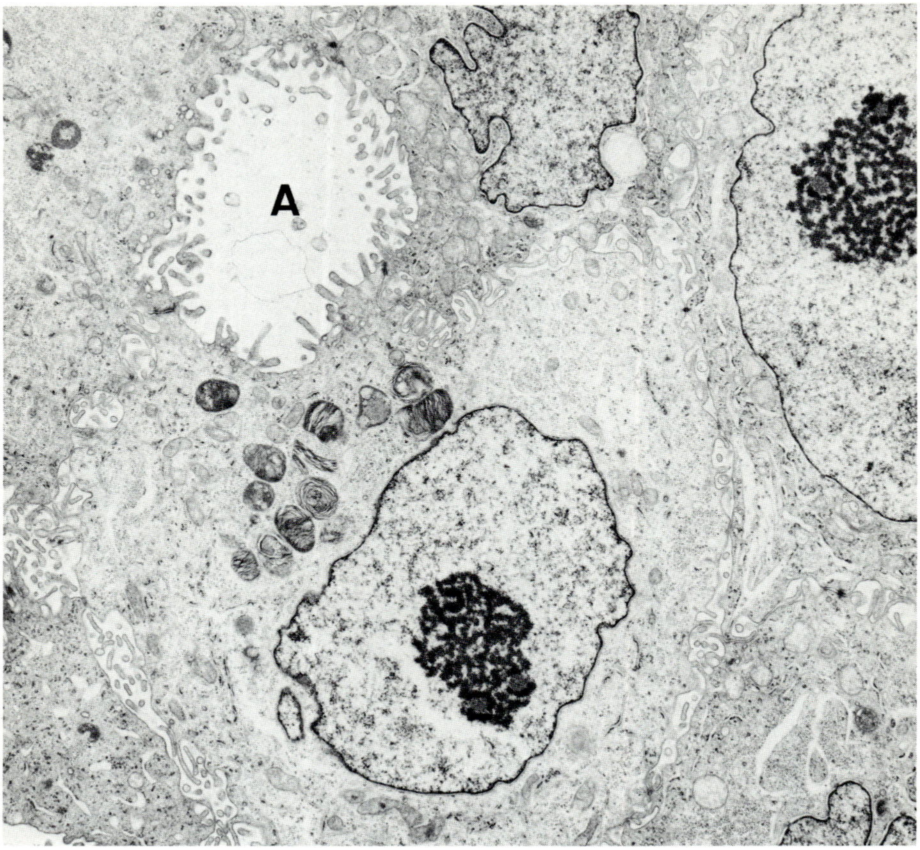

FIG. 18. Case 6. Neoplastic cells have formed an intercellular acinus (A). One contains numerous secretory granules. ×6,720.

rect, we feel that the more precise, original diagnostic impression will provide a better basis for comparing the outcome of different therapeutic measures.

The histogenetic classification of lung carcinomas used in the current study is based on the pulmonary epithelial cell types which have been shown to have the potential for mitotic division.[2-4,9,20,21,27,34] This proliferative capacity is necessary both for the repair of injured epithelium and for neoplastic hyperplasia. The cells with this replicative potential include basal cells, mucus secretory cells (goblet/small mucus granule cells), neuroendocrine secretory cells, Clara secretory cells, and type II alveolar secretory cells. The cases presented in this report were selected to illustrate the three cell types which are responsible for the peripheral adenocarcinomas we have studied; these three cell types are the Clara, mucus, and type II alveolar secretory cell. Their respective secretory products and staining affinities are summarized in Table 4.[8,19,26,29] Periodic acid-Schiff (PAS), with and without prior diastase treatment; alcian blue at pH 2.5 with prior hyaluronidase treatment; and mucicarmine are the routine stains performed on lung neoplasms in our laboratory.

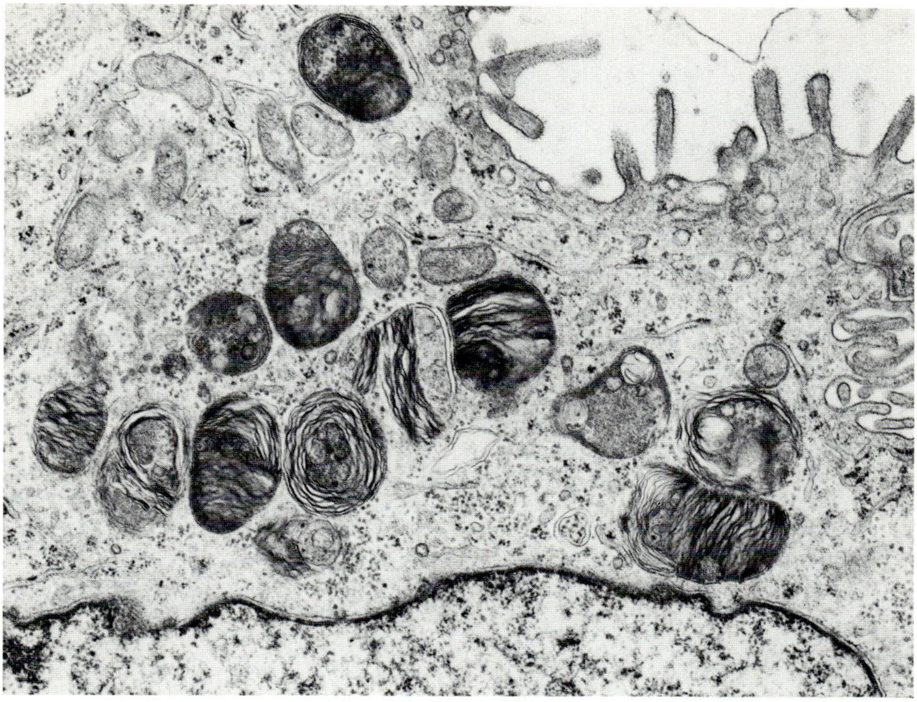

FIG. 19. Case 6. Higher-power magnification of Figure 18. Note typical lamellated phospholipid-rich secretory product. ×19,200.

The goblet/small mucus granule cell can be readily distinguished from the Clara cell and type II pneumocyte on the basis of its positive staining with mucicarmine and alcian blue. The histochemical distinction between the Clara cell and the type II pneumocyte can be more difficult; however, in our experience, the generally uniform, strong PAS staining of normal and neoplastic Clara cells contrasts with a more focal and weak staining of type II pneumocytes.

Clara cells are the primary secretory cells in the normal bronchiolar epithelium[7,8,17,29,31] (Figs. 21 and 22). They have abundant rough endoplasmic reticulum, prominent Golgi zones, and 0.3- to 0.6-μ-diameter secretory granules. These granules are located in the apical region of the cytoplasm and contain a uniformly dense, condensed secretory product. Biochemical studies indicate that the usual Clara cell secretory product is a mixture of phospholipid and carbohydrates strongly bound to a basic protein. Mucus is not formed under normal conditions, but can be produced by Clara cells as a reaction to a number of experimentally induced injuries.[28] Such a transformation in secretory product synthesis probably underlies the "mucus cell metaplasia" observed in a variety of human respiratory diseases, especially those associated with respiratory failure.[14] Following the conversion to mucus secretion, transformed Clara cells would be expected to contain either the uncondensed secretory product of goblet cells, the condensed product of small mucus granule cells, or both (Figs. 23 and 24). This stored

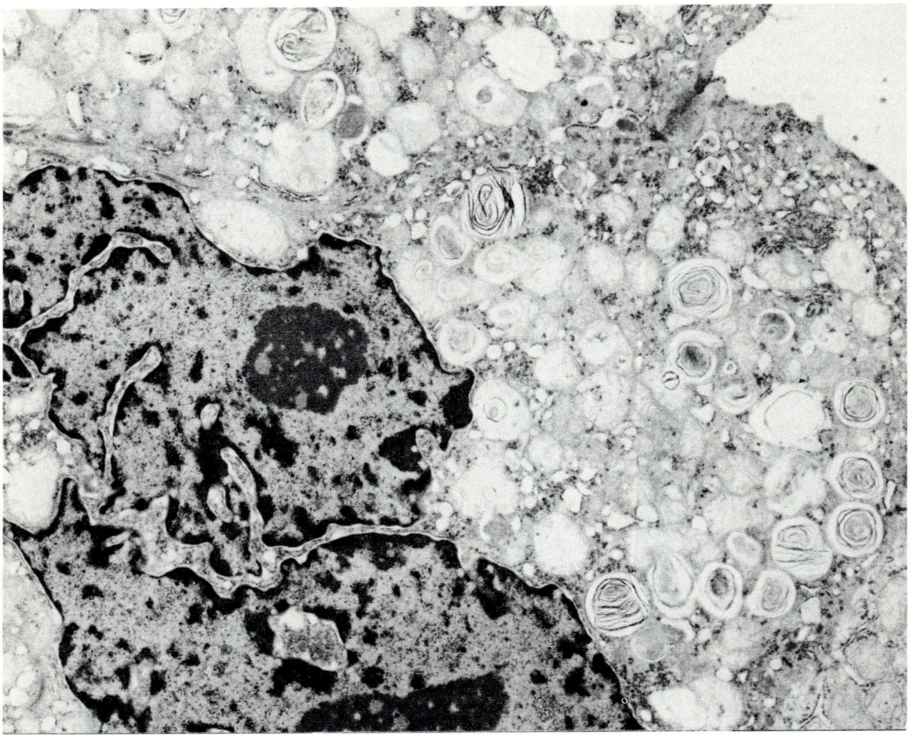

FIG. 20. Case 7. Neoplastic cells have lamellated phospholipid-rich secretory product. ×7,040.

mucus product, condensed or noncondensed, can be distinguished from typical Clara cell granules and from lysosomes by its affinity for acid mucin stains. Although we consider the apically oriented, mucin-stain-negative, condensed granule to be characteristic for Clara cells, we recognize that these morphologic criteria alone cannot distinguish Clara cell granules from lysosomes. We have not used methods for detecting acid phosphatase activity which would specifically identify lysosomal granules.

TABLE 4. Summary of Secretory Products and Staining Affinities

Cell Type	Cell Product With Diastase	PAS With Diastase	Alcian Blue	Muci-carmine	Luxol Fast Blue	Sudan Black
Clara Cell	Phospholipid-carbohydrate-basic protein	+	−	−	+	±
Goblet/small mucus granule	Primarily acid glycoprotein	+	+	+	−	−
Type II	Primarily phospholipid	±	−	−	+	+

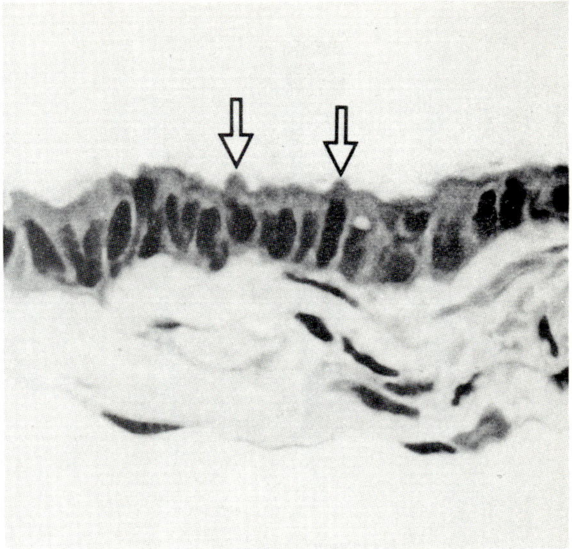

FIG. 21. Nonneoplastic bronchiolar epithelium. Note Clara cells (open arrows) with typical apical blebs distributed between ciliated respiratory epithelial cells.

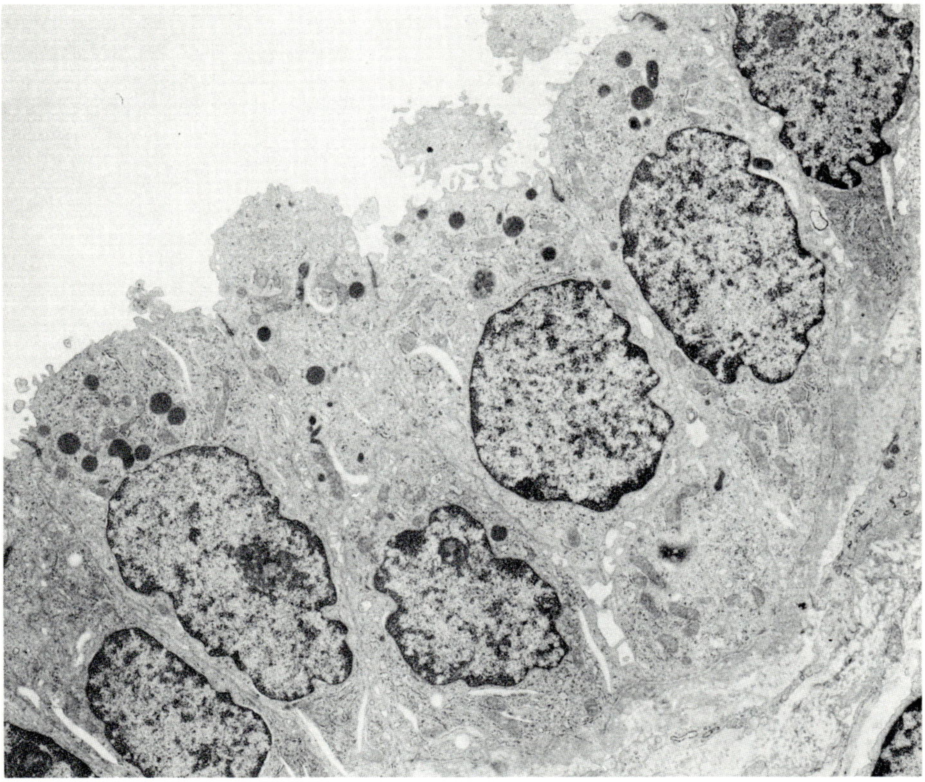

FIG. 22. Nonneoplastic, hyperplastic bronchiolar Clara cells with characteristic apically concentrated, electron-dense secretory granules. ×4,000.

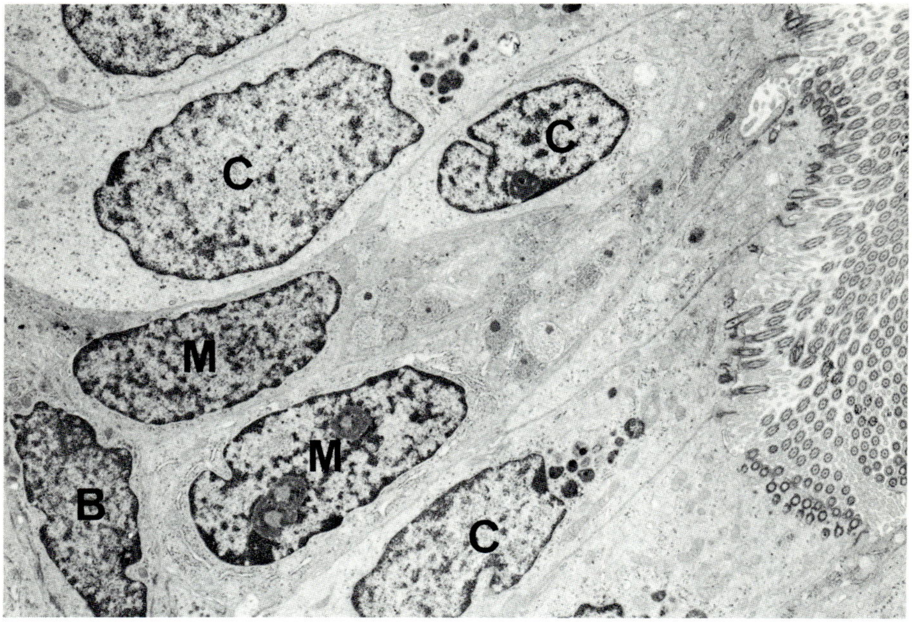

FIG. 23. Nonneoplastic bronchiolar epithelium. Located between ciliated cells (C) and basal cell (B), are two metaplastic mucus-producing cells (M). ×5,000.

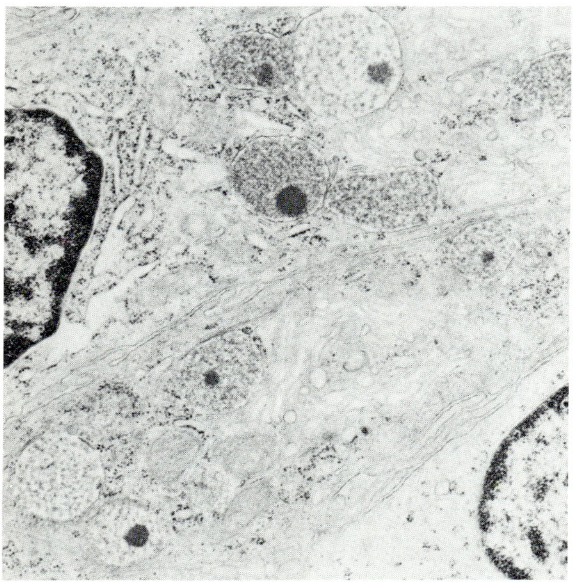

FIG. 24. Higher-power magnification of Figure 23. Metaplastic cells contain both flocculent and electron-dense secretory product. ×14,000.

Pulmonary neoplasms derived from Clara cells have been reported, usually as isolated case reports.[5,12,16,22,23,30] Their frequency is uncertain. In a series of 100 consecutive surgically resected lung neoplasms studied by light- and electron microscopy, only one was considered to have a Clara cell origin.[21] In another series of 25 pulmonary adenocarcinomas studied in a similar manner, 21 were considered to have a Clara cell origin.[13] The three cases we identified as Clara cell neoplasms were selected to illustrate the spectrum of histologic growth patterns; one (Case 1) appeared as a well differentiated bronchioloalveolar adenocarcinoma, another (Case 2) as a poorly differentiated adenocarcinoma, and the third (Case 3) as a large-cell undifferentiated carcinoma. All three of the neoplasms, irrespective of the histologic impression they gave, consisted of well-differentiated secretory cells with a histochemically and ultrastructurally typical Clara cell secretory product.

One of the three neoplasms we identified as being of Clara cell origin (Case 3) contained cytochemically and electron microscopically identifiable mucus storage granules in addition to Clara-type granules; this could be explained by the ability of Clara cells to synthesize both types of products under certain conditions. An interesting feature of one neoplasm (Case 2) was the striking abundance of endoplasmic reticulum, which focally formed whorled arrays characteristic of so-called ribosomal-lamellar complexes; these structural arrangements have been observed in a variety of pathologic conditions. The amount of smooth endoplasmic reticulum in these neoplastic cells was unusual for nonneoplastic human Clara cells, but is commonly noted in nonneoplastic rodent Clara cells.[17,31]

The major secretory cell type in the gas-exchange tissue of the lung is the alveolar type II pneumocyte (Figs. 25 and 26). This cell normally has abundant endoplasmic reticulum, prominent Golgi zones, and distinctive secretory granules. The granules consist of membrane-bound lamellated collections of phospholipid

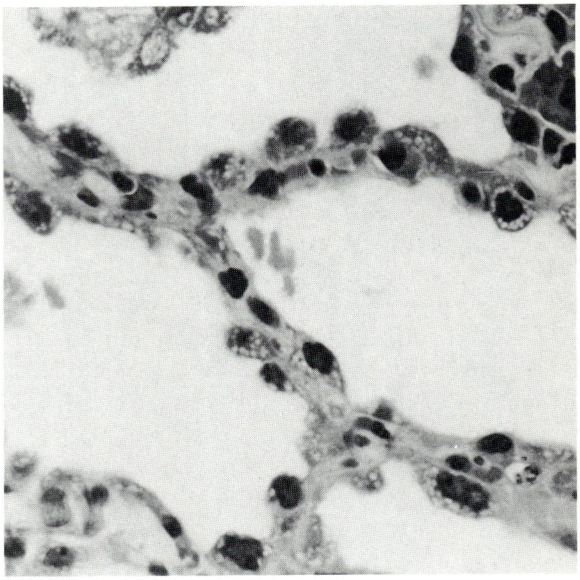

FIG. 25. Nonneoplastic, hyperplastic alveolar epithelial cells.

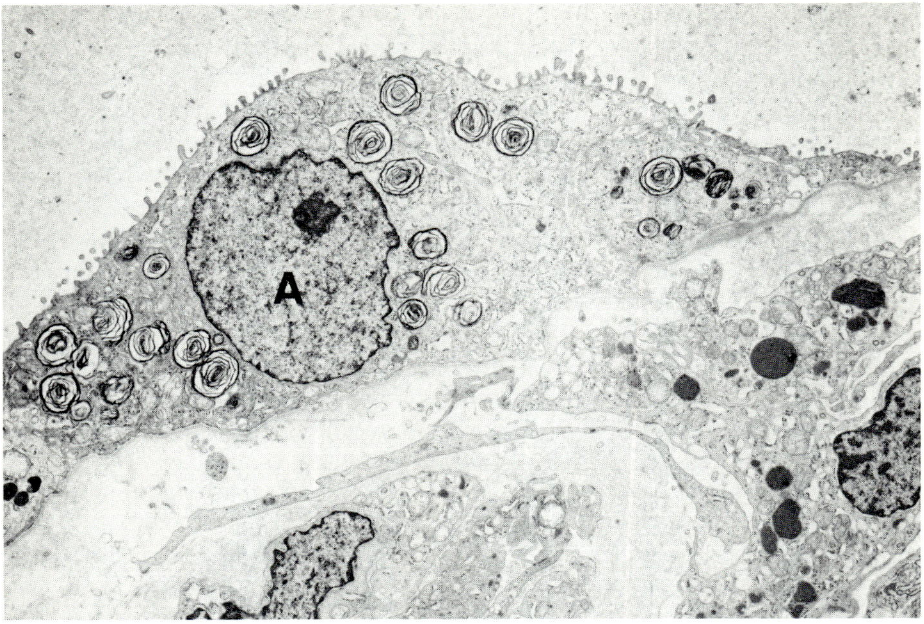

FIG. 26. Nonneoplastic, hyperplastic alveolar epithelial cell (A) with lamellated phospholipid-rich secretory product. ×4,400.

substances loosely bound to protein. The mature phospholipid secretory product may evolve from precursor multivesicular bodies.[10,32] The type II lamellar granule will generally stain with luxol fast blue and Sudan black for phospholipid material; however, PAS is generally weak and inconsistent in its staining intensity.

Pulmonary neoplasms derived from type II alveolar secretory cells have been reported, although the subject is controversial.[1,6,18,25] Several authors have suggested that there is no convincing proof of neoplastic type II secretory cells occurring in bronchioloalveolar growth patterns despite a number of isolated case reports to the contrary.[5,11,16,21] One report of neoplastic type II secretory cells in bronchioloalveolar growth patterns involved a case with apparent metastatic disease.[24] Some of the confusion surrounding the matter appears to stem from the difficulty in separating reactive type II hyperplasia from neoplastic type II hyperplasia. In this regard, we have frequently encountered an admixture of neoplastic cells and nonneoplastic type II cells at the edges of neoplasms. One of our current neoplasms (Case 3) illustrated this phenomenon and demonstrated junctional complexes between the two morphologically and biologically disparate cell types. The two neoplasms of type II secretory cells (Cases 6 and 7) cannot be considered atypical hyperplasias. Neither had a bronchioloalveolar growth pattern. Instead, the cells in both appeared as poorly differentiated carcinoma cells arranged in largely solid cell clusters. However, even though interpreted as being poorly differentiated histologically, both neoplasms contained moderately differentiated secretory cells.

In addition to Clara and type II secretory cells, mucus-producing cells have also been reported in peripheral adenocarcinomas, including those with bronchioloalveolar growth patterns. Our mucus-secretory neoplasm (Case 4) consisted of uniform cells with an abundant secretory product having a histochemical and morphologic similarity to the uncondensed mucus product in nonneoplastic, large-airway goblet cells. Another neoplasm (Case 5) consisted of less uniform cells having both condensed and uncondensed mucus storage granules as well as a variably prominent cytoskeletal apparatus. The spectrum of cytodifferentiation observed in the neoplastic cells of this neoplasm, with secretory cells at one end, structural cells at the other end, and transitional forms in between, is analogous to that observed in both reactive and neoplastic cell hyperplasia involving large-airway epithelium.[3,4,20,21,33]

Our findings generally parallel those of others who have studied peripheral adenocarcinomas by light and electron microscopy. Although histologic growth patterns did not distinguish these neoplasms histogenetically, the combined use of histochemical stains and electron microscopy provided such a distinction. This study reemphasizes the potential fallacy of predicting the degree of neoplastic differentiation solely on the basis of light-microscopically-detected growth patterns and cytology. Although we do not have sufficient follow-up information on most of the patients studied, we feel these discrepancies could result in an inappropriate estimate of prognosis. It must be appreciated that we selected these cases for their positive features. We have examined other peripherally located neoplasms with poorly developed histologic patterns and poorly differentiated neoplastic cell ultrastructure that have rendered their assignment to a histogenetic category either difficult and problematic or impossible. Most of these cases fall into the histologic classification of poorly differentiated small cell neoplasms and are the subject of another report now being prepared.

ACKNOWLEDGMENTS

The authors wish to express their appreciation to Florence Teshima and Jeri Krivacek for their technical assistance, and to Margie Perdue and Dawn Martin for preparation of the manuscript.

REFERENCES

1. Adamson JS, Senior R, Merril T: Alveolar cell carcinoma. Am Rev Respir Dis 100:550–557, 1969
2. Barrett LA, McDowell EM, Frank AL: Long-term organ culture of human bronchial epithelium. Cancer Res 36:1002–1010, 1976
3. Becci PJ, McDowell EM, Trump BF: The respiratory epithelium. II. Hamster trachea, bronchus, and bronchioles. J Natl Cancer Inst 61:551–561, 1978
4. Becci PJ, McDowell EM, Trump BF: The respiratory epithelium. IV. Histogenesis of epidermoid metaplasia and carcinoma in-situ in the hamster. J Natl Cancer Inst 61:577–586, 1978
5. Bedrossian CW, Weilbaecher DG, Bentinck DC: Ultrastructure of human bronchioloalveolar cell carcinoma. Cancer 36:1399–1413, 1975
6. Bonikos DS, Hendrickson M, Bensch KG: Pulmonary alveolar cell carcinoma. Am J Surg Pathol 1:93–108, 1977

7. Clara M: Zur Histobiologie des Bronchulepithels. Z Mikrosk Anat Forsch 41:321–347, 1937
8. Cutz E, Conen PE: Ultrastructure and cytochemistry of Clara cells. Am J Surg Pathol 1:93–108, 1977
9. Evans MJ, Johnson LV, Stephens RJ: Renewal of the terminal bronchiolar epithelium in rat following exposure to NO_2 or O_3. Lab Invest 35:246–257, 1976
10. Goldenberg VE, Buckingham S: Pilocarpine stimulation of granular pneumocyte secretion. Lab Invest 20:147–158, 1969
11. Greenberg SD, Smith MW, Spjut HF: Bronchiolo-alveolar carcinoma-cell of origin. Am J Clin Pathol 63:153–167, 1975
12. Jacques J, Currie W: Bronchiolo-alveolar carcinoma: A Clara cell tumor? Cancer 40:2171–2180, 1977
13. Kimula Y: A histochemical and ultrastructural study of adenocarcinoma of the lung. Am J Surg Pathol 2:253–264, 1978
14. Korpick RJ, Pratt PC, Asmundson T: Pathologic findings in respiratory failure: goblet cell metaplasia, alveolar damage and myocardial infarction. Ann Intern Med 72:189–197, 1970
15. Kreyberg L: Histological typing of lung tumors. In International Histological Classification of Tumors, No. 1. Geneva, World Health Organization, 1967, pp 1–28
16. Kuhn C: Fine structure of bronchiolo-alveolar cell carcinoma. Cancer 30:1107–1118, 1972
17. Kuhn C, Callaway LA, Askin FB: The formation of granules in the bronchiolar Clara cells of the rat. J Ultrastruct Res 49:387–400, 1974
18. Lieber M, Smith B, Szakal A, et al.: A continuous cell line from a human lung carcinoma with properties of type II alveolar epithelial cells. Int J Cancer 17:62–70, 1976
19. Maeda M, Kotake Y, Seike Y, et al.: Secretory cells of pulmonary surfactant. A comparative histochemical study of Clara cells and granular pneumocytes. Med J Osaka Univ 25:1–22, 1974
20. McDowell EM, Barrett LA, Glavin F, et al.: The respiratory epithelium. I. Human bronchus. J Natl Cancer Inst 61:539–549, 1978
21. McDowell EM, Mclaughlin JS, Merenyi DK: The respiratory epithelium. V. Histogenesis of lung carcinomas in the human. J Natl Cancer Inst 61:587–606, 1978
22. Montes M, Alder RH, Brennan JC: Bronchiolar apocrine tumor. Am Rev Resp Dis 93:946–950, 1966
23. Montes M, Binette JP, Chaudhry AP, et al.: Clara cell adenocarcinoma. Light and electron microscopic studies. Am J Surg Pathol 1: 245–253, 1977
24. Morningstar WA, Hassan MV: Bronchiolo-alveolar carcinoma with nodal metastases. Am J Surg Pathol 3:273–278, 1979
25. Nash G, Langlinais PC, Greenwald KA: Alveolar cell carcinoma. Cancer 29:322–326, 1972
26. Niden AH: Bronchiolar and large alveolar cell in pulmonary phospholipid metabolism. Science 158:1323–1324, 1967
27. Parkinson DR, Stephens RJ: Morphological surface changes in the terminal bronchiolar region of NO_2-exposed rat lung. Environ Res 6:31–51, 1953
28. Reid L, Jones R: Bronchial mucosal cells. Fed Proc 38:191–196, 1976
29. Roth J: The Clara cell and the pulmonary surfactant system. Light and electron microscopic studies on the function of Clara cells. Exp Pathol 8:305–313, 1973
30. Sidhu GS, Forrester EM: Glycogen-rich Clara cell-type bronchiolo-alveolar carcinoma. Cancer 40:2209–2215, 1977
31. Smith P, Heath D, Moosavi H: The Clara cell. Thorax 29:147–163, 1974
32. Sorokin SP: A morphologic and cytochemical study of the great alveolar cell. J Histochem Cytochem 14:884–892, 1966
33. Trump BF, McDowell EM, Glavin F: The respiratory epithelium. III. Histogenesis of epidermoid metaplasia and carcinoma in-situ in the human. J Natl Cancer Inst 61:563–575, 1978
34. Witschi H: Proliferation of Type II alveolar cells: A review of common responses in toxic lung injury. Toxicology 5:267–277, 1976

INFLAMMATION OF THE TESTIS, EPIDIDYMIS, PERITESTICULAR MEMBRANES, AND SCROTUM

GREGOR MIKUZ AND IVAN DAMJANOV

The testis, the male gonad, has a unique anatomic and physiologic status in the body, and many of the pathologic conditions involving this organ can be explained and fully understood only in view of the basic anatomic and physiologic premises concerning it.[1,2] Among the main characteristics of the testis that play an important role in the pathogenesis of various inflammatory conditions are the following:

1. Scrotal location. The testis is located in the scrotum and is closely enveloped by the tunica vaginalis; the scrotum secures the temperature needed for normal spermatogenesis, which is several degrees lower then the normal body temperature. On the other hand, the lower temperature of the testis may play an important role in some infections. It has been hypothesized that the frequent involvement of the testes by *Mycobacterium leprae* in lepromatous leprosy may be due to the lower temperature provided by the scrotum.[3] The scrotal location and the mobility of the testis make it highly vulnerable to trauma, compression, avulsion, and torsion.[4]
2. Close proximity of the testis to the epididymis and spermatic cord, and the continuity of the testicular and epididymal tubules and ducts. The testis, epididymis, and spermatic cord form a functional unit and are in direct continuity. Any infection of the testis could involve the other scrotal structures as well. The infection may spread through the lumen of the ducts, lymphatics, or blood vessels, or directly through the tissues and along the membranes.[5] Since the vas deferens communicates freely with the lower urinary tract, and urethrovasal reflux may occur,[6,7] it is quite obvious that the intraluminal spread of retrograde infection forms an important basis of both epididymal and testicular inflammation.
3. Existence of the blood–testis barrier.[8] The germ cells inside seminiferous tubules are sequestered and isolated from the rest of the body by a selectively permeable basement membrane and the closely apposed sustentacular (Sertoli) cells. The tight junctions between the Sertoli cells protect the germ cells from toxic

substances in the interstitial fluids, and also impede the contact of endogenous germ-cell-specific antigens with the immune system of the body. The blood–testis barrier plays an important role in the pathogenesis of autoimmune orchitis[9] and in the evolution of immunologically mediated testicular changes in patients whose testicular integrity has been altered, e.g., after vasectomy.[10]

INCIDENCE AND PREVALENCE OF ORCHITIS

The real incidence and prevalence of orchitis are unknown[5]; the inflammation is often asymptomatic and subclinical. In patients with systemic disease, signs of orchitis may be overshadowed by symptoms pertaining to other organs. Testalgia is a clinical sign of orchitis, and swelling of the testes in patients suffering from acute viral disease is most likely due to viral orchitis.[11] However, without a tissue diagnosis and other corroborating evidence, these data are only rough estimates of the prevalence and incidence of orchitis.

ETIOLOGY AND CLASSIFICATION OF EPIDIDYMO-ORCHITIS

Inflammatory diseases involving the testis and epididymis may be classified according to several criteria: According to its duration, the disease may be classified as acute, chronic, or recurrent. According to its etiology, the disease may be due to infectious agents (bacteria, viruses, spirochetes, etc.), autoimmune mechanisms, or physicochemical causes, or may be nonclassifiable, or "idiopathic." According to the anatomic location of the inflammation, the disease may be classified as orchitis, epididymitis, funiculitis, or periorchitis, although more often than not, more than one intrascrotal structure is involved.

Inflammation of the epididymis and testis is rarely isolated, and most often occurs as either a manifestation of a genitourinary tract inflammation or of a systemic disease.

Infectious Epididymo-orchitis

Infectious agents may reach the testis and epididymis in the blood, through the lymphatics, through the seminiferous canals, and in extremely rare cases along the tunica vaginalis testis or through the skin of the scrotum.[5,17] Blood-borne infection is common in viral and spirochetal diseases, but may occur in bacterial diseases as well. Bacterial and mycoplasmal infections of the urogenital tract reach the epididymis and testis through the seminiferous ducts and the lymphatics of the funiculus spermaticus.

Blood-borne infections tend to affect the testis more than the epididymis, whereas the intracanalicular lymphogeneous infections tend to affect the epididymis more extensively than the testis, with notable exceptions to this rule.

An ascending infection is most likely due to the reflux of infected urine from the urethra into the ejaculatory ducts and into the ductus deferens.[6,7] The existence of urethro-ejaculatory duct reflux has been disputed by some authorities and it is questionable whether it exists in healthy individuals.[12] On the other hand, substantial documentation for this pathogenic route of infection has been provided, especially in patients suffering from chronic infection of the urinary tract, in patients following instrumentation, and in patients with chronic obstruction of the bladder-neck area and neurogenic bladder.[12] Children with congenital malformations of the urethra, posterior urethral valves, and anovesical malformations may also have urethro-ejaculatory duct reflux and thus have a greater-than-average predisposition to bacterial epididymo-orchitis.[17-18,28]

Bacterial Infections. *Escherichia coli* is the most common bacterial pathogen isolated from the lower genitourinary tract or directly from the epididymis of men over the age of 35 diagnosed as having acute epididymitis.[16] *Neisseria gonorrheae* is the most common bacterial pathogen in patients younger than 35 years of age. Many other bacteria have been isolated and identified as etiologic agents in acute epididymo-orchitis, most notably Gram-negative bacteria such as *Aerobacter aerogenes, Pseudomonas,* and *Klebsiella.*[13,16] *Streptoccocus, Staphylococcus, Pneumococcus,* and other Gram-positive cocci have also been isolated in many cases of suppurative epididymitis and orchitis.[15,16,27] Epididymitis has also been recorded in several cases of meningococcal and *Haemophilus influenzae*[17,19] sepsis. Orchitis is a common complication of brucellosis, and is especially common in infections due to *Brucella melitensis.*[20] Epididymo-orchitis due to *Mycobacterium tuberculosis* was previously a relatively common disease and is today still seen in miliary tuberculosis and as a part of urogenital tract infections.[21,22] Lepromatous leprosy often involves the testis.[23] There are three well-documented cases of testicular abscesses caused by *Salmonella.*[24-26] All of the cases discussed above, although ostensibly rare, suggest that epididymo-orchitis may be caused by most, if not all, currently known human bacterial pathogens.

Uroplasma urealyticum has been isolated from the urine of the several patients with epididymitis. Since cultures of epididymal aspirates did not grow this microorganism, it is not clear whether *Uroplasma* may indeed reach the epididymis and cause epididymitis.

Experimental Bacterial Orchitis. The evolution of experimental bacterial orchitis was studied sequentially by Mikuz.[5] The inflammation begins as interstitial edema, followed by accumulation of polymorphonuclear leukocytes in the intertubular spaces. During this "interstitial phase" of orchitis, the Sertoli cells undergo focal necrosis and, 48 hours after the onset of the infection, the blood-testis barrier seems to have been irreversibly damaged (Figs. 1 and 2). The breakdown of the blood-testis barrier is a direct consequence of Sertoli cell necrosis and the increased permeability of the seminiferous tubules, which is most likely mediated by chemical byproducts of inflammation. During the second, "intratubular phase" of inflammation, the leukocytes invade the seminiferous tubules. Bacteria also enter the seminiferous tubules and are phagocytized by the Sertoli cells and the invading polymorphonuclear and mononuclear phagocytes (Fig. 1). The phagocytes ingest not only the bacteria but also the spermatozoa and the degenerating testicular cells.

The necrotic cells, bacteria, and leukocytes seen in the "intratubular phase" of

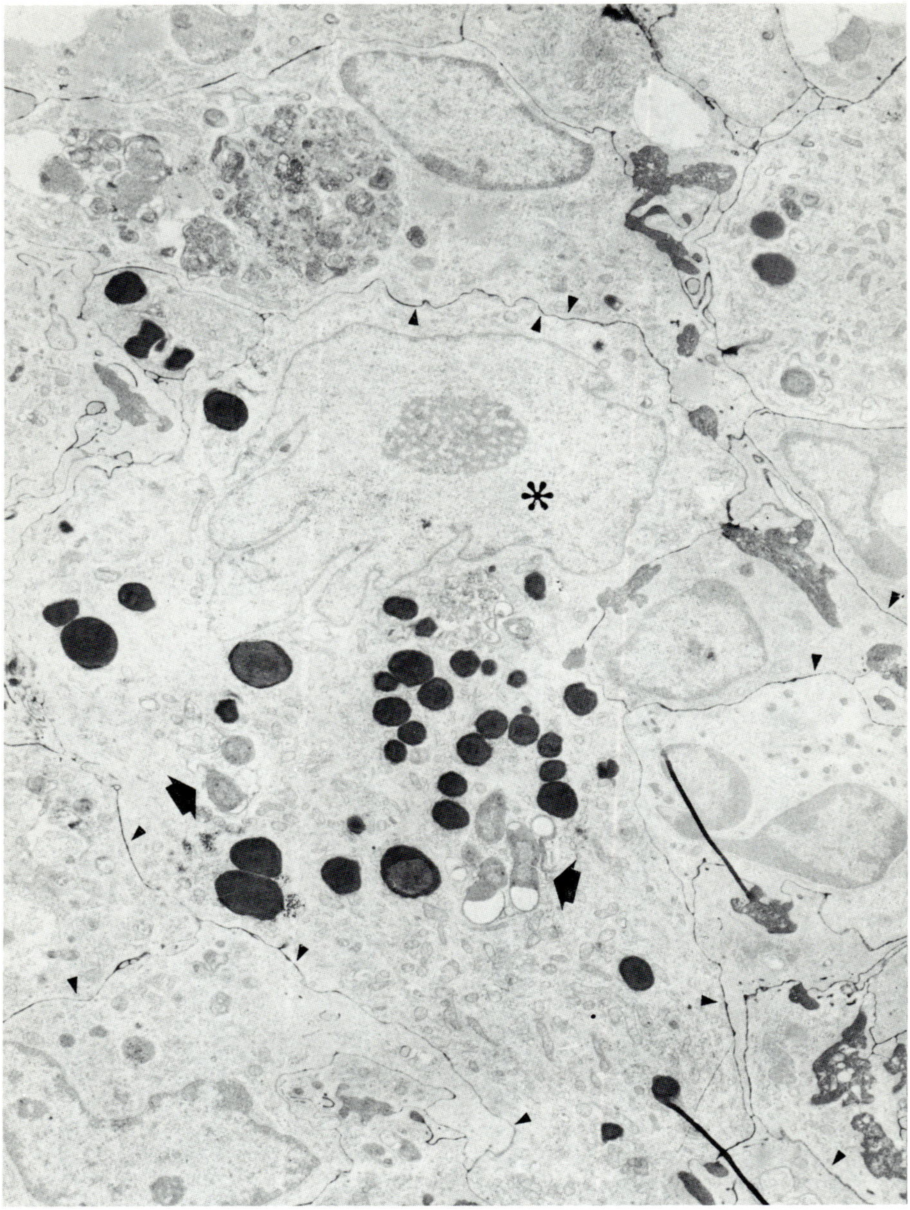

FIG. 1. Electron microphotograph of experimental bacterial orchitis in the guinea pig. The Sertoli cell marked with an asterisk is surrounded by numerous inflammatory cells. In the cytoplasm of the Sertoli cell, there are phagosomes and bacteria (arrow) and numerous residual bodies. The breakdown of the blood–testis barrier allows the entry of the electron-dense marker lanthanum in between the cells (small arrowheads). ×1,800.

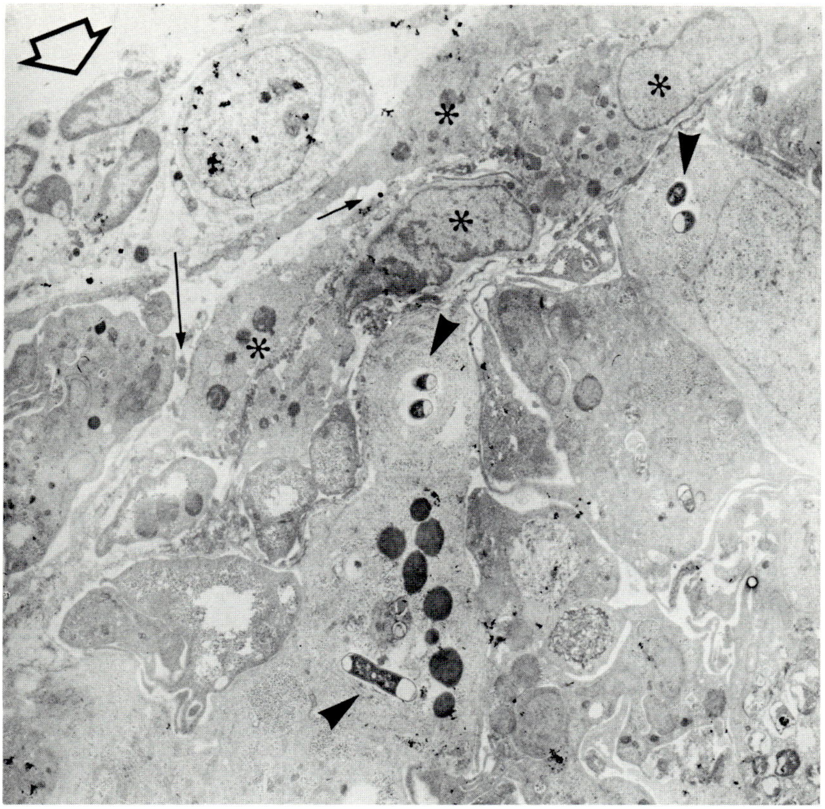

FIG. 2. Electron microphotograph of experimental bacterial orchitis in the guinea pig. The photograph illustrates the breakdown of the tubular wall in the early stages of the inflammation. The myoid cell (asterisk) is swollen. The thin arrows indicate the slits formed owing to disruption of the tubular basement membrane. The short arrow indicates the inflammatory cells in the interstitial spaces. The cytoplasm of the Sertoli cells contains bacteria (arrowheads). ×1,800.

experimental bacterial orchitis are discharged through the seminiferous tubules into the rete testis and thence reach the epididymis and ductus deferens. The seminiferous tubules will thus, after some time, appear "empty," and the "late interstitial phase" of the inflammation will be evidenced only by the thickening of the tunica propria and the interstitium between the seminiferous tubules (Fig. 3). The myoid cells of the tunica propria transform into fibroblasts and produce large amounts of peritubular collagen. The peritubular fibrosis obviously impairs the passage of nutrients into the lumen of the seminiferous tubules and hinders the regeneration of the germinal epithelium. It also promotes the degeneration of remaining Sertoli cells. Finally, most of the testis will be replaced with fibrous tissue, and only scarce foci of spermatogenesis will be preserved.

During experimental bacterial orchitis, the Leydig cells show increased eosinophilia and granularity of their cytoplasm. Ultrastructurally the smooth endoplasmic reticulum appears vesiculated and dilated, and the mitochondria show

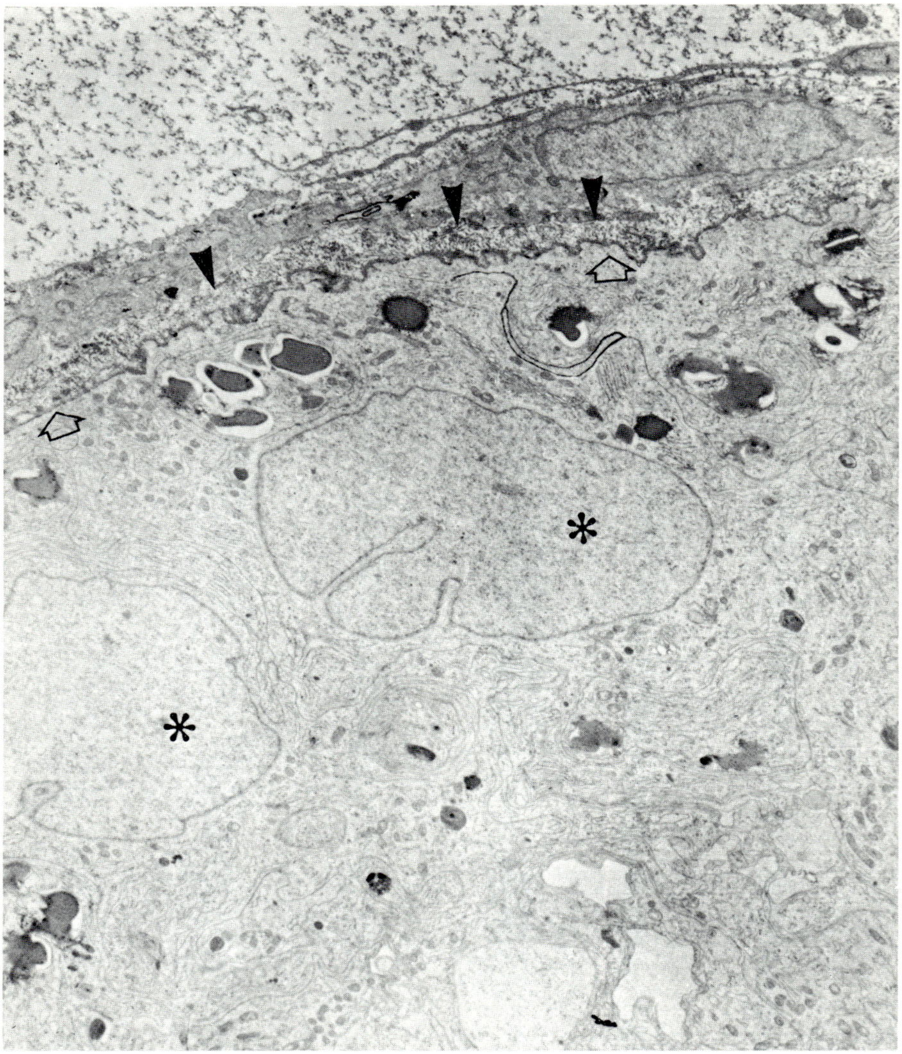

FIG. 3. Experimental infectious orchitis in the guinea pig. In the later stages of the inflammation, the tubules contain only Sertoli cells (asterisks). Note residual bodies in the cytoplasm of the Sertoli cells. The basement membrane of the tubule (empty arrows) is thickened. Arrowheads point to the increased amount of collagen surrounding the basement lamina. ×2,200.

degenerative changes. Some authors have suggested that the Leydig cells may act as facultative phagocytes, but the ultrastructural studies of Mikuz[5] do not lend support to this claim.

Experimental bacterial orchitis is mostly invariably accompanied by broad zones of parenchymal necrosis and thrombosis of small and large testicular vessels. It has been suggested that the widespread necrosis of testicular parenchyma, in analogy with the changes seen in papillary necrosis of the kidney, is due to the combined effects of inflammation and ischemic necrosis.

MORPHOLOGY OF SUPPURATIVE EPIDIDYMO-ORCHITIS

The acute inflammation leads to enlargement and swelling of the testis and epididymis.[17] The tunica albuginea is tense and may be covered with fibrin. The parenchyma of the testis is yellowish-brown and does not string with ease. Aggregates of pus and well-formed abscesses may be seen within short periods of time after the onset of infection (Figs. 4 and 5). Persistent suppurative inflammation will

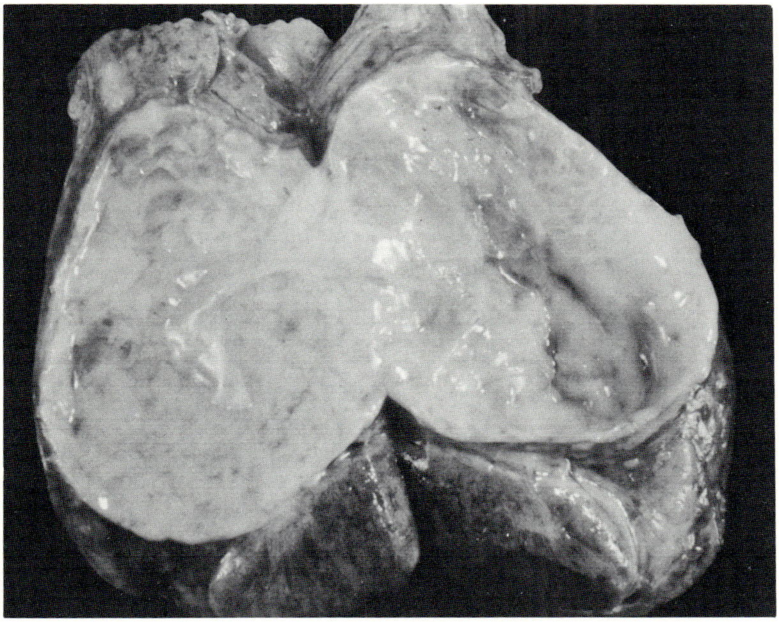

FIG. 4. Acute suppurative epididymitis. Extremely dilated epididymis filled with pus.

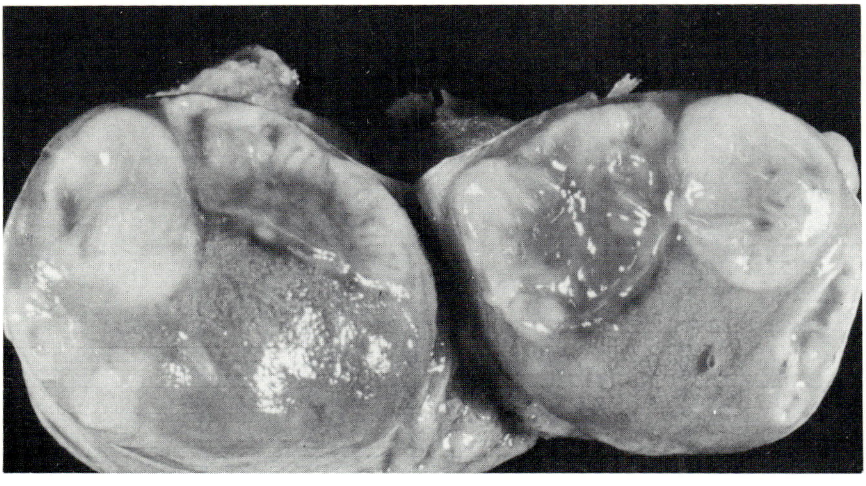

FIG. 5. Multiple abscesses in the testes.

cause destruction of the testicular parenchyma, which will be followed by the formation of granulation tissue and fibrosis. In long-standing infectious suppurative orchitis, the tunica albuginea is thickened and adherent to the tunica vaginalis. The subcapsular parenchyma is usually replaced by fibrous scarring, whereas the central areas contain pus and parenchymal debris. Chronic testicular abscesses may drain through fistula tracts to the surface of the scrotal skin, or may involve the contralateral side of the scrotum and the other testis.

The acutely inflamed epididymis is swollen, red, and usually covered with fibrin. The wall of the epididymis is thickened and the lumen may contain pus (Fig. 6). Inflammation will often lead to the formation of fistula tracts between the epididymis and the peritesticular space, or cause an overt rupture of the ductus epididymis. Extravasation of pus from the lumen of the epididymis is usually accompanied by the extravasation of sperm. Long-standing inflammation will thus show signs of suppuration as well as granulation tissue and sperm granuloma formation. Obliteration of the lumen of the epididymis and squamous metaplasia (Fig. 7) of the epididymal epithelium are often found in the reparative phase that follows suppurative epididymitis.[17]

TUBERCULOSIS

Tuberculosis of the testis and epididymis is almost invariably secondary to infection in some other part of the body, most often in the genitourinary tract.[21] *Mycobacterium tuberculosis* reaches the epididymis by intracanalicular or lym-

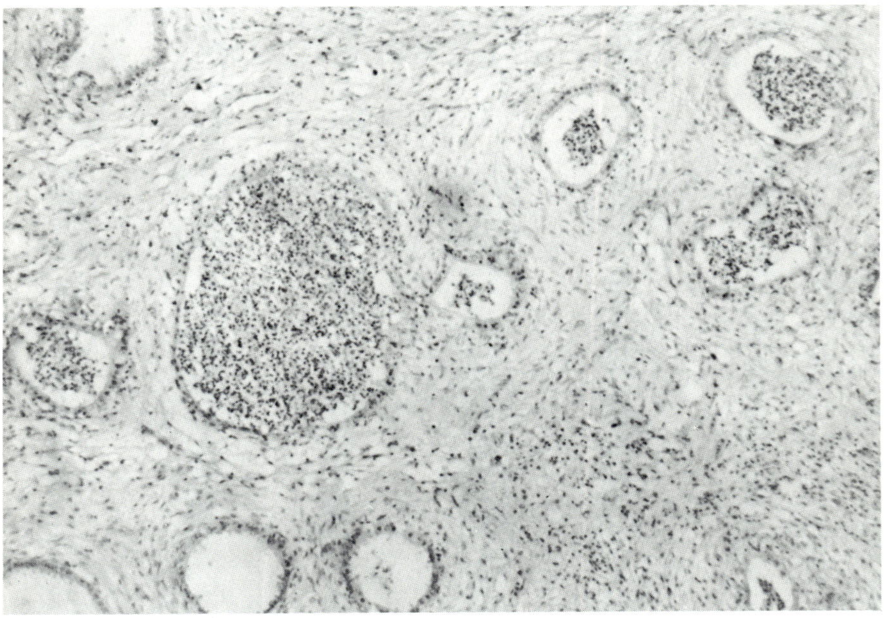

FIG. 6. Acute suppurative epididymitis. Note the large aggregates of pus within the lumen and in the swollen interstitial spaces. ×63.

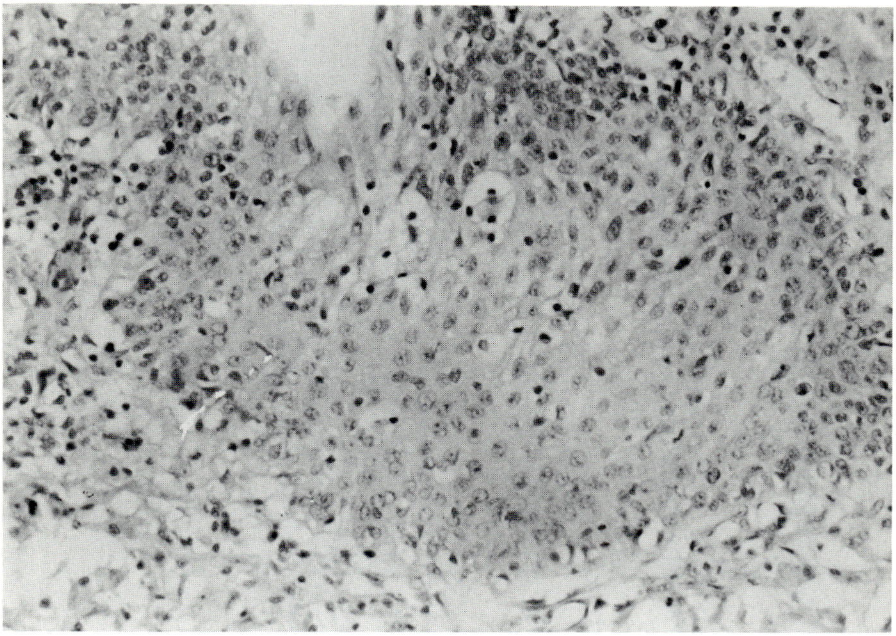

FIG. 7. Squamous metaplasia of chronic epididymitis. ×160.

phogenous routes from the prostate and seminal vesicles; blood-borne infection during miliary tuberculosis is rare. Tuberculous epididymitis occurs most often in mid-life and is very rare in children.[29] It is believed that the disease in children is due to hematogenous dissemination from distant foci rather than from the lower genitourinary tract, which usually shows no evidence of tuberculosis.

Tuberculosis begins as an epididymitis and the infection spreads secondarily to the testis.[17] The epididymis is the seat of the most prominent pathologic alterations, and is typically dilated, thickened, and "sausage-like." Testicular involvement is seen only in advanced, long-standing infections (Fig. 8). Microscopic and macroscopic caseating granulomas are seen in the wall of the epididymis, in the septula testis, and along the ductus deferens. In later stages of the disease, there is copious caseation, since the process tends to produce more exudation than fibrosis.[5]

LEPROSY

Orchitis is a common feature of lepromatous leprosy. Grabstald and Swan[23] studied 66 cases and found evidence of testicular involvement in all 38 patients suffering from lepromatous leprosy, but in none of the patients with tuberculoid or borderline leprosy. Later Karat et al.[30] showed that orchitis may be found in borderline leprosy. The orchitis is usually bilateral, although the degree of involvement may vary from one side to the other. Occasionally testicular leprosy may be the presenting sign of the disease and the biopsy may establish the diagnosis.[3] It has been suggested that the scrotal temperature, which as noted earlier is lower than the

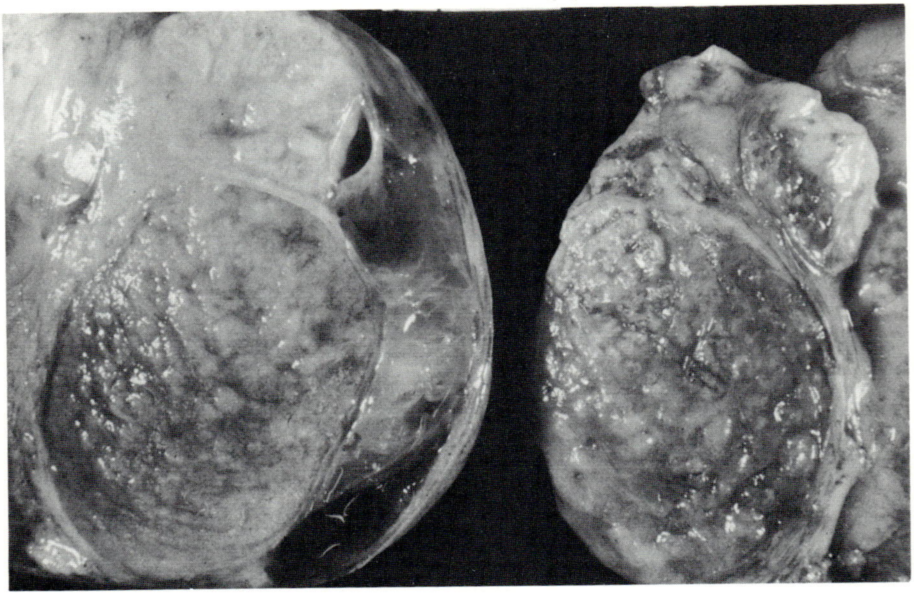

FIG. 8. Bilateral tuberculous epididymo-orchitis.

temperature of the rest of the body, may provide ideal conditions for the growth of the leprosy bacillus, but the real reasons for the frequent testicular involvement in leprosy are not known.

Grabstald and Swan[23] have recognized three phases of lepromatous orchitis: (1) vascular; (2) interstitial; and (3) obliterative. In the first phase, the disease is characterized by the perivascular infiltration of lymphocytes and vacuolated histiocytes. The histiocytes, known as Virchow's or lepra cells, contain acid-fast leprosy bacilli. In the second phase, there is marked obliterative endarteritis accompanied by interstitial fibrosis and atrophy of the seminiferous tubules. Diffuse fibrosis characterizes the third phase of the disease. Leprosy bacilli are most conspicuous in the second phase, and are hard to find or completely absent from the tissue in the obliterative stage of orchitis.

VIRAL INFECTIONS

Orchitis may develop in many systemic viral infections. Mumps virus is probably the viral pathogen most affecting the testis,[31-34] but subclinical orchitis may frequently pass unrecorded in other viral infections.[14] Testalgia, as a presumptive sign of orchitis, was thus recorded in 5 of 68 adults during an epidemic of rubella, but it remains to be determined whether this clinical symptom indeed reflects testicular inflammation or is just a nonspecific manifestation of viremia[11] (Fig. 9).

In addition to mumps, the following viruses have been isolated or serologically demonstrated in patients with clinically documented orchitis: Coxsackie virus types

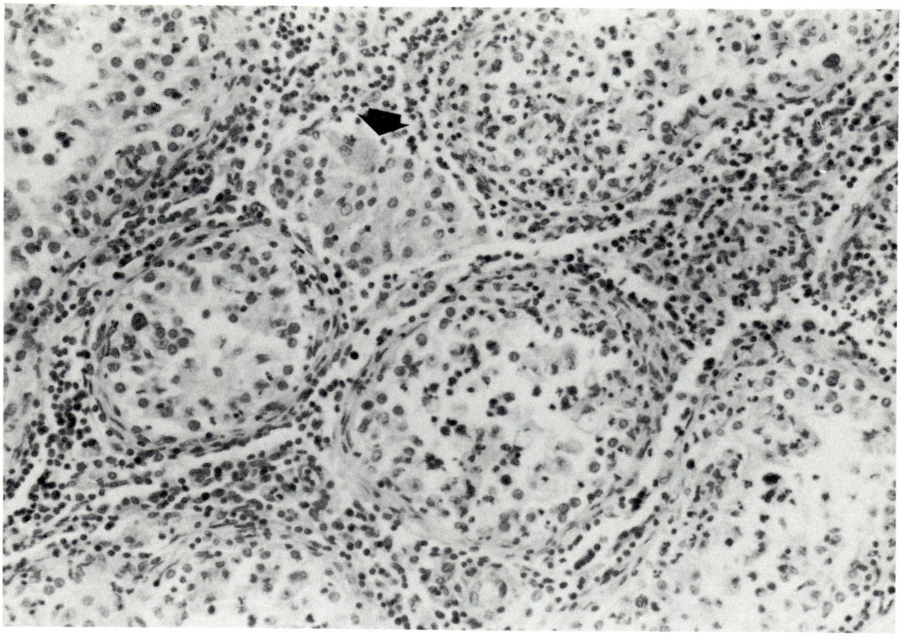

FIG. 9. Nonspecific orchitis considered to be of viral etiology. Note the interstitial and intratubular inflammatory cells accompanied by loss of germinal epithelium and preservation of the Leydig cells (arrow). ×160.

1 to 5, infectious mononucleosis virus, lymphocytic choriomeningitis, phlebotomus fever, adenovirus, bat salivary gland virus (a B-group arbovirus), influenza, dengue, smallpox, varicella and vaccinia viruses, echovirus (types 6, and possibly 9 and 11) and rubella.[35-44] Orchitis was also recorded in a case of mucocutaneous lymph node syndrome of Kawasaki.[45]

Testicular involvement is usually part of the systemic viral infections noted above, and there is little evidence that any known human viral pathogen has a selective or exclusive organotropism for the testis. The only exception to this statement could be the mumps virus, which seems to involve selectively the salivary glands, pancreas, testis, and brain.[46]

Testicular and epididymal involvement is common in adult mumps infection but uncommon in prepubertal patients. Orchitis was recorded in 20 percent of adults and only 1 percent of children suffering from mumps. Orchitis is bilateral in 16 percent and is accompanied by epididymitis in 85 percent of all patients showing signs of testicular involvement.[31-34] Epididymitis without testicular disease is rare.[47]

The classical morphologic studies of human mumps orchitis were done in the 1940s by Gall[48] and Charny and Meranze.[49] These authors have shown the focal nature of the inflammation and have described the sequential phases of the disease. During the initial stages of inflammation, interstitial edema is the most obvious finding. In this phase the blood vessels are congested and usually surrounded by cuffs of lymphocytes. Congestion and increased permeability of the blood vessels

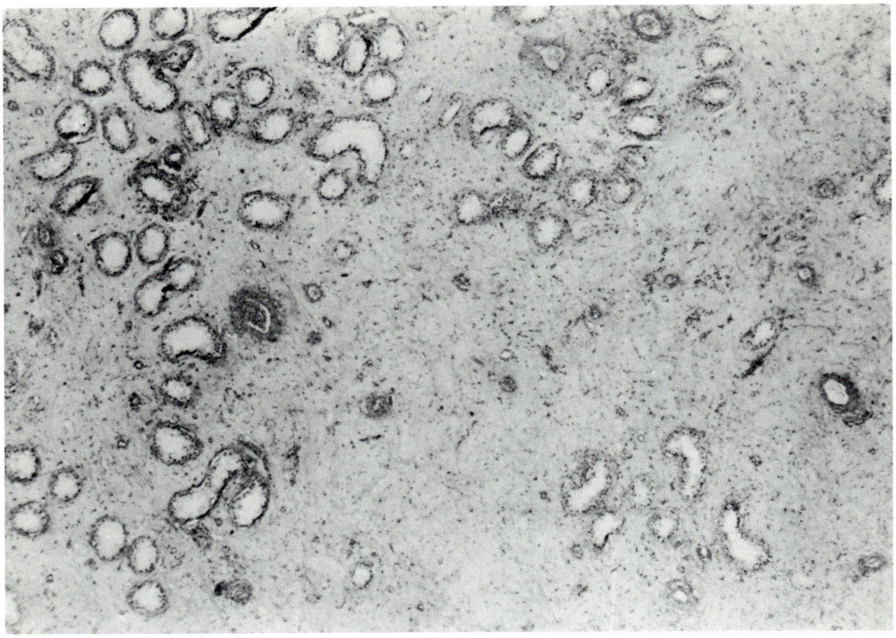

FIG. 10. Interstitial fibrosis and tubular atrophy following extensive mumps orchitis. ×25.

lead to focal interstitial hemorrhage and the exudation of fibrin and leukocytes. The germinal epithelium degenerates but the Sertoli and Leydig cells show little evidence of attrition. Repair is heralded by the interstitial deposition of collagen, concentric peritubular fibrosis, and tubular atrophy. Focal testicular fibrosis is the usual residue of mumps orchitis (Fig. 10).

Infertility due to the loss of germinal epithelium is a well-documented consequence of adult mumps infection.[49] The estimates on the prevalence of this complication vary. Werner[32] claims that half of all patients with mumps orchitis have signs of testicular damage, but the study of Petersdorf and Bennett[50] found testicular atrophy and azoospermia in only 22 percent of convalescents. Bartak et al.[51] followed up 124 patients and found severe oligospermia and azoospermia in early convalescence, but normospermia reappeared in two-thirds of patients with unilateral mumps orchitis and in a third of those with bilateral involvement. Aiman et al.[52] have found that mumps virus damages the Leydig cells, leading to the impaired secretion of androgens, but not affecting the secretion of estrogens. This probably accounts for the development of gynecomastia and contributes to the clinically apparent testicular atrophy recorded in some of the previous studies.

CHLAMYDIAL INFECTION

Two recent studies have indicated that *Chlamydia trachomatis* may be one of the most common causes of nonbacterial epididymitis, especially in young adults.[13,53]

The infection is transmitted sexually and the epididymal inflammation is often, but not always, accompanied by urethritis and prostatitis.

SYPHILIS

Syphilitic orchitis occurs in two forms: interstitial and gummatous.[5,17] With the advent of chemotherapy, gummas of the testis have become a medical rarity. Interstitial orchitis is a feature of both congenital and acquired syphilis and is the usual form of syphilitic inflammation seen today. The inflammation is characterized by perivascular and interstitial round-cell infiltration of the testis, followed by obliterative endarteritis and peritubular fibrosis (Fig. 11). These changes lead to tubular atrophy and aspermatogenesis. Diffuse fibrosis is the hallmark of the later stages of the disease. The epididymis is not affected.

FUNGAL INFECTIONS

Fungal infections of the testis and epididymis are extremely rare.[17] Thus, only a single case of testicular histoplasmosis is on record, despite the high prevalence of histoplasmosis in many parts of the world.[54] *Actinomyces* has been isolated from internal female genital organs[55] and is a known cause of scrotal skin infection,[56] but the testis and the epididymis appear to be spared. Only nine cases of testicular actinomycosis have been reported so far.[17]

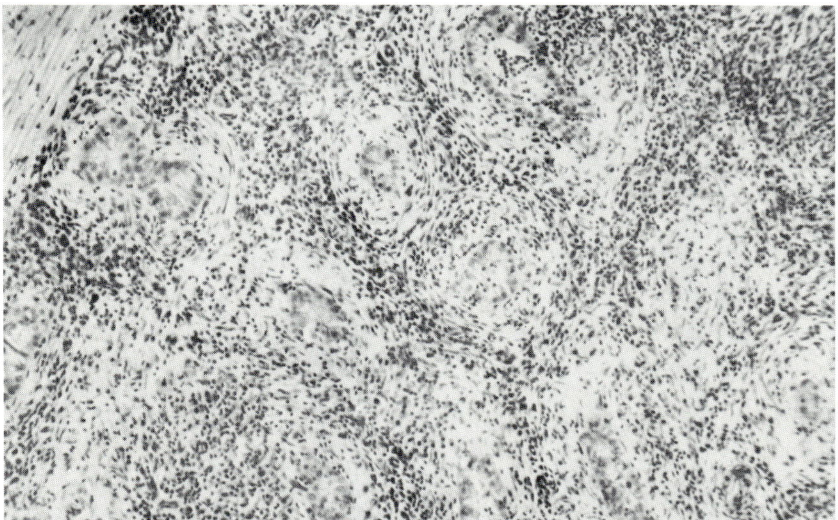

FIG. 11. Interstitial syphilitic orchitis. Note the dense round-cell infiltration of the interstitial spaces and peritubular fibrosis. ×100.

PARASITIC INFECTIONS

There are no exact accounts on the prevalence of parasitic epididymo-orchitis. *Wuchereria bancrofti* and *Schistosoma haematobium* are the most common pathogens in endemic areas.[17]

ALLERGIC ORCHITIS

The immunization of animals with homologous testicular extracts leads to the development of allergic autoimmune orchitis. According to Tung and Alexander,[57] the main histologic features of experimental autoimmune orchitis are: (1) aspermatogenesis; (2) mononuclear cell infiltration of the interstitial spaces, seminiferous tubules, and vessels; and (3) polymorphonuclear leukocytic infiltration of the efferent ducts, epididymis, and vas deferens. Orchitis develops due to a combined B-and T-cell immune response, but the exact role of the two components of the immune system is not fully understood. Orchitis may be transmitted from sensitized to pristine animals by adoptive lymphocyte transfer.[58] Vasectomy[59] and neonatal thymectomy[60] will induce allergic orchitis in some rat strains, but not in others, suggesting that a genetic predisposition regulates the onset of the disease. Some animals, most notably rabbits, appear to be extremely sensitive, and develop postvasectomy autoimmune orchitis more often than other species.[61] Vasectomized men often have a high titer of antisperm antibodies, but these antibodies seem to produce few morphologic changes.[10]

Autoimmune, allergic orchitis has been known to exist in humans, but the disease has not been fully characterized.[5] Interstitial orchitis has been described in conjunction with aspermatogenesis and sperm granulomas of the epididymis.[62-63] Taylor et al.[64] have studied patients with azoospermia and oligospermia, and have described three forms of immune injury, displaying the following changes: (1) linear deposits of IgG, IgM, C_3 and C_{1q} along the basement membrane of the seminiferous tubules; (2) granular deposits of IgG and C_3 in the walls of small testicular vessels; and (3) mononuclear infiltrates in the interstitial spaces (Fig. 12). The pathogenesis of human autoimmune orchitis remains obscure but, as in animals, the disease most probably has a multifactorial nature. On the other hand, deposits of immunoglobulins and complement may be found in chronic orchitis of unknown origin (Figs. 13 and 14), and this finding does not necessarily imply an autoimmune etiology of orchitis.

VASCULITIS

Vasculitis involving the testicular and epididymal blood vessels has been described in periarteritis nodosa, rheumatic arteritis, and Henoch-Schönlein purpura.[17,65] Clinically, common symptoms include testicular and epididymal swelling or pain. Vasculitis should be included in the differential diagnosis of acute scrotal diseases such as epididymo-orchitis, torsion and trauma of the testis, and rare forms of

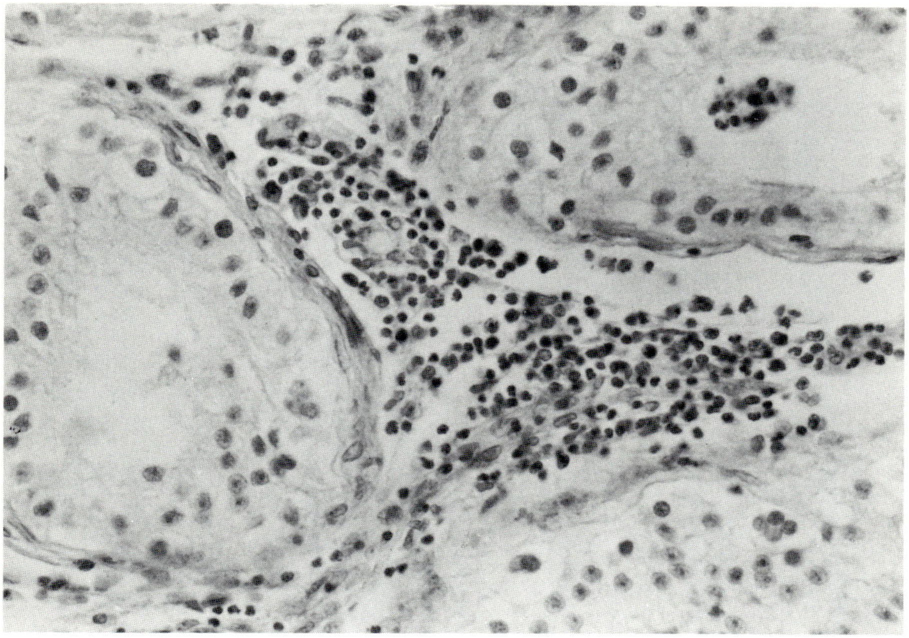

FIG. 12. Interstitial orchitis in an infertile patient. Note the interstitial lymphoplasmacytic cellular infiltration and the absence of intratubular spermatogenesis. ×250.

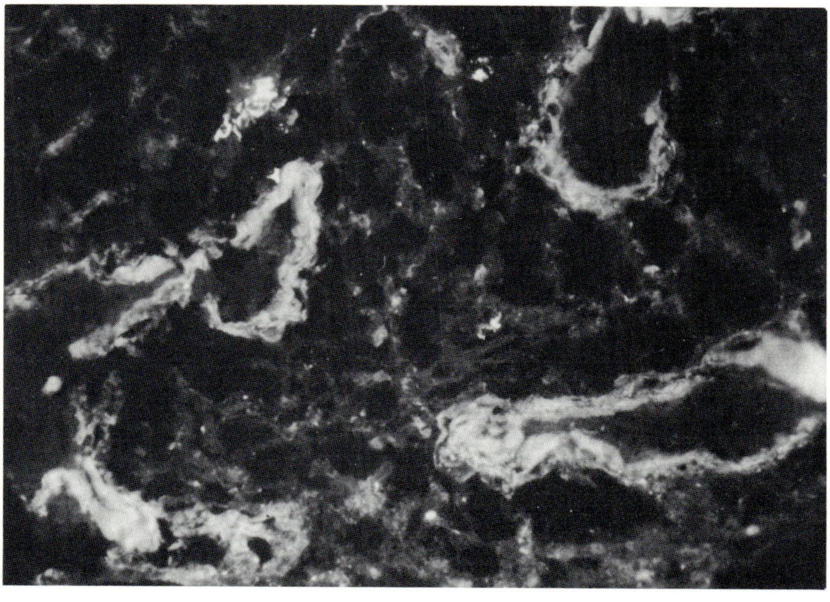

FIG. 13. Deposits of C_3 along the thickened basement membrane of the seminiferous tubules in a patient with unilateral orchitis. Immunofluorescence microscopy. ×100.

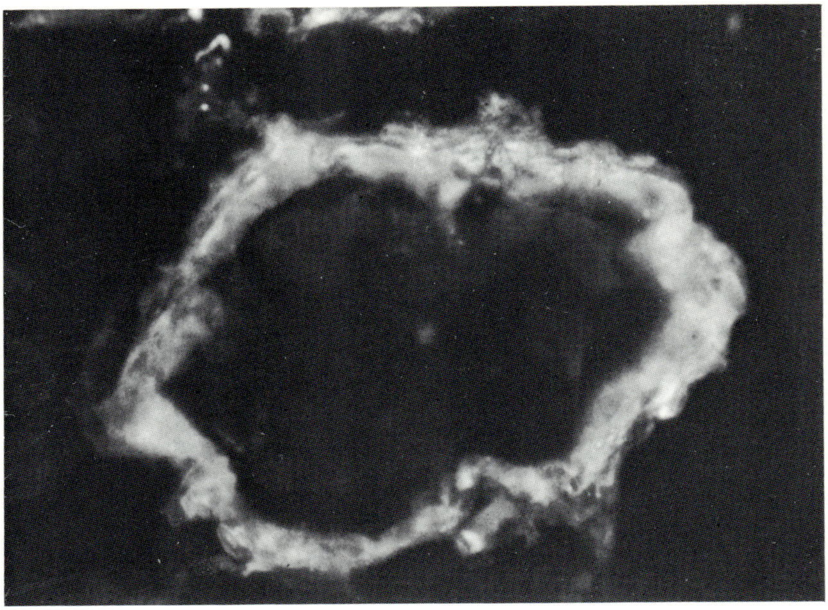

FIG. 14. Deposits of IgG along the basement membrane of the seminiferous tubules demonstrated by immunofluorescence microscopy. ×320.

testicular infarction and hemorrhage.[66,67] Morphologically, testicular vasculitis does not differ from vasculitides in other organs (Fig. 15). Ischemic necrosis occurs rarely because of the anastomosing collaterals between the terminal intratesticular arteries. Interstitial hemorrhage occurs in Henoch-Schönlein purpura (Figs. 16, 17).

GRANULOMATOUS ORCHITIS

The terms granulomatous orchitis and malakoplakia[68-75] have been used interchangeably to denote a form of testicular inflammation characterized by diffuse mononuclear infiltration of the entire organ, first described in 1926 by Grunberg.[68] The testis is enlarged and indurated; the tunica albuginea is thickened. The cut surface is grayish-white and homogenous or nodular owing to the accentuated prominence of the septula testis (Fig. 18). The lesion is usually unilateral and, because of its gross resemblance to seminoma, has often been clinically mistaken for a testicular tumor. In a review of 1,200 testicular masses resected with the presumptive diagnosis of neoplasia, 17 cases (5.1 percent) turned out to be granulomatous orchitis.[17] Similar experience was reported from the Armed Forces Institute of Pathology in Washington, D.C.[76]

Histologically, the testis in granulomatous orchitis is infiltrated with macrophages, plasma cells, lymphocytes, and scattered polymorphonuclear and eosinophilic leukocytes. The infiltrates surround and permeate the seminiferous tubules, which are usually devoid of germinal epithelium and sperm (Figs. 19 and

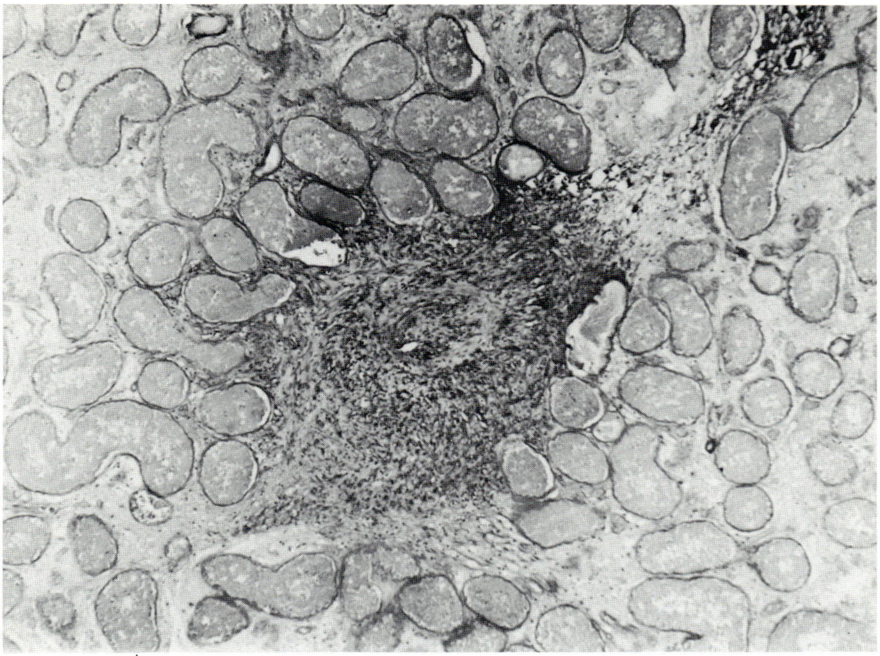

FIG. 15. Polyarteritis nodosa with focal necrotizing orchitis undergoing fibrosis. ×40.

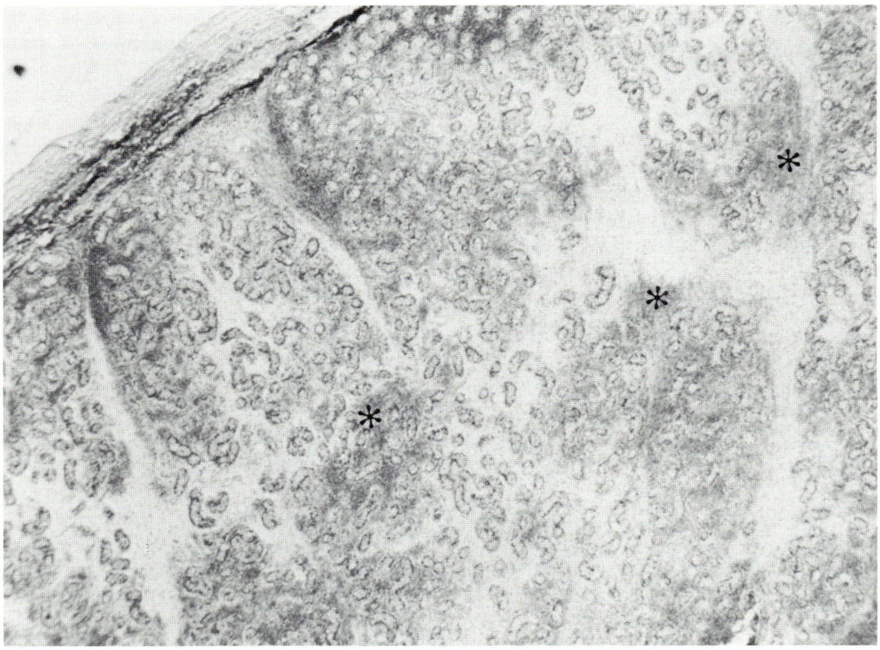

FIG. 16. Focal parenchymal hemorrhages due to vasculitis of Schönlein-Henoch purpura. The hemorrhagic areas are indicated by the asterisks. ×250. (From Mikuz et al.: Pathol Res Pract 165:323, 1979. Courtesy of Gustav Fischer Verlag.)

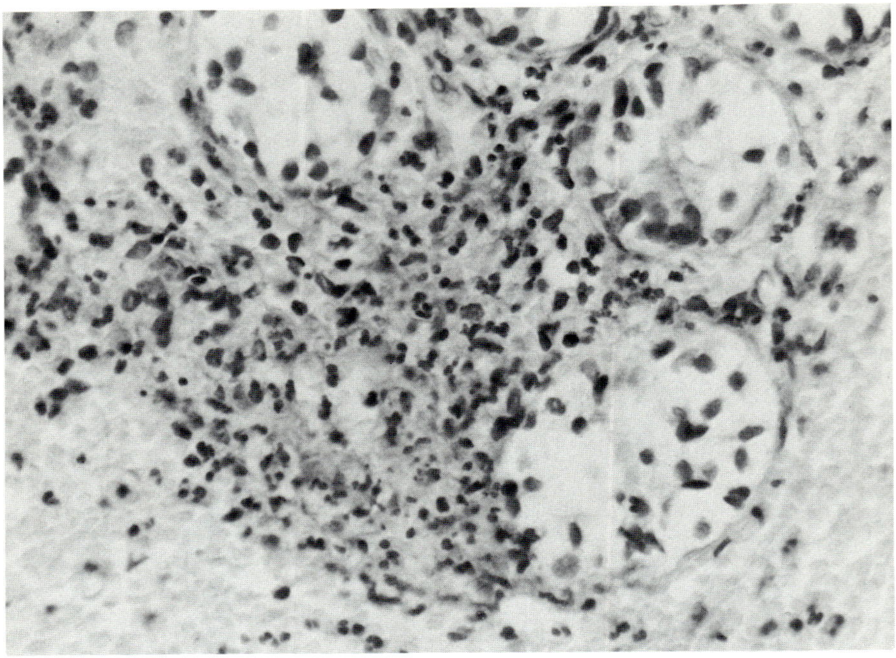

FIG. 17. Leukoclastic vasculitis of Schönlein-Henoch purpura. ×400. (From Mikuz et al.: Pathol Res Pract 165:323, 1979. Courtesy of Gustav Fischer Verlag.)

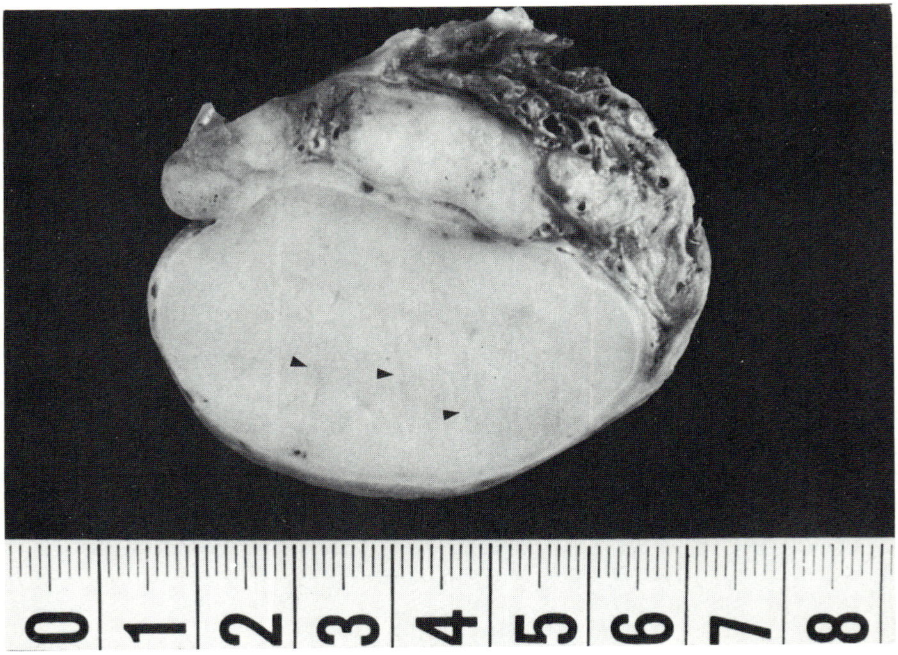

FIG. 18. Gross appearance of granulomatous orchitis in contrast to testicular tumors in this condition, the septa of the testis (arrowheads) are still preserved.

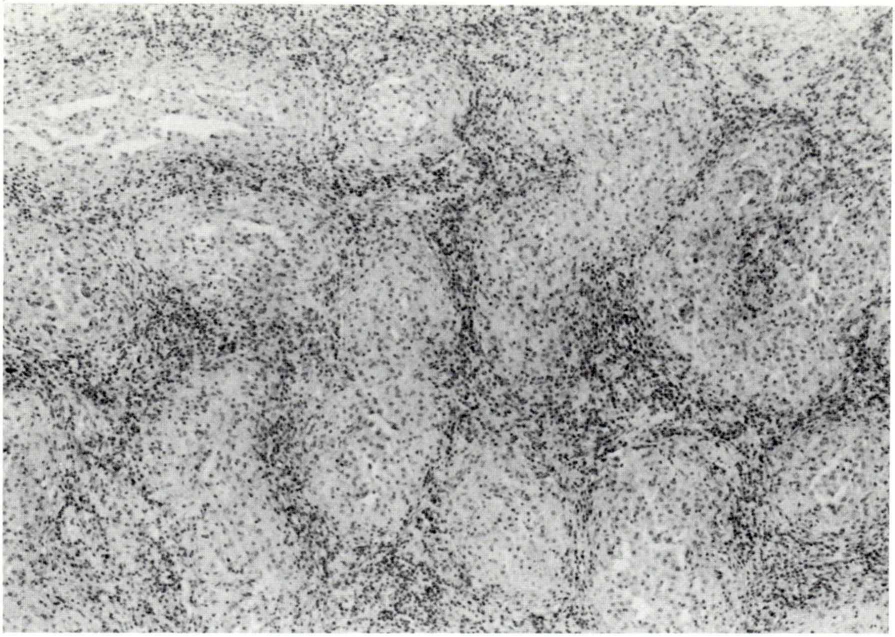

FIG. 19. Granulomatous orchitis. The outines of the tubules are still preserved. The tubules contain numerous mononuclear macrophages. In the interstitial spaces there are plasma cells and lymphocytes. ×40.

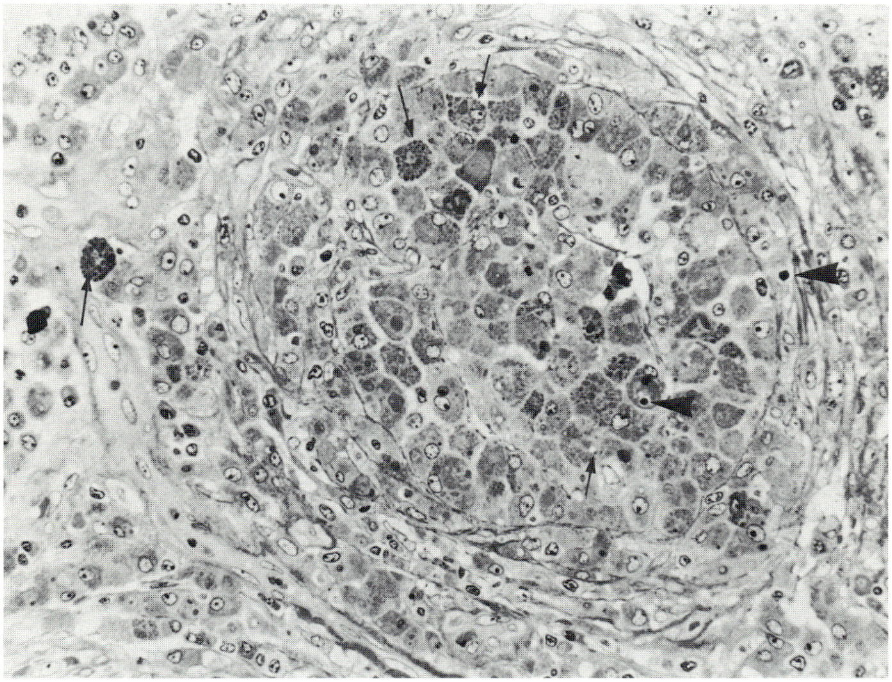

FIG. 20. Granulomatous orchitis. Note numerous macrophages distributed within and outside the tubules (arrows). Many macrophages contain intracytoplasmic bodies (arrowheads). ×250. (From Mikuz: Virchows Arch Abt A 360:223, 1973. Courtesy of Springer-Verlag.)

20). The macrophages have abundant cytoplasm which often contains "bulls-eye"-shaped calcospherites, the so-called Michaelis-Gutmann bodies (Fig. 21). Mononuclear cells within the tubules were initially thought to represent phagocytic Sertoli cells, but recent electron microscopic studies have proven beyond any doubt that these cells are also macrophages[70,74] (Fig. 22). Some of these macrophages contain engulfed bacteria (Fig. 23), and the prevailing evidence indicates that granulomatous orchitis is in most instances caused by bacterial pathogens, or is in some way related to a bacterial infection. The exact pathogenesis of granulomatous orchitis is not clear, although it seems that the disease develops more often in immunodeficient individuals than in the general population. Current hypotheses suggest that malakoplakia may be causally related to the malfunction of macrophages.[77] Experimentally, Csapo et al.[78] have induced testicular malakoplakia with extracts of denatured *E. coli* injected directly into the testis.

Bunzli[69] has described three morphologic forms of granulomatous orchitis: the classic form, the fibrosing form, and the megalocytic form. The megalocytic form ("large cell inflammation") corresponds to typical malakoplakia and is hallmarked by the predominance of large eosinophilic histiocytes. In the classic and fibrosing type of granulomatous orchitis, there were fewer macrophages, but more plasma cells and lymphocytes, and the interstitial fibrosis was more pronounced than in the megalocytic form of inflammation. It is not clear whether the various forms of orchitis represent phases in the evolution of the same disease process or whether one is dealing with pathogenetically distinct lesions.

Malakoplakia may involve the epididymis together with the testis. Isolated epididymal malakoplakia has also been recorded.[79]

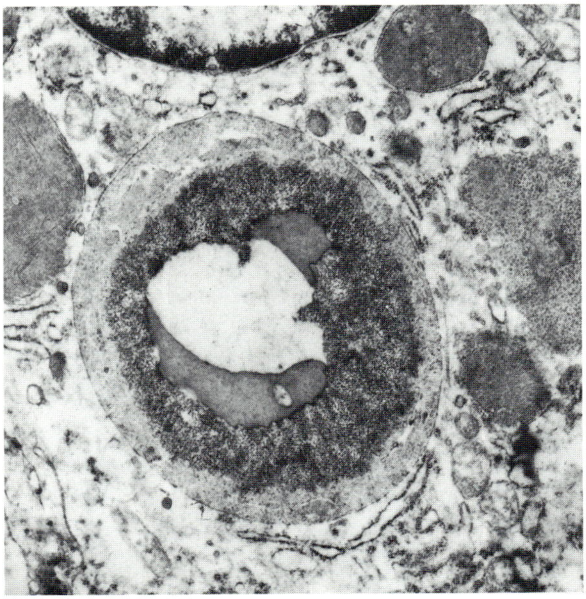

FIG. 21. Intracytoplasmic calcospherites corresponding to Michaelis-Gutmann bodies. ×23,000.

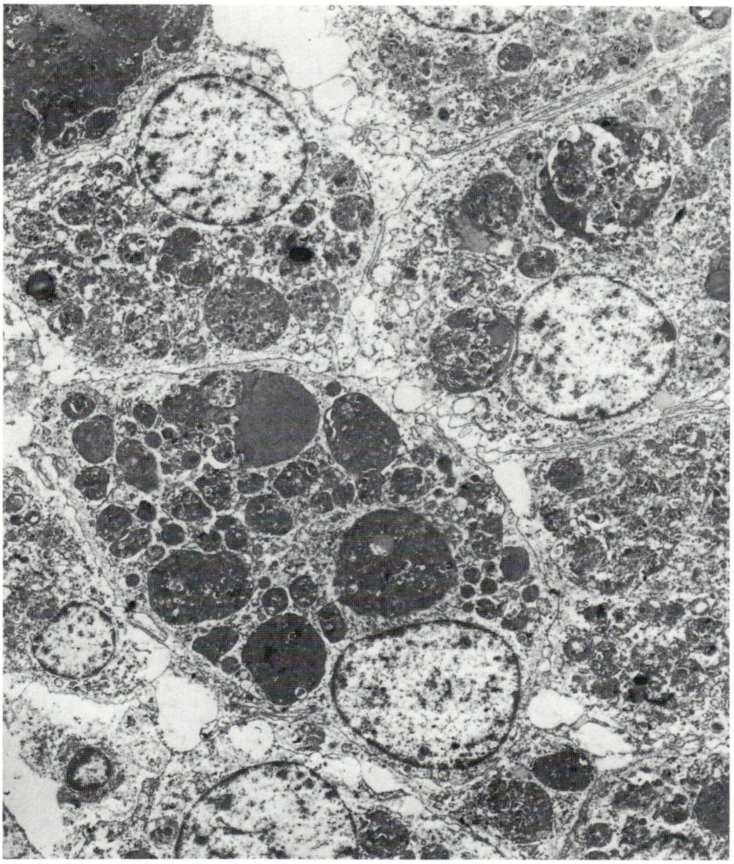

FIG. 22. Granulomatous orchitis. Ultrastructure of inflammatory cells indicates that these cells are macrophages and that their cytoplasm is filled with numerous phagolysosomes. ×1,800. (From Mikuz: Virchows Arch Abt A 360:223, 1973. Courtesy of Springer-Verlag.)

SARCOIDOSIS

Genital involvement occurs in approximately 5 percent of all patients with systemic sarcoidosis.[80] Sarcoid granulomas are usually multifocal, but the epididymis appears to be the most common seat of intrascrotal disease.[81] Only three cases of isolated testicular sarcoidosis are on record.[82] Biopsy of the lesion is indicated in order to exclude other infectious granulomas and tumors.

SPERM GRANULOMA

Sperm granulomas develop in response to the presence of sperm in the interstitial spaces of the epididymis and funiculus spermaticus, and only exceptionally in the testis itself.[63,83-85] Initally, the extravasation of sperm elicits a pleomorphic

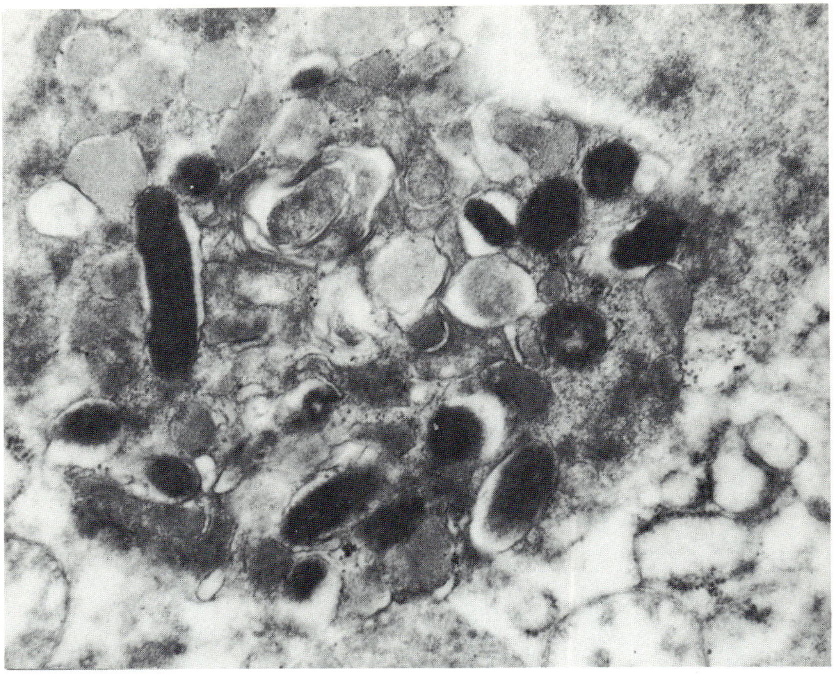

FIG. 23. Granulomatous orchitis. Phagolysosomes from inflammatory cells contain partially degraded bacteria. × 19,000. (From Mikuz: Virchows Arch Abt A 360:223, 1973. Courtesy of Springer-Verlag.)

phagocytic reaction followed by the formation of granulomas composed of macrophages and giant cells[17] (Fig. 24). With the progression of time, the granulomas become less cellular and more fibrotic. In late stages of the disease, the granulomas are replaced by fibrous scars which may or may not contain clumps of spermatozoa.

Kupfer and Buschmann[83] have examined 250 autopsies and found sperm granulomas in 2.6 percent. Extravasated sperm, without evidence of granuloma formation, were found in an additional 10 percent of cases. This indicates that extravasation of sperm is not the sole factor responsible for the formation of granulomas. Sperm granulomas occur more often in patients with a past history of trauma, vasectomy, chronic epididymitis, or granulomatous orchitis than in the population at large. It is thought that sperm granulomas represent a combination of a foreign-body-type reaction and an autoimmune response to sperm antigens.[5,17]

LIPID GRANULOMAS

Lipid-containing granulomas localized in the scrotum are caused either by endogenous or exogenous lipids.[17,86] Cholesterol granuloma destroying and replacing a part of the testis was reported by Lin et al.[87]; the authors thought that the granuloma was a late consequence of intratesticular hemorrhage, but its real cause

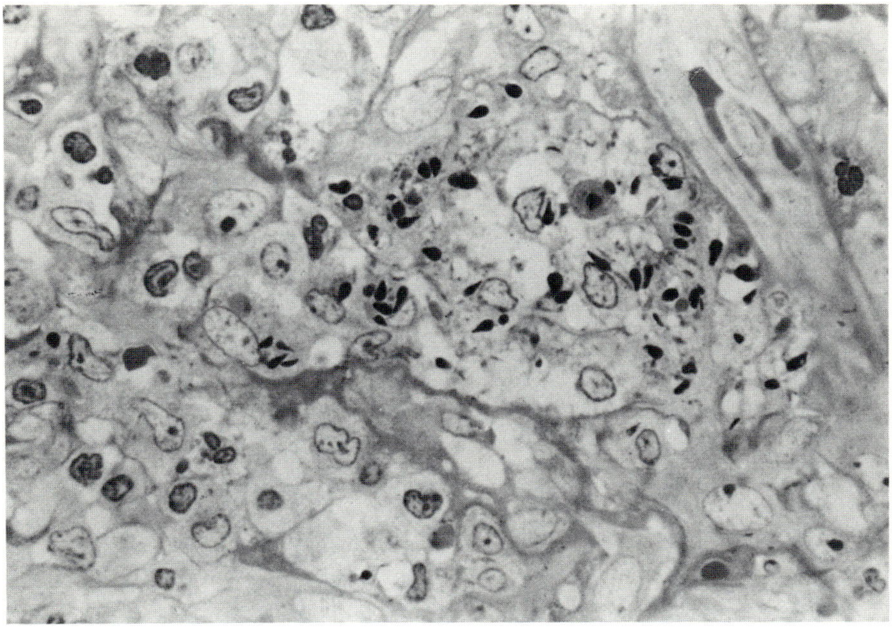

FIG. 24. Sperm granuloma. One may recognize sperm heads in between the macrophages. ×800.

could not be determined. Sclerosing lipogranulomas of the scrotum, testes, and external genitalia have been reported following the injection of mineral oils.[88] Scrotal fat necrosis, leading to the formation of distinct peritesticular nodules, has been described in prepubertal boys.[89] The lesion is most likely related to trauma and has not been reported in adults, since the adult scrotal wall does not contain fat tissue.

PERITESTICULAR GRANULOMAS, FIBROSIS, AND CALCIFICATIONS

Inflammation of the testis and epididymis may spread into the peritesticular tissues and cause periorchitis, vaginalitis, or funiculitis[5,17] (Figs. 25 and 26). Isolated vaginalitis is rare, and is mainly due to infection of a hydrocele or an incarcerated scrotal hernia.

Meconium vaginalitis is a form of sterile inflammation of the tunica vaginalis that occurs in utero as part of a chemical peritonitis caused by the meconium.[90,91] After birth, the processus vaginalis obliterates, and the meconium enclosed in the tunica becomes organized into fibrotic, partially calcified scrotal nodules.

Glove-powder granulomas of the tunica vaginalis following abdominal surgery were described by Pugh and Stringer.[92]

Nodular periorchitis, also known under the name of multifocal fibrous pseudotumor of the testicular tunica, or periorchitis proliferans, is a peculiar form of chronic inflammation of the tunica vaginalis and tunica albuginea.[93] Both tunics are thickened and covered with nodules on their surface. The nodules are composed

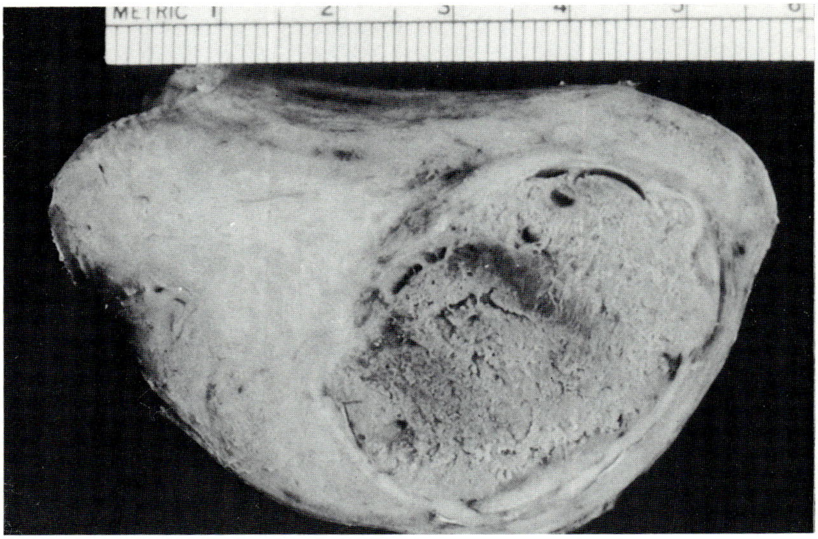

FIG. 25. Chronic periorchitis.

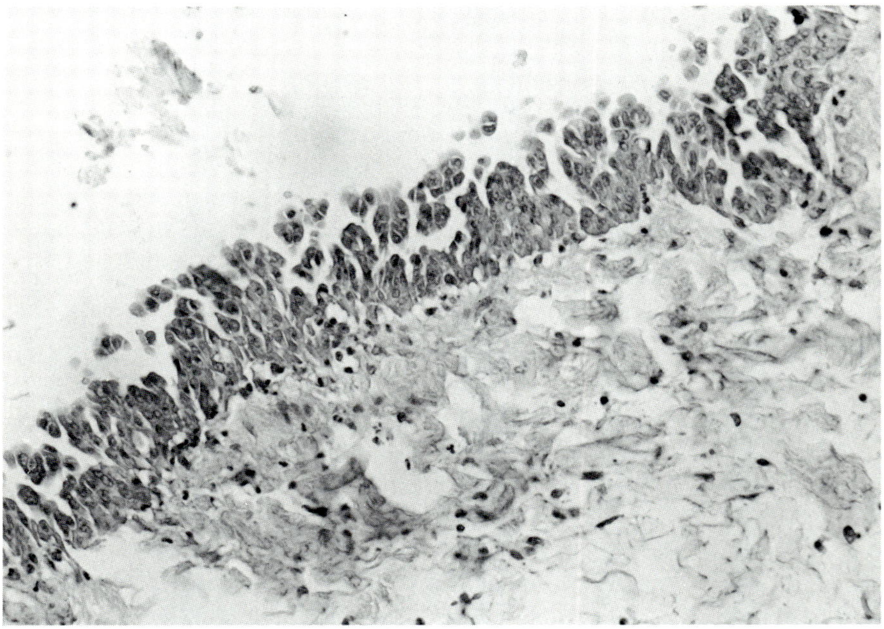

FIG. 26. Chronic inflammation of the tunica vaginalis with a marked proliferation of the mesothelial cells. ×320.

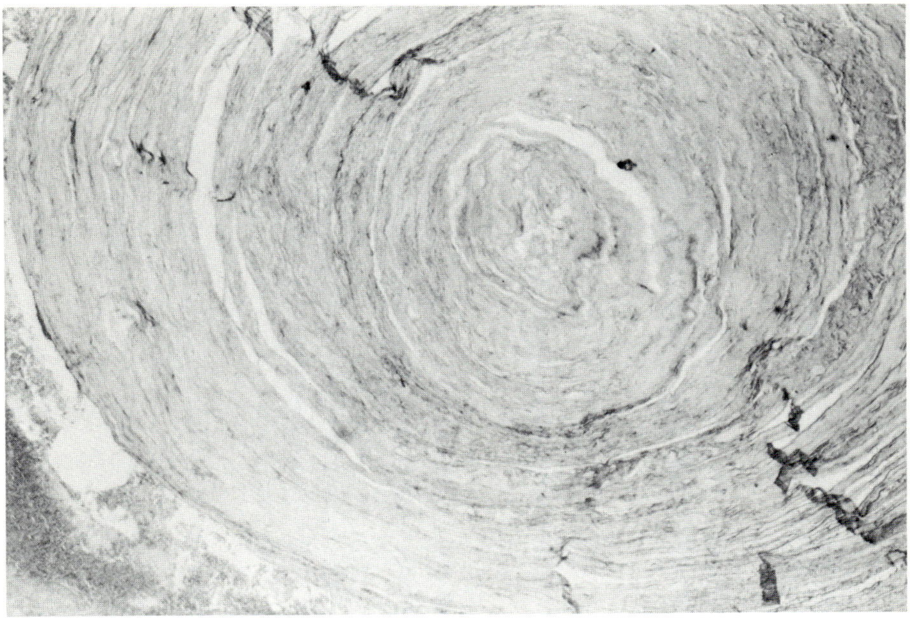

FIG. 27. Nodular periorchitis. The nodule is composed of concentrically layered fibrous tissue. ×25.

of dense, collagenous connective tissue, with focal lymphocytic and plasmacellular infiltration. In later stages, the nodules contain dystrophic calcifications. Nodules attached to the tunica with fibrous stalks may detach and give rise to free bodies floating in the periorchic space. These free bodies consist of concentric lamellae of hyalinized collagen. The etiology of nodular periorchitis is not known: 30 percent of patients have a past history of trauma or inflammation, and 45 percent have a hydrocele (Fig. 27).

Constrictive albuginitis is an obscure degenerative disease involving the tunica albuginea.[94] The testes are small and firm and the patients are usually sterile. Constrictive albuginitis seems to be distinct from the nonspecific testicular fibrosis described by Honore.[95] The latter disease presents with testicular enlargment, and was thought to represent the end-stage of chronic lymphedema due to a hypothetical congenital deficiency of lymphatics in the peritesticular tissue.

REFERENCES

1. Johnson AD, Gomes WR (eds): The Testis, Vols I–IV. New York, Academic Press, 1972–1977
2. Steinberger A, Steinberger E (eds): Testicular Development, Structure, and Function. New York, Raven Press, 1980
3. Akhtar M, Ali MA, Mackey DM: Lepromatous leprosy presenting as orchitis. Am J Clin Pathol 73:712, 1980

4. Williamson RCN: Torsion of the testis and allied condition. Br J Surg 63:465, 1976
5. Mikuz G: Orchitis. Morphologische und funktionelle Untersuchungen bei Versuchstieren und beim Menschen. In Bargmann W, Doerr W (eds): Normal and Pathological Anatomy, Vol 36. Stuttgart, Georg Thieme Verlag, 1978
6. Kiviat MD, Shurtleff D, Ansell JS: Urinary reflux via the vas deferens. Unusual cause of epididymitis in infancy. J Pediatr 80:476, 1972
7. Megalli M, Gursel E, Lattimer JK: Reflux of urine into the ejaculatory ducts as a cause of recurring epididymitis in children. J Urol 108:978, 1972
8. Neaves, W.B.: The blood testis barrier. In Johnson AD, Gomes WR (eds): The Testis, Vol IV. New York, Academic Press, 1977, p 126
9. Tung KSK: The nature of antigens and pathogenetic mechanisms in autoimmunity to sperm. In Edidin M, Johnson MH (eds): Immunobiology of Gametes. Cambridge, Cambridge University Press, 1977, p 157
10. Alexander NJ, Anderson DJ: Vasectomy: Consequences of autoimmunity to sperm antigens. Fertil Steril 32:253, 1979
11. Preblud SR, Dobbs HI, Sedmak GV, et al.: Testalgia associated with rubella infection. South Med J 73:594, 1980
12. Williams CB, Litvak AS, McRoberts JW: Epididymitis in infancy. J Urol 121:125, 1979
13. Harnisch JP, Alexander ER, Berger RE, et al. Aetiology of acute epididymitis. Lancet 1:819, 1977
14. Riggs S, Sanford JP: Viral orchitis, N Engl J Med 266:990, 1962
15. Shapiro ST, Breschi LC: Acute epididymitis in Vietnam: Review of 52 cases. Milit Med 138:643, 1973
16. Holmes KK, Berger RE, Alexander ER: Acute epididymitis: Etiology and therapy. Arch Androl 3:309, 1979
17. Morgan AD: Inflammation and infestation of the testis and paratesticular structures. In Pugh RCB (ed): Pathology of the Testis. Oxford, Blackwell, 1976, p 79
18. Haahr J, Sparrevohn S: Epididymitis in children. Acta Paediatr Scand 60:248, 1971
19. Davis WH, Scardino PL: Meningitis presenting as epididymitis. South Med J 65:936, 1972
20. Hunt AC, Bothwell PW: Histological findings in human brucellosis. J Clin Pathol 20:267, 1967
21. Ross JC, Gow JG, St. Hill CA: Tuberculous epididymitis. A review of 170 patients. Br J Surg 48:663, 1961
22. Steinhauser K, Wurster K: Die Nebenhodentuberkulose im Wandel der Zeit. Urologe [A] 14:6, 1975
23. Grabstald H, Swan LL: Genitourinary lesions in leprosy: With special reference to problems of atrophy of testes. JAMA 149:1287, 1952
24. Mitchell RG, Oxon BM: Urinary tract infections caused by salmonellae. Lancet 1:1092, 1965
25. Kostalas G, Thomas E: Orchitis and testicular abscess formation as implication of Salmonella virchow gastroenteritis. Med J Aust 2:769, 1973
26. Ackley A, Pickens R: Salmonella virchow testicular abscess. J Urol 122:267, 1979
27. Mittemeyer B, Lennox KW, Borski AA: Epididymitis: A review of 610 cases. J Urol 95:390, 1966
28. Wesson, M.B.: Epididymitis, facts and fancies. Med Clin North Am 43:1645, 1959
29. Karpouzas J, Papahatzi-Kalmanti M, Benetos S, Xipolita A: Tuberculous epididymo-orchitis. Case report. Helv Pediatr Acta 33:453, 1978
30. Karat ABA, Job CK, Karat S: Erythema nodosum leprosum in borderline leprosy. Int J Lepr 35:17, 1967
31. Werner CA: Mumps orchitis and testicular atrophy. I. Occurrence. Ann Intern Med 32:1066, 1950
32. Werner CA: Mumps orchitis and testicular atrophy. II. A factor in male sterility. Ann Intern Med 32:1075, 1950
33. Lyon RP, Bruyn HB: Mumps-epididymo-orchitis. JAMA 196:736, 1966

34. Bjorvatn B: Mumps virus recovered from testicle by fine-needle aspiration biopsy in cases of mumps orchitis. Scand J Infect Dis 5:2, 1973
35. Swann NH: Epidemic pleurodynia, orchitis and myocarditis in an adult due to Coxsackie virus, group B. Type 4. Ann Intern Med 54:1008, 1961
36. Craighead JE, Mahoney EM, Carver DH, et al.: Orchitis due to Coxsackie virus group B. Type 5: Report of a case with isolation of virus from the testes. N Engl J Med 267:498, 1962
37. Ralston LS, Saiki AK, Powers WT: Orchitis as a complication of infectious mononucleosis. JAMA 173:1348, 1960
38. Wolnisty C: Orchitis as a complication of infectious mononucleosis: Report of a case. N Engl J Med 266:88, 1962
39. Naveh Y, Friedman A: Orchitis associated with adenoviral infection. Am J Dis Child 129:257, 1975
40. Sulkin SE, Burns KF, Shelton DF, Wallis C: Bat salivary gland virus: infections of man and monkey. Tex Rep Biol Med 20:113, 1962
41. Habel K, Utz JP: Mumps. Pediatr Clin North Am 7:979, 1960
42. Lewis JM, Utz JP: Orchitis, parotitis and meningoencephalitis due to lymphocytic choriomeningitis virus. N Engl J Med 265:776, 1961
43. Welliver RC, Cherry JD: Aseptic meningitis and orchitis associated with echovirus 6 infection. J Pediatr 92, 239–240, 1978
44. Hanid TK: Infectious mononucleosis complicated by hydrocele. Br Med J 2:706, 1977
45. Connolly KD, Timmons D: Epididymo-orchitis in Kawasaki disease. Arch Dis Child 54:728, 1979
46. Beard CM, Benson RC, Kelalis PP, Elveback LR: The incidence and outcome of mumps orchitis in Rochester, Minnesota, 1935 to 1974. Mayo Clin Proc 52:3, 1977
47. Gall AE: The histopathology of acute mumps orchitis. Am J Pathol 23:637, 1947
48. Charny CW, Meranze DR: Pathology of mumps orchitis. J Urol 60:140, 1948
49. Scott LS: Mumps and male fertility. Br J Urol 32:183, 1960
50. Petersdorf RG, Bennett IL Jr: Treatment of mumps orchitis with adrenal hormones. Arch Intern Med 99:222, 1957
51. Bartak V, Skalova E, Nevarilova A: Spermiogram changes in adults and youngsters after parotitic orchitis. Int J Fertil 13:226, 1968
52. Aiman J, Brenner PF, MacDonald PC: Androgen and estrogen production in an elderly man with gynecomastia and testicular atrophy after mumps orchitis. J Clin Endocrinol 50:380, 1980
53. Berger RE, Alexander ER, Monda GD, et al.: Chlamydia trachomatis as a cause of acute "idiopathic" epididymitis. N Engl J Med 298:301, 1978
54. Monroe MJ: Granulomatous orchitis due to Histoplasma capsulatum masquerading as sperm granuloma. J Clin Pathol 27:929, 1974
55. Hager WD, Majmudar B: Pelvic actinomycosis in women using intra-uterine contraceptive devices. Am J Obstet Gynecol 133:60, 1979
56. Sarosdy MF, Brock WA, Parsons CL: Scrotal actinomycosis. J Urol 121:756, 1979
57. Tung SK, Alexander NJ: Autoimmune reactions in the testis. In Johnson AD, Gomes WR (eds): The Testis, Vol IV. New York, Academic Press. 1977, p 491
58. Tung KSK, Unanue ER, Dixon FJ: Pathogenesis of experimental allergic orchitis. I. Transfer with immune lymph node cells. J Immunol 106:1453, 1971
59. Bigazzi PE, Kosuda LL, Harnick LL: Sperm autoantibodies in vasectomized rats of different inbred strains. Science 197:1282, 1977
60. Lipscomb HL, Gardner PJ, Sharp JG: The effect of neonatal thymectomy on the induction of autoimmune orchitis in rats. J Reprod Immunol 1:209, 1979
61. Bigazzi PE, Kosuda LL, Hu KC, Andres GA: Immune complex orchitis in vasectomized rabbits. J Exp Med 143:382, 1976
62. Rumke P: Autospermagglutinins. Cause of infertility in men. Ann NY Acad Sci 124:696, 1965

63. Glassy FJ, Mostofi FK: Spermatic granulomas of the epididymis. Am J Clin Pathol 26:1303, 1956
64. Taylor TA, Scott DG, Anderson CK, et al. Immunological studies of testicular tissue in oligoazoospermic patients. J Urol 50:419, 1978
65. Mikuz G, Hofstadter F, Hager J: Testis involvement in Schoenlein-Henoch purpura. Pathol Res Pract 165:323, 1979
66. Fernicola AR: Idiopathic hemorrhagic infarction of the testis in the newborn. J Urol 72:230, 1954
67. Kuchemann K: Totale Hodennekrose mit extramedullarer Myelopoese und Megakaryocyteninfiltration bei einem Fall von Osteomyelosklerose. Verh Dtsch Ges Pathol 53:373, 1969
68. Grunberg H: Uber drei ungewohnliche Falle von chronischer Orchitis unter dem klinischen Bilde eines Hodentumors. Frankfurt Z Pathol 33:217, 1926
69. Bunzli HF: Formen granulomatoser Orchitis. Virchows Arch [Pathol Anat] 345:33–44, 1968
70. Mikuz G: Elektronenmikroskopische Untersuchung an zwei Fallen granulomatoser Orchitis. Virchows Arch [Pathol Anat] 360:223–234, 1973
71. Spjut HJ, Thorpe JD: Granulomatous orchitis. Am J Clin Pathol 26:136, 1956
72. Fajardo LF, Dueker GE, Kosek JC: Light and electron microscopic observations on granulomatous orchitis. Invest Urol 6:158–169, 1968
73. Rinaudo P, Damjanov I, Stoesser B: Malacoplakia of testis. Int Urol Nephrol 9:249, 1977
74. Brown RC, Smith, BH: Malacoplakia of the testis. Am J Clin Pathol 47:135, 1967
75. Kruger R, Schulte-Wissermann H, Luchtrath H: Immunohistologische Befunde am Hoden bei granulomatoser Orchitis. Dtsch Med Wochenschr 98:2215, 1973
76. Mostofi FK, Price EB: Tumors of the Male Genital System. Washington DC, Armed Forces Institute of Pathology, 1973
77. Damjanov I, Katz SM: Malakoplakia. Pathol Annu 16(2):103, 1981
78. Csapo T, Kuthy E, Lantos J, Ormos J: Experimentally induced malakoplakia. Am J Pathol 79:453, 1975
79. Green WO: Malacoplakia of the epididymis without testicular involvement. The first reported case. Arch Pathol 86:538, 1968
80. Rudin L, Megalli M, Mesa-Tajeda R: Genital sarcoidosis, Urology 3:750, 1974
81. Mikhail JR, Mitchell D, Dyson JL: Sarcoidosis with genital involvement. Am J Resp Dis 106:465, 1972
82. Opal SM, Pittman DL, Hofeldt FD: Testicular sarcoidosis. Am J Med 67:147, 1979
83. Kupfer, M Buschmann G: Spermieninvasion und Granulome des Nebenhodens. Frankfurter Z Pathol 74:742, 1965
84. Cullen TH, Vess HJ: Sperm granulomata of the testis. Br J Urol 38:202, 1966
85. Kisbenedek L, Nemeth A: Granulomatous orchitis and sperm granuloma. Int Urol Nephrol 7:141, 1975
86. Philips DEH: Lipid granulomata of the testis and epididymis. Br J Urol 33:448, 1961
87. Lin JI, Tseng CH, Marsidi PJ, Bais VC: Cholesterol granuloma of right testis. Urology 14:522, 1979
88. Arduino LJ: Sclerosing lipogranuloma of male genitalia. J Urol 82:155, 1959
89. Macbeth WAAG, Douglas BS: Fat necrosis in the scrotum. N Z Med J 67:409, 1968
90. Fries JW, Talbot BS: Scrotal calcification due to meconium peritonitis. J Urol 73:1059, 1955
91. Berdon WE, Baker DH, Becker J, deSanctis P: Scrotal masses in healed meconium peritonitis. N Engl J Med 277:585, 1967
92. Pugh JI, Stringer P: Glove powder granuloma of the testis. Br J Surg 60:240, 1973
93. Gilchrist KW, Benson RC Jr: Multifocal fibrous pseudotumor of testicular tunics. Urology 14:285, 1979
94. Shafik A: Constrictive albuginitis: Report of 3 cases. J Urol 122:269, 1979
95. Honore LH: Nonspecific testicular fibrosis manifested as testicular enlargement. Clinico-pathologic study of nine cases. Arch Surg 113:814, 1978

CLINICAL AND PATHOLOGIC STUDY OF APONEUROTIC (EPITHELIOID) SARCOMA

MARIA DABSKA AND TADEUSZ KOSZAROWSKI

Soft-tissue sarcomas present one of the most difficult differential diagnostic problems in tumor pathology. The proper diagnosis of a soft-tissue neoplasm may sometimes be difficult if not impossible to make, even if it is based on a surgical specimen. On the other hand, the best treatment and the exact prognosis in any soft-tissue neoplasm depend, to a considerable extent, on the accuracy of histopathologic evaluation. The pathologist's personal experience with the microscopic and clinical aspects of mesenchymal tumors is an important factor in diagnosis.

This chapter presents a review of our recent clinical and pathologic experience with epithelioid sarcoma (aponeurotic sarcoma); we hope that it will underscore some of the known characteristics of this unusual sarcoma and help in defining its true biologic nature and behavior.

In 1948, Laskowski, who was always fascinated by soft-tissue tumors, was concerned by a peculiar, distinctive, but previously unidentified malignant tumor in the soft tissues of the palm of a 27-year-old man (Fig. 1). This was the first in a series of tumor cases that Laskowski later called aponeurotic sarcomas. One of us (T.K.) treated the patient by local excision of the tumor, and he remained free of disease for more than 20 years. Beginning with this case, Laskowski undertook a prospective clinicopathologic study of aponeurotic sarcoma which we joined in 1952.

In 1960, at the Ninth Congress of the Polish Oncological Society, held in Wroclaw, Laskowski presented his first clinicopathologic observations, based on seven cases of aponeurotic sarcoma. The series was published in 1961[1] and was translated into English in 1970,[2] shortly after Laskowski's death. In that same year the lesion became more widely known as epithelioid sarcoma, following Enzinger's paper[3] based on a retrospective study of 62 cases. Since that time, more than 90 new cases of epithelioid sarcoma have been reported in the world literature.[4-17]

There is no doubt that this sarcoma, from the clinical viewpoint, is rare and very unusual. And, with respect to morphology, it is one of the most confusing

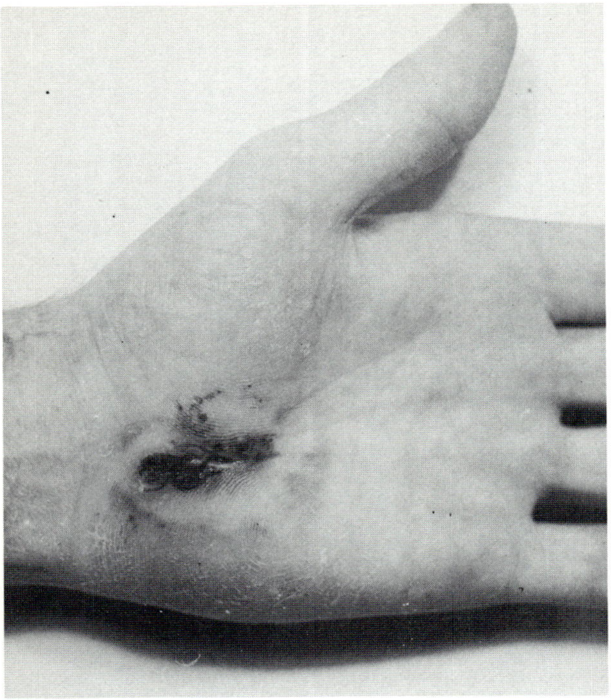

FIG. 1. Case 1. The neoplasm appears not as a tumor but as a subcutaneous thickening of hard consistency. The overlying skin shows discoloration, with a hemorrhagic field in the center after trauma to the lesion.

neoplasms in human pathology; it is noteworthy that epithelioid sarcoma was described in the past by a multiplicity of diagnoses.[3, 18-21] Enzinger's paper lists 20 malignant and 11 benign diagnoses originally made in the cases he studied. However, a pathologist familiar with this entity should have no great difficulty in dealing with it.

Our experience with consultative cases clearly shows that epithelioid sarcoma needs to be better known, especially by clinicians. The clinical behavior of the tumor is often unpredictable, with cure likely only if the lesion is recognized early in its course. This may be achieved if the tumor is small and localized, permitting adequate surgical excision, as shown in a few of our cases. Unfortunately, epithelioid sarcoma usually presents in a form resembling a posttraumatic, nonspecific, indolent lesion which can remain for a long time without being suspected as a malignant growth. Even when the regional lymph nodes are involved by metastasis, some clinicians are not aware that they are dealing with a highly malignant neoplasm.

CLINICAL FEATURES

Twenty-two cases of a relatively distinct histologic pattern of epithelioid (aponeurotic) sarcoma, assembled from our own and consultative cases, form the basis of this study. Included are the cases collected by Laskowski,[1] with further follow-up. It proved very important to have a longer period of observation in order to come to the conclusion that epithelioid (aponeurotic) sarcoma has an unpredictable and in most cases fatal clinical outcome.

Follow-up

Fourteen patients with epithelioid sarcoma were treated and followed up in the Surgical Clinic of the Institute of Oncology in Warsaw; the remaining patients were treated elsewhere. The pertinent clinical data are summarized in Table 1. Follow-up ranging from 1 to 28 years was obtained for the patients recorded in the Institute. Four of the 14 (28 percent) survived 20, 21, 21, and 26 years, respectively, without recurrence. One patient (Case 13) is living with a local recurrence of tumor, 1 year after excision of a primary tumor in the palm. This girl will soon have further surgery. Seven patients seen in consultation have been lost to follow-up at 2 to 3 years after treatment; since all had advanced disease when first seen, it is likely that the outcome in these cases was fatal.

Sex and Age

There were 8 females and 14 males. The age of the patients at the time of the initial surgical procedure ranged from 13 to 57 years. Eight patients were biopsied in the fifth, and six in the second decade of life. All were Caucasians.

Anatomic Location of Tumors

All but two tumors developed in an extremity, the volar aspect of either hand being the most favored site. Eleven tumors were found in the palm; the locations of these being the volar surface near the fingers, the mid-palm, the thenar eminence, and, in one case, the dorsal intermetacarpal. In three patients the distal part of the forearm was involved (the extensor surface in two and the mid-interosseous membrane in one). Of three lesions of the leg, one developed on the anterior surface below the knee, one on the posterolateral aspect, and one on the plantar part of the heel. Unusual presentations were a 3-cm tumor in the belly of the sternocleidomastoid muscle near the mastoid process, and a 6-cm mass deep within the gluteus maximus of the buttock that caused erosion of the iliac bone.

Trauma and Complaints

Sixteen patients reported previous injury at the site of the tumor. Some of these patients were manual workers. Repeated trauma to the hand was outstanding in four patients who were either farmers or laborers involved in digging (spade workers).

TABLE 1. Clinical Data on Aponeurotic (Epithelioid) Sarcoma from the Marie Curie-Sklodowska Institute of Oncology, Warsaw, Poland

Case	Sex, Age at Onset, Year of Diagnosis	Duration Prior to Initial Treatment	Primary Site (Size)	Therapy	Course	Death (Yr. From Onset of Symptoms)
			CASES TREATED AT INSTITUTE OF ONCOLOGY			
1	M, 27, 1948	5 Yr.	Palm, right hand (3 cm)	Local electro-excision	Well, 20.5 years	
2	M, 23, 1949	1 Yr.	Palm, left hand (2 cm)	Local excision. Local excision and electroexcision. Below-elbow amputation and axillary node dissection. Excision of one of multiple nodules on the head	Two local recurrences in 3 years after primary excision. Refused amputation. Recurrence 1954; electroexcision and, after 9 days, amputation with axillary nodes negative. Widespread metastases (skin of head and lungs) 1955. Widespread skin metastases 1956	8
3	F, 42 1953	1 Yr	Palm, left hand (4 cm)	Amputation of digits 3 and 4 and metacarpal bones	Well, 21 years after removal of the tumor with fingers and metacarpal bones	
4	M, 50 1955	3 Yr. 2 Yr.	Palm, right hand (2.5 cm)	Amputation of digits 3,4, and 5 and metacarpal bones and three carpal bones. Eight local excisions. Below-elbow amputation, chemotherapy, x-ray	Between 1955 and 1962 eight local recurrences and above-elbow amputation. Chemotherapy-arterial infusion. X-ray therapy in 1963 for axillary metastases	14
5	M, 46, 1958	14 Yr.	Palm, left hand (5 cm)	Amputation of digits 3,4, and 5 and metacarpal bones	Well 21 years after amputation and 35 yrs. after onset of symptoms	

6	M, 48, 1960	3 Yr.	Palm, left hand (4 cm)	Amputation of two fingers. Below-elbow amputation	After finger amputation in 1960, wide local recurrence. In 1961 amputation and in 1962 axillary node metastases; spread to shoulder, chest wall, lungs	6
7	F, 20, 1968	2 Yr.	Palm, right thumb (3 cm)	Excision. Axillary node dissection and local excision of recurrence (3 cm). Simple mastectomy, right breast. Wide excision of chest-wall skin	Treated initially as a "ganglion." 1969 excision of the recurrence and axillary dissection for positive nodes. 1972 multiple nodules in the breast: simple mastectomy. 1973 "en bloc" excision of multiple nodules in the chest wall and a metastasis from the scalp	7
8	F, 34, 1963	4 Yr.	Wrist, left volar (4 cm)	Local excision in 1963. Disarticulation in 1967	Multinodular dissemination in the whole arm with ulceration of the skin, 1967. 1969 widespread multinodular skin dissemination	8
9	M, 17, 1968	2 Yr.	Wrist, right volar (1 cm)	Local excision in 1968 and subcutaneous axillary metastases. Three local excisions of recurrences and axillary nodes. Disarticulation	First surgical treatment when 13 years. Reexcision of one recurrence and axillary nodes 5 weeks after primary. In 4 years, 3 recurrences. 1973 disarticulation. 1975 well, without evidence of disease. 1976 death from pulmonary metastasis	8
10	M, 20 1975	1.5 Yr.	Wrist, right volar (1.8 cm)	Local excision. Local excision of one of multiple disseminated nodules in the arm	Patient admitted for amputation: refused. In short time, unoperable involvement of the whole arm and axilla. Pulmonary metastases, death in 1978	5.5

(Continued)

TABLE 1. (Continued)

Case	Sex, Age at Onset, Year of Diagnosis	Duration Prior to Initial Treatment	Primary Site (Size)	Therapy	Course	Death (Yr. From Onset of Symptoms)
11	M, 42, 1972	1 Yr.	Mastoid insertion and belly of left sternocleidomastoid muscle	Radiotherapy: 5700 rads and wide excision. Chemotherapy	Wide dissemination, lung and brain metastasis	2
12	F, 48 1973	1.5 Yr.	Left buttock and bone involvement	Excision, recurrence	?	4.5
13	F, 19 1979	2 Yr.	Palm-finger (1.5 cm)	Excision, re-excision, recurrence	Living with small recurrence in the palm	
14	F, 48 1954	2 Yr.	Forearm, Right mid-interosseous membrane (6 cm)	Wide biopsy, radiotherapy ca. 5,000 rads	After x-ray therapy massive calcification of the whole tumor. Patient well. Follow-up 25 years, to 1980	
			CASES SEEN IN CONSULTATION BUT TREATED ELSEWHERE			
15	M, 34	3 Yr.	Left knee, posterior	Local excision	After surgery followed for two years. Lost to follow-up	
16	F, 48	Not known	Palm, right	Local excision	Lost to follow-up	

17	M, 57	2 Yr.	Heel, left plantar (1.5 cm)	Fungating small tumor. Patient cut it off. Local excision of the deep portion of the tumor and skin graft	After surgery, only 1 year observation: well
18	M, 19	1 Yr.	Palm, left hand	Incomplete local excision	After surgery, rapid growth of tumor. Lost to follow-up
19	F, 28	1.5 Yr	Knee, below anterior right (2 cm)	Local excision	Patient refused amputation. Seen at the Institute; lost to follow-up
20	M, 18	1.5 Yr.	Forearm, left (6 cm)	Local excision	Big local ulcerated recurrence. Lost to follow-up
21	M, 45	3 Yr.	Hand, right dorsum (2.5 cm)	Forearm amputation and axillary node dissection	After biopsy, amputation. The tumor was ulcerated. Nodes in the axilla were involved. Patient well, lost to observation after 2 years
22	M, 57	1 Yr.	Forearm, right size unknown	Excision: tumor not examined histologically. Local excision of small breast tumor	After excision of the forearm tumor a metastasis appeared at 1 year in the breast. Patient was living 3 years after second operation. Status unknown

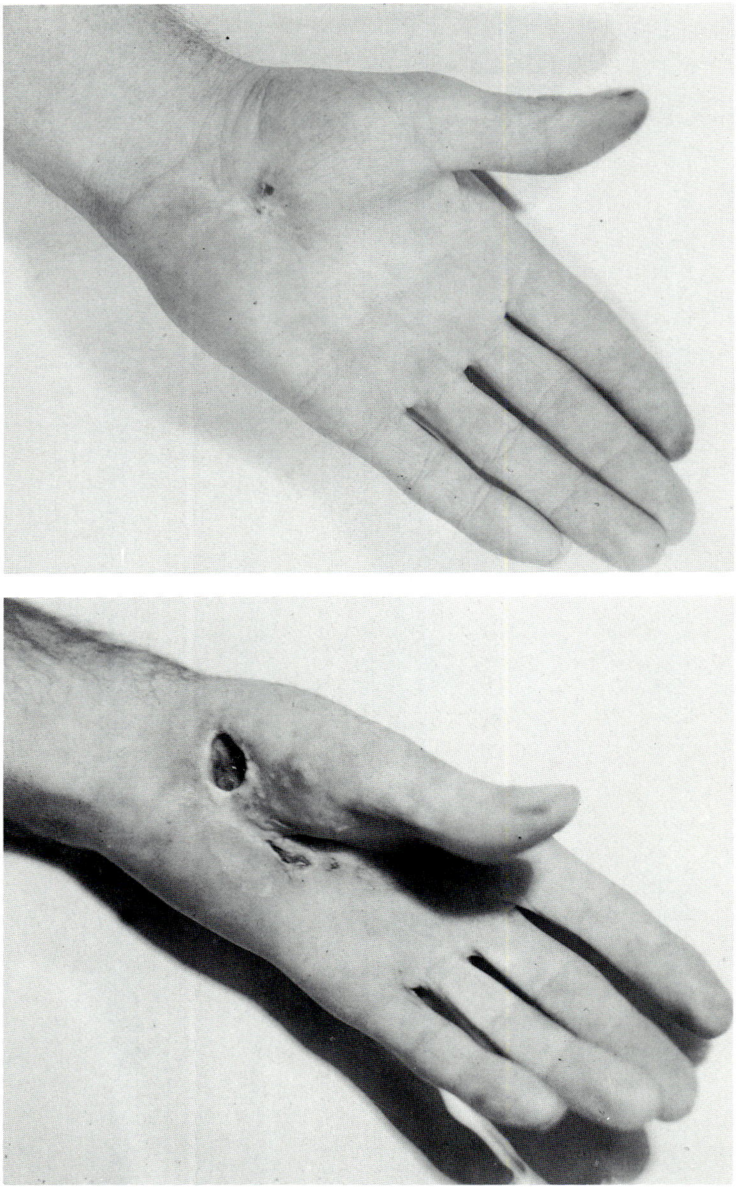

FIG. 2. Top. Case 2. First recurrence after electrocoagulation of the tumor, showing only a thickening of the soft tissues and a constricted scar in the overlying skin. **Bottom.** Case 2. The same hand 3 years later (second recurrence) showing an oval, deep ulcer with hard, sharply outlined borders, small fissures in the palmar region, and contracture of the fingers.

Five patients reported the rapid appearance of an ulcer after injury to an area that had had diffuse induration for years (Figs. 2 Top and Bottom). Of the 22 patients, only 7 complained of severe pain connected with the neoplasm. In four patients with arm injuries, the arm was edematous, and in two of these the pain was of such degree that neurotomy was required. Generally, when the area of the lesion was small, no complaints were recorded even when there was ulceration. Later in the course of the disease, sensory changes appeared together with deep ulceration and contractures of the fingers (Fig. 3).

Physical Findings

The lesions appeared to start in one of two ways: some presented as a small, rather localized nodule situated deep in the soft tissues, covered by intact skin; others formed an ill-defined area of flat induration (Fig. 1) confined at first to the skin. On the palm, this latter development took the form of a kind of diffuse plaque, usually wooden-hard and indolent. All patients initially had a single nodule or plaque.

The size of the lesion was known in 19 cases, and ranged from 1 to 6 cm. Most of the lesions were between 2 and 4 cm in their greatest diameter.

Of particular note is the fact that patients with either type of lesion usually had, at some stage of the disease, a characteristic cleft in the skin, having sharply

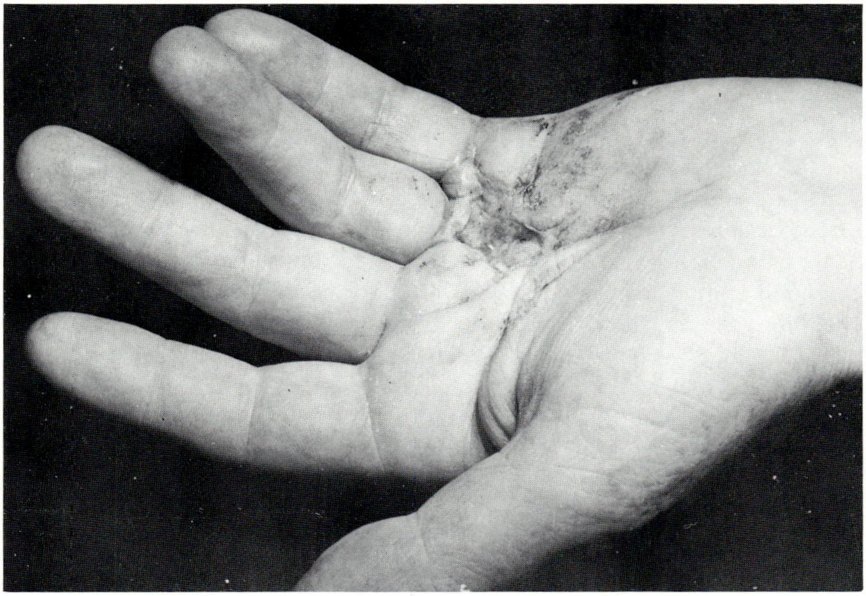

FIG. 3. Case 5. After amputation of the fingers and metacarpal bones, resulting in a "small hand", this patient is living and well 35 years after the onset of symptoms. Nonspecific ulceration with contracture of the fingers is to be seen.

cut margins and discharging serous fluid. Shortly, the cleft was transformed into a large ulceration with an indurated bottom and margins (Figs. 4 Top and Bottom). It was remarkable that even in such advanced stages of the lesion, some clinicians did not suspect the neoplastic character of the disease.

Clinical Course

Both forms of the sarcoma usually grew slowly. Regional or distant metastases appeared later, sometimes after years. In three cases, however, the clinical course was rapid, leading to death in from 1 to a few years.

The average duration of the clinical symptoms before medical attention was 1 to 3 years. One patient delayed seeking medical care for 14 years.

For a long time the exact clinical course of epithelioid sarcoma was unclear to us, and we were of the opinion that the sarcoma appeared exclusively on the palm. Later it became apparent that the tumor may involve the lower extremity and other parts of the body. Laskowski did not know that this sarcoma may manifest itself as multiple small nodules in the skin of the whole arm, arising from the subcutis and deeper parts of the extremity during the occult propagation of the neoplasm. The first example of this unusual clinical course of epithelioid sarcoma came to our attention for the first time late in 1967; it was observed in Case 8, a woman operated upon elsewhere for a 4-cm tumor localized to the volar aspect of her left wrist. One year later she noticed slight edema of the whole arm and the gradual appearance of multiple small nodules, some of them disintegrating superficially and discharging proteinaceous material. The patient was observed and conservatively treated by dermatologists for an unknown skin disease for a year. She was then seen by us in consultation. Two biopsies done at the dermatologic clinic were not conclusive. A biopsy performed at our Institute showed the characteristic pattern of aponeurotic sarcoma, although the clinical picture (Fig. 5) was very different from that in our previous experience with this neoplasm.

The patient underwent a disarticulation of the arm. Dissection of the amputated extremity revealed that the recurrent tumor situated in the palmar aponeurosis diffusely infiltrated and encased all tendons of the flexor digitorum muscle, obliterating the mid-palmar spaces, and was firmly attached to the periosteum of the carpal bones. Neoplastic tissue was present deep in the sectioned forearm and upper arm, as well as superficially in the subcutis and cutis. The sarcoma grew diffusely, enveloping nearly all tendons and vascular and nerve sheaths with a fine, translucent, gelatinous ‘‘muff’’ of grayish-white, grayish-pink, or cherry-red color. In some places, however, the sarcoma grew in a multinodular manner, the nodules being from 0.5 to 1.5 cm in greatest diameter. Some tendons passing through the tumorous area were movable, but others were fixed by infiltrating tumor masses. Superficial nodules, especially those located in the subcutis, were firmer than those lying deeper and were commonly grayish-tan or grayish-yellow in color. The nodules situated in the corium were elevated above the skin surface, some of them simulating ‘‘mole hills’’ and some presenting as somewhat collapsed, small tumors, usually with a central ulcer on the top of the elevated skin. In some places the nodules were confluent (Fig. 5). Unfortunately,

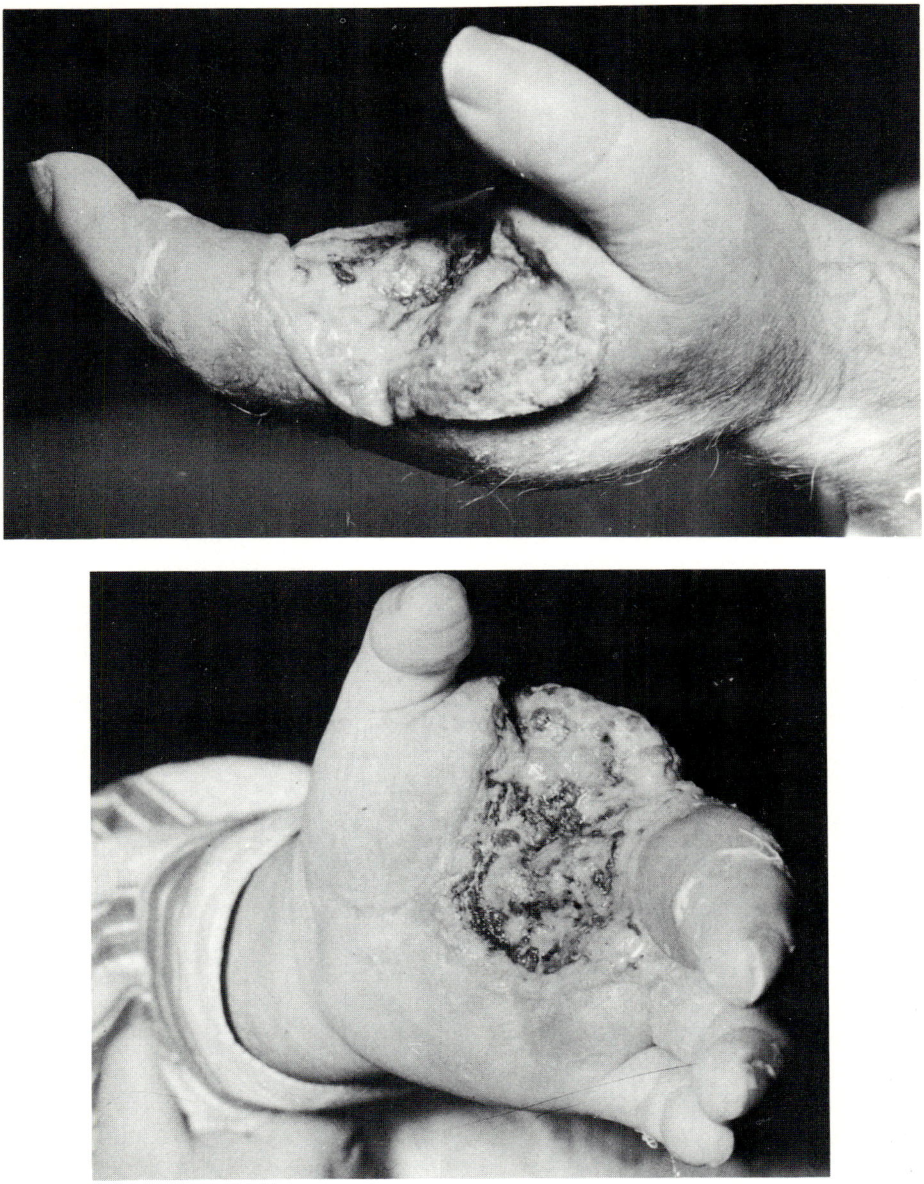

FIG. 4. Case 6. **Top and Bottom.** After amputation of the index finger a large ulceration of the skin and soft tissues is to be seen owing to persistent tumor. There are sharply outlined and punched-out borders. The nodular tumor tissue is covered with fibrin and necrotic debris.

the patient died 3 years after treatment, 8 years from the onset of the tumor. An autopsy was not done but the last clinical examination revealed evidence of brain metastases and dissemination of the neoplasm in the skin of the trunk.

Another case also illustrated to us the fact that epithelioid sarcoma tends to grow—from a primary tumor mass situated distally in the extremity—proximally

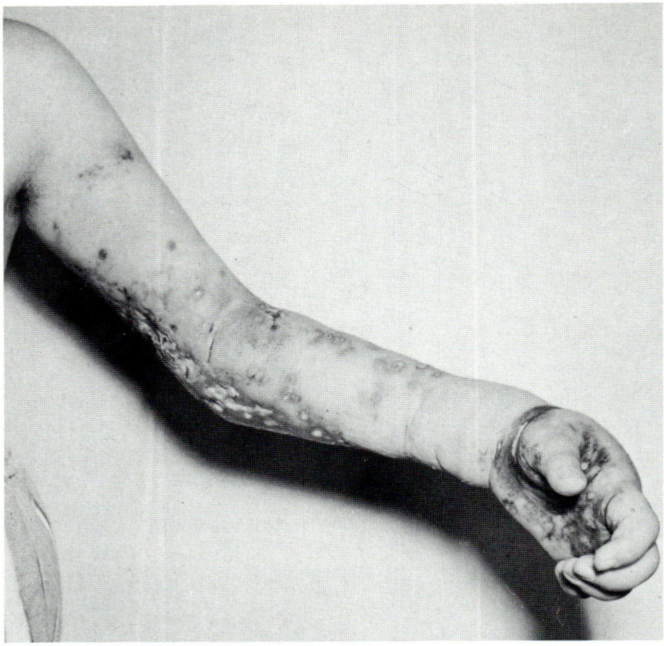

FIG. 5. Case 8. This sarcoma, which originally began as a small nodule in the volar aspect of the wrist, subsequently grew proximally along synovial sheaths and tendons to the axilla, with massive edema of the extremity and multinodular skin involvement.

along the fascial planes, tendons, and sheaths of vessels and nerves up to the axilla. This patient was 13 years of age when he had local excision of a lesion on the right wrist (Case 9). After three local recurrences appeared within 5 years, the extremity was amputated at our Institute. The patient was then well for nearly 4 years, but rapidly deteriorated and died in 1976 of massive metastases to both lungs. The biopsy specimen in this case had the same gross picture as in the former case (see Fig. 9).

Case 7 also deserves special attention because of the unusual manner of tumor spread. When first seen the patient was 20 years old. She came to us with a recurrence in the thumb of her right hand; 1 year earlier, a deeply situated tumor had been locally excised elsewhere from the same hand. At the time of admission to the Institute, an axillary lymph node was enlarged. The patient was treated with a wide local excision of the recurrent tumor and an axillary lymph node dissection. In both surgical specimens typical epithelioid sarcoma was found. The patient was well for about 4 years until multiple, round, painless nodules were found in her right breast. In the patient's opinion these were slowly enlarging and multiplying. The clinical diagnosis was "possibly multiple fibroadenomas of the breast" and a decision was made for biopsy with frozen-section examination. When this revealed epithelioid sarcoma in the breast, a simple mastectomy was done. On palpation and on the cut surface of the breast, numerous ill-defined, rounded tumors were found. These resembled fibroadenomas and were located mainly in the outer upper quadrant, close to the pectoralis fascia. The sarcoma appeared to have involved the breast by direct spread from metastatic deposits in the axilla; it grew along the broad plane of the pectoralis fascia, extending into the mammary gland along fascial septa. Soon after the mastectomy, a multinodular recurrence appeared in the chest wall. The patient died of multiple metastases in both lungs and the scalp 7 years after the onset of the disease. In this case the extremity remained free of disease except for the initial primary site and metastatic disease in the axilla. Spread along the fascia occurred from the metastatic focus rather than from the primary site.

PATHOLOGIC FEATURES

Gross Appearances

As emphasized above, the most conspicuous feature on the cut surface was the nodular character of growth of the sarcoma. This was most striking in cases in which the tumor was situated deep in the tendons, in the muscles, or in the subcutis. Both primary and secondary ("satellite") nodules were closely attached to the fibrous structures: aponeuroses, tendons, tendon sheaths, vessels, and nerve sheaths. Primary tumors consisted of a main mass accompanied by small sprouts or satellite nodules. These primary complexes measured from 2 to 8 cm in greatest diameter. The tumor tissue was grayish-tan, yellow-tan, or even whitish in color. In the dermis the tumor was less nodular in appearance, less circumscribed, and rather irregular in contour.

The neoplastic tissue we saw was usually hard in consistency, in some cases woody hard. Small tumors of 0.5 to 1.5 cm, dispersed from the primary, and especially those small tumors that grew perpendicular to the axilla along tendons and fibrous tissues investing nerves and vessels, were rather soft in consistency and glistening. This striking capacity of the neoplasm to grow in a multinodular manner within and along various fibrous anatomic structures resulted in multifocal skin lesions of the entire involved extremity, and caused extensive edema (Fig. 5). Sometimes it was hard to distinguish between satellite nodules and lymph nodes involved by the sarcoma.

Microscopic Features

The microscopic features of epithelioid sarcoma were well illustrated by Enzinger[3] and by Prat et al.[21] This discussion will be concerned mainly with the cytologic peculiarities of the neoplasm.

At lower-power magnification, the tumor is multifocal and the lesions exhibit central necrosis. Foci situated in the subcutis, in close apposition to one another, form geographic patterns created by fields of necrosis. Necrosis is also prominent within the centers of some separate nodules, giving them a granulomatous appearance. In some instances small nodules show the pattern of a granuloma, owing to a centrally located, delicate network of dilated blood capillaries. In fascia and tendons, tumor cells grow in bands or fascicles and in single-cell patterns bearing a close resemblance to the infiltrative mode of spread of a breast carcinoma (see Fig. 10).

CELL TYPES

Epithelioid sarcoma in our series was a pleomorphic neoplasm. It is obvious that the wide spectrum of its cytologic features contributed, in the past, to the difficulty in making the proper diagnosis of this neoplasm.[3,21] Five distinct cell types were observed, as follows:

1. *Stem cells.* These were small and lymphocyte-like, with a plump, dark-stained nucleus and a scanty rim of cytoplasm. They were sparse and merged easily with other types of cells (Fig. 6).
2. *Intermediate cells.* These were somewhat larger than stem cells, and were polyhedral in shape (Fig. 6). Located close to these cells were transition forms from stem to intermediate and epithelioid cells. The cytoplasm of the intermediate cells was eosinophilic and was more abundant than in the stem cells. The nuclei of the intermediate cells were vesicular, and a single nucleolus appeared in some of them. In Figure 6 is to be seen an alveolar pattern reminiscent of the pattern of alveolar rhabdomyosarcoma.

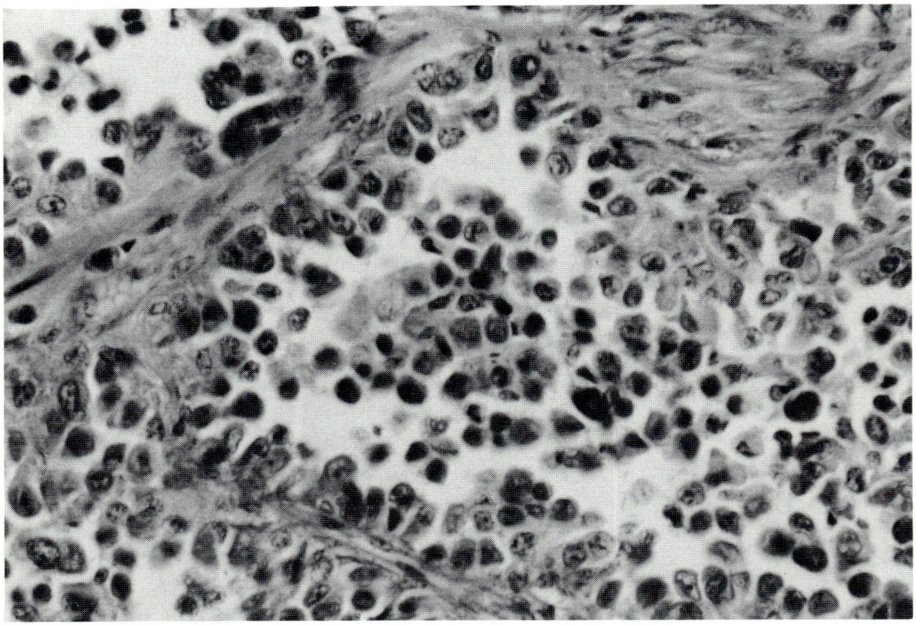

FIG. 6. Alveolar pattern of epithelioid sarcoma, bearing a close resemblance to alveolar (embryonal) rhabdomyosarcoma. Small, scattered stem and intermediate cells are to be seen. H&E. ×200.

It is to be stressed that epithelioid cells constituted the widest range of cell populations, varying from plump and ovoid to polyhedral and pleomorphic cells. They varied in size from moderate to very large cells.

3. *Epithelioid cells.* These occurred in several variants: (1) *"Myogenous" cells* were large cells resembling the strap-shaped pleomorphic cells of rhabdomyosarcoma (Fig. 7). The cytoplasm of these cells, when stained with H & E, was outstandingly eosinophilic. The pleomorphism of the cells, the longitudinal fibrillar appearance of their cytoplasm, the prominence of pale nuclei, and their multinucleation resembled the features of malignant rhabdomyoblasts. There was considerable variation in the shape and size of those cells. However, most "myogenous" cells, unlike true malignant rhabdomyoblasts, have no sharply outlined cytoplasm. (2) *"Ganglion"-like cells* constituted a striking variant of epithelioid cells (Fig. 8); they showed well-preserved cytoplasmic membranes with short but evident cytoplasmic processes. Their nuclei were prominently vesicular, demonstrating hyperchromasia and indented membranes. Multinucleated forms with bright-red nucleoli were a constant feature of these cells, in which respect the cells resembled the characteristic polygonal but benign-looking cells of proliferative myositis. It is possible that the ganglion-like cells represent modified malignant fibroblasts. (3) *"Melanoma"-like cells* represented another variant of epithelioid cells (Fig. 9). The cytoplasm of these cells was abundant, vitreous, and pink-to-red when stained with H & E. Block-shaped, with well-preserved cell membranes, the melanoma-like cells resembled those of epithelioid malignant melanomas. The nuclei were prominent, vesicular, often demon-

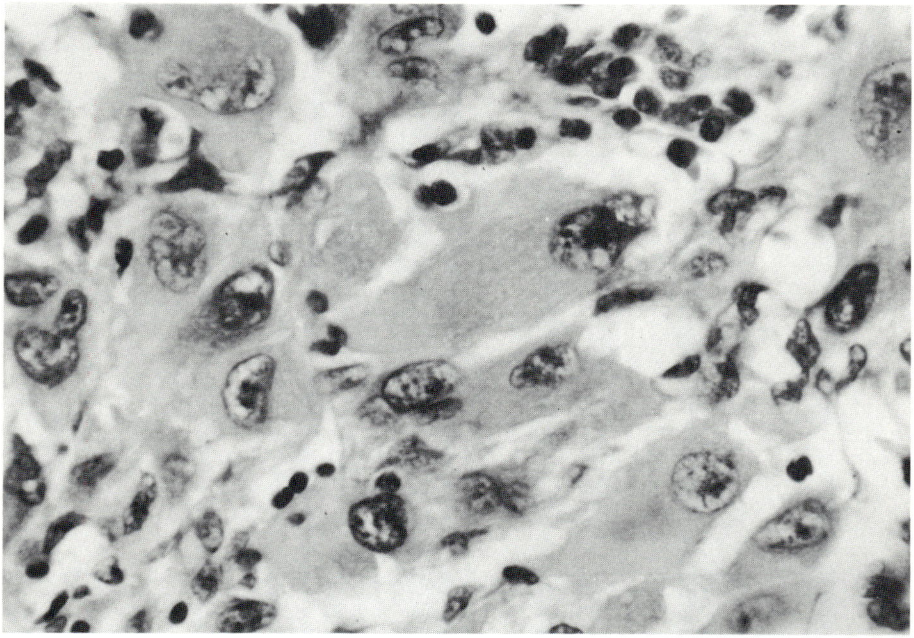

FIG. 7. Large "myogenous" cells compatible with malignant rhabdomyoblasts. H&E. ×400.

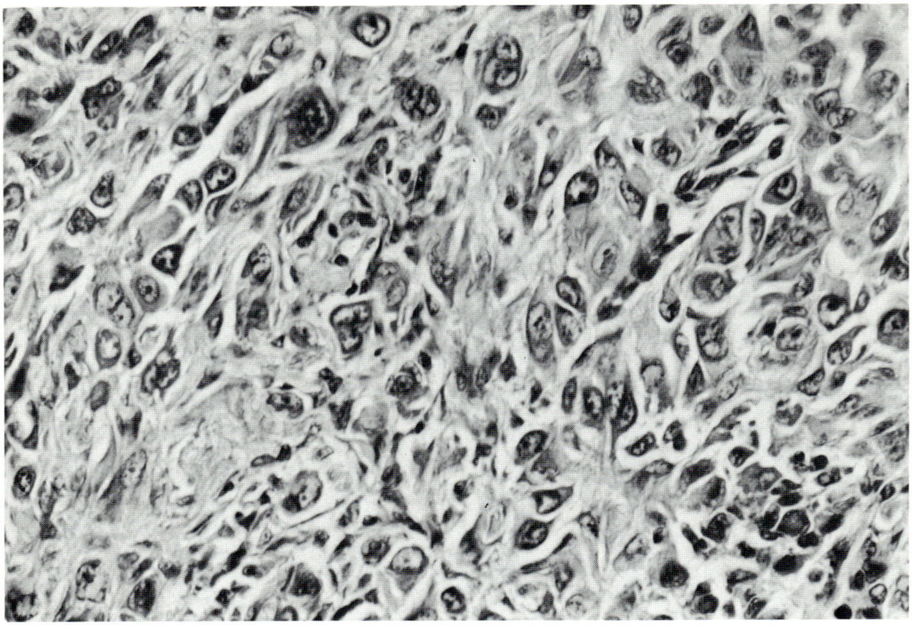

FIG. 8. "Ganglion"-like cells in an epithelioid sarcoma, bearing a close resemblance to cells seen in progressive myositis. However, the malignant morphologic appearance of these cells is obvious. H&E. ×200.

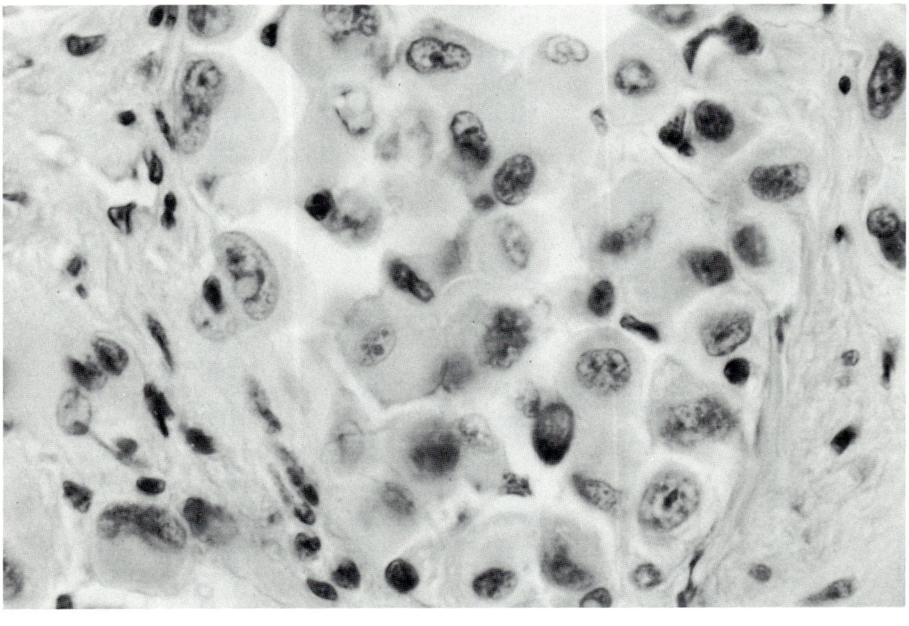

FIG. 9. The pattern of this epithelioid sarcoma is suggestive of a malignant melanoma. The cell boundaries are sharply outlined, and a deeply acidophilic, abundant cytoplasm is an outstanding feature. H&E. ×400.

strated multinucleation, and had indented membranes. One or more nucleoli, cyclamen in color, were prominent. (4) *"Carcinoma"-like cells* are illustrated in Figure 10. They were usually polyhedral, moderate in size, and some mimicked the growth pattern of undifferentiated squamous cell carcinoma or mammary carcinoma (Fig. 10).

The tendency toward elongation of the various types of epithelial-looking cells was in some places very outstanding, especially where an active fibrous-tissue proliferation appeared around the neoplastic nodules.

4. *Spindle cell variants* were also observed. These cells varied much in size, shape, and growth pattern. There were places where they formed compact fascicles and bands (Fig. 11). They sometimes occurred in interlacing bundles, reminiscent of the pattern seen in fibrosarcoma. Some spindle cells showed a conspicuous fibromatous appearance as a result of the extensive production of collagen fibers by the neoplasm (Fig. 12). Trichrome staining in such cases usually demonstrated dense, birefringent collagen. Quite frequently, transitions between epithelioid cells and spindle cells were noted, and fine collagen fibers also encircled individual epithelioid cells. Some fibroblastic elements of the neoplasm were well differentiated and merged with a large amount of collagen or with hyalinized fields. A loosely arranged spindle-cell pattern is shown in Figure 13. Hyperchromasia, multinucleation, and high mitotic activity were prominent features of these spindle cells. There were also polygonal cells merging imperceptibly with the spindle cells, so that sharp delineation between the spindle and epithelioid cells was not always possible (Fig. 14).

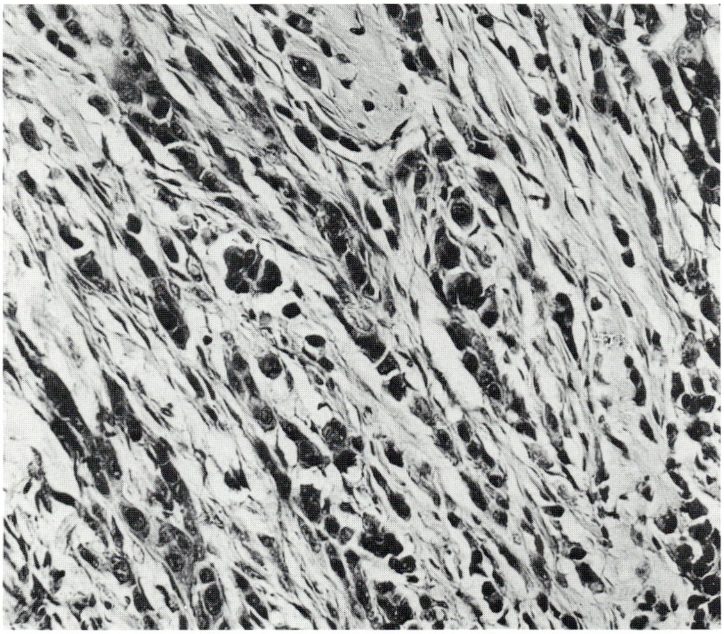

FIG. 10. The cells of epithelioid sarcoma are arranged in a cord-like pattern, mimicking a breast carcinoma. H&E. ×200.

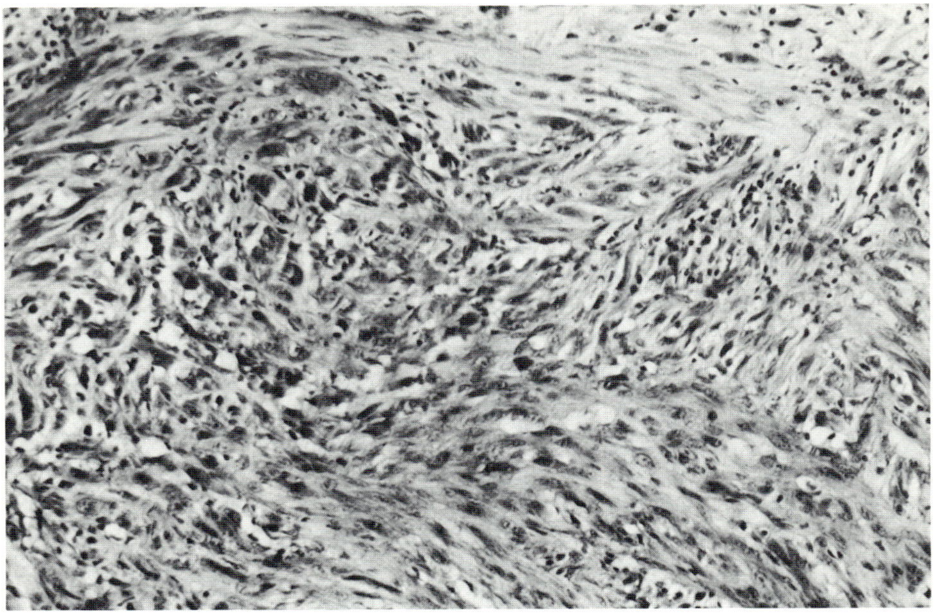

FIG. 11. Fibrosarcomatous appearance in epithelioid sarcoma. H&E. ×200.

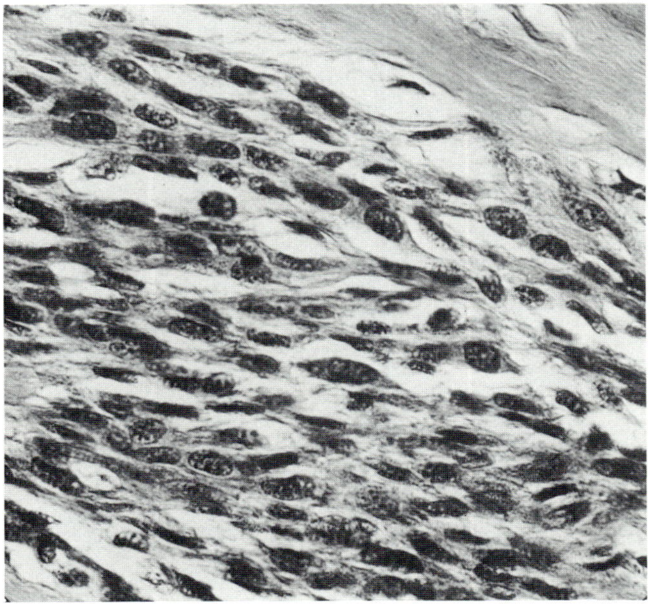

FIG. 12. Spindle cells of epithelioid sarcoma in a loose arrangement, showing abundant collagen production in the upper corner. H&E. ×250.

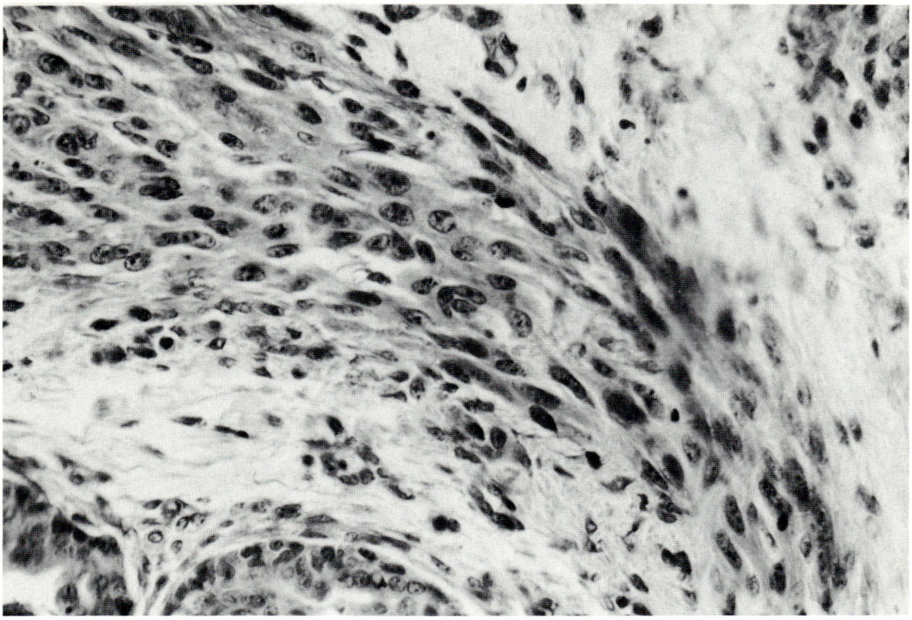

FIG. 13. Spindle cells of epithelioid sarcoma invading the stroma of the breast (Case 7). At the bottom, fragments of proliferating duct epithelium are shown. H&E. ×200.

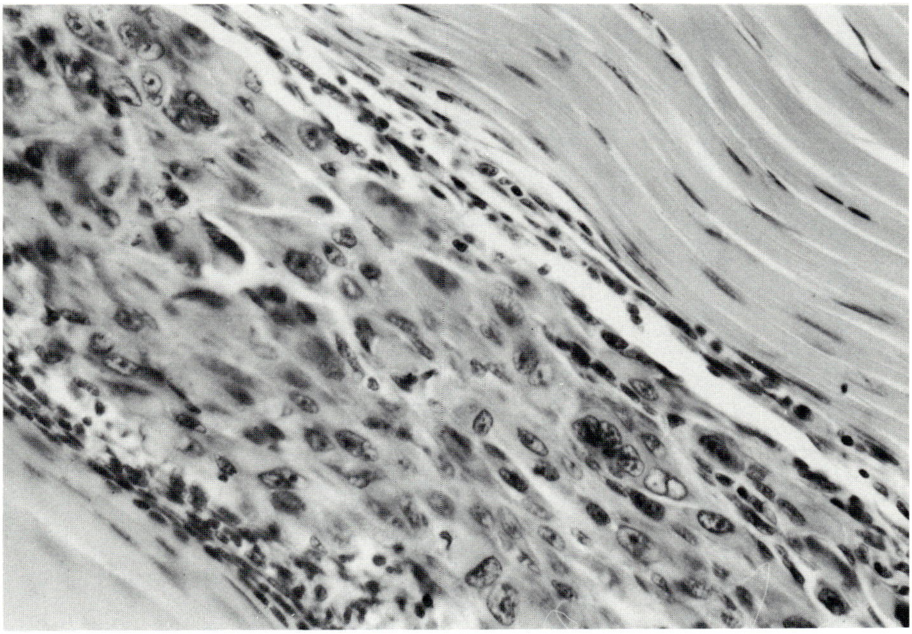

FIG. 14. Case 9. Cords of elongated epithelioid cells infiltrating a big tendon. H&E. ×200.

5. *Cells with clear cytoplasm.* These were sparse, and were seen only in two cases; they were moderate in size and ovoid or polyhedral, with sharply outlined cell boundaries and a vesicular, haphazardly located nucleus. A water-clear cytoplasm gave these cells an appearance reminiscent of plant cells.

STROMAL CHANGES

Fibrosis and hyalinization were evident to a variable degree in all cases (Fig. 15). In foci of fibrosis and hyalinization, the cytoplasmic margins of cells were indistinct and blurred, giving the tumor cells a syncytial appearance. Not infrequently, fingerlike processes of fibrous tissue extended peripherally, involving the adventitia of vessels.

Myxoid changes were to be seen, especially in the subepidermal spaces (Fig. 16). Stains for acid mucopolysaccharides were positive in the tumor stroma but not in the tumor cells. Intracytoplasmic lipid droplets have been found in exceptional cases of epithelioid sarcoma, around necrotic fields.

Calcification in the form of psammoma bodies was only occasionally noted and appeared to be the result of degeneration of some cell clusters, but was rarely noted in recurrent tumors. Hemosiderin deposition was inconspicuous in most cases. Cartilage or bone formation was observed only in Case 14, an unusual epithelioid sarcoma which will be described elsewhere, in detail.[31] The sarcoma in

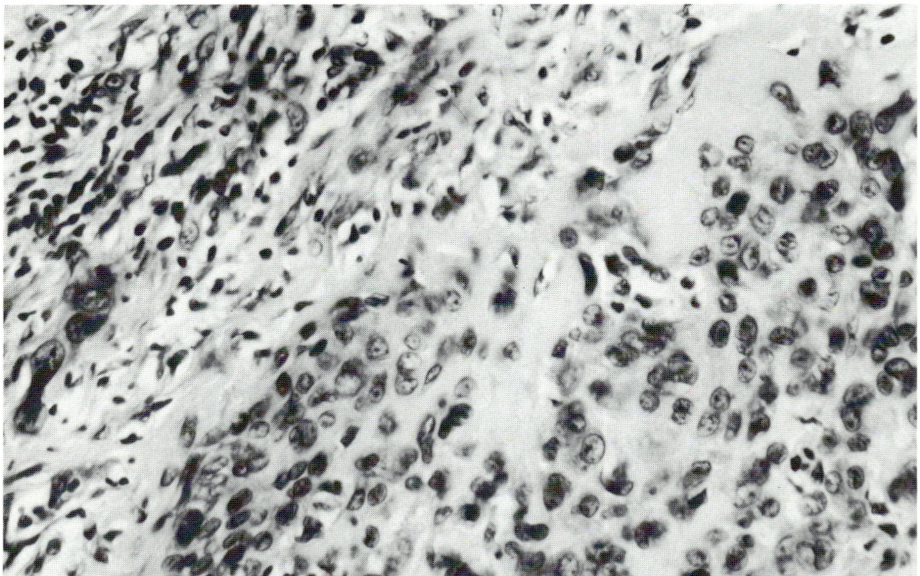

FIG. 15. Extensive hyalinization within stem and intermediate cells, creating loss of cellular cohesion and blurring of cytoplasmic margins. H&E. ×200.

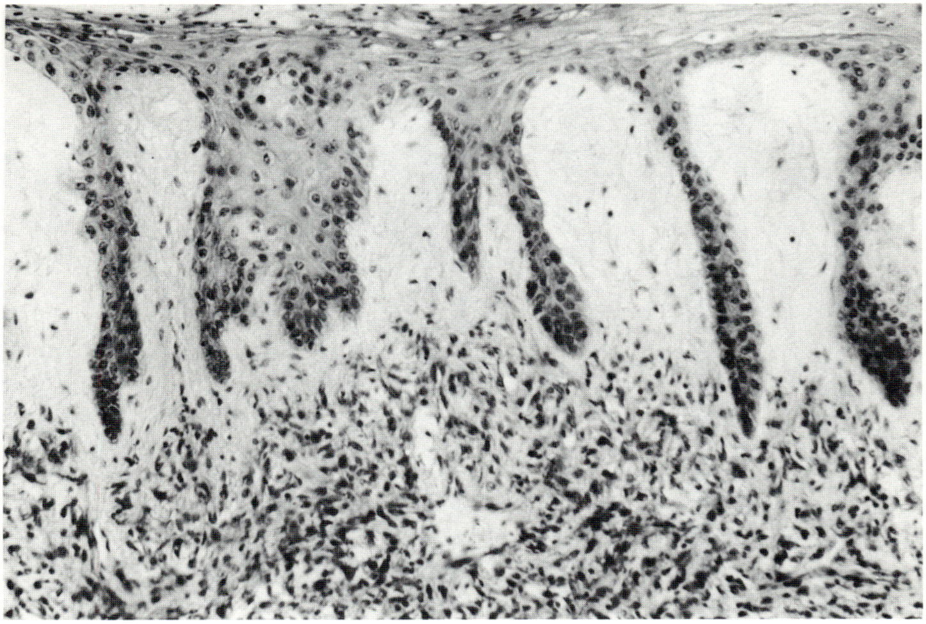

FIG. 16. Elongation of rete pegs and subepidermal edema in a case of massive whole-arm involvement. H&E. ×150.

this case involved the mid-interosseous membrane of the forearm and underwent massive calcification as the result of x-ray treatment. The patient remains well more than 26 years after the onset of the disease. Epithelioid sarcoma involving the breast by extension from metastasis in the axilla (Case 7) caused extensive proliferation of the mammary duct epithelium. No vascular invasion was found in eight cases. Nerve sheath involvement was prominent in nine cases.

Tumor metastatic to the lymph nodes, subcutaneous tissues, or soft tissues was, for the most part, composed of epithelioid cells. These cells often showed an arrangement that resembled poorly differentiated squamous cell carcinoma (Fig. 17), nonspecific granuloma, or malignant melanoma.

DATA FROM ELECTRON MICROSCOPY

Relatively little work has been done on the ultra-structure of epithelioid sarcoma. Only recently has the electron microscope been used on a large scale to investigate the histogenesis of this neoplasm. The entire scope of epithelioid sarcoma is not yet defined, and the nature of the cellular constituents of the tumors in the disease has not yet been generally agreed upon.

Ultrastructural studies in epithelioid sarcoma have yielded contradictory results[22-28]; some investigators are inclined to put epithelioid sarcoma into the group of synovial sarcomas, while others claim that the tumor represents a differentiation toward histiocytes and fibroblasts. Gabbiani et al.[23] and Akiyama et al.[28] postulate

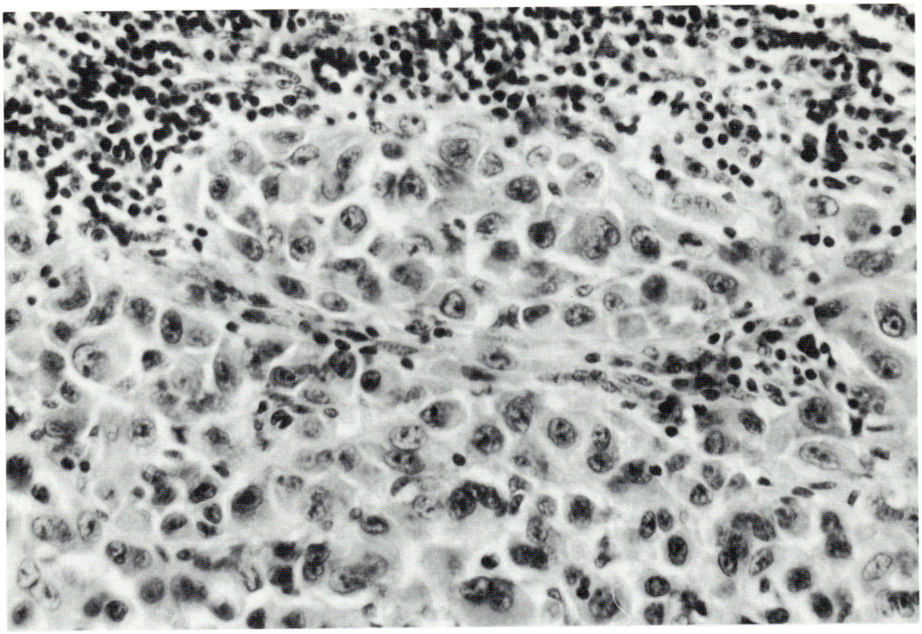

FIG. 17. Lymph node metastasis, showing a pattern reminiscent of poorly differentiated squamous carcinoma. H&E. ×250.

the existence of a third type of cell (called by us the "stem" cell) which, in their opinion, is a small, primitive progenitor cell that differentiates into epithelioid and spindle cells. Akiyama et al. expressed the view that the sarcoma cells in epithelioid sarcoma seem to be of histiocytic origin, suggesting that both cell types are derived from one undifferentiated mesenchymal cell. In contradistinction to this, Gabbiani et al. doubted the histiocytic origin of epithelioid sarcoma, favoring a synovial origin for this neoplasm. Hajdu et al.[29] included epithelioid sarcoma in a group of soft-tissue neoplasms labeled "tendosynovial tumors."

An interesting finding has been reported by Medenica et al.[26] Using the electron microscope, they found lymphocytic infiltrates which formed close contacts with neoplastic cells, and came to the conclusion that the slow tendency of epithelioid sarcoma to metastasize might be related to a high efficacy of lymphocyte-mediated defenses against this neoplasm.

Our own electron microscopic studies, done in two cases, will be recorded in detail elsewhere.[30,31] In general, our findings are similar to those from the literature. Clear and dark cells have been found, including scattered small aggregates of lymphocyte-like, round, undifferentiated cells. A scanty rough endoplasmic reticulum (RER), inconspicuous Golgi zones, few mitochondria, numerous intracytoplasmic microfilaments, some lipid droplets, and lysosomes, desmosomes, and maculae adherentes between spindle cells and junctional complexes have been noted.

DISCUSSION

Our clinicopathologic experience with epithelioid sarcoma, together with all of the accumulated information from the literature, does not preclude new developments with regard to this neoplasm. Clinical observations and follow-up on living patients continue to reveal new, exuberant aspects in the natural potential and biology of the neoplasm. The list of sites of primary tumors and the distribution of metastases continues to enlarge. In fact, epithelioid sarcoma has been found recently in such unexpected places as the vulva[32-34] and penis.[35-36] Moreover, Ratnam and Naik,[37] in Zambia, described a case of epithelioid sarcoma which clinically resembled sporotrichosis. Schiffman[38] has described the unique coexistence of epithelioid sarcoma and synovial sarcoma in the same knee. The author noted that while this might be relevant to the histogenesis of epithelioid sarcoma, he could not rule out simple coincidence.

The recurrence rate of epithelioid sarcoma is high and, on the basis of our experience with the data from the literature, ranges from 70 to 80 percent. The neoplasm usually recurs locally before metastasizing, and the metastatic rate is variable (20 to 40 percent).

Early, wide local excision should be the treatment of choice for epithelioid sarcoma before lymph node metastases develop. However, one patient from our series (Case 11) died of blood-borne metastasis without clinical evidence of lymph node involvement. Another patient died of lung metastasis after a primary lesion in the hand was cured. Extensive chest-wall involvement and lung metastases arose from axillary metastases (Case 7).

Comparison of the results of various surgical procedures is difficult to make. Wide local excision, especially in the hand, is sometimes ineffective owing to anatomic limitations. Radical surgery should be applied in all cases when there is doubt about the effectiveness of local treatment. Radiation therapy seems to us of little value. Too few cases have been treated by chemotherapy to evaluate the usefulness of this modality.

Most of our cases thus far studied seem to have had a similar, slowly progressive course, with 9 of 14 patients for whom follow-up information was available, having died of disease. Undoubtedly, a better understanding of the natural history of epithelioid sarcoma will generate more effective local treatment and better survival rates.

In view of the unsettled question of the histogenesis of epithelioid sarcoma, the exact cell origin of this neoplasm is still uncertain, and is the subject of further investigation. The authors are of the opinion that the tumors in the disease arise from a small, primitive mesenchymal cell related to fibroblastic elements of the fascia, aponeuroses, and tendinous insertions. In the course of differentiation, this cell may represent a modified fibrohistiocytic cell.

The etiology of the tumors in epithelioid sarcoma is also unknown, and it is debatable whether trauma may play a role in their genesis.[1,21,39] One often finds a history of injury in recorded cases, and manual workers, as first shown by Laskowski,[1] constitute a large percentage of patients with this tumor.

REFERENCES

1. Laskowski J: Sarcoma aponeuroticum. Nowotwory 11:61–67, 1961
2. Laskowski J: Aponeurotic sarcoma. Polish Med J 10:12–17, 1971
3. Enzinger FM: Epithelioid sarcoma. A sarcoma simulating a granuloma or a cancer. Cancer 26:1029–1041, 1970
4. Mackenzie DH: Two types of soft tissue sarcoma of uncertain histogenesis. Br J Cancer 25:458–461, 1971
5. Heppenstall RB, Yvars MF, Chung SMK: Epithelioid sarcoma. Two case reports. J Bone Joint Surg 54A:802–806, 1972
6. Nelson FR, Craford BE: Epithelioid sarcoma. A case report. J Bone Joint Surg 54A:798–801, 1972
7. Males JL, Lain KC: Epithelioid sarcoma in XO/XX Turner's syndrome. Arch Pathol 94:214–216, 1972
8. Santiago J, Feinerman LK, Lattes R: Epithelioid sarcoma: A clinical and pathologic study of nine cases. Hum Pathol 3:133–147, 1972
9. Soule EH, Enriquez P: Atypical fibrous histiocytoma, malignant fibrous histiocytoma, malignant histiocytoma, and epithelioid sarcoma. A comparative study of 65 tumors. Cancer 30:128–143, 1972
10. Linell F, Myhre-Jensen O, Osteberg G, Carstam N: Epithelioid sarcoma. Review and report of two cases. Acta Pathol Microbiol Scand (A) 236:21–26, 1973
11. Seemeyer TA, Dionne PG, Tabah EJ: Epithelioid sarcoma. Can J Surg 17:37–42, 1974
12. Bryan RS, Soule DH, Dobyns JH, et al.: Primary epithelioid sarcoma of the hand and forearm. A review of thirteen cases. J Bone Joint Surg 56A:458–465, 1974
13. Kuchemann K: Epithelioid sarcoma. Beitr Pathol Bd 155:84–89, 1975
14. Lo HH, Kalisher L, Faix JD: Epithelioid sarcoma: Radiologic and pathologic manifestations. Am J Radiol 128:1017–1020, 1977
15. Smolianikov AV: Epithelioid sarcoma. Arch Pathol 40:8–13, 1978
16. Pilla G, Pagani PA, Boriani S: Epithelioid sarcoma (Review of the literature and case report). Chir Organi Mov 64:99–103, 1978
17. Boyes JG, Marroum MC: Epithelioid sarcoma of hand and forearm. Hand 10:302–305, 1978
18. Berger L: Synovial sarcomas in serous bursae and tendon sheaths. Am J Cancer 34:501–508, 1938
19. DeSanto DA, Tennant R, Rosahn PD: Synovial sarcomas in joints bursae and tendon sheaths. A clinical and pathological study of 16 cases. Surg Gynecol Obstet 72:951–981, 1941
20. Bliss BO, Reed RJ: Large cell sarcomas of tendon sheath. Malignant giant cell tumors of tendon sheath. Am J Clin Pathol 49:776–781, 1968
21. Prat J, Woodruff JM, Marcove RC: Epithelioid sarcoma: an analysis of 22 cases indicating the prognostic significance of vascular invasion and regional lymph node metastasis. Cancer 41:1472–1487, 1978
22. Fisher ER, Horvat B: The fibrocytic derivation of so-called epithelioid sarcoma. Cancer 30:1074–1084, 1972
23. Gabbiani G, Fu YS, Kaye GI, et al.: Epithelioid sarcoma. A light and electron microscopic study suggesting a synovial origin. Cancer 30:486–498, 1972
24. Bloustein PA, Silverberg SG, Waddell WR: Epithelioid sarcoma. Case report with ultrastructural review, histogenetic discussion and chemotherapeutic data. Cancer 38:2390–2400, 1976
25. Patchefsky AS, Soriano R, Kostianovsky M: Epithelioid sarcoma. Ultrastructural similarity to nodular synovitis. Cancer 39:143–152, 1977
26. Medenica M, Casas C, Lorincz AL, Van Dam DP: Epithelioid sarcoma. Ultrastructural observation of lymphoid cell-induced lysis of tumor cells. Acta Derm Venereol (Stockh.) 59:333–339, 1979

27. Szadowska A: Value of ultrastructural studies in the diagnosis of malignant soft tissue tumors. Pol Tyg Lek 34:1249–1251, 1979
28. Akiyama T, Honda T, Mori M, Yoshida H: A case of epithelioid sarcoma. J Dermatol (Tokyo) 6:309–315, 1979
29. Hajdu SI, Shiu MH, Fortner JG: Tendosynovial sarcoma: A clinicopathological study of 136 cases. Cancer 39:1201–1217, 1977
30. Pietrow D, Dabska M, Jeziorska M: Ultrastructure of epithelioid sarcoma. Nowotwory (In press).
31. Dabska M, Buraczewski J: An unusual case of epithelioid sarcoma of the mid-interosseous membrane of the forearm eradicated by x-ray treatment (26-year follow-up). Nowotwory (In press).
32. Piver MS, Tsukada Y, Barlow J: Epithelioid sarcoma of the vulva. Obstet Gynecol 40:839–842, 1972
33. Gallup PG, Abell MR, Morley GW: Epithelioid sarcoma of the vulva. Obstet Gynecol (Suppl.) 48:14–17, 1976
34. Hall DJ, Grimes MM, Goplerud DR: Epithelioid sarcoma of the vulva. Gynecol Oncol 9:237–246, 1980
35. Moore SW, Wheeler JE, Hefter LG: Epithelioid sarcoma masquerading as Peyronie's disease. Cancer 35:1706–1710, 1975
36. Iossifides I, Ayala AG, Johnson DE: Epithelioid sarcoma of the penis. Urology 14:190–191, 1979
37. Ratnam AU, Naik KG: Epithelioid sarcoma. A case report. Br J Dermatol 99:451–453, 1978
38. Schiffman R: Epithelioid sarcoma and synovial sarcoma in the same knee. Cancer 45:158–166, 1980
39. Jefferiss CD, Caldwell RA: Epithelioid sarcoma. Case report of a young musician's hand. Hand 6:208–210, 1974

SOFT TISSUE SARCOMAS

Classification and Treatment (A Symposium)

GERALD FINE, STEVEN I. HAJDU,
DONALD L. MORTON, FREDERICK R. EILBER,
HERMAN D. SUIT, AND SHARON W. WEISS

1. What guidelines should be recommended for the biopsy of a soft-tissue tumor? Are there situations in which clinical features may influence the type of biopsy? Is needle biopsy appropriate? Should a frozen section be performed? How reliable is incisional biopsy for classification and grading? Are there data on the frequency with which diagnoses made by incisional biopsy are altered (change in classification and/or grade) when the entire tumor is available for study?

Dr. Fine: Since the therapy of a soft-tissue mass is predicated on the nature of the tumor, it is imperative that one establish its histogenesis (if possible), histologic grade, and clinical stage prior to the institution of definitive therapy. Examination of representative tumor tissue is the goal of the biopsy, and the method of obtaining it—whether needle aspiration or incisional or excisional biopsy—will be influenced by the location and size of the tumor and the experience of the surgeon and pathologist.[1,2] Excision of the tumor will yield the greatest volume of tissue for examination, but unless the tumor is small and superficial, and in a location that will permit its removal with a good margin of "normal" tissue surrounding it, the excisional procedure is apt to open new avenues for local and distant tumor dissemination. Incisional biopsy of large tumors situated deep to the superficial fascia or fungating through the skin should be done to provide sufficient tissue for histogenetic classification and grading of the tumor, but is fraught with problems of tumor spillage, bleeding, etc. It is imperative that tumor tissue, and not just reactive or capsular tissue, be removed. Tissue showing the relationship of the tumor to the peripheral tissue may provide valuable information regarding the growth of the tumor, as in myositis ossificans versus osteogenic sarcoma. Needle or aspiration biopsy is the simplest method for obtaining tissue, but is least apt to provide histogenetic and grading information because of the size of the specimen and inexperience of the pathologist in interpreting such material.

Regardless of the biopsy method employed, it is imperative that the specimen removed be handled gently and promptly, with representative tissue being fixed quickly and appropriately for light- and electron microscopy and, if sufficient tissue is available, tissue being quick-frozen for storage and use in cytochemical techniques requiring unfixed tissue.

Frozen-section diagnosis can be used for verifying the presence of tumor tissue in a biopsy specimen, and in the institution of immediate definitive therapy. The latter will depend upon the quantity of material obtained for examination and the pathologist's experience in interpreting this type of preparation.

I am unaware of studies comparing the accuracy of tumor classification and grading from the examination of aspiration biopsies or from paraffin and frozen sections of incisional biopsies with paraffin sections of resected tumors. I believe there would be greater accuracy of histogenetic classification and tumor grading using paraffin sections of incisional biopsies than from aspiration biopsy or frozen sections. Influencing factors would be the size of the biopsy specimen, the type and size of the tumor, the quality of the section, and the experience of the pathologist. Differences in histologic grading and/or classification in examining paraffin sections of an incisional biopsy and tissue from the resected specimen most likely would result from inadequate tumor sampling (particularly in large tumors), or from poor-quality sections resulting from improper fixation, tissue processing, or staining of the biopsy. The simple failure of adequate eosin staining of cytoplasm may lead to failure of recognition of a rhabdomyosarcoma.

Dr. Hajdu: The biopsy of a previously undiagnosed soft-tissue tumor must be generous and representative. Minute tissue pieces are inadequate; as Senn[3] said: "The greatest blunders in diagnosis and treatment have been committed by surgeons through placing too great reliance on the microscopic examination of fragments of tumor-tissue." Whether a biopsy is to be an incisional or excisional biopsy must be decided by the operating surgeon, through consideration of the size, location, and clinical appearance of the tumor. I would also hope that the biopsy be done by a surgeon familiar with soft-tissue neoplasms.

I do not recommend needle biopsy as a diagnostic technique for previously undiagnosed soft-tissue tumors. The hazards of diagnosis of soft-tissue tumors from a needle aspirate are due to sampling errors and to the limited amount of histologic structure in the tissue fragments that may be in the aspirate. However, familiarity with the cytomorphology of soft-tissue tumors is useful when recurrence or metastasis are suspected. Familiarity with the cytomorphology can also be rewarding at the time of local resection of bulky soft-tissue sarcomas, when the operating surgeon is in need of assistance in order to assess the resection margins, especially bone margins. It is essential that the cytologic interpretation be made with full knowledge of the clinical history and prior diagnosis, and it is advisable to have all prior material available for comparison. If there is a dissimilarity between the prior tissue biopsy and cytologic material, then it may be best to rely on an open biopsy.[4,5] Of historic interest is that the first soft-tissue sarcoma diagnosed from an aspirate, interpreted by Surgeon General Woodward as "round celled sarcoma," was recorded by Hamilton.[5]

Frozen section of soft-tissue neoplasms should not be used for the sake of satisfying a curious surgeon or as a tool to frustrate pathologists. As far as I am concerned, a therapeutic decision based on a frozen section of a soft-tissue neoplasm should be discouraged. Undoubtedly there will always be situations in which the pathologist's services are required by the operating surgeon; nevertheless, the pathologist must find a way in which to communicate to the surgeon that frozen sections shall not be done; (1) unless the selection of a modality of treatment, e.g., amputation vs. wide excision, is influenced by the result of frozen section; and (2) unless the pathologist is fully informed about the clinical history, clinicopathologic findings, clinical diagnosis, and modality of surgical treatment contemplated in a given case.

Drs. Morton and Eilber: It is our feeling that a biopsy should be done only after a careful history and complete physical examination of the patient. It should be remembered that the purpose of a biopsy is to obtain tissue for accurate histopathologic interpretation, while at the same time causing as little tissue disruption as possible. The type of biopsy (incisional versus needle) does not appear to be a crucial factor for treatment outcome but excisional biopsy is contraindicated for all except small superficial sarcomas. It should be mentioned that needle biopsies are certainly appropriate if the pathologist in the institution is accustomed to reading and interpreting the tumor type on the basis of such small samples. We prefer an incisional biopsy, but it is mandatory that the surgeon doing the biopsy be well aware of the different operative procedures necessary to surgically extirpate tumors biopsied by incision, in order to place the biopsy incision where it can be completely excised with the definitive operation. Horizontal biopsy incisions in the extremity are mentioned only to be condemned; all biopsies should be done in a vertical manner. If the tumor is suspected of being malignant, sufficient tissue for diagnosis is all that is required from the biopsy. All too often the surgeon does an excisional biopsy of a very large, firm tumor only to find on pathologic examination that the tumor is malignant. The disturbance of tissue planes and the absence of the definitive mass makes a subsequent definitive surgical procedure much more difficult. We do perform frozen sections on biopsies to confirm that we have representative tissue and that the tumor is malignant. We do not rely on frozen section for an exact histopathologic diagnosis or to determine the grade of a tumor.

Exact information on the reliability of incisional biopsy for classification and grading is not clear. In our experience grading on the basis of an incisional biopsy has been accurate. Clearly, if a patient has a grade 3 tumor, regardless of whether there are grade 1 elements in the lesion, the overall prognosis and treatment must be based on the higher-grade classification. We have found that only 5 percent of biopsies will show a low-grade tumor, when, in fact, the histology of the resected specimens will indicate a lesion of higher grade. This grading difference occurs often in the neurofibrosarcomas, and histologic grading of these tumors is not too valuable. In several instances tumors have been called either benign neurofibroma or grade 1 neurofibrosarcoma, whereas at excision grade 3 elements were found.

Dr. Suit: The biopsy should be planned after the patient has had a complete history, physical examination, laboratory study, and radiographic evaluation. The radiographic evaluation of the primary site (suspected of being malignant) should include, as a minimum, soft-tissue films of the affected part, xerograms, and/or computerized body tomographic studies. In many instances arteriographic study is appropriate. The point here is that the evaluation of the lesion should be complete and comprehensive. The findings of these studies should be helpful in planning the site and character of the biopsy.

In general, the plan for biopsy of a soft-tissue tumor suspected of being a malignancy should be based on the following considerations: the object of the biopsy procedure is to provide adequate material to establish the histopathologic nature of the lesion, and to do this in a manner which will in no way compromise the ultimate definitive treatment of the patient should the lesion prove malignant. This means that the biopsy should be so sited and of such a length and character that if subsequent surgery is performed, the specimen with the biopsy scar can be readily excised in one procedure and that the requisite inclusion of the biopsy scar present no problems with the surgical resection, preparation of flaps, etc. The biopsy scar should be small, i.e., 1 to 2 cm; a longer incision is unnecessary, and a short scar presents minimal problems for the subsequent definitive treatment. Meticulous attention should be paid to hemostasis; the flow of blood along tissue spaces could reasonably be expected to carry with it tumor cells, and hence to spread tumor along previously uninvolved tissue planes. A short biopsy incision, closed with secure hemostasis, eliminates any requirement for drains and facilitates healing by primary intention. A small lesion, say of the order of 1 to 2 cm and which is considered to be benign or possibly malignant, could most reasonably be biopsied by an excisional approach. Again, the incisional scar should be small, and special attention should be paid to achieving hemostasis. A portion of the material obtained during the biopsy should be fixed in glutaraldehyde to permit electron-micrographic studies to be performed at a later time if indicated.

For virtually all primary sarcomas of soft tissue, my strong preference is that the patient have an incisional biopsy as described above, and that interpretations of paraffin sections be made available with respect to histopathologic type and histopathologic grade before planning the definitive treatment of the patient. A good specimen is required to prepare a first-quality paraffin section and to have some material for possible electron microscopic study. Needle biopsy specimens are not adequate for establishing the histologic type and grade of a sarcoma in an important proportion of attempts. A needle biopsy is appropriate only where the treatment would not be modified by the histologic diagnosis. This may obtain in some situations in which radical surgery or amputation is to be performed independent of the histology, and in which the only requirement is to establish that there is a mesenchymal sarcoma. This is most unusual in the treatment of a patient with a primary sarcoma. Needle biopsy is an entirely appropriate and reasonable method for the biopsy of suspected metastatic lesions for the purpose of confirming that the metastatic lesion is in fact malignant and probably of sarcomatous origin.

The planning of definitive treatment should be based on a paraffin section and not on a frozen section. Frozen-section material does not give an adequately high quality for determining the histopathologic type or grade of a tumor in virtually all instances. Nor are mistakes rare in the reading of frozen sections. For example, a lesion of low-grade malignancy may be read as benign and be the basis for inappropriate surgery.

Dr. Weiss: In my opinion the type of biopsy of a soft-tissue lesion is influenced by its size and location. Small or superficial lesions should be removed by excisional biopsy, whereas large or deeply situated tumors often lend themselves best to incisional biopsy. Obviously incisional biopsy may not always be representative of the lesion as a whole, but it does provide the most reasonable approach to the diagnosis of large lesions in which total excision would cause significant morbidity. Regardless of the approach used, care should be exerted to minimize contamination of the surrounding tissue and to plan the biopsy site in such a way that it can be totally removed by a definitive excision. I believe that, in contrast to the case for both excisional and incisional biopsy, the use of needle biopsy should be restricted. I often recall the analogy Dr. Lichtenstein drew between reading a needle biopsy and riding a bicycle with your hands tied behind your back, and prefer not to interpret such material for several reasons: The needle biopsy is less apt to be representative of the lesion as a whole and, therefore, may lead to errors in grading. Second, it may not yield sufficient tissue to perform special stains or electron microscopy in cases in which these procedures may be indicated. Finally, needle biopsy is particularly risky in certain types of soft-tissue lesion in which the pathologist relies heavily on the pattern of the overall lesion rather than on the features of the constituent cells. This is especially true of cellular forms of fasciitis characterized by large numbers of mitoses, and of neurilemomas possessing large, pleomorphic giant cells. Conversely, certain sarcomas may contain areas which, out of context, could be interpreted as benign. A good example of this is the myxoid malignant fibrous histiocytoma, which is often interpreted as a myxoma or nodular fasciitis when only small amounts of material are available. Therefore, I believe that needle biopsy is best reserved for: (1) patients who already have a diagnosis of tumor and in whom one merely wishes to confirm the presence or absence of tumor in a local or metastatic site; or (2) individuals who simply cannot undergo surgery. Once a biopsy is performed it is obviously necessary to perform a frozen section if definitive surgery is to be done at the same time. However, it is also appropriate if the surgeon wishes assurance that he has viable, lesional tissue.

2. Is a definitive histogenetic diagnosis of a soft-tissue sarcoma essential for the management of the tumor? Is it possible to do away with the histogenetic classification of soft-part sarcomas, and to replace this with a system of grading as a guide to prognosis and treatment? What features are

important for the grading and staging of soft-part sarcomas? Does the grade of a sarcoma change in the course of the disease? How often? Is this likely to be influenced by therapy?

Dr. Hajdu: It seems to me that everybody, from the time Virchow,[7] in 1858, introduced the term "histogenesis," has considered it important to establish the histogenesis of neoplasms. Ewing,[8] for example, wrote in the second edition of his book that "The final classfication of tumors must depend chiefly on histogenesis and structure." And Gilford,[9] in 1925, wrote that "without biological understanding of cancer we cannot hope for a real and lasting solution of the problem." It seems obvious that no progress can be made in therapy without knowing the histogenesis, cell type, and natural history of soft-tissue sarcomas. In not considering the histogenesis of soft-tissue sarcomas at the time of treatment selection, clinicians would be like a driver without a road map on a cross-country tour. Who would deny that the precise histogenetic diagnosis of highly radiosensitive neoplasms such as myxoid liposarcoma or embryonal rhabdomyosarcoma is not important? Would it be proper to ignore that certain neoplasms, e.g., epithelioid sarcoma, Kaposi's sarcoma, lymphangiosarcoma, and certain peripheral nerve tumors—owing to their histogenesis—have a tendency to be multifocal? Similarly, can it be ignored that such neoplasms as embryonal rhabdomyosarcoma, epithelioid sarcoma, and angiosarcoma quite readily metastasize to regional lymph nodes? Certainly not without grave consequences.

I think pathologists should be as precise as possible in their histogenetic subclassification of soft-tissue neoplasms and, as I state in my answer to question 4, they may have to rely on ultrastructural, histochemical, and light microscopic findings for such precision.[10]

Any attempt at the grading and staging of soft-tissue sarcomas must be made after the histogenesis and histologic type of the neoplasm have been established. Without considering the histogenesis and histologic type of soft-tissue sarcomas, one may end up by comparing apples with oranges. Admittedly there will always be a neoplasm that defies all attempts at subclassficiation, in which case it is perhaps justified to depend solely on the grade and stage of the neoplasm. Table 1 shows that the case fatality rate in soft-tissue sarcomas of identical stage varies according to histologic type.

Although soft-tissue neoplasms, just like epithelial neoplasms, can be benign or malignant, in situ soft-tissue sarcoma, a stage analogous to carcinoma in situ, is not recognized. Because the in situ or preinvasive form of soft-tissue sarcomas is not recognized, and because soft-tissue sarcomas vary significantly in structure and behavior, the grading and staging of soft-tissue sarcomas are necessary in order to express their malignant potentials.

The first grading system for soft-tissue sarcomas was introduced by Quick and Cutler[11] in 1927. Ewing,[12] in 1931, said that "the grade of potential malignancy is very important information." It is surprising to me now, looking back, that despite general agreement that there is a difference in the malignancy of soft-tissue sarcomas according to their histologic type, size, site, and degree of differentiation;[6,12,13]

TABLE 1. Case Fatality Rate of Soft-Tissue Sarcomas According to Histologic Type and Stage of Primary Tumor During a Period of 25 Years

Histologic Type	Total No. of Cases Staged*	Stage and Mortality in (%)*					
		I†	(%)	II†	(%)	III†	(%)
Malignant fibroblastic fibrous histiocytoma‡	130	1/76	(1)	7/42	(16)	11/12	(92)
Malignant histiocytic fibrous histiocytoma§	24	0/8	(0)	1/3	(33)	12/13	(92)
Malignant pleomorphic fibrous histiocytoma	125	0/9	(0)	12/32	(38)	60/84	(71)
Desmoid tumor	160	2/58	(3)	15/102	(15)	-	-
Fibrosarcoma‖	114	1/4	(25)	16/42	(38)	52/68	(76)
Tendosynovial sarcoma	120	1/3	(33)	26/66	(39)	48/51	(94)
Liposarcoma	220	1/9	(11)	26/98	(27)	75/113	(68)
Embryonal rhabdomyosarcoma	240	-	-	35/58	(60)	137/182	(75)
Pleomorphic rhabdomyosarcoma	88	-	-	12/21	(57)	62/67	(93)
Hemangiosarcoma#	30	1/6	(17)	7/8	(88)	15/16	(94)
Neurogenic sarcoma**	80	9/16	(56)	22/29	(76)	33/35	(94)
Total	1331	16/189	(8)	179/501	(36)	505/641	(79)

* Patients who were admitted with metastatic tumor are not included. Also excluded are 17 patients who had stage 0 tumor. Twelve of the 17 excluded patients had malignant fibrous histiocytoma and 5 patients had desmoid tumor. All 17 patients who had stage 0 sarcoma are alive and well.
† Numerator: died with disease; denominator: total number of patients.
‡ These are all dermatofibrosarcoma protuberans cases except for the 12 stage III tumors.
§ These are all malignant giant-cell tumors of soft tissue.
‖ Fibrosarcoma other than desmoid.
Kaposi's sarcoma is not included.
** Includes malignant collagenous and noncollagenous schwannomas.
(Reproduced from: Hajdu SI: Pathology of Soft Tissue Tumors. 1979. Courtesy of Lea and Febiger, publisher.)

the Soft Tissue Task Force of the American Joint Committee on Cancer Staging and End Result Reporting did not consider the anatomic site in its grading and staging scheme.[14]

In the staging system that I proposed[10] in 1979, soft-tissue sarcomas were classified according to histologic type, size, site, and histologic grade of the tumor. Once the size, site, and histologic grade are defined, the stage of the primary tumor can be estimated. I would like to point out that for the sake of simplicity and practical application, the sarcomas were graded either as low grade or high grade by considering their cellularity, differentiation, amount of stroma and necrosis, and number of mitosis. It should be noted that the number of mitotic figures is just one of the five factors that should be considered at the time of grading of any given sarcoma. The value of the mitotic count has been debated from the time Williams[15] pointed out in 1908 that "the nuclei of the cells of malignant tumors frequently originate mitoses." Unfortunately, the mitotic count is subjective and unreliable because certain nonneoplastic lesions, e.g., pyogenic granuloma, may have more mitotic figures than most of the fully malignant soft-tissue sarcomas.

In reference to the last part of this question, I say that in my experience most recurrent and metastatic soft-tissue sarcomas are more cellular, more vascular, and less differentiated than the corresponding primary neoplasms.

Dr. Fine: Over a period of years there has evolved a histogenetic classification of soft-tissue tumors based on growth pattern and cytology, the latter having been greatly augmented by electron microscopy. Such a classification has aided in the recognition of differences in biologic behavior among soft tissue neoplasms formerly inseparable because of their being grouped as spindle-cell, round-cell or pleomorphic sarcomas, and has resulted in a variable therapeutic approach to these neoplasms. The therapy of soft-tissue sarcoma has changed over the years, and no doubt will change further as advances are made in oncology, surgery, and radiotherapy.

But although the histogenetic classification of soft-tissue sarcomas should be pursued in order to obtain information regarding tumor response to various therapeutic modalities instituted singly or in combination, it is not the only nor the most important parameter at this time for the management of a soft-tissue neoplasm. As important, if not more so, is the grading and staging of the tumor. In most instances, once the diagnosis of sarcoma has been established, aggressiveness of the neoplasm, indicated by its histologic grade and clinical stage, will dictate the management in a particular case. A number of examples are supportive of this as follows:

First, the poorly differentiated neoplasm in which there is agreement as to its sarcomatous nature but disagreement as to its histogenesis. Management of the pleomorphic tumor formerly classified as a rhabdomyosarcoma or pleomorphic liposarcoma, and which is now considered by many as malignant fibrous histiocytoma, has not changed because of the change in thought regarding its histogenesis, but has changed with the grade and stage of the tumor. Second, a grade 3 spindle-cell sarcoma with focal hyalinized areas might be interpreted as fibrosarcoma, monophasic synovial sarcoma, or osteogenic sarcoma by different observers, but its management would be influenced by its grade and stage. There are exceptions to the above; the small round-cell tumors—embryonal rhabdomyosarcoma, neuroblastoma, malignant lymphoma, neurectodermal tumor, and extraskeletal Ewing's sarcoma—in which differences in response to chemotherapy and/or radiation therapy have made their recognition more meaningful.[16,17] Perhaps in the future therapeutic protocols may reveal differences in response among the various spindle-cell and pleomorphic sarcomas to various therapeutic modalities, making a histogenetic classification among these tumors more meaningful in their management.

A guide to prognosis and treatment could be developed on the basis of a grading and staging system for soft-tissue sarcomas, but the addition of a histogenetic classification to these two parameters provides a more complete approach to evaluation of the prognosis and treatment of these neoplasms. Support for this is found in the studies of Hajdu and that of the Soft Tissue Task Force.[14,35] Unless one is able to segregate neoplasms into as pure groups as possible, one cannot hope to gain reliable information concerning their response to various therapeutic modalities which are and will be employed singly or in combination.

The management and prognosis of soft-tissue neoplasms are predicated on their clinical behavior, which in turn is the result of an interaction of a number of factors (Fig. 1). It is apparent from past, and particularly from more recent studies, that the grading and staging of soft-tissue neoplasms are an important guide to their management and prognosis, just as it is in epithelial neoplasms. The features to be considered in the grading of soft-tissue tumors are those that have long been accepted: cell anaplasia or differentiation, frequency and abnormality of mitosis, and the quantity and maturity of tissues produced by the tumor, including fibrous tissue, cartilage, bone, and adipose tissue. Staging of the neoplasm should be combined with histologic grading in order to arrive at the most accurate appraisal of the tumor's potential. To be considered in staging are the size of the tumor and its relationship to the superficial fascia, its infiltrating qualities, its relationship to surrounding tissues such as nerve, bone and other organs, and its spread to regional lymph nodes and distant sites. But while grading has been a part of the study of soft-tissue neoplasms for a number of years, the value of combined grading and staging has more recently been emphasized.

Spontaneous histologic changes occur during the course of mesenchymal neoplasms, but I believe that these are infrequent and are often difficult to establish to everyone's satisfaction. The changes in long-standing primary and locally recur-

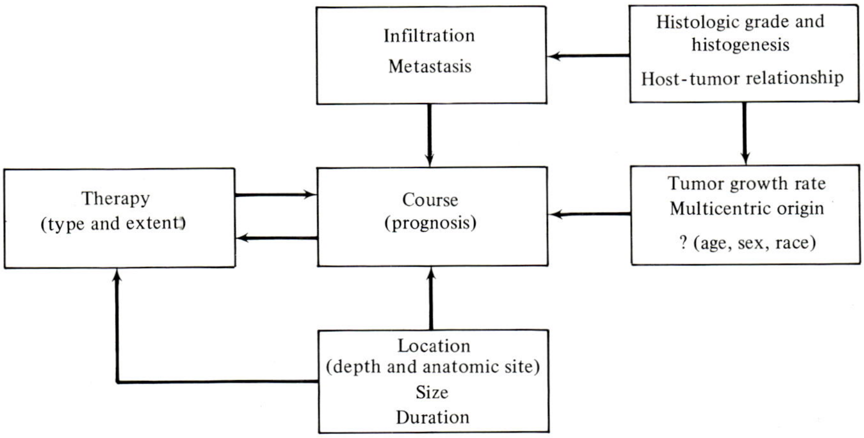

FIG. 1. Factors influencing the clinical course and therapy of soft-tissue sarcomas.

rent growths have been of three types: (1) dedifferentiation from benign to malignant as in the change of myositis ossificans to osteogenic sarcoma, of neurofibroma to neurofibrosarcoma, of lipoma to liposarcoma, of desmoid to fibrosarcoma, and of a variety of benign mesenchymal bone tumors to sarcoma; (2) change from a low-grade to a higher-grade malignancy as in the so-called parosteal osteoma (parosteal osteogenic sarcoma) to osteogenic sarcoma of higher-grade malignancy or of differentiated fibrosarcoma (grade 1) to grade 3 fibrosarcoma; and (3) changes in histologic type as seen among the tenosynovial sarcomas.[18-21] In some cases metastases may differ, at least in part, from the primary tumor. Evidence of differentiation, as in the rhabdomyoblastic, chondroid, or osseous tumors; change in histologic type, as seen in the tenosynovial sarcomas and dedifferentiation, as in classical sacrococcygeal chordoma to an anaplastic spindle-and giant-cell tumor, may all occur. Among soft-tissue sarcomas, histologic changes resulting from chemotherapy and/or radiotherapy apparently have had little investigation, judging from the lack of published material on this subject. The effect of x-irradiation on normal tissue, its role in the production of soft tissue and bone sarcomas secondary to the therapy of carcinoma, and its influence in the malignant transformation of a variety of benign mesenchymal bone lesions have been observed.[18,20,21]

Dr. Weiss: There is little question that a valid system of grading for sarcomas is greatly needed as part of a general staging system. Unfortunately it is not yet possible to abandon our current histogenetic classification of sarcomas in favor of a grading system, for two reasons:

First there is no universally accepted grading system. Many clinicians and pathologists probably have inferred that such a system exists, as a result of the recent publication, by the Soft Tissue Task Force, on the staging of sarcomas. However, the authors of this paper are careful to point out that their determination of grade was an "assessment of malignancy by an experienced pathologist *based on histological and other features of the tumor*."[14] The major obstacle in devising a grading system has been that there are no histologic features equally applicable to all sarcomas in assigning a grade. For example, mitotic figures may constitute the most important histologic feature in determing the grade of most fibrosarcomas, but may be less emphasized in evaluating malignant fibrous histiocytomas, and are essentially meaningless in evaluating rhabdomyosarcomas. Moreover, some tumors, such as the epithelioid sarcoma, are difficult to grade reliably and are perhaps best segregated altogether from other forms of sarcoma.

The second problem in utilizing any grading system is that we currently do not have sufficient data to know whether sarcomas of comparable grade and stage have the same behavior and therapeutic response regardless of their histogenetic type. Some studies suggest that this may be true; however, additional data are needed before grading can supplant a histogenetic classification.

For the present, both a histogenetic category and an attempted grade would seem to be the most appropriate method of diagnosing sarcomas. However, it should be emphasized that not all sarcomas can be classified. In our experience about 10 percent of sarcomas are too poorly differentiated to permit their classification. In such instances it is usually sufficient to indicate whether a tumor is of high or low grade—a judgement usually made on the basis of a combination of cellularity, mitotic activity, and pleomorphism. This distinction usually provides sufficient information to the clinician to permit therapy to be instituted.

Dr. Suit: Although the histopathologic grade is the single most important determinant of prognosis that can be gleaned from the histologic study of a biopsy specimen, information regarding the histogenetic diagnosis is valuable in planning treatment. Although certain tumors—such as embryonal or alveolar rhabdomyosarcoma—are almost always high-grade with the probability of metastatic disease hence being inferable from knowing either the histopathologic type or the grade of the lesion, there are tumors which histologically may be assessed as low-grade but nonetheless have a high potential for metastatic disease and an ultimate fatal outcome. This would particularly include the angiosarcomas.[14] Certain sarcomas may be quite low-grade or innocent-appearing histopathologically, i.e., just barely distinguishable from a simple angioma on a histologic basis, but may nonetheless exhibit a high tendency to metastasis. The clinican may be provided important information regarding patterns of likely spread if the histogenetic diagnosis is given. For example, malignant schwannoma is a tumor that is more likely to infiltrate along nerve trunks, and hence the distinction between malignant schwannoma and a fibrosarcoma would be valuable. The distinction between a malignant synovioma and a fibrosarcoma around the wrist would cause concern about the likely extent of tumor along tendon sheaths in the former but not in the latter, even though the tumor were low-grade. As another example, epithelioid sarcomas have an unusually high tendency to metastasize to regional lymph nodes.[22] The first task of the pathologist is to provide the best statement of the histogenetic diagnosis, and the next and most important task is to estimate the histopathologic grade of a tumor. This is because the grade of malignancy is the best guide to the frequency of development of metastatic disease.

In order to assess the histopathologic grade of a soft-tissue sarcoma, the pathologist should have first-quality histologic slides with appropriate stains, and access to the block in order to prepare special stains as indicated. The determination of histopathologic grade requires that the pathologist review several sections and consider all histologic features of the tumor. These include cellularity, the abundance of extracellular material, cellular and nuclear pleomorphism, mitotic index, pattern of infiltration into adjacent tissues or structures, and presence of necrosis. The grading of a sarcoma is to an important degree a subjective assessment of the total appearance, and not just of one or two parameters. One of the more important parameters, and the one which is quantitative, is the mitotic index. It would be unusual to classify a lesion with a mitotic count of less than 8 to 10 per 10 high-power fields (HPF) as grade 3. Similarly, a lesion with a mitotic count of less than 1 per 10 HPF is not likely to be classed as grade 2. However, there is considerable overlap in mitotic index for the various grades. For example, a lesion might exhibit 5 mitotic figures per 10 HPF but be classed as grade 3 if the lesion were quite cellular with extensive pleomorphism, necrosis, etc. In contrast, a tumor with a mitotic count of 5 per 10 HPF could be read as grade 1 if the cells were near normal in appearance (minimal pleomorphism), no necrosis, etc. A further consideration in the interpretation of mitotic index is that the mitotic count depends not only upon the proliferative activity of the tumor in vivo, but also the manner in which the specimen is handled, particularly the time between resection and fixation. If there is a long period between resection and fixation, cells may complete the mitotic process, leading to an artificially low mitotic index.

The staging of soft-part sarcomas depends not only on histopathologic grade but on the size of the lesion, the pattern of infiltration into adjacent structures, and the presence of disease in regional lymph nodes or distant sites. Tumor size determines whether the T stage is T1 (<5 cm) or T2 (≥ 5 cm). The primary lesion should be examined for evidence of invasion of major vessels, nerves, or bone, which would mean that the lesion is T3. I do not accept a positive bone scan as proof of the invasion of bone by a tumor. Invasion of bone is diagnosed only upon clear evidence of bone destruction on bone films or CT scan. Invasion of nerves or vessels can best be determined at surgery, viz., it is quite difficult to distinguish between the invasion of nerve by a tumor and the effects of pressure by a growing tumor even from a careful neurologic examination. CBT and/or arteriographic studies may be helpful in demonstrating complete encasement of a vessel by tumor, hence making it a stage T3 tumor. Radiographic evidence must be unambiguous in order to justify upstaging to T3. To classify a patient as N1 requires histologic proof of metastasis to the regional node. Demonstration of a distant metastatic lesion by clinical or radiographic examination puts the patient in stage M1. If there is only one metastasis demonstrated, this should be confirmed histologically. This is stated because an occasional case will be incorrectly staged as M1, and not given the appropriate therapy for a true M0 lesion.

Although the frequency with which a sarcoma changes its character during the course of the disease cannot be stated, it is not rare for a recurrent lesion to be diagnosed as a soft-tissue sarcoma at the site from which a previously benign lesion was resected. This may be so for fibro- or neurofibroma particularly. Further, a recurrent lesion may be of higher grade than the primary. For example, a grade 2 lesion may recur and be a grade 3. The more likely sequence is for the recurrent lesion to be of the same character as the primary lesion. However, the fact that some tumors do recur at a higher grade is a strong stimulus for making every effort toward successful treatment at the first attempt.

Drs. Morton and Eilber: Generally speaking, the most important single factor appears to be the grade of a soft-tissue sarcoma rather than its histogenesis. We mention this only because in our experience there is at least a 30 percent difference of opinion as to the exact histogenesis of various types of soft-tissue sarcomas. Also, the results of retrospective analysis from the American Joint Committee on Staging and End Results appear to indicate that the most influential prognostic factor is the tumor grade rather than its exact histogenesis. The only exceptions to this would be certain types of sarcomas that uniformly carry a poor prognosis and which therefore should be treated with a multimodality approach from the beginning. These types of tumors include synovial sarcomas, adult rhabdomyosarcomas, neurofibrosarcomas, and epithelioid sarcomas. In our experience, epithelioid sarcoma has been a particular problem in that it tends to spread longitudinally for great lengths, with normal intervening tissue. Although this characteristic is shared somewhat by all sarcomas, it has in our hands been a particular problem with epithelioid sarcomas, making it necessary to design the operative procedure for this neoplasm so as to encompass these "skip" areas of normal-appearing intervening tissues both proximally and distally, in order to encompass all areas of potential disease.

We do not feel that it is possible to do away with the histologic classification of soft-tissue sarcomas, since there are some particular histogenetic types of sarcomas that carry a bad prognosis irrespective of grade. However, if one were to treat all sarcomas as if they were highly malignant, regardless of grade, according to our combined-modality preoperative approach, then the histologic classification of soft-tissue sarcomas would become less important. We do not advocate this approach, however, since there are other histologic types of sarcomas that have limited malignant potential and are curable by adequate surgical excision.

In soft-tissue sarcomas, changes in grade have not been reported with any frequency. We have seen patients with osteogenic sarcoma metastatic to the lungs in which biopsy shows the metastasis to be a very poorly differentiated tumor, but in whom, following adriamycin and high-dose methotrexate therapy, the lesion has calcified. Histology would also show the primary osteosarcoma to be very undifferentiated. However, this has not been our experience with the soft-tissue tumors.

3. Does the behavior of soft-tissue sarcomas of apparently similar histogenesis differ among children and adults?

Dr. Weiss: It has been assumed by many that certain soft-tissue sarcomas of childhood enjoy a far better prognosis than their adult counterparts. This generalization has been fostered by several early papers documenting the excellent clinical course of children with "liposarcomas,"[23] "hemangioendotheliomas,"[24] and "histiocytic" tumors.[25] However, by current diagnostic standards, many of these lesions would probably be considered benign. For instance, the lesions reported by Kauffman and Stout[23] as childhood liposarcomas are probably for the most part lipoblastomas. The hemangioendotheliomas are cellular hemangiomas of infancy, and the histiocytic tumors embrace a number of lesions. In fact, there are relatively few sarcomas that occur with sufficient frequency in both children and adults to allow reliable comparisons of their behavior. Neuroblastoma and rhabdomyosarcoma, the two most common childhood sarcomas, are rare in adults.* Malignant fibrous histiocytoma and liposarcoma, the two most common adult sarcomas, rarely occur in the pediatric age group. Perhaps the only histologically comparable tumor occurring in both children and adults and which has been extensively studied is the fibrosarcoma. In this instance there is reasonably convincing evidence that young children with this tumor have a better prognosis than adults. In our experience[26] the so-called infantile fibrosarcoma, despite its presentation as a

*Pleomorphic or adult forms of rhabdomyosarcoma are currently classified as malignant fibrous histiocytoma since they consistently lack evidence, by light- and electron microscopy, of muscle differentiation.

massive enlargement of an extremity, carries a 5-year survival of over 80 percent as compared to 5-year survivals in adult fibrosarcoma that average about 40 percent,[27] depending on certain factors.

Thus, the striking phenomenon in comparing childhood and adult soft-tissue sarcomas lies not so much in differences or similarities in the behavior of comparable sarcomas, but rather in the interesting observation that these two groups develop histologically different types of tumors having little overlap with one another.

Dr. Hajdu: My experience with childhood soft-tissue sarcomas other than embryonal rhabdomyosarcoma, is limited, but it is perhaps worthwhile to point out that in our review[28,29] of tendosynovial sarcomas, we found that the 5-year disease-free survival of children is better (70 percent) than that of adults (40 percent), and that we know that today, embryonal rhabdomyosarcoma in children is a highly curable disease while in adults it carries a 75 percent mortality.[10]

Dr. Suit: This is a very difficult question because of the small number of tumor types that occur with high frequency in both the child and the adult. For example, rhabdomyosarcoma is common in children but most uncommon in adults (age 25 years or greater). Fibrosarcomas are not rare in children and are one of the more common sarcomas of soft tissue in the adult. There are data indicating a better survival among the younger patients with this tumor. Suit et al. reviewed the experience at the Massachusetts General Hospital in the treatment of childhood fibrosarcoma and neurofibrosarcoma by radiation therapy and conservative surgery: the disease-free survival at 1 to 7 years after treatment was 9/9 and 14/24 for patients <21 and ≥ 21 years of age, respectively.[30] This means that more of the older patients developed local regrowth or distant metastasis (there were three young patients each at stages I, II, and III). This better survival rate among young patients with fibrosarcoma has been reported by others.[31]

Dr. Fine: The question of behavioral differences among soft-tissue sarcomas of similar histogenesis in children and adults, with the exception of rhabdomyosarcoma, is difficult to assess because of their infrequency in children and the paucity of published 5-year survival data.[32] It would appear that there is no difference among the various sarcomas that are of similar histogenesis, histologic grade, and stage. Even the data regarding embryonal rhabdomyosarcoma, which is more frequent in children and has been reported to have a poorer 5-year survival rate than the pleomorphic rhabdomyosarcoma which is more frequent in adults, is open to question.[33,34] This difference is not borne out by the data of Hajdu,[35] and it would appear that reevaluation must be undertaken, since it is likely that a number of the pleomorphic rhabdomyosarcomas previously reported would now be classified as malignant fibrous histiocytomas. It is also questionable whether behavioral differences in the sarcomas—if they indeed do exist—can be attributed solely to age differences of the patients, since embryonal rhabdomyosarcoma occurs more commonly in the head and neck and pelvic and retroperitoneal regions—sites less amenable to surgical extirpation of the tumor. In a study of embryonal rhabdomyosarcoma outside of the head and neck region, 5-year survivors who were free of tumor were children, most of whose tumors were in surgically accessible areas—the buttock and the extremities. The adults succumbed to their tumor early in its course, but the location of the tumor was not designated.[36]

Drs. Morton and Eilber: It is our opinion that the tumors in adults and children clearly differ. Rhabdomyosarcoma of childhood is exquisitely sensitive to radiation and vincristine-adriamycin-cyclophosphamide (VAC) chemotherapy, whereas adult rhabdomyosarcomas are not. As far as the other soft-tissue sarcomas are concerned, we do not feel that there is enough information to say that there is a vast difference between the two age groups. With regard to rhabdomyosarcomas, we believe this distinction has to do both with the difference in histogenesis and anatomic location. Rhabdomyosarcomas in children are much more common in the head and neck areas, whereas rhabdomyosarcomas in adults more often occur in an extremity.

4. Does electron microscopy play a primary role in the diagnosis of sarcomas? In what situations do special stains provide useful information?

Dr. Fine: Electron microscopy is a useful procedure in the histogenetic classification of neoplasms, allowing one to discern cell structure that is unidentifiable or questionable at the light-microscopic level. Electron microscopy is helpful in distinguishing poorly differentiated neoplasms, such as sarcomas from poorly differentiated carcinoma, amelanotic melanoma, and other neuroectodermal tumors, and in clarification of the identity of a variety of neoplasms—myogenous, schwannian, histiocytic, tenosynovial, liposarcomatous, and granular cell (alveolar soft part sarcoma, granular cell myoblastoma, and paraganglioma), and neuroblastoma, Ewing's tumor, chordoma, chondrosarcoma, and osteogenic sarcoma. While electron microscopy has proven to be a useful adjunct in tumor classification, it must be used in conjunction with light microscopy in order to be of maximum value. The extent of examination and the degree of tumor differentiation have always been important in classification by light-microscopy, and are equally if not more important in classification by electron microscopy.

The role of histologic stains other than the almost universally employed H&E preparation in the diagnosis and classification of tumors is both inversely and directly related to the experience of the pathologist. Generally speaking, the greater one's experience with the histology of neoplasms, the less one must rely on special techniques for their diagnosis, but by the same token, the more experience one has with special staining procedures, the more helpful these are apt to be. Whether special stains are needed for the classification of a particular neoplasm depends on a variety of factors in addition to the observer's experience and training. Proper classification of a tumor differentiated to the point of forming tissue such as osteoid, cartilage, or striated muscle, or having such characteristic growth patterns as the biphasic appearance of the synovial sarcoma, requires only H&E-stained sections, providing the quantity of tissue for examination and the quality of the preparations are satisfactory. It is the spindle-cell, myxoid, pleomorphic, round-cell, and organoid granular-cell tumors devoid of the previously mentioned characteristics that are most likely to require the use of special stains for identification of their histogenesis. The use of special stains in the identification of soft-tissue sarcomas is more complex than might appear, since poorly differentiated entodermal and ectodermal neoplasms must also occasionally be considered in the differential diagnosis, making it essential for one also to be cognizant of the staining characteristics of these neoplasms. A variety of staining procedures are available, some of which are nonspecific in their mode of action, and others of which are specific histochemical stains. Generally speaking it is only the postitive reaction that has the greatest significance, but since a positive reaction may be found in a variety of tumors, one must, as in many other situations, correlate the findings with the histology.[37]

Stains for reticulin fibers led to the recognition of an epithelial and sarcomatous growth pattern of neoplasms—the epithelial and glial growths having little supportive reticulum and/or collagen compared to the abundance and intimate relationship of these latter two components with the tumor cells in mesenchymal growths. However, with greater experience, it became clear that the all-or-none rule did not apply—mesenchymal growths were found not only to have a sarcomatous pattern, but also to have an epithelial or mixed epithelial-sarcomatous pattern. The morphology of the reticulin fibers has been useful in distinguishing various spindle-cell tumors. The straight, wire-like appearance of these fibers in schwannian and smooth-muscle growths contrasts with the twisted, kinked reticulin that entwines individual cells, whether they be fibrocytes or facultative histiocytes.

The trichrome and phosphotungstic acid-hematoxylin (PTAH) stain may be assets in the identification of smooth- and skeletal-muscle tumors. However, caution must be exercised in interpreting these stains since the cytoplasmic dyes employed are not specific for myofibrils, and the degree of cytoplasmic coloration will be affected by the type and quality of the fixation, as well as to some degree by the technician in performing the stain. Any cytoplasm that stains red with the trichrome or blue with the PTAH stain is not myogenous.

Nerve-fiber stains may be a great asset in distinguishing the neuroblastoma from other small, round-cell tumors, such as Ewing's sarcoma, embryonal rhabdomyosarcoma, malignant lymphoma, anaplastic small-cell carcinoma, and other neuroectodermal tumors.

The periodic acid-Schiff (PAS) stain with and without prior diastase digestion of the section can provide useful information for differentiating some neoplasms. The variable amount of diastase-labile polysaccharide that may be present in a variety of carcinomas and soft-tissue sarcomas limits the usefulness of the PAS reaction in tumor diagnosis. Diastase-labile polysaccharide of embryonal rhabdomyosarcoma and Ewing's sarcoma has been considered an aid in their differentiation from the negative-staining neuroblastoma, malignant lymphoma, and anaplastic small-cell carcinoma. More detailed recent studies demonstrating glycogen in 3 of 38 electron-microscopically-proven neuroblastomas of varying differentiation further limits the value of the PAS stain in the diagnosis of small round-cell tumors.[38] Diastase-stable polysaccharide can also be found in a variety of neoplasms, and its variation in quantity and shape can be useful in tumor classification. The crystalline and abundant irregular granular polysaccharide found, respectively, in the alveolar soft-part sarcoma and granular-cell myoblastoma serve to distinguish these two tumors from one another and from other tumors that may be histologically similar, including paraganglioma, alveolar rhabdomyosarcoma, amelanotic melanoma, and granular renal-cell carcinoma.

Stains for acid mucopolysaccharide (mucicarmine, alcian blue, and colloidal iron), when used at different pH's with and without prior bovine testicular hyaluronidase digestion, can be helpful in separating epithelial tumors from sarcomas and in distinguishing histologically similar sarcomas from one another. Positive stromal staining is found in carcinomas and sarcomas—generally more so in the latter, but cytoplasmic staining, with the exception of the mesothelioma, is indicative of an epithelial neoplasm. The stability of the stromal acid mucopolysaccharide in cartilaginous tumors and some synovial sarcomas to bovine testicular hyaluronidase has proven useful in separating these neoplasms from other, morphologically similar neoplasms.

Silver stains other than those for demonstrating reticulin fibers are important in separating nonmesenchymal growths that may mimic sarcoma. The argentaffin and argyrophilic reactions may prove useful in distinguishing melanoma from sarcoma, by demonstrating small amounts of melanin undetected in the H&E preparation. Argyrophilic reactions are valuable in distinguishing the positive-staining paraganglioma and neuroectodermal tumors from the negative-staining alveolar soft-part sarcoma, the granular-cell myoblastoma, and the granular variety of renal-cell carcinoma.

The use of lipid stains to identify poorly differentiated liposarcomas from other varieties of sarcoma and even from undifferentiated carcinoma must be done with caution, since lipid may be found in a variety of neoplasms. When taking into consideration the amount of lipid present, and the type of cell in which it is found, the lipid stain is an asset in distinguishing liposarcoma from other mesenchymal neoplasms.

The methyl green-pyronine stain used in conjunction with ribonuclease digestion can be useful in distinguishing mesenchymal tumors which are more commonly rich in cytoplasmic ribonucleic acid (RNA), such as Burkitt's lymphoma, osteogenic sarcoma, and plasma-cell myeloma, from histologically similar tumors that have little cytoplasmic RNA.

Histochemical enzymatic reactions are helpful in tumor classification. Dopa oxidase activity within tumor cells is a useful and highly specific means of identifying amelanotic melanoma masquerading as a sarcoma, provided, of course, that the enzyme is present. A positive naphthol-As-D-chloroacetate esterase reaction may prove invaluable in distinguishing an immature granulocytic sarcoma from other varieties of round-cell sarcoma. Adenosine triphosphatase activity in tumor cells can be useful in distinguishing rhabdomyosarcoma[39] from other sarcomas, and the presence of alkaline phosphatase may be useful in separating osteogenic sarcoma from other spindle-cell varieties of sarcoma, particularly when osteogenesis is not overt.

The newest aid in histogenetic classification is the employment of immunohistochemical techniques utilizing fluorescein- or peroxidase-labeled antibodies to detect cellular myosin, actin, myoglobin, and factor VIII, in order to establish the myogenous or endothelial origin of a soft-tissue tumor.[40-42]

Dr. Hajdu: Despite numerous reports on the ultrastructure of soft-tissue neoplasms studied with the electron microscope, the way in which this instrument is used today in most laboratories is limited with regard to the primary diagnosis of sarcomas. However, I agree that careful consideration of the ultrastructural features of soft-tissue sarcomas occasionally complements observations made with the light-microscope, and that the electron microscope is occasionally a useful instrument in the assessment of undifferentiated sarcomas. For example, the demonstration of primitive sarcomeres in undifferentiated rhabdomyosarcoma, the visualization of longitudinal myofilaments with fusiform dense areas in undifferentiated leiomyosarcoma, or the localization of neurofilaments and neurotubules in peripheral nerve tumors are important, and cannot be ignored in the histogenetic classification of soft-tissue neoplasms. But perhaps the most important role of the electron microscope is in the differential diagnosis of tonofilament-containing spindle-cell carcinomas and myofibroblast-containing mesenchymal neoplasms. Furthermore, the accurate demonstration of neurosecretory granules or melanosomes is often impossible without ultrastructural examination.

Among the most important contributions to the ultrastructure of soft-tissue sarcomas are the articles written by Stembridge et al.,[43] Fine and Horn,[36] Gabbiani et al.,[44] Morales et al.,[45] Rosai et al.,[46] Taxy and Battifora,[47] and Kindblom and Save-Soderbergh.[48] After reviewing these articles and studying the ultrastructure of a number of soft-tissue neoplasms, I recently put together a table on the most pertinent structures that one may encounter under the electron microscope (Table 2).

The contributions of Mallory, Cajal, and Masson to the better understanding of soft-tissue neoplasms through the use of special or histochemical stains are well known to all of us. In the assessment of connective tissue neoplasms I see little use for special stains other than trichrome, reticulin, PAS, and alcian blue. Also, there are no more than a handful of histochemical stains that are valuable in the differential diagnosis of soft-tissue sarcomas. It is perhaps truer in the case of soft-tissue sarcomas than in any other neoplasms that if one is not able to make a diagnosis from good H&E-stained slides through considering the neoplastic cells and their pattern of growth, that the special stains will be of little help in the majority of such cases.

Drs. Morton and Eilber: In our experience, electron microscopy has not played a major role in the diagnosis of soft tissue sarcomas. Often such tumors are very undifferentiated, and electron microscopy has been of very little clinical assistance.

Dr. Suit: At biopsy, a piece of the specimen should be fixed in glutaraldehyde in case there is a requirement for electron microscopy to assist in the determination of the histogenetic diagnosis of the sarcoma. This may be valuable in discriminating between rhabdomyosarcoma and unclassified or poorly differentiated sarcomas of other origin, and stems from the ability of electron microscopy to pick out myofibrils. A related problem is the differential diagnosis of fibrosarcoma from

TABLE 2. Ultrastructural Features of Soft-Tissue Sarcomas

Tumor	Features
Malignant fibrous histiocytoma	Extensive RER, free polyribosomes, Golgi complexes, cytoplasmic vacuoles, glycogen-like particles, dense bodies, abundant lysosomes, cytoplasmic filopodia
Fibrosarcoma	Prominent RER, richly collagenous stroma
Tendosynovial sarcoma	Junctional complexes, microvilli-lined lumina, absence of basement membrane, fibroblast-like cells prominent in RER and glycogen, phagocytic epithelioid cells containing sparse RER
Liposarcoma	Intracytoplasmic lipid droplets, glycogen, compressed cytoplasmic organelles
Leiomyosarcoma	Myofibrils with associated pinocytotic vesicles, arranged cytoplasmic actin filaments, basement membranes, dense plaques, dense bodies
Rhabdomyosarcoma	Thick and thin myofilaments and myofibrils
Hemangiopericytoma	Cytoplasmic microfibrils, pinocytotic vesicles, glycogen, basement membrane, or fragments of basement membrane
Hemangiosarcoma	Cytoplasmic microfibrils, pinocytotic vesicles, basement membrane, tight junctions, Weibel-Palade bodies
Malignant schwannoma	Long interdigitating cytoplasmic processes, intact or fragmented basement membrane, long-spaced collagen, remnants of "pi" granules, microtubules, clumps of glycogen, occasional dense bodies
Alveolar soft-part sarcoma	Intracytoplasmic granules and crystals

RER = rough endoplasmic reticulum.

leiomyosarcoma: the demonstration of muscle fibrils within the rhabdomyosarcoma cell would establish the diagnosis of rhabdomyosarcoma.

Dr. Weiss: In our consultation work we have generally utilized special stains rather liberally but electron microscopy selectively in reaching diagnoses. The combination of good H&E-stained slides and a few relevant special stains either establishes the diagnosis or significantly limits the possibilities in most cases. Clearly, certain situations dictate the use of specific special stains. For instance, the distinction of carcinomas from mesotheliomas usually requires the use of an alcian blue (with and without hyaluronidase) stain coupled with mucin stains, and the Masson trichrome stain is routinely used in our laboratory to document either smooth-muscle or skeletal-muscle differentiation within a tumor. However, the stain that we have employed successfully in a more general fashion has been the periodic acid-Schiff (PAS) stain for glycogen. This stain is both easy to perform and to interpret, although it should be recalled that glycogen can be lost from poorly preserved tissue, and can also be increased in cells surrounding areas of

TABLE 3. Cytoplasmic Staining for Glycogen in Soft-Tissue Tumors

Glycogen Positive	Variable	Glycogen Negative
Leiomyosarcoma	Carcinoma	Malignant fibrous histiocytoma
Chondrosarcoma	Liposarcoma	Malignant schwannoma
Clear-cell sarcoma	Epithelioid sarcoma	Fibrosarcoma
Melanoma	Angiosarcoma	Synovial sarcoma
Rhabdomyosarcoma		Neuroblastoma
Extraskeletal Ewing's sarcoma		

tissue necrosis. As shown in Table 3, soft-tissue tumors can be divided into those that are usually glycogen-negative and those usually glycogen-positive (with a few showing variable staining). As a result of this property the PAS stain is useful in narrowing down certain diagnostic alternatives, and may be helpful in evaluating:

1. Pleomorphic tumors in which the differential diagnosis might include carcinoma, melanoma, pleomorphic leiomyosarcoma, and malignant fibrous histiocytoma.
2. Round-cell tumors such as neuroblastoma, rhabdomyosarcoma, and extraskeletal Ewing's sarcoma.
3. Spindle-cell neoplasms in which the suspected diagnosis rests between a smooth-muscle and a neural tumor.

Depending on the results of the PAS stain, additional stains may be required. For instance, in situation 1, above, a positive glycogen stain usually eliminates the diagnosis of malignant fibrous histiocytoma, but would necessitate additional stains for mucin, melanin, or myofibrils.

In contrast to special stains, electron microscopy has not played a primary role in the diagnosis of soft-tissue sarcomas, but has usually served as a confirmatory procedure once the diagnosis has been suggested by light-microscopy. However, there are a few circumscribed situations in which electron microscopy has played a key role. Its greatest use has been realized in the differential diagnosis of round-cell sarcomas of childhood, such as rhabdomyosarcoma, neuroblastoma, and Ewing's sarcoma. In situations in which the light microscopic appearance of the tumor is quite similar, the presence of specific ultrastructural "markers" can establish the diagnosis. For example, the presence of thick and thin filaments or Z-band material establishes the diagnosis of rhabdomyosarcoma, while small, dense core granules within cytoplasmic processes are characteristic of neuroblastoma in this setting. Although there are no features specific for Ewing's sarcoma, the absence of the foregoing features, coupled with the presence of large amounts of cytoplasmic glycogen, strongly suggest this diagnosis over the two foregoing ones. To a lesser extent electron microscopy may provide useful information in the evaluation of pleomorphic tumors in adults. Usually the question asked is whether the tumor is a carcinoma, melanoma, or pleomorphic sarcoma. While we have not found electron microscopy useful in making the distinction between various types of pleomorphic sarcomas, it can sometimes suggest to us whether a tumor is more likely to be epithelial or mesenchymal, on the basis of the size and frequency of desmosome-like attachments as well as on the basis of specific organelles such as melanosomes or mucin droplets.

The success of electron microscopy in diagnosis obviously depends greatly on the ability to narrow down the diagnostic alternatives and then to systematically search for specific ultrastructural features that will strongly favor one diagnosis over another. In summary, I think electron microscopy is still in a "fact-finding" stage in soft-tissue pathology. We are still in the process of learning the full range of ultrastructural features of the diagnostic categories defined by light-microscopy. For this reason electron microscopy has proved useful only in a few circumscribed areas, but in time it may be expanded to include a wider variety of problems.

> 5. Malignant fibrous histiocytoma has become an increasingly popular diagnosis. What criteria are required for this diagnosis? Is this a meaningful clinicopathologic entity or is it a potpourri of mesenchymal tumors?

Dr. Weiss: Although there is no histologic feature that is ultimately diagnostic of the malignant fibrous histiocytoma, we believe that there are a set of criteria which, when properly applied, define a reasonably homogeneous group.[49,50] First, malignant fibrous histiocytomas are relatively pleomorphic sarcomas. This implies that intermediate or borderline lesions such as the dermatofibrosarcoma protuberans (which obviously fulfill some of the following criteria) be excluded. Second, such tumors must contain a mixture of fibroblast-like and histiocyte-like cells. The proportions of fibroblast-like and histiocyte-like cells vary, as can the degree of pleomorphism. A storiform pattern is often present but is by no means specific for malignant fibrous histiocytomas. There is also a striking tendency for these tumors to contain inflammatory elements, xanthoma cells, and siderophages. Finally, tumors considered as malignant fibrous histiocytomas should show no specific features of differentiation apart from collagen production and phagocytosis. This last criterion is, in my opinion, one of the most important, and excludes other pleomorphic sarcomas, such as pleomorphic liposarcoma, which may have areas indistinguishable from a malignant fibrous histiocytoma.

Defined in such a way, the malignant fibrous histiocytomas emerge as a group of lesions which have a rather characteristic clinical setting. They occur principally during late adult life, in the proximal portion of the extremities and in the retroperitoneum. Biologically the majority are high-grade sarcomas, with a propensity to recur and metastasize in about half of all cases. Their ability to metastasize can be correlated with their location (i.e., depth) in soft tissue when first diagnosed.

Unfortunately, we have, in our consultation material, repeatedly seen a variety of lesions misdiagnosed as malignant fibrous histiocytoma, and errors of this type undoubtedly contribute to the impression that this diagnosis does not represent a meaningful entity. Most such errors are the result of putting undue emphasis on a particular histologic criterion without evaluating the lesion as a whole. For instance, cellular examples of nodular fasciitis exhibiting a storiform pattern are frequently confused with malignant fibrous histiocytoma. Likewise, anaplastic carcinomas metastatic to soft tissue provide a treacherous mimicry of malignant fibrous histiocytoma. In such cases it is necessary for the pathologist to use all of the resources available to him or her (e.g., special stains, electron microscopy, extensive tumor sampling) in order to exclude epithelial differentiation not immediately apparent on routine H&E-stained sections.

It is my belief that if this diagnosis is conscientiously made, the concept of the malignant fibrous histiocytoma is a useful one to pathologists and clinicians despite the fact that questions concerning the histogenesis of this tumor are still unanswered.

Dr. Hajdu: If the number of articles published in recent years on fibrous histiocytomas is considered as the true indicator of the incidence of these neoplasms, one would get the impression that every other soft-tissue neoplasm was a fibrous histiocytoma. It is also true that if the term fibrous histiocytoma were used indiscriminantly, many neoplasms could be called fibrous histiocytoma because, in poorly differentiated neoplasms of almost any type, it is not rare to find areas with features commonly seen in fibrous histiocytomas, e.g., a storiform pattern, pleomorphism, and phagocytic activity.

I for one believe that there are at least three major microscopic forms of fibrous histiocytoma: fibroblastic, histiocytic, and pleomorphic (Fig. 2). Fibroblastic fibrous histiocytomas are predominantly composed of slender, noncollagenous fibroblastic cells arranged in a storiform pattern. The histiocytic fibrous histiocytomas are predominantly composed of histiocytic round forms and epulis-type multinucleated giant cells; the pleomorphic forms contain, in addition to the foregoing elements and patterns, foam cells, multinucleated Touton giant cells, and bizarre multinucleated giant cells.

I am certain that it will take some time to convince everybody that there is a place in our nomenclature for fibrous histiocytomas, but it should be remembered that the term fibrous histiocytoma should be reserved for neoplasms that are predominantly composed of embryonal, undifferentiated forms of fibrous-histiocytic cells.[10]

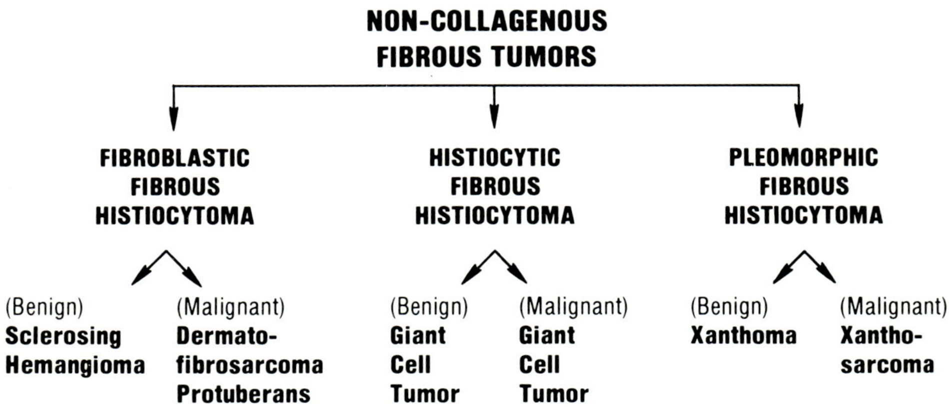

FIG. 2. Subclassification scheme of fibrous histiocytomas (From Hajdu SI: Pathology of Soft Tissue Tumors. 1979. Courtesy of Lea & Febiger, publisher.)

Drs. Morton and Eilber: In our experience, malignant fibrous histiocytoma is a meaningful clinical entity. Although it may in fact be a potpourri of mesenchymal tumors, we have found it to be a very aggressive, highly malignant, mainly grade-3 tumor that deserves a different therapy regimen than do the low-grade malignancies.

Dr. Fine: The variation in cytology and growth pattern that may be observed in the tumors considered to be of histiocytic derivation makes it difficult to keep the group "pure," since one or more of the features ascribed to this type of tumor can be found to varying degrees in a number of other soft-tissue neoplasms. The storiform or cartwheel arrangement of the spindle-cell component most often and characteristically found in dermatofibrosarcoma protuberans is the hallmark of the histiocytic lesion, but this pattern may be mimicked to varying degrees in a variety of other neoplasms, including schwannian, smooth-muscle, and fibroblastic (sclerosing) liposarcoma. Other features important in making the diagnosis of a histiocytic tumor are the lipid-laden foam cells in nonnecrotic areas, admixed with non-lipid-containing tumor cells, the presence of multinucleated (osteoclastic-epulis or Touton type) giant cells, bizarre lobulated or binucleated giant cells, and occasionally a mononuclear cell population resembling that in malignant lymphoma. The quantity of stroma is variable and may be related to individual cells or to groups of tumor cells; it is generally delicate staining as reticulin in silver preparations, but collagen may be present, particularly in those tumors with a spindle-cell population. Stromal changes, whether myxomatous, vascular, or infiltrated with neutrophils, may be a prominent aspect of some of the histiocytomas, and may simulate, respectively, the myxoid liposarcoma, hemangiopericytoma, or an inflammatory process. This variability in morphologic and cytologic appearance has given rise to the variety of names used for this neoplasm—fibrous histiocytoma, fibrous xanthoma, pleomorphic fibrous histiocytoma, atypical fibrous histiocytoma, histiocytoma, myxoid fibrous histiocytoma, and inflammatory histiocytoma.[49-52] As with any classification of neoplasms, it is difficult to keep a particular group pure, and differences of opinion undoubtedly do exist regarding the placement of some tumors in the histiocytic category rather than in other soft-tissue tumor classifications. But while this group of soft-tissue tumors may well be contaminated with other varieties of sarcoma, it is worthwhile to continue to retain it for those mesenchymal growths having one or more of the above features—preferably more than one—so that information can be obtained regarding the response of these growths to various therapeutic modalities and prognosis.

6. Can and should the well-differentiated fibrous growths—fibromatosis and well-differentiated fibrosarcoma—be distinguished from one another, and are the distinctions of clinical importance?

Dr. Hajdu: Yes, these distinctions are of great clinical importance. And, because of this, we must attempt—although it is often difficult or impossible—to distinguish fibromatoses from well-differentiated fibrous growth such as desmoid tumors.

The controversy surrounding fibromatoses and desmoid tumors dates back to Peiffer[53] and Nichols,[54] who felt that desmoid tumors should not be called sarcomas. Our experience[10] with desmoid tumors shows that despite occasional overlapping histopathologic features of fibromatoses and desmoid tumors, the differential diagnosis of these neoplasms is not too difficult if adequate material is available for histopathologic examination (Table 4). Desmoid tumors are more homogenous and collagenous fibrous lesions than are fibromatoses. Characteristically, desmoid tumors occur in young adults, and are deeply seated, solitary, bulky, and pseudoencapsulated, and are most commonly found in the trunk, proximal part of the extremity, and head and neck areas. They have a high rate of recurrence (64 percent) after local excision, may cause death (11 percent) by local extension into vital organs and, rarely, may metastasize.[10]

On the other hand, fibromatoses most frequently affect infants and children. These nonneoplastic proliferative lesions may occur anywhere in the body, but are most commonly found in the distal part of the extremities, the mediastinum, and the retroperitoneum. They are usually subcutaneous or submucosal in location, and may be multiple. Despite their infiltrative nature they are self-limited and rarely recur after excision with clear margins.[10]

Dr. Fine: Controversy regarding the designation of well-differentiated fibrous growths as fibromatosis or differentiated fibrosarcoma appears to be a matter of lack of agreement as to whether the criteria separating them should be histologic or both histologic and clinical, and whether or not the designation sarcoma should be reserved for those tumors that have the capacity to produce distant metastases. More cellular fibrous growths, particularly those that are musculoaponeurotic, i.e., the desmoid tumors, whether abdominal or extraabdominal, appear to provide the

TABLE 4. Distinguishing Features of Fibromatoses and Desmoid Tumors

	Fibromatoses	Desmoid Tumors
Average age of patient	Younger than 20 years	Older than 20 years
Most common anatomic site	Hand, foot, and digits	Trunk, head, and neck
Average size	Less than 5 cm	More than 5 cm
Location	Superficial	Deep
Growth pattern	Nonencapsulated, proliferative, and inflammatory	Pseudoencapsulated, infiltrative, and destructive
Histopathology	Partly collagenous, cellular, myxoid, and haphazardly arranged	Collagenous, hypercellular, sclerosing, and uniformly arranged
Rate of recurrence	Low	High

greatest point of contention.[10] Looking at the history of such lesions one finds that there have been two factions—one supporting a benign classification and the other a low-grade malignant classification—for years. Some observers have served in both camps, switching from the malignant to the benign over the course of years. Stout was one of the latter; in 1954 he put forth the concept of fibromatosis,[55] including in this group the differentiated, infiltrative fibrous growths that have a variable collagen content and lack the cytologic features of malignancy, including scanty or no mitotic activity. Although they may exhibit an aggressive clinical behavior, often with recurrences, these growths lack the capacity to metastasize, and Stout therefore believed that they should not be designated as sarcomas. To add to the confusion regarding this duality of terminology, Stout stated in a 1961 paper that about 0.5 percent of the fibromatoses metastasized, and in an illustration of a case which was cellular and had no mitoses, the caption read "fibromatosis (or differentiated fibrosarcoma)."[57]

The histologic differentiation of well-differentiated fibrous growths—fibromatosis and well-differentiated fibrosarcoma (grade I)—presents a problem not unfamiliar among mesenchymal tumors, i.e., leiomyoma and differentiated leiomyosarcoma. The microscopic separation of these growths is based on their degree of cellular atypia, mitotic activity, and collagen content. With the possible exception of the mitotic count, these criteria are subjective, and their interpretation may well vary among observers. Even the degree of mitotic activity considered by different pathologists to be indicative of malignancy is variable. Ackerman and Rosai[56] consider a mitotic activity of greater than 1 per high-power field (HPF) to be a feature of malignancy in the differentiated fibrous tumors, while other authors have accepted a lower count as being indicative of sarcoma. Regardless of the subjectivity of these criteria, data from studies of fibrous tumors indicate that there are differences in behavior that can generally be correlated with the histologic grade of the tumor. Even among the better-differentiated fibrosarcomas (grade I), a 5-year mortality of 12 to 27 percent[14,58] has been observed, which is in contrast to the behavior reported for the fibromatoses, including the musculoaponeurotic group.[59] For those reported abdominal and extraabdominal desmoid tumors that have metastasized and behaved clinically contrary to the majority of similar tumors,[10] one might ask whether the desmoid tumors (fibromatoses) that gave rise to these might have undergone a malignant transformation, as has been reported by others.[60,61]

Regardless of the terminology one wishes to employ for these differentiated fibrous tumors, the recommended therapy is wide local excision to prevent local recurrence.

Drs. Morton and Eilber: The clinical differentiaton of fibromatoses from well-differentiated fibrosarcoma is probably not of significant clinical import. Both of these diseases and conditions need to be treated by complete, wide surgical resection, with consideration given for adjuvant radiotherapy. The distinction between the two conditions in terms of their definitive surgical therapy is that of a high grade 3 undifferentiated fibrosarcoma and a grade 1, well-differentiated tumor.

Dr. Suit: The distinction between aggressive fibromatosis and well-differentiated sarcoma is practical on a histopathologic basis. Furthermore, this is of great importance clinically because of the fact that the fibromatoses do not metastasize, whereas low-grade fibrosarcomas do metastasize, although with low frequency. This has important implications for management policy. Recurrence of fibromatosis is not an ominous sign, whereas the recurrence of fibrosarcoma is associated with an increased risk of development of metastasis.[62,63] This means that the requirement to achieve cure at the first treatment is not absolute for fibromatosis, but that treatment for fibrosarcoma must be radical, with all reasonable efforts made to achieve cure at the first treatment. Recurrence of fibromatosis is not inevitable even though the surgical margins of excision may have been very close or uncertain, whereas for fibrosarcoma in this situation recurrence is highly likely and further treatment is required. The patient with a fibrosarcoma—even of grade 1—should be subjected to a comprehensive and radical course of treatment and this should not be delayed. The intention should be to achieve permanent control of the primary tumor process on the first treatment. For fibromatosis, I think it is reasonable to follow a more moderate course, and that if the patient has had an initial but nonoptimal resection, viz., all gross tumor has been removed but with close or questionable margins, that it would be reasonable to observe the patient. If the growth process recurred, definitive treatment should be planned at that time using surgery, surgery and radiation, or radiation alone. One special feature of the fibromatoses is that following successful radiation therapy regression is very slow, although complete and permanent regression will be achieved. It is usual for the regression to continue for 1 to 2 years after the completion of the radiation therapy. For the great majority of these lesions, surgery alone should be the treatment, and excellent results can be expected. However, a small proportion will be so sited that resection with secure margins is unlikely or resection may not be technically feasible. In these situations radiation therapy can be most valuable. Successful treatment of a desmoid tumor by radiation has been well documented.[64,65] At the MGH, 11 patients have been treated by radiation and followed for 1 to 7 years. The radiation dose level has been approximately 6,500 to 7,000 rads over 7 to 8 weeks. There has been one local failure and this was in a nine-year-old child who presented with recurrent desmoid (after multiple surgical procedures) extending from the submental region to the suprasternal notch. Because of age and anatomic location, the dose was limited to 5,100 rad. The mass did regress, but at 2.5 years recurred; this was the only lesion in this series given less than 6,000 rad.

Dr. Weiss: Well-differentiated fibroblastic growths can be histologically divided into two categories: fibromatosis and well-differentiated fibrosarcoma. Since in practice the therapy of these two lesions is often identical, there is a tendency in some centers to consider the two lesions as part of the same spectrum. However, I believe that the patient's interests are best served if fibromatosis is separated from fibrosarcoma. There are several points of difference that warrant this separation.

First, the two lesions are quite distinct histologically, and only rarely are transitional tumors observed. Fibromatosis represents the more differentiated lesion. It is recognized by the presence of cells which closely resemble normal fibroblasts, and have a delicate but irregular nuclear membrane, indistinct cytoplasmic borders, few mitotic figures, and abundant interstitial collagen. The lesions may be so differentiated as to resemble a reactive fibroblastic process. On the other hand, the well-differentiated fibrosarcoma is a qualitatively different lesion. The cells have a more hyperchromatic nucleus with chromatic clumping, more distinct cytoplasmic borders, and mitotic figures; and while the amount of interstitial collagen varies, it is usually less striking than in fibromatosis.

Second, the behavior of the two lesions differs. Lesions designated as fibromatosis have a limited potential for autonomous growth. While they often recur following surgical excision, they have neither a capacity for metastasis[66] nor a capacity for transformation into a fibrosarcoma. In fact, the rare familial incidence, occasional bilaterality of palmar and plantar lesions, postpartum occurrence of abdominal lesions, and very rare instances of spontaneous regression of lesions designated as fibromatoses have suggested that these growths may not represent true neoplasms. While I do not agree with this contention, it is clear that their behavior contrasts with that of the well-differentiated fibrosarcoma, which has not only a capacity to recur but also to metastasize in a small but definite number of cases. Finally, in view of the nonmetastasizing nature of fibromatosis, I think one can adopt a more flexible approach to its treatment. Although both fibromatosis and fibrosarcomas are ideally treated by excision with wide surgical margins, I believe that fibromatosis represents one situation in which one is justified in performing a less than radical excision in order to salvage a limb, provided that a subsequent recurrence will not jeopardize the patient's chance for curative surgery. This temporizing or conservative approach can be rationalized on the grounds that the nature of the underlying disease does not put us in a position of having to decide between "limb and life."

> 7. What general principles should be observed in the treatment of soft-part sarcomas? How are these guidelines altered by the anatomic location of the tumor? Surgery, chemotherapy, and radiation, both alone and in combination, have been recommended for the treatment of soft-part sarcoma. Given a soft-part sarcoma of the lower extremity, what therapeutic recommendations should be considered, and what factors influence the choice among these alternatives? What are the results obtained with the recommended treatment (including expected frequency of local recurrence or pulmonary metastases)? Is it necessary to resect from origin to insertion the muscle that is minimally involved by a small, low-grade tumor, e.g., of the malignant fibrous histiocytoma type?

Dr. Suit: The principles to be followed in treatment of the patient with a soft-tissue sarcoma are: (1) there should be a complete history and physical examination, with comprehensive laboratory and radiographic evaluation. Of special importance are the evaluation of the pattern of local extension, involvement of regional nodes, and for presence of distant metastasis. The assessment of the primary lesion is usually assisted in a most important manner by CT study in addition to a xerogram and possibly an arteriogram. In some instances ultrasound scans may be entirely adequate. CT studies have been most valuable in assessing the extension of tumor between muscles or along muscle bundles, through foramena, to encase neurovascular bundles, to invade bone, etc. (2) After the diagnostic work-up has been completed, the patient's problem should be presented to a multidisciplinary group of physicians who are concerned with and interested in this group of tumors. The biopsy should be planned if it has not already been obtained; and preferably the biopsy should be done by a surgeon who will participate in the definitive treatment of the patient. (3) After staging of the tumor (GTNM), the multidisciplinary group should develop a treatment strategy designed to meet the particular needs of the individual patient. (4) The object of the primary treatment is to achieve eradication of the tumor and to do this with a minimum morbidity (cosmetically, anatomically, and functionally). The patient should then be appraised of the approach which is judged to be the most likely to be successful, the risk of morbidities associated with such treatment, and some details of the alternate modalities.

There is currently an intensive effort to employ treatments which minimize the anatomic, cosmetic, and functional loss to the patient as a result of radical surgery, particularly where this means amputation. These more conservative approaches (conservative surgery and radiation therapy with or without chemotherapy) yield disease-free survival results which approach closely those that would be expected for amputation alone.[67,68] As such, they represent an entirely reasonable first-line approach to the patient with soft-tissue sarcoma of the extremity. I think that the patient should be informed that for lesions of an extremity, amputation probably has a small but real advantage in terms of local control. This pertains only for lesions of the distal thigh, leg, ankle, and foot, or the distal upper arm, elbow, forearm, hand, and wrist. That is, for such locations, the local control results of amputation should be as high as is currently feasible. The difference between amputation and the conservative approach with respect to local control should be only a few percentage points, particularly for small lesions. For example, of 25 patients treated at the MGH by surgery and radiation therapy for primary soft-tissue sarcomas which were <5 cm in diameter, there have been no local failures during follow-up periods of 1 to 8 years. Results are slightly less good for the treatment of recurrent sarcomas and for larger lesions (primary or recurrent). For lesions near the groin or shoulder girdle, it is not clear that amputation offers the best method of treatment. The lesions at these sites are often large (≥ 5 cm). Even radical amputation is associated with a worthwhile proportion of stump recurrences, and hence procedures other than hindquarter or forequarter amputation can be considered. For example, at Memorial Hospital, amputation yielded an 18 percent local failure rate.[62] The combination of preoperative radiation therapy followed by resection may be a better approach.[69] More data from longer follow-up examinations are essential to an evaluation of the efficacy of these conservative approaches to this group of sarcomas.

In planning a treatment strategy, there is often included a major chemotherapeutic component. Specific allowance must be made for the impact of the chemotherapy, radiation therapy, and surgery on the overall tolerance and specific tissue-site tolerance of each treatment modality. Additionally, there needs to be an appreciation of the quantitative change in tolerance to one modality that is caused by another. Unless consideration is given to making "appropriate" adjustment of the aggressiveness with which each modality is administered, the patient may be severely overtreated.

A further principle in the management of soft-tissue sarcoma patients is the inclusion in the initial treatment strategy consideration of rehabilitation or physical therapy. This is often valuable in achieving minimal functional loss.

It is not necessary to resect from origin to insertion the muscle which is minimally involved by a small low-grade tumor as for example, malignant fibrohistiocytoma type. Results from radiation therapy and surgery for T1 lesions (less than 5 cm in diameter) and of grade I or II at the Massachusetts General Hospital fail to justify comprehensive coverage of the entirety of the affected muscle. As cited above, for small primary lesions treated by radiation therapy and surgery, local failures or marginal failures have not been seen. These patients have had less than comprehensive coverage of the affected muscle, i.e., fields covering much less than the origin to insertion. Usually for small, grade 1 to 2 lesions, the treatment field extended 10 to 12 cm above and below the area of known involvement or beyond the surgical field if seen postoperatively. For lesions which are of high grade, are large, extensively invading muscles, or recurrent, it is reasonable to treat more comprehensively perhaps the entirety of the affected muscle from the origin to the insertion. I do not know of firm support for this statement. In the instance of rhabdomyosarcoma, the entirety of the affected muscle should be treated (by surgery or radiation). There is certainly an increase in morbidity by treating or operating on the affected muscle from its origin to insertion; hence, the need for this greater radicalism should be justified by future clinical investigation.

Drs. Morton and Eilber: General principles for the treatment of soft-part sarcomas include nonviolation of the tumor or spillage of the tumor cells, complete resection of all biopsy and needle tracks, and a wide surgical resection well beyond the pseudocapsule of the tumor. In general, this procedure involves resection of the tumor at least one fascial plane beyond the structure of origin. If the tumor lies in fat, the resection involves at least a 6-cm margin in all directions. If the tumor is in a particular, identifiable muscle group, the resection must include the muscle from its origin to its insertion. These guidelines for resection are not altered by the anatomic location of the tumor—the same principles used for the extremities are used in the head and neck or retroperitoneum. However, the head and neck and retroperitoneum do present certain anatomic constraints, although the resection principles are the same. In general, these tumors, in any location, can be removed from an adjacent artery by dissection in the subadventitial plane or subneural plane of an adjacent major nerve. From our experience, adventitium or perineurium are, in general, effective barriers to the spread of the tumor, and dissection beneath these planes is usually possible without local recurrence when the combined-modality approach of preoperative therapy is used.

The primary treatment for soft-part sarcomas is individualized and, although many factors are considered, certainly the clinical stage of the tumor is very important. If the patient already has metastatic disease, recommendations for treatment are tempered by the palliative intent of therapy. Therefore, we will confine our remarks to those patients who have no evidence of distant metastases by chest x-ray and whole-lung tomography.

The primary treatment is surgical resection. Although there are many different types of surgical procedures, in this instance we are discussing either a radical local excision or an amputation. The results from either of these treatments appear to be equal and, therefore, the choice should be the patient's. If the tumor is well differentiated, it is our impression that a radical local excision, if anatomically feasible, is adequate for local control. If the pathologic margins are close, postoperative radiation therapy of 5,000 rads is advised.

Patients with a high-grade sarcoma, regardless of size or location, are treated preoperatively with chemotherapy and irradiation. Our protocol calls for intra-arterial adriamycin delivered over 3 consecutive days, followed by 3,500 rads of radiation, then a radical local surgical procedure. In a consecutive series of 85 patients, the overall local control rate with this protocol has been 98 percent, with only one local recurrence. It appears from the literature and other reports that an equally effective regimen of treatment may be radical local excision and post-operative irradiation to 5,000 or 6,000 rads.

The role of adjuvant chemotherapy following surgical resection is controversial. The results from the American Joint Committee on Staging and End Results indicate that the 5-year survival with a grade 3 or 4 clinicopathologic stage III or IV tumor is between 10 and 30 percent. However, it has become clear that these results were based on treatment with surgery alone, from which the recurrence rate averaged 30 percent. It is unclear whether combination surgery, radiation, and chemotherapy given to the primary tumor, and improved local control, will ultimately affect local recurrence and survival for these patients. The question of whether adjuvant chemotherapy is indicated is the subject of several ongoing studies. Clearly, the most effective chemotherapeutic agent is adriamycin. There are several prospective studies now underway to determine whether additional adjuvant chemotherapy following complete surgical resection will improve the patient's overall survival rate.

If a soft-part tumor originates in a clearly defined muscle, our policy is to remove the entire muscle, from origin to insertion, and encompassing the adjacent muscular fascial planes. Although there are no data to support this concept absolutely, it would seem to be a valid principle of therapy. If one is resecting three-fourths of a specific muscle group, the functional results are identical to those for the entire muscle group from origin to insertion. In patients with extremity sarcomas, it is often difficult to identify, either pre- or intraoperatively, the specific muscle of origin with certainty.

Dr. Hajdu: Being a pathologist, I hesitate to write anything on the modality of treatment for soft-tissue sarcomas, but I think that in most cases it is still true today what was said by Hunter[70] in 1794, that "a surgeon ought not to be contented with removing merely the indurated or actually diseased part, but that he should also take away some portion of the surrounding substance." Another way of saying this is that cancer, including soft-tissue sarcomas, should be removed with clear surgical margins. Whether the best modality of treatment is wide excision, monobloc soft-part resection, or amputation must be decided by a competent surgeon on the basis of the size, anatomic site, histologic grade, and histologic type of the sarcoma.[71,72] My surgical colleagues tell me that amputation does not offer any significant improvement in survival, and that they resort to amputation only when the sarcoma cannot be removed by less aggressive surgical therapy.[28,58,71] I personally feel that there is still a place for the old saying that "it is better to be alive without one leg than to die with two legs." Whether pre- or postoperative irradiation and/or chemotherapy will be applied must be decided by considering the above factors as well as the natural history of the tumor.

I do not know whether the approach to muscle-group resection has changed recently, but in 1958, according to Bowden and Booher,[73] two highly skilled surgeons, "when resection of soft parts is feasible for the removal of a sarcoma, it includes wide ablation of surrounding grossly normal tissue, removal of entire muscle bundles at points of origin and insertion."

Although the treatment of a number of soft-tissue sarcomas has improved dramatically during the last 10 years as a consequence of combining well-planned surgery with irradiation and chemotherapy, the unpredictable sensitivity of many soft-tissue sarcomas to irradiation and chemotherapy must be kept in mind at the time of selection of the best modality of therapy.[74]

8. Are there data that strongly support the concept that immunomodulation can alter the efficacy of the host reaction against a soft-part sarcoma?

Drs. Morton and Eilber: There are data that strongly support immunomodulation by *Bacille Calmette-Guérin* (BCG), *C-parvum,* or tumor-cell vaccine in soft-tissue sarcomas. Morton et al.[77] demonstrated clearly that immunization with a cultured tumor cell vaccine can evoke a host immunologic response in terms of antibody and cytotoxic lymphocyte production. The efficacy of these antibodies, in terms of their benefit for overall prognosis, has not yet been established. Ongoing clinical trials are investigating whether immunotherapy added to chemotherapy or immunotherapy added to surgical resection has a significant influence on overall survival. At present, these immunologic agents must remain as experimental therapy.

Dr. Hajdu: I am convinced that soft-tissue sarcomas, because of their morphologic diversity, variability in behavior, insidious spread, and lack of tumor-specific antigen, pose one of the most formidable challenges to immunotherapists.[78]

Despite attempts with various modalities of immunotherapy, including nonspecific immunostimulation, as with Coley's toxin and *Corynebacterium parvum*;[79] tumor-specific immunization, as with irradiated sarcoma cell lysates in combination with the injection of *Bacille Calmette-Guérin*;[80] or adoptive immunization, as with immunocompetent lymphocytes or the administration of transfer factor and interferon, the immunotherapy of soft-tissue sarcomas remains highly investigational. According to Sinkovics,[81] immunotherapy may temporarily delay the progression of certain sarcomas, but it is doubtful whether BCG or any other modality of immunotherapy added to the conventional modalities of treatment—surgery, irradiation, and chemotherapy—will be capable of altering the course of the disease. Although the results are disappointing, I feel that the immunotherapy or perhaps the chemoimmunotherapy of metastatic soft-tissue sarcomas, under controlled conditions, is worthy of vigorous pursuit, because conventional modalities of treatment almost invariably fail.[75,76]

Dr. Suit: Unfortunately for studies of the human tumor, the data from studies for effective immunomodulation do not support the contention that important improvement in local control or disease-free survival is achieved through use of the so-called immunopotentiators—BCG and *C. parvum.*

CONCLUDING COMMENTS

Dr. Fine:

QUESTION 2. There can be no doubt that tumor histogenesis provides valuable information regarding the clinical behavior and therapeutic response of soft-tissue sarcomas. However, other factors that may influence the course of these tumors must not be overlooked, and we must recognize that their management can and should be undertaken in those cases in which the histogenetic classification is uncertain. The interplay of factors that may influence the clinical behavior of a sarcoma makes it difficult to assess the importance of any one of these factors, i.e., histogenesis, since many tumor characteristics (histologic grade, tumor site, tumor size and duration, and modality and extent of therapy) must be considered in investigating the importance of histogenesis in the course of soft-tissue neoplasms. The influence of histogenesis indicated by Dr. Hajdu in Table 1 should be interpreted with caution. The significance of the data for stage I and II tumors is more difficult to evaluate, and the role of histogenesis is more suspect in stage I and II than in stage III tumors, since there are three substages in each of the first two stages. This affords a greater likelihood of not having uniformity with regard to tumor size, depth, and histologic grade among the different histogenetic categories. Furthermore, while there are some impressive differences in mortality rate among the histogenetically different stage III sarcomas, a critical analysis makes one reconsider the influence of histogenesis. This is particularly important among those tumors whose classification involves possible differences of opinion. The malignant pleomorphic fibrous histiocytoma and the pleomorphic liposarcoma which, as Dr. Weiss indicated, may be confused histologically, have mortalities of 71 percent and 68 percent, respectively, and the less likely confused fibrosarcoma and embryonal rhabdomyosarcoma have mortalities differing little from one another—76 percent and 75 percent, respectively—as well as from the previous two tumors. The mortality of 94 percent for tenosynovial sarcoma versus that of 76 percent for fibrosarcoma is impressive, but the difference between the tumors for which there is apt to be conflict of opinion regarding their histogenesis—namely, the monophasic spindle-cell synovial sarcoma and the fibrosarcoma—is another matter. The 5-year mortality rate of 74 percent given by Hajdu[28] for monophasic spindle-cell synovial sarcoma of greater than 5 cm diameter differs only slightly from the 76 percent figure for stage III fibrosarcoma listed in Table 1. Furthermore, among stage III pleomorphic rhabdomyosarcoma, hemangiosarcoma, neurogenic sarcoma, and the malignant histiocytic and malignant fibroblastic fibrous histiocytoma, one notes no significant mortality difference, albeit their histogenesis is different. While Table 1 suggests a relationship between tumor histogenesis and mortality, it seems to me that a more pronounced and clearer correlation between tumor stage and mortality is indicated.

Dr. Suit's comments regarding mitotic activity in tumor grading are pertinent. I am particularly intrigued by the statement that an artificially low mitotic index may be the result of completion of the mitotic process owing to a delay in fixation of the tissue. I wonder if he has any data to support such a statement? If completion of mitotic activity is postulated during this period, might not other cells be expected to begin division?

QUESTION 3. While Dr. Stout's reports of lipoblastic, angiomatous, and histiocytic tumors in children may have included some benign growths by today's standards, there can be no doubt from photomicrographs and the clinical course of a number of cases in each group of tumors that he was dealing with malignant tumors. But the small number of cases and the brief follow-up for many of these tumors makes comparison with adult sarcomas insignificant. Even the stated differences in behavior of fibrosarcoma and synovial sarcoma in children are questionable when one evaluates the data critically. It seems that the apparent differences may be the result of not comparing tumors of similar grade and stage and the extent of surgery in these two age groups. The 80 percent survival that Dr. Weiss quotes among children with fibrosarcoma differs from the 40 to 60 percent quoted by Pritchard and Soule[27] and by others. But one must remember that the adult figures include all grades of fibrosarcoma, while the childhood data include a number of cases that may belong within the group of fibromatosis or grade I fibrosarcoma. These large and bulky tumors were superificial, often treated by amputation, and in many cases were followed for less than 5 years. If one compares the 80 percent survival figure with the 5-year survival in grade I fibrosarcoma in adults,[58] there is little difference.

The 70 percent and 40 percent 5-year survival, respectively, among children and adults with synovial sarcoma given by Dr. Hajdu is impressive, but one must ask whether the tumors represented by these figures were of similar histologic type, grade, and size, and if the treatment was similar. As Dr. Hajdu has pointed out, we must not compare apples with oranges. In Dr. Hajdu's publication on synovial sarcoma in children,[29] a 67 percent 5-year survival free of disease included only the 12 cases operated on initially at Memorial Hospital. The 12 cases that had been treated elsewhere initially, and which presented with recurrence or metastases, had a 54 percent 5-year survival, but these patients were not free of disease. Only 9 of the 23 (39 percent) children followed were free of tumor after 5 years—a figure not significantly different from the 40 percent 5-year survivals among adults.

QUESTION 6. It seems from the participants' replies to this question that there is agreement that fibromatosis should be separated from the well-differentiated fibrosarcoma, but I do not believe it has been clearly defined how this is done on a purely histologic basis. Nor do I believe that we are of a unified opinion regarding the classification of the desmoid-type tumor as fibromatosis or fibrosarcoma. It appears that we again have two camps—Dr. Hajdu in the fibrosarcoma camp and Drs. Weiss, Suit, and myself in the fibromatosis camp. But it seems that we all agree that the complete removal of the tumor should be attempted, and that this certainly need not be done as aggressively as with fibrosarcomas of higher grade, particularly when the tumor occurs in sites in which wide excision cannot be accomplished without sacrificing an extremity or affecting a vital function. But while I share the views of the other participants in this symposium regarding the need for classification and grading of the fibrous tumors and the separation of the potentially metastasizing tumors from the nonmetastasizing ones, I continue to feel frustrated by an incapability of making this distinction among many of the well-differentiated fibrous growths. I take solace in Stout's statement, in his paper on fibrosarcoma in infants and children,[82] that fibrosarcoma is difficult to distinguish from fibromatosis. Among his 23 cases, he found that mitotic activity varied from 0 to 19 per 50 HPF (a rate not considered by some as indicative of sarcoma among fibrous tumors), and that cellular anaplasia was minimal or absent in many of the tumors. The two tumors that metastasized—one in the palm with axillary node metastasis and the other a tumor of the foot which metastasized to the back—showed, respectively, 0 and 1 mitosis per 50 HPF and little or no cellular anaplasia.

Dr. Hajdu: I am delighted that members of the panel agreed that the biopsy of soft-tissue neoplasms must be generous and representative. It seems to me that we also agree that the specific classification of primary soft-tissue neoplasms as to type and histologic grade should be attempted on technically adequate paraffin sections, after careful examination of the neoplastic cells and their pattern of growth, and not on frozen sections or specimens obtained by needle biopsy. I liked very much Dr. Weiss's analogy between the bicyclist and the aspirator.

I firmly believe that the anatomic site has an influence on the morphology as well as on the prognosis of soft-tissue neoplasms.[10,82,83] According to my experience, the anatomic site should be considered together with the size, histologic type, and histologic grade in the staging or prognostication of soft-tissue sarcomas.[10,28,72,84,85,86]

I do not share Dr. Suit's view on the importance of the mitotic index in grading as he summarized it in his answer to question 2. In my experience the number of mitotic figures must be viewed in combination with at least four other factors in order to find the most appropriate designation for the histologic grade (Table 5). Dr. Fine's table (Fig. 1) shows elegantly the interaction of various factors that may influence the behavior of soft-tissue sarcomas. It is perhaps important to reemphasize that there is, unfortunately, no magic formula for the grading of soft-tissue sarcomas. My experience, as well as that of Drs. Weiss and Fine (see their answers to question 2), shows that soft-tissue sarcomas of comparable grade and stage exhibit different behavior depending on their histologic type and histogenesis (Table 1). How could we ignore, despite its innocuous appearance, the ominous nature of monophasic synovial sarcoma.[10,28,29]

I am aware of the current tendency to classify all or most pleomorphic sarcomas, especially pleomorphic rhabdomyosarcoma, as malignant fibrous histiocytoma. It is often difficult or impossible to establish the histogenesis of soft-tissue

TABLE 5. Factors to be Considered in Histologic Grading of Soft Tissue Sarcomas

Low Grade	High Grade
Hypocellular	Hypercellular
Much stroma	Minimal stroma
Minimal necrosis	Much necrosis
Good maturation	Poor maturation
Mitosis $<5/10$ HPF	Mitosis $>5/10$ HPF

(From Hajdu SI: Pathology of Soft Tissue Tumors, 1979. Courtesy of Lea & Febiger, publisher.)

neoplasms, especially in consultation practice, as Dr. Weiss pointed out. However, if one works together with the operating surgeon and carries out a proper gross dissection, with generous sampling of the specimen for routine as well as special studies, longitudinal or cross-striated myofilaments as well as embryonal myoblasts can be detected in most pleomorphic myosarcomas.

I agree with the remarks expressed by the pathologist members of the panel that the greater the pathologist's experience with the histologic appearance of neoplasms, the less he or she must rely on special techniques for their diagnosis. Of course, dependence on high-quality H&E-stained sections should not prevent us from searching for histochemical or immunologic markers and specific ultramicroscopic structures.

I do not like to disagree with a fellow pathologist, but I must point out that Dr. Weiss's definition of malignant fibrous histiocytomas, in discussing question 5, as having to "clearly be pleomorphic sarcomas" is at variance with the definition of Stout and Lattes, who defined fibrous histiocytomas as "embryonal forms of fibroblastic neoplasms." Whether we like a definition or not, we are not entitled to change it. For example, we all know that cystosarcoma phyllodes is not a sarcoma in the overwhelming majority of cases, but we still use the term in the same way in which it was introduced by Johannes Muller.

I would also like to take issue with Dr. Weiss's statement that "borderline lesions such as dermatofibrosarcoma protuberans be excluded" from the group of fibrous histiocytomas. First of all, I do not consider dermatofibrosarcoma protuberans as a borderline lesion. Our experience with these neoplasms at Memorial Sloan-Kettering Cancer Center shows that they are capable of metastasizing and that they kill about 10 percent of the patients in whom they occur.[10] Second, pleomorphic and multinucleated cells are produced, in most instances, by the fusion of mononucleated forms. Therefore, just by plain logic, if there are pleomorphic and giant-cell-forming fibrous histiocytomas, there must be fibrous histiocytomas composed of mononucleated and nonpleomorphic round or spindle-shaped facultative fibroblasts—the so-called tissue histiocytes. I admit that the subdivision of fibrous histiocytomas as it is shown in Figure 2 is schematic and arbitrary, but it is the result of many years of speculation, thinking, and searching for an explanation.[5,10,82,83] If proof is presented that I erred in my concept in reference to fibrous histiocytomas, I am willing to revise myself. Until then, however, I would like to remind all of us of the statement of Claude Bernard that "A fact in itself is nothing. It is valuable only for the idea attached to it, or for proof which it furnishes."

I am pleased that most of the panelists agreed that attempts should be made to distinguish desmoid tumor (low-grade fibrosarcoma) from fibromatosis (a non-neoplastic lesion). Although it is not always possible to distinguish these two entities purely on the basis of their histologic appearance, the typical desmoid tumor can be recognized without too much difficulty.

Contrary to Dr. Morton's and Dr. Eilber's feeling that "the clinical differentiation (of fibromatosis and desmoid tumor) is not of significant clinical import," my experience supports the views held by Dr. Suit and Dr. Fine that distinction between fibromatosis and desmoid tumor is of great importance clinically, because fibromatoses rarely recur and do not metastasize, whereas desmoid tumors frequently recur, are locally destructive, and may metastasize.[10,58,72,84]

In reference to the treatment of soft-tissue sarcomas, my impression is that, as we make progress in the better understanding of the histogenesis and natural history of mesenchymal neoplasms, there will be significant improvements in multimodal therapy, and that the frequency of recurrence and metastases will be minimized by prompt and appropriate therapy.[72,75,76,81]

As a final note, I would like to thank the editors of the *Pathology Annual* for their invitation to contribute to this discussion. It is reassuring that despite occasional controversies and the diverse backgrounds of members of the panel, there was agreement on all important and practical matters.

Drs. Morton and Eilber: We believe that the most important guidelines for the management of soft-tissue sarcomas are as follows:

1. Incisional biopsy and definitive pathologic diagnosis should be obtained prior to surgical extirpation of the soft-tissue mass. The biopsy incision should be made along the long axis of the extremity, not transversely.
2. Since these are rare neoplasms, the average surgeon is unlikely to have much experience in their management. Therefore, we believe that the results of therapy are apt to be improved if patients with soft-tissue neoplasms are referred to regional centers that have multidisciplinary teams experienced in their management.
3. The results of limb-salvage procedures using our technique of preoperative, intraarterial chemotherapy combined with radiation therapy have produced recurrence and survival rates equal or superior to those achieved by amputation. Therefore, we believe that this combined-modality approach should be considered in all patients in whom amputation is contemplated.

Dr. Suit: The influence on the observed mitotic count of the time between removal of the specimen and its fixation has been discussed in several articles. This was reviewed by Scully, wherein evidence shows, at least for some tumor systems, that the mitotic count may decrease appreciably at a time greater than 1 hour after excision.[87,88]

Dr. Weiss: Soft-tissue sarcomas are rare tumors and it is clear that meaningful information regarding their pathogenesis and optimum therapy will come only through close cooperation between the clinician and the pathologist, and in turn through the cooperation of centers treating large numbers of affected patients. However, in reading the responses it is evident that there are still problems to overcome before we can set about the task of large prospective studies.

First, it will be necessary to agree on a standard system of classification for the soft-tissue sarcomas, one that is not only easy for the pathologist to use reproducibly, but one which reflects the current state of thinking regarding these tumors. The responses to some questions underscore the fact that classifications differ and, therefore, it is difficult to compare the experience of one center with that of another. For instance, the question concerning differences between childhood and adult tumors to some extent reflects the bias of whether pleomorphic or adult rhabdomyosarcomas exist, or whether all or most are examples of malignant fibrous histiocytoma. It has been our experience that true rhabdomyosarcomas occurring in adults are exceedingly rare and can be discounted from a practical point of view. Dr. Hajdu's comments on this question also illustrate other differences among pathologists. At the Armed Forces Institute of Pathology we do not use the term tendosynovial sarcoma as a diagnostic entity, since it embraces so many different entities (clear-cell sarcoma, epithelioid sarcoma, synovial sarcoma) which seem worthy of separate designations. Moreover, Dr. Hajdu's classification of malignant fibrous histiocytoma is at variance with ours, which includes four subtypes (storiform-pleomorphic, giant-cell, myxoid, and inflammatory), the latter two having a better prognosis than the first two. Finally, Dr. Hajdu uses the term "desmoid" as synonymous with "grade 1 fibrosarcoma" and his answer consequently addresses differences between desmoids and certain benign fibroblastic lesions. On the other hand, I, along with others, consider desmoids as separate from fibrosarcoma and, therefore, our answers deal with the differences between desmoids and conventional fibrosarcoma.

A second problem confronting us is the requirement for a systematic grading system. It is reassuring that despite the major thrust toward devising such a system, most of us acknowledge that the foundation of a grading system resides in a sound histogenetic classification. As indicated by several contributors, some information is clearly lost if a histologic classification is totally abandoned. Moreover, pathologists run a definite risk of overdiagnosing reactive lesions or benign tumors if each time they approach a soft-tissue lesion it is with an inviolate set of histologic criteria aimed at grading a malignancy. Each case must be approached systematically, with the first decision being whether it is neoplastic, the second concerning its line of differentiation, and the third its grade, depending on the most appropriate set of criteria for that cell line. The task of defining these criteria will hopefully be successfully addressed in the near future by the American Joint Committee for the Staging of Soft Tissue Tumors.

Finally, only when the first two problems have been surmounted will it be possible to compare adequately large numbers of carefully matched patients in a prospective study in order to solve the third problem, which is the optimum mode of therapy for these tumors.

REFERENCES

1. Lattes R: The pathological diagnosis of soft tissue tumors. Seventh National Cancer Conference Proceedings. Philadephia, J.B. Lippincott, 1972, pp 869–872
2. Pack GT, Ariel IM: Tumors of the Soft Somatic Tissues. New York, Hoeber-Harper, 1958, pp 63–64
3. Senn N: The Pathology and Surgical Treatment of Tumors. Philadelphia, W.B. Saunders, 1900
4. Hajdu SI, Hajdu EO: Cytopathology of Sarcomas and Other Nonepithelial Malignant Tumors. Philadelphia, W.B. Saunders, 1976
5. Hajdu SI, Melamed MR: The diagnostic value of aspiration smears. Am J Clin Pathol 59:350–356, 1973
6. Hamilton JB: Lectures on Tumors from a Clinical Standpoint, ed 2, Detroit, G.S. Davis, 1892
7. Virchow R: Die Cellularpathologie in ihrer Begrundung auf physiologische und pathologische Geweblehre. Berlin, A. Hirschwald, 1858
8. Ewing J: Neoplastic Diseases, ed 2, Philadelphia, W.B. Saunders, 1922
9. Gilford H: Tumors and Cancers. A Biological Study. London, Selwyn and Blount, 1925
10. Hajdu SI: Pathology of Soft Tissue Tumors. Philadelphia, Lea & Febiger, 1979
11. Quick D, Cutler M: Neurogenic sarcoma: A clinical and pathological study. Ann Surg 86:810, 1927
12. Ewing J: Causation, Diagnosis and Treatment of Cancer. Baltimore, Williams and Wilkins, 1931
13. Stout AP: Pathological aspects of soft part sarcomas. Ann NY Acad Sci 114:401, 1964
14. Russell W, Cohen J, Enzinger F, et al.: A clinical and pathological staging system for soft tissue sarcomas. Cancer 40:1562, 1977
15. Williams WR: The Natural History of Cancer. New York, W. Wood and Company, 1908
16. D'Angio GJ, Evans A: Soft tissue sarcomas. In Bloom HJG, Lemerle I, Neidhardt MK, Voute PA (eds): Cancer in Children. Clinical Management. New York, Springer-Verlag, 1975, pp 217–241
17. Donaldson MH: Treatment of neuroblastoma. Seventh National Cancer Conference Proceedings. Philadelphia, J. B. Lippincott, 1972, pp 605–609
18. Dorfman HD: Malignant transformation of benign bone lesions. Seventh National Cancer Conference Proceedings. Philadelphia, J. B. Lippincott, 1972, pp 901–914
19. Hajdu SI: Pathology of Soft Tissue Tumors. Philadelphia, Lea & Febiger, 1979, pp 192–193
20. Jaffe HL: Tumors and Tumorous Conditions of the Bones and Joints. Philadelphia, Lea & Febiger, 1958, pp 491–497
21. Pack GT, Ariel IM: Tumors of the Soft Somatic Tissues. New York, Hoeber-Harper, 1958, pp 45–50
22. Prat J, Woodruff, JM, Marcove R: Epithelioid sarcoma. An analysis of 22 cases indicating the prognostic significance of vascular invasion and regional lymph node metastases. Cancer 41:1472–1487, 1978
23. Kauffman SL, Stout AP: Lipoblastic tumors of children. Cancer 12:912, 1959
24. Stout AP: Hemangioendothelioma: A tumor of blood vessels featuring vascular endothelial cells. Ann Surg 118:445, 1943
25. Kauffman SL, Stout AP: Histiocytic tumors (fibrous xanthoma and histiocytoma) in children. Cancer 14:469, 1961
26. Chung EB, Enzinger FM: Infantile fibrosarcoma. Cancer 38:729, 1976
27. Pritchard DJ, Soule EH, Taylor WF, Ivins JC: Fibrosarcoma: A clinicopathologic and statistical study of 199 tumors of the soft tissue of the extremities and trunk. Cancer 33:888, 1974
28. Hajdu SI, Shiu MH, Fortner JG: Tendosynovial sarcoma. A clinicopathologic study of 136 cases. Cancer 39:1201–1217, 1977

29. Lee SM, Hajdu SI, Exelby PR: Synovial sarcomas in children. Surg Gynecol Obstet 138:701, 1974
30. Suit HD: Soft tissue sarcomas: Radiotherapy applications (excluding rhabdomyosarcoma). Proceedings of CCIRC Symposium on Sarcomas of Soft Tissue and Bone in Childhood. J. Natl Cancer Inst (In press)
31. Soule EH, Pritchard DJ: Fibrosarcoma in infants and children. A review of 110 cases. Cancer 40:1711–1721, 1977
32. Pack GT, Ariel IM: Tumors of the Soft Somatic Tissues. New York, Hoeber-Harper, 1958, pp 681–693
33. Linschild RL, Soule EH, Henderson ED: Pleomorphic rhabdomyosarcomata of the extremities and limb girdles. A clinicopathological study. J Bone Joint Surg 47A:715–726, 1965
34. Pack GT, Eberhart WF: Rhabdomyosarcoma of skeletal muscle. Surgery 32:1023–1064, 1952
35. Hajdu SI: Pathology of Soft Tissue Tumors. Philadelphia, Lea & Febiger, 1979, p 46
36. Lawrence W Jr, Jegge G, Foot FW Jr: Embryonal rhabdomyosarcoma. A clinicopathological study. Cancer 17:361–376, 1964
37. Fine G, Horn RC Jr: Soft tissue tumors: Aids in differential diagnosis. Pathol Annu 4:211, 1969
38. Yunis EJ, Agostini RM Jr, Walpusk JA, Hubbard JD: Glycogen in neuroblastomas. A light and electron-microscopic study of 40 cases. Am J Surg Pathol 3:313, 1979
39. Sarnat HB, deMello DE, Siddiqui SY: Diagnostic value of histochemistry in embryonal rhabdomyosarcoma. Am J Surg Pathol 3:177, 1979
40. Koh S, Johnson WW: Antimyosin and antirhabdomyoblast sera. Their use for the diagnosis of childhood rhabdomyosarcoma. Arch Pathol 104:118, 1980
41. Morales AR, Fine G, Nadji M: Cardiac myxoma. Immunohistochemical evidence for an endothelial origin. Hum Pathol 12:896, 1981
42. Mukai K, Rosai J, Hallaway BE: Localization of myoglobin in normal and neoplastic human skeletal muscle cells using an immunoperoxidase method. Am J Surg Pathol 3:373, 1979
43. Stembridge VA, Luibel FC, Ashworth CT: Soft tissue sarcomas: Electron microscopic approach to histogenetic classification. South Med J 57:772, 1964
44. Gabbiani G, Fu YS, Gordon I, et al.: Epithelioid sarcoma. A light and electron microscopic study suggesting synovial origin. Cancer 30:486, 1972
45. Morales AR, Fine G, Pardo V, Horn RC: Ultrastructure of smooth muscle tumors with a consideration of the possible relationship of glomangiomas, hemangiopericytomas and cardiac myxomas. Pathol Annu 10:65, 1975
46. Rosai J, Summer HW, Kostianovsky M, Perez-Mesa C: Angiosarcoma of the skin. A clinicopathologic and fine structural study. Hum Pathol 7:83, 1976
47. Taxy JB, Battifora H: Malignant fibrous histiocytomas: An electron microscopic study. Cancer 40:254, 1977
48. Kindblom LG, Save-Soderbergh J: The ultrastructure of liposarcoma. Acta Pathol Microbiol Scand (Section A) 87:109, 1979
49. Weiss SW, Enzinger FM: Myxoid variant of malignant fibrous histiocytoma. Cancer 39:1672, 1977
50. Weiss SW, Enzinger FM: Malignant fibrous histiocytoma: An analysis of 200 cases. Cancer 41:2250, 1978
51. Roques AWW, Horton LWL, Leslie J, Buxton-Thomas MS: Inflammatory histiocytoma in the left upper abdomen with a leukemoid blood picture. Cancer 43:1800, 1979
52. Soule EH, Enriquez P: Atypical fibrous histiocytoma, malignant fibrous histiocytoma, malignant histiocytoma and epithelioid sarcoma. A comparative study of sixty-five tumors. Cancer 30:128, 1972
53. Peiffer C: Die Desmoide der Bauchdeiken und ihre Prognose. Beitr Klin Chir 44:334, 1904

54. Nichols RW: Desmoid tumors. A report of 31 cases. Arch Surg 7:277, 1923
55. Stout AP: Juvenile fibromatoses. Cancer 7:953, 1954
56. Ackerman LV, Rosai J: Surgical Pathology ed 5. St. Louis, C. V. Mosby, 1974, pp 1116–1122
57. Stout AP: In DePalma AF (ed): The Fibromatoses. Clinical Orthopedics. Philadelphia, J. B. Lippincott, 1961, pp 11–17
58. Castro EB, Hajdu SI, Fortner JG: Surgical therapy of fibrosarcoma of extremities. Arch Surg 107:284, 1973
59. Enzinger FM, Shiraki M: Musculo-aponeurotic fibromatosis of the shoulder girdle (extra-abdominal desmoid). Cancer 20:113, 1967
60. Donald JM, Caylor HD: Fibrosarcoma developing in a desmoid. Ann Surg 89:631, 1929
61. Soule EH, Scanlon, PW: Fibrosarcoma arising in an extra-abdominal desmoid tumor—Report of a case. Mayo Clin Proc 37:443, 1962
62. Cantin J, McNeer GP, Chu FC, Booker RJ: The problem of local recurrence after treatment of soft tissue sarcoma. Ann Surg 168:47–53, 1968
63. Van der Werf-Messing B, Van Unnik JAM: Fibrosarcoma of the soft tissues. Cancer 18:1113–1123, 1965
64. Suit HD, Russell WO: Radiation therapy of soft tissue sarcomas. Cancer 36:759–764, 1975
65. Hill DR, Newman H, Phillips TL: Radiation therapy of desmoid tumors. Am J Roentgenol 117:84–89, 1973
66. Enzinger FM, Shiraki M: Musculoaponeurotic fibromatosis of the shoulder girdle (extra-abdominal desmoid): analysis of 30 cases followed 10 or more years. Cancer 20:1131, 1967
67. Suit H, Russell WO, Martin RG: Sarcoma of soft tissue: clinical and histopathologic parameters and response to treatment. Cancer 35:1478–1483, 1975
68. Morton DL, Eilber FR, Weisenburger TH, et al.: Limb salvage using preoperative intra-arterial Adriamycin and radiation therapy for extremity soft tissue sarcomas. Aust NZ J Surg 48:56–59, 1978
69. Suit HD, Proppe KH, Mankin HJ, Wood WC: Preoperative radiation therapy for sarcoma of soft tissue. Cancer (In press)
70. Hunter J: A Treatise on the Blood, Inflammation and Gunshot Wounds. London, G. Nicol, 1794
71. Shiu MH, Magill GB, Hopfan S: Recent Trends in Treatment of Soft Tissue Sarcomas. In Hajdu S: Pathology of Soft Tissue Tumors. Philadelphia, Lea & Febiger, 1979
72. Shiu MH, Hajdu SI: Management of soft tissue sarcoma of the extremity. Semin Oncol 8:172–179, 1981
73. Bowden L, Booher RJ: The principles and technique of resection of soft parts for sarcoma. Surgery 44:963, 1958
74. Sordillo PP, Helson L, Hajdu SI, et al.: Malignant schwannoma—Clinical characteristics. Survival and response to therapy. Cancer 47:2503–2509, 1981
75. Sordillo PP, Hajdu SI, Magill GB, et al.: Effect of desacetyl vinblastine amide (DVA)[1] against human sarcomas heterotransplanted in nude mice. Cancer Clinical Trials 3:391–394, 1980
76. Sordillo PP, Magill GB, Shiu MH, et al.: Adjuvant chemotherapy of soft-part sarcomas with Alomad (S4). J Surg Oncol 18:345, 1981
77. Morton D, Saxton RE, Irie RF: unpublished data
78. Sethi J, Hirshaut Y: Complement-fixing antigen of human sarcomas. J Natl Cancer Inst 578:489, 1977
79. Israel L, Edelstein R: Nonspecific immunostimulation with Corynebacterium parvum in human cancer. In Immunological Aspects of Neoplasia. Baltimore, Williams and Wilkins, p 485, 1975
80. Townsend CM, Eilber FR, Morton DL: Skeletal and soft tissue sarcomas. Treatment with adjuvant immunotherapy. JAMA 236:2187, 1976
81. Sinkovics JC: Immunotherapy of human tumors. Pathobiol Annu 8:241, 1978

82. Stout AP: Fibrosarcoma in infants and children. Cancer 15:1028–1040, 1962
83. Hajdu SI: The paradox of sarcomas. Acta Cytol 24:373–383, 1980
84. Hajdu SI, Lemos L, Kozakewich H, et al.: Growth patterns and morphology of human soft tissue sarcomas in nude mice. Cancer 47:90–98, 1981
85. Yazdi HM, Hajdu SI: Non-myogenic soft tissue sarcomas in children. (In preparation)
86. Cody HS, Turnbull AD, Fortner JG, Hajdu SI: The continuing challenge of retroperitoneal soft tissue sarcomas. Cancer 47:2147–2152, 1981
87. Bullough WS: Mitotic activity in the tissues of dead mice, and in tissues kept in physiological salt solution. Exp Cell Res 1:410–420, 1950
88. Scully RE: Mitosis counting-1. Hum Pathol 7:481–482, 1976

DEVELOPING CARCINOMA (DYSPLASIA) OF THE URINARY BLADDER

WILLIAM M. MURPHY AND MARK S. SOLOWAY

Contemporary interest in premalignant lesions of the urothelium began in 1952, with the publication of Melicow's report of multifocal "hyperplasia" in grossly normal areas of urinary bladders removed for carcinoma.[1] Subsequently, studies by Schade and Swinney documented areas of "atypia" in cystoscopically normal urothelium obtained by random mucosal biopsy in 86 percent of 100 patients being followed for bladder cancer.[2,3] These results were similar to those of Eisenberg, who called the lesions "atypical hyperplasia."[4] More recently, comparable abnormalities have been found by Koss[5] and Farrow[6] after complete mapping of the urothelia of total-cystectomy specimens.

Concurrently, experimental model systems of bladder cancer were being developed. Studies by Erturk,[7,8] Ito,[9,10] Druckrey,[11] Hicks,[12] and others indicated that transitional cell carcinomas could be induced in rodents by a variety of chemicals. The tumors tended to grow rather slowly, and evidently developed via either hyperplasia followed by dysplasia or through dysplasia alone.[13] These early experiments were primarily designed to establish that bladder cancer could be induced by carcinogens, and reference to the pathologic features of premalignant lesions tended to be cursory. Nevertheless, both experimental and clinical observations described pathologically recognizable, albeit clinically obscure, precursors of both papillary and flat bladder carcinomas, and led to the currently held concept that bladder cancer arises through a field-change phenomenon in which grossly visible lesions represent only the most florid components of the carcinogenic process.

A variety of terms have been used to describe the changes of developing urothelial carcinoma; atypia, atypical hyperplasia, and dysplasia are most often cited. None of these terms is totally adequate to describe the observed changes, yet it seems advisable to adhere to one or another of these terms rather than to introduce completely new names, all of which would have their own peculiar inadequacies. For the purpose of this presentation, the lesions of developing urothelial carcinoma will be called dysplasias. Although the temptation to extrapolate directly from the morphologic changes described in the uterine cervix should be avoided, the term dysplasia is firmly established in the medical nomenclature, has a more restricted definition in common medical usage than does "atypia," has been applied to both cells and tissue, and generally connotes a premalignant condition.

CLINICAL FEATURES

Urothelial dysplasia is a relatively recently and still rather inadequately defined entity. As recognition of the lesions defined by this term increases and diagnostic terminology crystallizes, knowledge of their incidence, symptomatology, and biologic significance will expand. Undoubtedly, some of our concepts will require revision. The disease is multifocal and is most often encountered in patients being followed for bladder cancer; the frequency with which it has been documented varies considerably (22 to 86 percent),[3,4,14,15] and is probably related to host factors as well as to the frequency of examination and adequacy of sampling. Although constantly present in bladders removed for widespread or intractable carcinoma, dysplastic epithelium is also found in random or selected mucosal biopsies from patients with previously resected superficial bladder cancer and no apparent clinical disease.[5,6,16] Most patients with urothelial dysplasia are middle-aged males without urinary tract infection who complain of frequency, dysuria, and/or hematuria; however, symptoms specific to urothelial dysplasia have not yet been identified. The lesions cannot at present be localized endoscopically, but recent refinements in fiberoptics, allowing texture (e.g., granularity) as well as color discrimination, promise increased recognition in the future. Furthermore, although dysplastic cells exfoliate into the urine, the criteria for their interpretation have not yet been completely elucidated, so that a definitive diagnosis of the disease rests on histologic identification.

The biologic potential of urothelial dysplasia has not been completely determined. Preliminary evidence from clinical sources indicates that it represents developing urothelial carcinoma. In a retrospective review of flat urothelium adjacent to resected superficial bladder cancers, Althausen et al.[14] found that 9 of 25 patients with dysplasia had developed invasive carcinomas during a 5-year follow-up. Murphy et al.,[16] in a prospective study of selected mucosal biopsies from patients being followed for bladder cancer, documented recurrences in 11 of 29 (38 percent) patients after the appearance of premalignant lesions, as compared to only 5 of 32 (16 percent) individuals with normal mucosae at these selected sites.

PATHOLOGY

The urothelium can be evaluated in terms of 10 characteristics:

1. Number of cell layers. The number of cell layers depends upon the degree of distention of the bladder at the time tissue is removed. In properly prepared sections, there are from four to seven cell layers.[17] Although common in experimental animals, an increase in the number of cell layers is not a constant

feature of developing carcinoma in humans. The basal and intermediate cells are morphologically similar; the superficial cells are cytologically, histologically, and ultrastructurally distinct.[18] The superficial cells form a single continuous layer along the luminal surface of the epithelium, and are highly specialized to form surface membrane. These cells often have tetraploid chromosomal numbers[19] (Fig. 1). Ultrastructural studies have indicated that they are not present in invasive tumors and may not be involved in the carcinogenic process.[20,21]

2. Polarity. Normal basal and intermediate cells are slightly columnar, with their long axes perpendicular to the basal lamina. Their nuclei are ovoid, with a similar orientation. Superficial cells may be columnar but are usually flat with their nuclei oriented parallel to the basal lamina. During carcinogenesis, the basal and intermediate cells become polygonal with round nuclei, so that normal polarization is lost.
3. Denudation. Urothelial cells are tightly cohesive. Extensive denudation may occur after mechanical trauma, topical chemotherapy, or in areas of carcinoma in situ. Such denudation is not a feature of dysplasia.

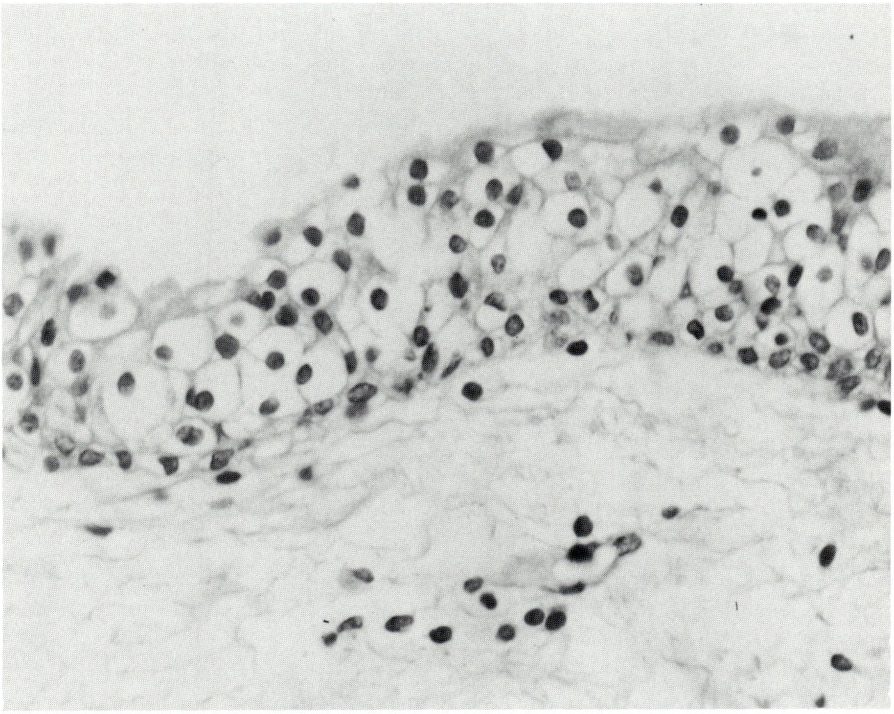

FIG. 1. Normal urothelium. This slightly tangential section of normal human urothelium accentuates the superficial cells. These cells often contain mucin as well as glycogen, and rarely have complete clearing of their cytoplasm. In this area, the nuclei are not reactive, and are therefore only slightly larger than the nuclei of the underlying basal and intermediate cells. Note the cytoplasmic clearing, lack of nuclear crowding, and relatively uniform size of the nuclei. The underlying lamina propria is rich in thin-walled blood vessels. H&E. ×512.

4. Cytoplasmic clearing. Basal and intermediate cells often appear to have clear cytoplasm. This is the result of dissolution of their glycogen during fixation and processing. Lack of cytoplasmic clearing is readily identified at low magnification and may be the first indication of a urothelial abnormality such as dysplasia.
5. Nuclear size. Basal and intermediate urothelial cells have small nuclei of uniform size. During the early phases of developing carcinoma, these nuclei increase to at least twice normal size. In the late phase, nuclear size is more variable; the nuclei of superficial cells may be bizarre but the nuclear-to-cytoplasmic (N:C) ratios of these cells remain low. Changes in superficial cell nuclei are not helpful in the evaluation of developing carcinoma.
6. Nuclear crowding. In normal tissue, sectioned at 2 to 4 μ, the nuclei are centrally located and widely spaced. One of the earliest indications of cellular hyperplasia is the tendency of the nuclei to crowd together so that their borders apparently overlap. While focal nuclear overlapping may occur in sections cut at 6 to 8 μ, this process is more pronounced in dysplasia.
7. Nuclear notching. Indentations in nuclear borders can be seen in normal as well as degenerating cells. These notches are more prominent among the cells of developing carcinoma. When viewed en face they appear as creases. Dysplastic cells usually contain only one or two nuclear notches, the remaining contours being convex. The presence of numerous nuclear notches is indicative of degeneration.
8. Chromatin pattern. The granularity and distribution of chromatin depend upon many factors and vary among laboratories. In our preparations, normal nuclear chromatin tends to accentuate the nuclear borders. Elsewhere it is evenly distributed and so fine that individual grains are difficult to discern. During developing carcinoma, nuclear chromatin becomes more granular but remains evenly distributed. As the cells develop into malignant elements, the chromatin becomes coarsely granular and tends to be irregularly distributed.
9. Nucleoli. Depending upon the type of preparation, numerous small, angular nucleoli can be identified in normal urothelial cells. The presence of large nucleoli indicates increased cellular activity. In developing carcinoma, this is a feature of advanced lesions.
10. Mitoses. Mitoses are rare in normal urothelium. Their presence indicates increased cellular activity but is not necessarily suggestive of carcinogenesis.

None of the above features are exclusive to dysplasia, and the pathologist should always attempt to study and compare areas considered to represent normal urothelium before rendering a diagnosis.

Dysplasia describes a spectrum of abnormalities between normal urothelium and carcinoma in situ (CIS). As with many histologic processes, these lesions can be divided into three degrees of morphologic severity—mild, moderate, and severe (or slight, moderate, and marked). Lesions of the lowest grade must be distinguished from reactive, regenerative, and/or reparative epithelium. Abnormalities of the highest grade must be differentiated from unequivocal carcinoma. Since similar names have been applied to well-defined morphologic changes in developing carcinoma of the uterine cervix, it is tempting merely to extrapolate on a one-for-one basis, and to define dysplasia of the urothelium in terms of lesions of similar names in the uterine cervix. However, both intuition and the scanty available clinical evidence caution against this approach.

A recent study using the N-butyl-N-(4-hydroxybutyl) nitrosamine (BHBN) model system in Wistar rats serves to emphasize the pitfalls in defining urothelial dysplasia through the terms employed for cervical carcinoma.[22] These inbred animals were given a known carcinogen, and their bladders were studied at regular intervals during the development of carcinoma. Three stages of developing cancer could be recognized. The earliest histologic lesions (mild dysplasia) were characterized by a slight increase in the number of cell layers, cellular and nuclear enlargement, sharp angulations (notches) of the nuclear borders, and a finely granular, evenly distributed chromatin (Fig. 2). Large nucleoli were not apparent, and mitoses were rare. As time progressed and the next stage of morphologic severity (moderate dysplasia) occurred, more cells were involved but the morphologic changes did not differ significantly in type from those of the early phase (Fig. 3). Nuclei of dyplastic cells continued to be large but not larger than those of cells in the early lesions. Nuclear notching and crowding were more prominent and mitoses more easily identified than in the early lesions, but this prominence related almost entirely to increased numbers of involved cells. The cellular chromatin remained

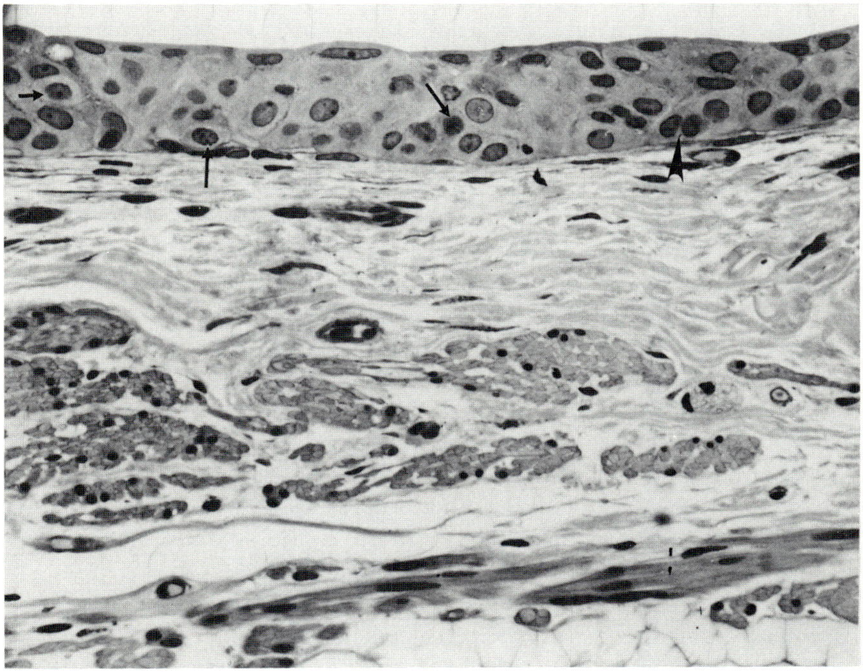

FIG. 2. Mild dysplasia in rat urothelium. Note the slight nuclear crowding (arrowhead) in this section cut at 2.5 μ. Many, but not all, nuclei have notches in their borders (arrows). There is slight disorientation of nuclei as well as variability in nuclear size. PAS. $\times 512$.

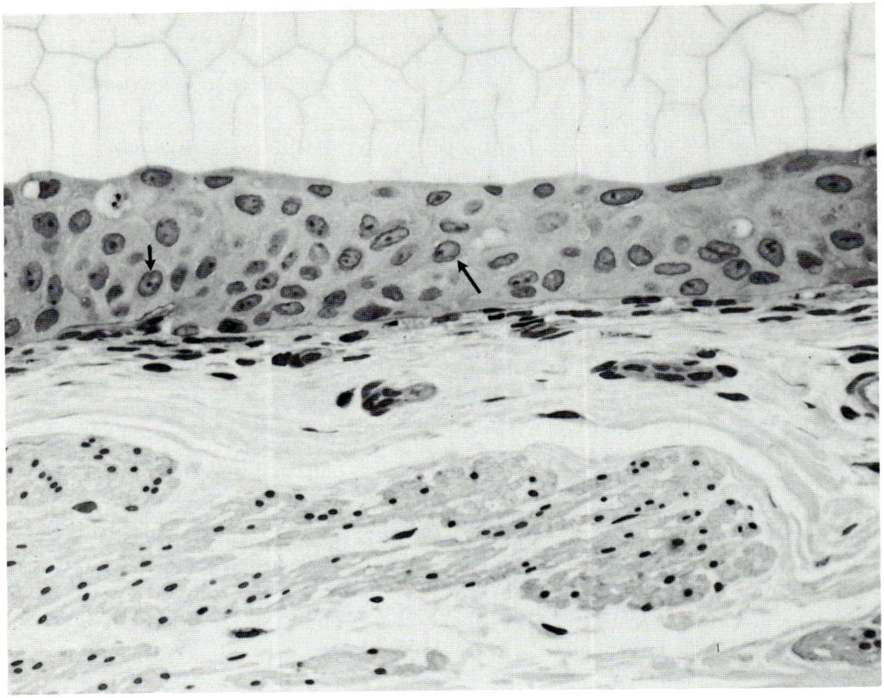

FIG. 3. Moderate dysplasia in rat urothelium. The increased nuclear size, nuclear crowding, and nuclear notching (arrows) in Figure 2 are more prominent here. In addition, there is an increase in the number of cell layers and a slight increase in the granularity of the nuclear chromatin. A few, small nucleoli are present. PAS. ×512.

finely granular and evenly distributed, although a few cells began to exhibit a coarser, more irregular chromatin pattern. As with early lesions, large nucleoli were uncommon. During this period, papillary tumors composed of cells similar to those in the flat areas began to appear. Late lesions (severe dysplasia) differed from early and intermediate phases both in degree and type of cellular involvement (Fig. 4). Both cells and nuclei became smaller and more numerous. Macronucleoli and mitoses were prominent. The chromatin became more coarsely granular and irregularly distributed. In some areas, small foci of microinvasion occurred, even though maturation was evident in the overlying epithelium. During this period, frank carcinoma was developing in other areas. The cells composing the invasive tumors were similar morphologically to those in the adjacent flat, noninvasive epithelium.

Of course the results of controlled carcinogenesis in experimental animals cannot be used to define the lesions of spontaneously developing carcinoma in humans. They do, however, serve to underscore the proposition that the various grades of dysplasia differ qualitatively as well as quantitatively, that the spectrum of histologic abnormalities should not be arbitrarily divided into three equal parts, that the

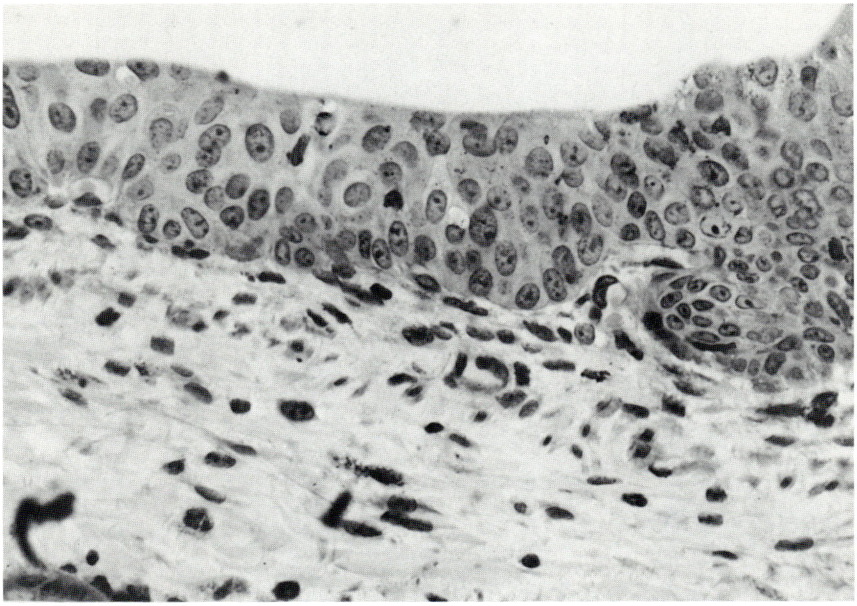

FIG. 4. Severe dysplasia in rat urothelium. In this photograph, the changes of moderate dysplasia on the left blend into those of severe dysplasia in the center and right. Note the coarsely granular, irregularly distributed chromatin and prominent nucleoli in the severely dysplastic areas. PAS. ×512.

cellular features of a dysplasia may be more important than the histologic pattern in determining biologic potential, and that invasive carcinoma can arise prior to replacement of the entire overlying epithelium with tumor cells.

On the basis of the foregoing experimental and clinical data, the histologic features of urothelial dysplasia can be described.

Dysplasia—mild and moderate. This is a multifocal, flat urothelial lesion first recognized at low magnification by the lack of cytologic clearing (vacuolization) of its cells (Fig. 5). An increase in the number of cell layers, i.e., greater than seven, is unusual, although five to seven cell layers are common. The basal and intermediate cells are larger than those in adjacent normal areas. The nuclei are large and more spherical than ovoid, so that there appears to be a loss of cellular polarization. Increased numbers of nuclei with apparent nuclear crowding are prominent. On closer inspection, the nuclei have one or two angular indentations (notches) in their borders. Viewed en face, these irregularities appear as creases (Fig. 6). The remaining nuclear contours are smooth and convex, in contrast to the nuclei of degenerative cells, which have numerous crenelations associated with shrunken, concave contours. The chromatin of dysplastic nuclei, when compared to that of adjacent normal elements, is more granular and does not tend to aggregate along and accentuate the nuclear borders (Fig. 7). One or several

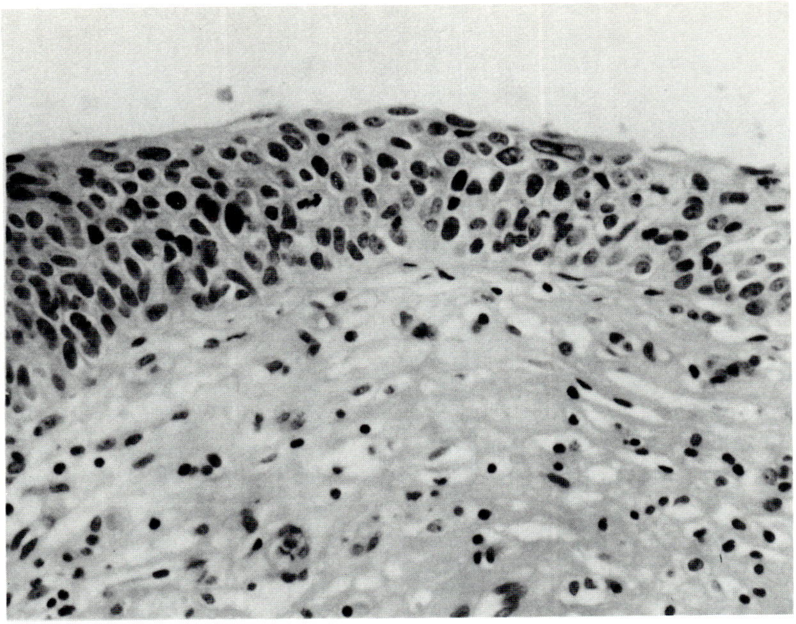

FIG. 5. Dysplasia in human urothelium. At low magnification, there is loss of cytoplasmic clearing and nuclear crowding in this section cut at 4 to 6 μ. H&E. ×320.

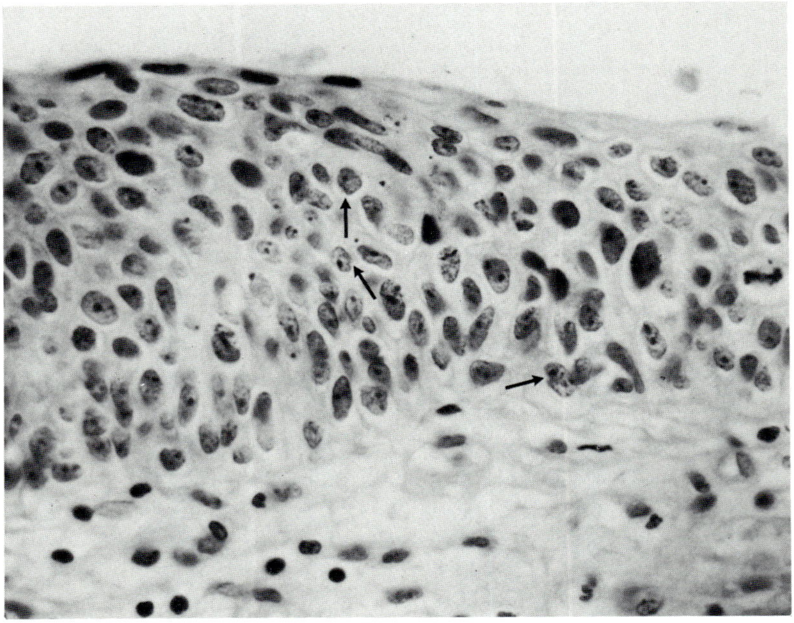

FIG. 6. Higher magnification of Figure 5. There are numerous nuclear notches (arrows). A few nuclei contain small nucleoli. A mitosis occurs on the right side of the photograph. Although indicative of increased cellular activity, mitoses are not a distinguishing feature of dysplasia. H&E. ×512.

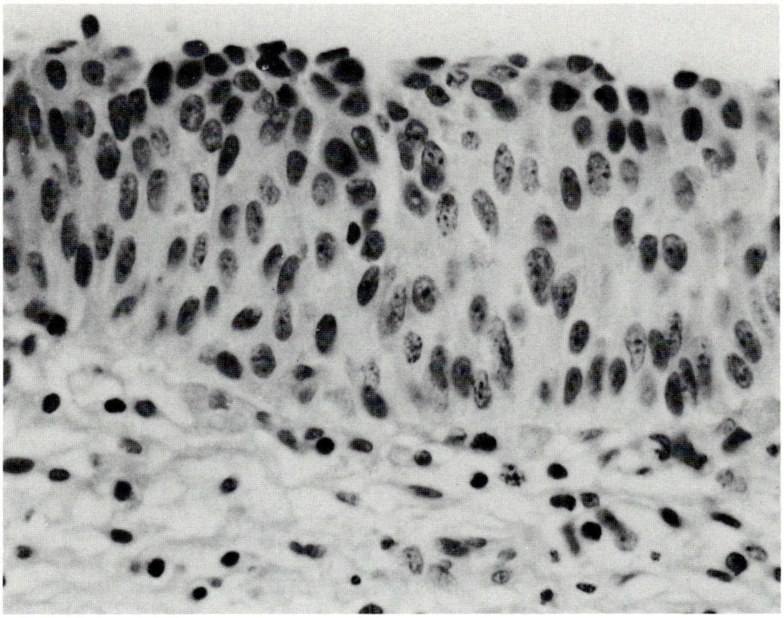

FIG. 7. Dysplasia in human urothelium. Note the uniformly distributed, finely granular chromatin in these cells. The chromatin is more granular than that in the experimental animals but not as coarse as in the severe dysplasia illustrated in Figure 8.

nucleoli may be identified, depending upon the method of tissue preparation, but they are small and angular. Mild dysplasia can be separated from moderate dysplasia, but the distinction is a matter of degree rather than of kind. Although this difference may become important in the future, at present there seems little justification for emphasizing it. Mitoses, though often present, are not a distinguishing feature of urothelial dysplasia. Superficial cells form a continuous layer of epithelium over dysplastic areas.

Dysplasia—severe. This comprises a markedly abnormal urothelium that bears a closer resemblance to carcinoma in situ than to mild-moderate dysplasia. At low magnification the cells are large and often hyperchromatic, with homogeneous cytoplasm and increased N:C ratios. An increase in the number of cell layers is not a constant feature of severe dysplasia, nor is nuclear crowding (Fig. 8). At high magnification, increased nuclear size, notching, and pleomorphism are readily observed. The chromatin tends to be coarsely granular and may be irregularly distributed. Large nucleoli are the rule. Mitoses are common but not a necessary diagnostic feature.

Severely dysplastic cells are usually intermixed with elements of lesser severity, and are covered by superficial cells. In contrast to the cells of carcinoma in situ, the abnormal cells tend to be more cohesive and do not occupy the full thickness of the epithelium. However, this distinction may have more morphologic than biologic significance, since invasion may proceed from severe dysplasia prior to the development of a characteristic in situ pattern (Fig. 9).

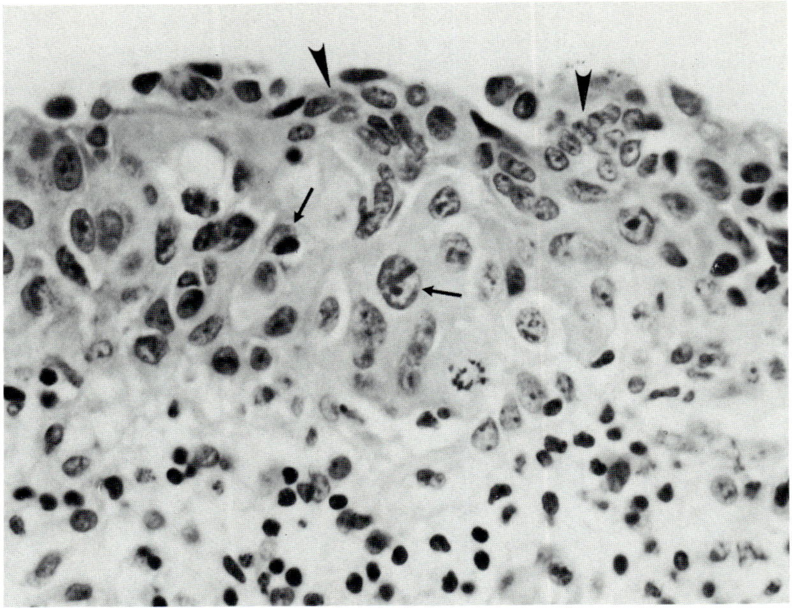

FIG. 8. Severe urothelial dysplasia. The severely dysplastic cells occupy the lower layers of the epithelium. In this section, these cells are large, with abundant eosinophilic cytoplasm, but such cells may also be smaller with higher N:C ratios. The distinguishing features are the coarsely granular, irregularly distributed chromatin and large nucleoli (arrows). Note the overlying, less dysplastic cells (arrowheads). H&E. ×512.

PITFALLS IN HISTOLOGIC DIAGNOSIS

Although severe dysplasia may be variably interpreted as malignant or benign, it is readily recognized as a significant abnormality. The major problems in histologic interpretation in this area involve the mild–moderate lesions. The urothelium lining the ureters, renal pelves, bladder neck, and urethra is normally composed of larger cells with less cytoplasmic clearing than that of the bladder proper (Fig. 10), and epithelium from these areas may resemble dysplasia at low magnifications. The absence of significant nuclear abnormalities such as crowding, notching, and finely granular chromatin should lead to the correct diagnosis. A similar caution applies to the evaluation of urothelium overlying lymphoid follicles (cystitis follicularis), although the cause of slight cellular atypia among these cells is unclear. Non-dysplastic cells that have been mechanically compressed and/or those lining crypts may appear larger and more crowded than normal (Fig. 11). The diagnosis of urothelial dysplasia should not rest solely on such areas.

Nuclear atypicalities are not uncommon among cells in Brunn's nests or cystitis glandularis. While such changes may reflect real lesions, especially in patients receiving radiation and/or topical chemotherapy, they may also be secondary to growth abnormalities related to local inflammation and obstruction. Reactive or reparative urothelium may resemble dysplasia upon cursory inspection; large cells with increased nuclear size, nuclear notching, and granular chromatin may be seen in both lesions (Fig. 12). Lack of nuclear crowding, relatively low N:C ratios, and

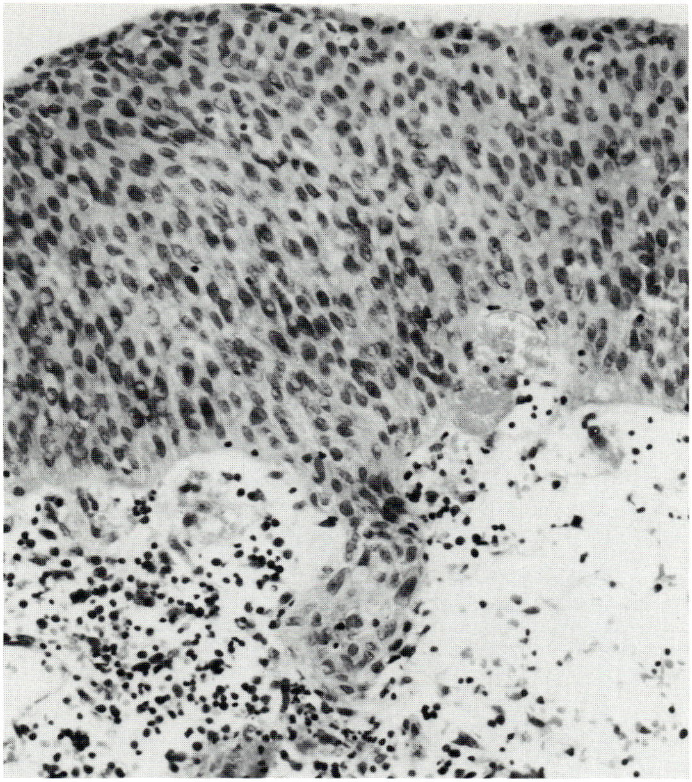

FIG. 9. Focal invasion of the lamina propria may occur in the absence of a full-thickness neoplastic change. In this section, from the lateral bladder wall, a finger-like projection of neoplastic urothelial cells extends into the lamina propria. Note the apparent maturation, manifested by a decrease in N:C ratios, loss of nucleoli, and decreased nuclear size, of the cells as they approach the surface. H&E. ×205.

the presence of prominent nucleoli tend to distinguish reactive or reparative lesions from dysplasia. The factors that might alter urothelium are myriad and poorly understood. Therefore, whenever possible, one should, prior to rendering a diagnosis, compare normal urothelium to those areas considered to be dysplastic.

URINARY CYTOLOGY

Urinary cytology may be a valuable tool in the identification and follow-up of patients with urothelial dysplasia. As the cellular features of low-grade neoplasms become better delineated, it will be but a small further step to recognize the changes of dysplasia. Controlled studies on experimental animals indicate that dysplastic cells can be recognized, but that they are not prone to exfoliate in great numbers.[22] Such cells apparently can be distinguished by their increased nuclear size, nuclear notching, and granular chromatin (Fig. 13). The confounding factors—repair, mechanical artifact, and degeneration—noted upon histologic evaluation are even

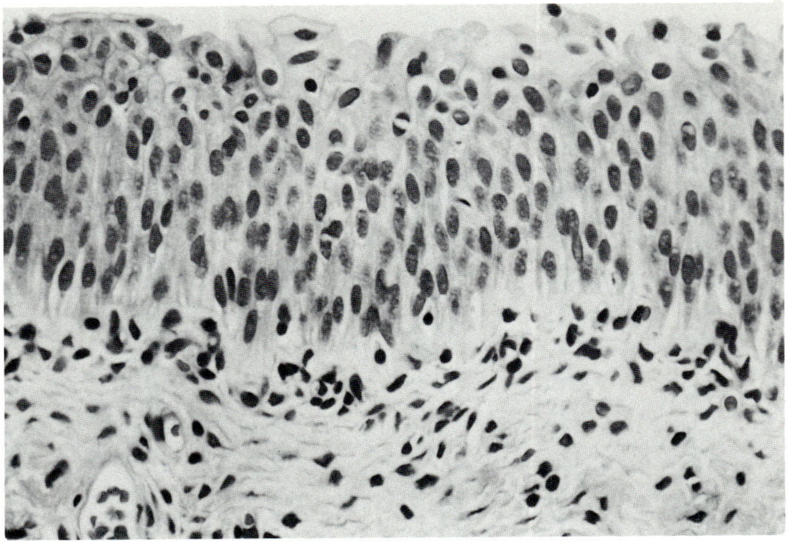

FIG. 10. Normal urothelium from the bladder neck. Despite the slight electrocautery artifact in this section, one can note the lack of cytoplasmic clearing and the apparent hyperplasia, as well as nuclear crowding. The uniformity and normal polarity of the nuclei as well as their chromatin pattern are not characteristic of dysplasia, however. H&E. ×320.

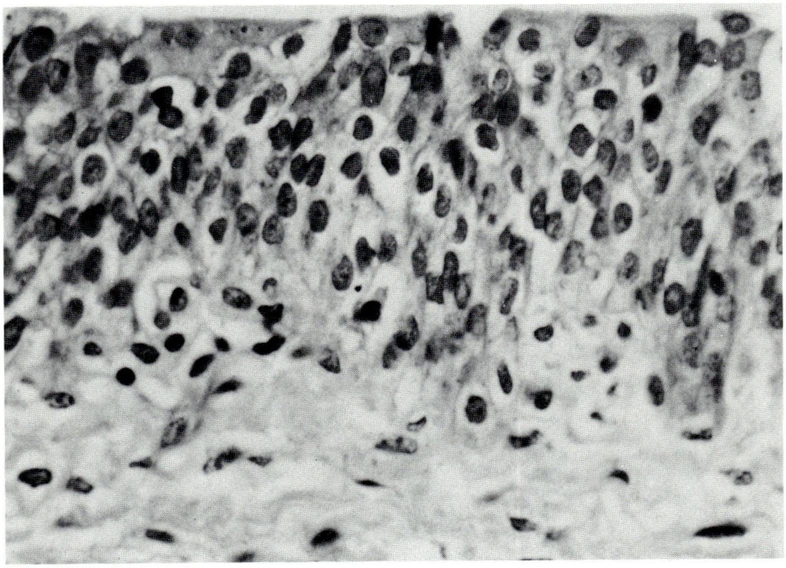

FIG. 11. Epithelium lining a crypt. While these cells may well be dysplastic, slight nuclear crowding and an apparent increase in chromatin granularity can result from compression. The diagnosis of dysplasia should not rest solely on cells in crypts. H&E. ×512.

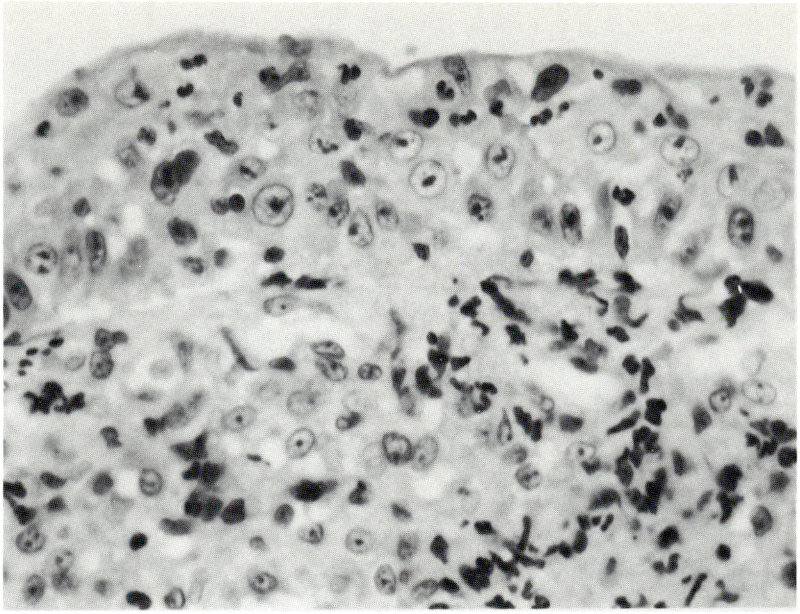

FIG. 12. Urothelial regeneration and repair. The low N:C ratios, regular nuclear borders, and prominence of nucleoli distinguish this lesion from dysplasia. Also, note the presence of numerous neutrophils in the epithelium. While not diagnostic, this finding is more common in urothelial regeneration than in dysplasia. H&E. ×512.

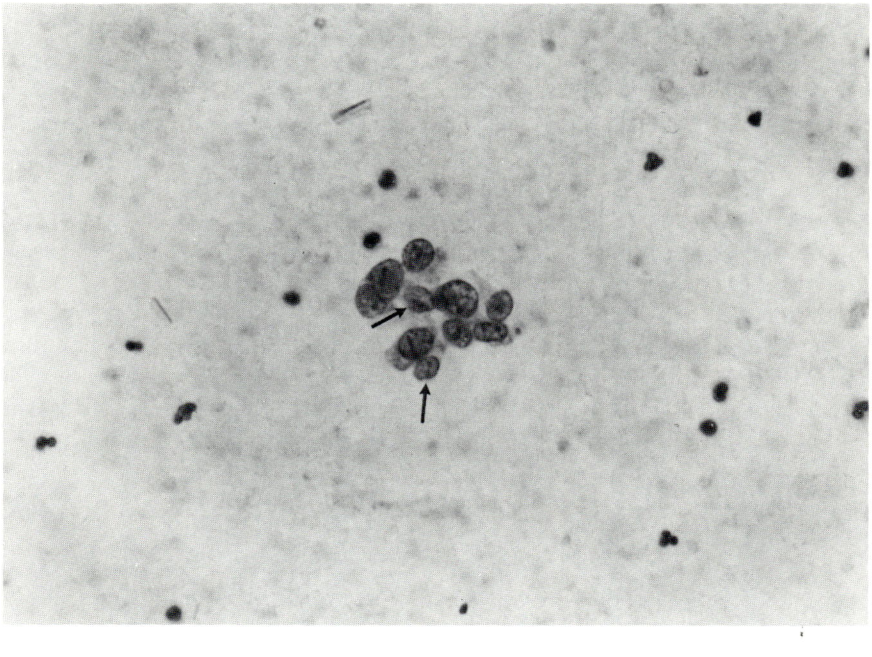

FIG. 13. Dysplastic cells in voided urine. Although nuclear notches (arrows) are difficult to discern in this two-dimensional representation, the chromatin granularity is prominent. Also note the increased N:C ratios. EA50. ×512.

more troublesome when only a small number of loosely aggregated cells are available for study.

Nevertheless, in a recently completed analysis of our clinical material, using definitions established from work in experimental animals, the cytologic diagnosis of urothelial dysplasia was found to identify a population of patients with significant urothelial disease.[23] Of the 1,554 urinary specimens examined during the period of study, 77 (5.0 percent) contained dysplastic cells. Among the 48 patients involved, 29 (60.4 percent) either had or were being followed for cancer. Eight of these patients had histologically documented dysplasia. Dysplasia in the absence of previous or coincident cancer occurred in an additional 12.5 percent, so that overall, dysplastic lesions were histologically documented in 29.2 percent of patients with dysplastic cells in their urinary specimens. These results are encouraging, especially since all patients with dysplastic cells were not biopsied, and since the abnormal areas were not endoscopically apparent. However, much more work will be required in this area before the cytologic diagnosis of urothelial dysplasia can be added to the armamentarium of the practicing pathologist.

ELECTRON MICROSCOPY AND BIOLOGIC MARKERS

Not surprisingly, little work specifically related to urothelial dysplasia has been done in the areas of electron microscopy and biologic markers. However, ultrastructural analyses of both human and experimentally induced developing carcinoma have been reported. One of the earliest morphologic events of developing urothelial carcinoma is the loss of surface microridges and their replacement by pleomorphic microvilli[12,24] (Fig. 14). The asymmetrical unit membrane becomes symmetrical and a surface glycocalyx forms.[25] The cells begin to lose their cohesion and deep clefts appear.[24] With freeze-fracture techniques, a reaggregation of protein molecules in the lipid layer of cell membranes can be identified.[26]

Studies using the specific red-cell adherence test to determine the presence of ABO isoantigens on dysplastic urothelium have been equivocal;[27] this relates at least in part to the difficulty of identifying dysplastic elements. Urothelial cells produce carcinoembryonic antigen (CEA) in varying amounts, but almost nothing is known of the relationship of this potential biologic marker to dysplasia. Nor, apparently, is measurement of urinary CEA useful as an adjunct to the diagnosis of dysplasia.[28] Dysplastic epithelium has a significantly increased lactic dehydrogenase V/I isoenzyme ratio;[29] the chromosomal complement of the epithelium is unknown.

RADIATION AND CHEMOTHERAPY

Systemic and topical chemotherapy as well as external radiation can all induce urothelial changes resembling those of dysplasia[30,31]; these changes have been documented both in experimental animals and in humans. Similar abnormalities can be seen after a variety of nontherapeutic procedures, including catheterization alone.[31] The cellular changes are not specific to any known agent. With rare excep-

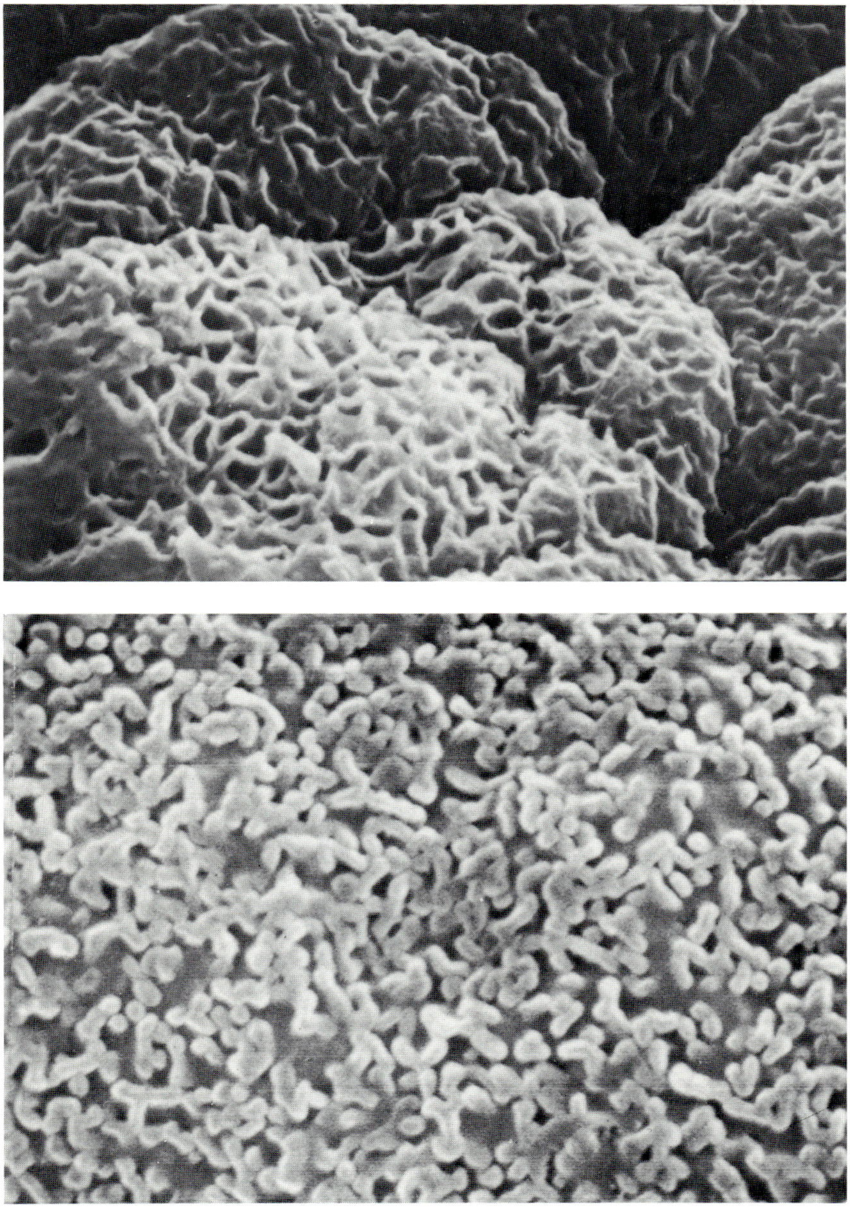

FIG. 14. Top. Normal surface microridges in a scanning electron micrograph (SEM) of a Wistar rat bladder. ×11,000. **Bottom.** Pleomorphic microvilli in the bladder of a Wistar rat during carcinogenesis. ×20,000.

tions, lesions related to radiation, drugs, and/or instrumentation can be readily distinguished histologically from those of urothelial dysplasia. Fortunately, such lesions are usually confined to superficial cells. When basal and intermediate cells are involved, the atypicalities are localized to individual elements and are seldom widespread (Fig. 15).

THE UROLOGIST'S APPROACH TO DYSPLASIA

Over the last few years, urologists have become sensitive to the possibility of dysplasia and/or carcinoma in situ in patients with irritative bladder symptoms not readily explained by inflammatory conditions such as cystitis, prostatitis, and the trigonitis-urethritis syndrome. If dysplasia is initially indicated by urinary cytology, bladder biopsies should be planned at the time of complete endoscopic examination. Endoscopy should be preceded by excretory urography to delineate completely the upper urinary tracts. Assuming that no lesions are found either in the upper tracts or in the bladder, selected biopsies should be obtained lateral to each ureteral orifice, in the posterior midline, and from the dome; in the male, a cold cup biopsy from the prostatic urethra should also be considered. Biopsies should be obtained even if the selected sites appear endoscopically normal. The diagnosis of dysplasia by cytology, whether or not confirmed by histologic examination, should not call for therapeutic intervention. Careful follow-up, including endoscopy, cytology, and even selected site biopsies to rule out a more serious lesion are recommended.

Far more commonly, dysplasia is discovered in a patient with a previous or coincident bladder tumor whose ''normal'' mucosa has been biopsied as part of an initial or follow-up examination. The diagnosis of dysplasia in these circumstances may lead to repeat biopsies at regular intervals, intravesical chemotherapy, or both. In a patient with concurrent superficial bladder tumors, a finding of dysplasia will usually lead to intensive intravesical chemotherapy following resection of the cystoscopically visible lesions. It should be emphasized that no universal standard of treatment for dysplasia has as yet been accepted by urologists, and that the pathologist should discuss his or her findings with the clinician to ensure appropriate therapy. Follow-up should include excretory urography and endoscopy plus cytology and biopsy. The interval at which these studies should be performed varies, but most urologists reevaluate every 3 to 6 months; these examinations are done primarily for the early detection of more serious lesions. In institutions with a strong emphasis on urinary cytology, invasive procedures may be done at less frequent intervals.

DISCUSSION

The concept that invasive carcinoma of the urothelium may develop through a series of morphologically recognizable stages is widely accepted. The biologic potential of any particular phase is incompletely understood, but mounting evidence indicates that the lesions described here are premalignant. Urothelial

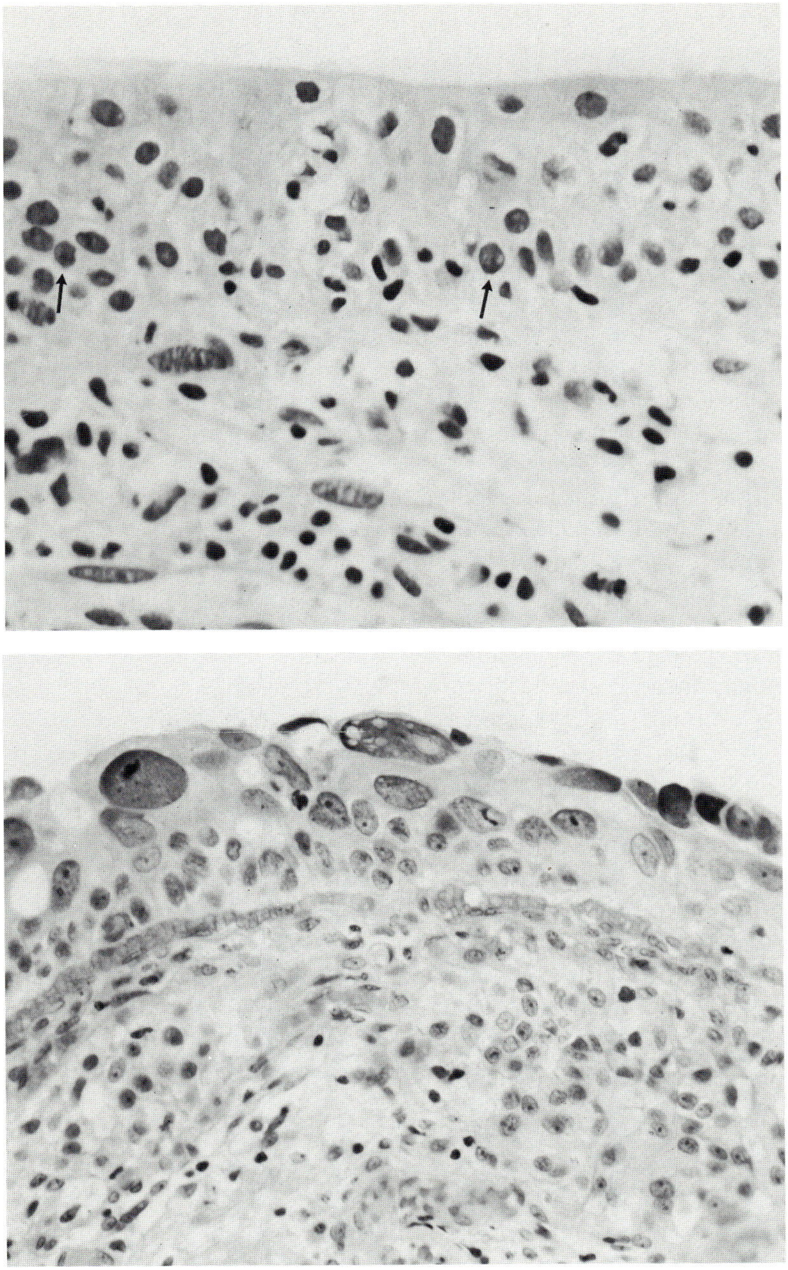

FIG. 15. Top. The effect of radiation on normal urothelium. Fine cellular detail is obscured by the radiation damage. Individual nuclei may have the features of dysplasia (arrows) but they are intermixed with more normal elements. H&E. ×512. **Bottom.** Urothelium after treatment with thiotepa. The major effect of this drug is epithelial denudation. Less often, bizarre nuclear changes in superficial cells are identified. Note that the superficial cells affected by the drug can be easily distinguished from the underlying dysplastic intermediate and basal cells. H&E. ×320.

dysplasia bears a superficial resemblance to the premalignant abnormalities of similar names in the uterine cervix.[32] It precedes as well as accompanies papillary and/or invasive cancer. Indeed, when bladders containing papillary or invasive neoplastic lesions have been thoroughly examined, dysplasia has been found in almost every case.[5,6,33] Most importantly, recent clinical studies indicate that patients whose bladders exhibit dysplasia are at an increased risk of developing new tumors, some of which may be invasive.[14,16]

It is to be expected that in any area of pathology as new as urothelial dysplasia, conflicts with established dogma and controversies over the interpretation of emerging data will exist; the inadequacy of the nomenclature connected with this condition has already been discussed. A more fundamental problem is the conflict between established definitions and conceptual themes arising from current clinical and experimental studies. From long usage, papillary tumors of the urothelium have been regarded as neoplasms, and variation in their cellular features have been graded according to increasing degrees of severity. From a conceptual standpoint, however, the cells of grade 1 papillary carcinoma differ little from those of flat, mild–moderate dysplasia. One might argue that a more credible scheme would be to classify urothelial abnormalities as papillary carcinoma grades 1, 2, and 3, and flat carcinoma (or carcinoma in situ) grades 1, 2, and 3.[34,35] Yet despite the simplicity and intellectual appeal of such a system, it cannot be implemented without a major overhaul of the data base—including the results of treatment—for bladder cancer. Papillary and invasive urothelial carcinomas are readily identified endoscopically and easily followed, and have been studied for decades. Flat urothelial lesions are cystoscopically obscure, relatively difficult to detect during follow-up, and only recently recognized as distinct pathologic entities. Should we then treat papillary and flat lesions similarly? Few would recommend such a step, although it would follow logically from the classification scheme described above. Should moderate dysplasia be labeled CIS grade 2, the danger of inappropriate therapy is obvious.

The proper attitude toward urothelial dysplasia has received little attention. Should it be viewed as a benign disease that marks a "disturbed" epithelium responding abnormally to carcinogenic stimuli, and which is therefore more prone to develop clinical carcinoma? Or are the dysplastic lesions themselves part of a neoplastic process which, if untreated, will eventuate in carcinoma? If we may benefit from observations made during 30 years of intensive study of the uterus, elements of both theories may apply. The spectrum of urothelial dysplasia may include lesions of such severity as to suggest that they are already malignant morphologically if not biologically; severe dysplasia as defined here may be an example of this. Conversely, abnormalities of the opposite end of the spectrum lack the cellular features of malignancy, and although morphologically benign when sampled, may have the capacity to become malignant. This may be manifested either by progression through a more advanced, in situ stage or by invasion without further dedifferentiation. Until further information becomes available we have chosen to recognize both the morphologic innocence as well as the biologic potential for malignancy of early lesions, and have classified them together as mild–moderate dysplasia. In contrast, both experimental studies and morphologic analysis indicate that severe dysplasia is closely akin to carcinoma in situ. The recognition of only two grades of premalignant flat urothelium tends to separate low-grade, possibly reversible lesions from high-grade, probably irreversible ones, and should not only facilitate the identification but encourage the diagnosis of these abnormalities by practicing pathologists.

While knowledge of the biology, course, and prognosis of urothelial dysplasia is accumulating, there is a need for a widely accepted system of nomenclature and classification for this condition. The one proposed and illustrated here is very similar to one explored by the collaborating pathologists of the National Bladder Clinical Collaborative Group A.[36] Using a given set of definitions, the author and nine other pathologists participated in a Delphi study* to determine if individuals from various institutions could agree on a set of cellular features that would describe the grades of dysplasia. There were three rounds, during which each pathologist examined and diagnosed 24 representative sections, discussed his finding with the group, and reevaluated the material in the light of any new knowledge gained. The results established that substantial agreement was possible in this area. Eighteen of the 24 examples were bracketed within one degree of morphologic severity by at least 9 of the 10 participating pathologists. Among the six instances in which a 90 percent concensus could not be achieved, 80 percent agreement occurred in two; three sections depicted changes in cystitis glandularis; and one apparently illustrated two lesions. Acceptance of a standard classification will form the basis for future observations and comparison of results among institutions. Perceived flaws in the concepts embodied in this scheme will foster further research. There is an urgent need to quantitate the types of observed cell changes and to better correlate the degrees of dysplasia with prognosis. Meanwhile, developing carcinoma of the urothelium, whether termed dysplasia, atypia, or atypical hyperplasia, can and should be recognized and recorded. Patients with these lesions should be systematically but not necessarily aggressively evaluated and followed. The discovery of new biologic markers and the refinement of established tests will, hopefully, open additional avenues of understanding.

CONCLUSIONS

Urothelial dysplasia is a premalignant condition usually involving multiple sites in the bladder and upper collecting system. The diagnosis is suspected clinically in patients with irritative bladder symptoms who have no evidence of urinary tract infection. The lesions cannot be localized endoscopically and are almost always found in random or selected biopsies from apparently normal mucosa. Cytology is useful in detection of the lesions, but a definitive diagnosis depends upon tissue studies. Urothelial dysplasia comprises a spectrum of morphologic changes from normal to unequivocal carcinoma. Mild changes must be distinguished from reactive/reparative states, whereas severe abnormalities may already be biologically malignant. Histologic criteria for diagnosis of the condition have been outlined

*See the chapter by Nagy, Frable, and Murphy: "Classification of Premalignant Urothelial Abnormalities," pp 219–233.

and, if the vagaries of nomenclature can be overcome, pathologists can learn to recognize these changes and agree on a workable classification scheme. Urologists are increasingly aware of urothelial dysplasia and are beginning to incorporate urinary cytology and selected site biopsies into their initial and follow-up evaluation regimens. At present, a pathologic diagnosis of dysplasia should lead to careful follow-up and, in some cases, intravesical chemotherapy. Aggressive treatment, including cystectomy, is not indicated.

REFERENCES

1. Melicow MM: Histological study of vesical urothelium intervening between gross neoplasms in total cystectomy. J Urol 68:261, 1952
2. Schade ROK, Swinney J: Pre-cancerous changes in bladder epithelium. Lancet 2:943, 1968
3. Schade ROK, Swinney J: The association of urothelial atypism with neoplasia. J Urol 109:619, 1973
4. Eisenberg RB, Roth RR, Schweinberg MH: Bladder tumors and associated proliferative mucosal lesions. J Urol 84:544, 1960
5. Koss LG, Tiamson EM, Robbins MD: Mapping cancerous and pre-cancerous bladder changes. JAMA 227:281, 1974
6. Farrow GM, Utz DC, Rife CC: Morphological and clinical observations of patients with early bladder cancer treated with total cystectomy. Cancer Res 36:2495, 1976
7. Erturk E, Price JM, Morris JE, et al.: The production of carcinomas of the urinary bladder in rats by feeding N-[4-(5-nitro-2-furyl)-2-thiazolyl] formamide. Cancer Res 27:1996, 1967
8. Erturk E, Cohen SM, Price JM, et al.: Pathogenesis, histology, and transplantability of urinary bladder carcinomas induced in albino rats by oral administration of N-[4-(5-nitro-2-furyl)-2-thiazolyl] formamide. Cancer Res 29:2219, 1969
9. Ito N, Hiasa Y, Tamai A, et al.: Histogenesis of urinary bladder tumors induced by N-butyl-N-(4-hydroxybutyl) nitrosamine in rats. GANN 60:401, 1969
10. Ito N, Matayoshi K, Arai M, et al.: Effect of various factors on induction of urinary bladder tumors in animals by N-butyl-N-(4-hydroxybutyl) nitrosamine. Gann 64:151, 1973
11. Druckrey H, Preussmann R, Ivankovic S, et al.: Auslesende Erzeugung von Blasenkrebs an Ratten durch dibutyl und N-butyl-N-butanol (4)-nitrosamin. Z Krebsforsch 66:280, 1964
12. Hicks RM, Chowaniec J: Experimental induction, histology, and ultrastructure of hyperplasia and neoplasia of the urinary bladder epithelium. Int Rev Exp Pathol 18:199, 1978
13. Kunze E, Schauer A, Schatt S: Stages of transformation in the development of N-butyl-N-(4-hydroxybutyl) nitrosamine-induced transitional cell carcinomas in the urinary bladder of rats. Z Krebsforsch 87:139, 1976
14. Althausen AF, Prout GR Jr, Daly JJ: Non-invasive papillary carcinoma in situ. J Urol 166:575, 1976
15. Soloway MS, Murphy WM, Rao MK, et al.: Serial multiple site biopsies in patients with bladder cancer. J Urol 120:57, 1978
16. Murphy WM, Nagy GK, Rao MK, et al.: "Normal" urothelium in patients with bladder cancer. Cancer 44:1050, 1979
17. Koss LG: Tumors of the Urinary Bladder. Washington, D.C., Armed Forces Institute of Pathology, 1975, pp 1–7
18. Firth JA, Hicks RM: Interspecies variation in the fine structure and enzyme cytochemistry of mammalian transitional epithelium. J Anat 116:31, 1973

19. Levi PE, Cooper EH, Anderson CK, et al.: Analyses of DNA content, nuclear size and cell proliferation of transitional cell carcinoma in man. Cancer 23:1074, 1969
20. Fulker MJ, Cooper MD, Tanaka T: Proliferation and ultrastructure of papillary transitional cell carcinoma of the human bladder. Cancer 27:71, 1971
21. Newman J, Hicks RM: Detection of neoplastic and preneoplastic urothelia by combined scanning and transmission electron microscopy of urinary surface of human and rat bladders. Histopathology 1:125, 1977
22. Murphy WM, Irving CC: The cellular features of developing carcinoma in murine urinary bladder. Cancer (In press)
23. Murphy WM, Crabtree WN: The cytology of urothelial dysplasia. Acta Cytol (In press)
24. Jacobs JB, Arai M, Cohen SM, et al.: Early lesions in experimental bladder cancer: scanning electron microscopy of cell surface markers. Cancer Res 36:2512, 1976
25. Hicks RM, Wakefield JStJ: Membrane changes during urothelial hyperplasia and neoplasia. Cancer Res 36:2502, 1976
26. Pauli BU, Friedell GH, Weinstein RS: Topography and numerical densities of intramembrane particles in chemical carcinogen-induced urinary bladder carcinomas in Fischer rats. Lab Invest 39:565, 1978
27. Weinstein RS, Alroy J, Farrow GM, et al.: Blood group isoantigen deletion in carcinoma in situ of the urinary bladder. Cancer 43:661, 1979
28. Murphy WM, Vandevoorde JP, Rao MK, et al.: The clinical value of urinary carcinoembryonic antigen-like substances in urothelial cancer. J Urol 118:806, 1977
29. Bredin HC, Daly JJ, Prout GR Jr: Lactic dehydrogenase isoenzymes in human bladder cancer. J Urol 113:487, 1975
30. Koss LG: Diagnostic Cytology and Its Histopathologic Bases, ed 2. Philadelphia, J.B. Lippincott, 1968, pp 413–418
31. Murphy WM, Soloway MS, Lin CJ: Morphological effects of thio-TEPA on mammalian urothelium: changes in abnormal cells. Acta Cytol 22:550, 1978
32. Patten SF Jr: Diagnostic Cytopathology of the Uterine Cervix, ed 2, revised. New York, S. Karger, 1978, pp 115–207
33. Soto EA, Friedell GH, Tiltman AJ: Bladder cancer as seen in giant histologic sections. Cancer 39:447, 1977
34. Friedell GH, Bell JR, Burner SW, et al.: Histopathology and classification of urinary bladder carcinoma. Urol Clin North Am 3:53, 1976
35. Mostofi FK, Sesterhenn I: Carcinoma in situ of bladder. Abstract presented at the American Urological Association, San Francisco, May 1980
36. Nagy GK, Frable WJ, Murphy WM: The classification of premalignant urothelial abnormalities: A Delphi study of the National Bladder Clinical Collaborative Group A. Pathol Annu 17(1):219, 1982

CLASSIFICATION OF PREMALIGNANT UROTHELIAL ABNORMALITIES

A Delphi Study of the National Bladder Cancer Collaborative Group A

GEORGE K. NAGY, WILLIAM J. FRABLE, AND WILLIAM M. MURPHY

Since the early studies of Melicow,[7] bladder cancer has been increasingly recognized as a field-change phenomenon wherein endoscopically detectable tumors represent only a part of the neoplastic process. In patients with bladder cancer, a systematic search frequently reveals grossly normal urothelium to be histologically abnormal.[6] Experimental studies have demonstrated that carcinoma of the bladder can progress through several stages of morphologic evolution, from subtle, barely recognizable changes to invasive tumors.[4] Little is known about the biologic behavior, clinical importance, and natural history of these lesions which deviate from normal structure but fall short of being in situ carcinoma.

Over the past several years, the Central Pathology Laboratory of the National Bladder Cancer Collaborative Group A has collected over 5,000 urothelial biopsies and 250 cystectomy specimens according to a standard protocol.[9,10] Microscopic urothelial abnormalities were frequently encountered in this material. Since prolonged and careful follow-up information is available for the cases from which these biopsies come, they seem particularly suitable for studying the following important questions:

1. Is it possible to establish histologic criteria for such subtle urothelial morphologic changes that will permit different pathologists, using these criteria, to classify individual cases in reproducible manner?

This study was supported by Public Health Service Grant CA 15490 from the National Cancer Institute through the National Bladder Cancer Project.

TABLE 1. Coded Diagnostic Terms

Code	Diagnostic Term
B	Normal/benign
M0	Hyperplasia
M0.5	Atypia, not otherwise classified
M1	Atypia/dysplasia, mild
M2	Atypia/dysplasia, moderate
M3	Atypia/dysplasia, severe
M4	Carcinoma in situ

2. Is such a classification clinically meaningful, i.e., will cases classified in different divisions of the system have different natural histories when measured by clinical parameters (e.g., length of survival, "recurrence" rate, etc.)?

The present study was undertaken to investigate the first question.

MATERIALS AND METHODS

Study Set

The lesions under study were depicted in a set of 26 colored 35-mm photomicrographs (transparencies) illustrating the entire range of histologic urothelial abnormalities, from very slight changes to noninvasive carcinoma. During the study, two cases were judged to contain early invasive cancer; these were not used in the analysis. Thus, only "flat" and "noninvasive" lesions were considered.

Classification System

Since terminology itself (atypia or dysplasia, for example), can evoke emotional responses among pathologists, the definitions used for the lesions being studied were given number codes and discussed in these terms (Table 1). A category indicating lesser abnormality which could not be classified according to the submitted definitions was included ("M 0.5"); participants were encouraged, however, to use this code sparingly. A set of histologic definitions was set up for each proposed category and was circulated among the participating pathologists. After preliminary discussions, a final outline was established (Tables 2 to 7), and thereafter, every participating pathologist was requested to use this admittedly arbitrary classification system in evaluating the photomicrographs.

The number of categories in this system (one for probable non-premalignant changes, three for probable premalignant changes, and one for outright neoplastic changes without invasion) might appear unnecessarily high. However, since the

TABLE 2. Guidelines for Interpretation of Flat, Noninvasive Lesions of Urothelium (Histology)

Terms	Definitions
Urothelial thickening	At least eight nuclear layers present in areas sectioned perpendicular to the basal lamina.
Polarization	A. Normal: The basal cells are columnar. Almost all nuclei, except those in the superficial layer, are arranged perpendicular to the basal layer and/or the surface. B. Altered: The nuclei of intermediate cells are no longer arranged with their long axes perpendicular to either the surface or the basal lamina. This disorientation varies in degree. In general, more loss of polarity occurs in more severe lesions.
Nuclear crowding	A focal increase in number of nuclei per unit space. Often this is manifested by overlapping of nuclei in relatively thin sections (4 μ). Nuclear crowding probably reflects increases in nuclear-cytoplasmic ratios. Care should be taken to avoid interpretation of cells in invaginated areas, crypts, or areas of compression.
Nuclear border irregularity	Angular indentations of nuclear border with tendency toward lobulation of nuclei. The indentations may vary from one to three and may be so marked that the nuclei appear folded. In general, more severe lesions have more nuclear irregularity.
Increased nuclear size	Nuclei larger than those of normal intermediate cells. There is some variation in nuclear size and shape among cells.
Chromatin	Evaluation of the chromatin structure is very subjective. The apparent composition and distribution are dependent upon fixation and staining. Nevertheless, some guidelines in the interpretation of chromatin are offered. A. Normal: Very finely granular (dusty) with a tendency toward peripheral concentration. B. Abnormal: The granules are more distinct and may be either fine or coarse. As the lesion becomes more severe, the chromatin tends to be less peripherally concentrated and more irregularly distributed throughout the nuclei.

clinical usefulness of such a system should be determined by later follow-up, "splitting" seemed to be preferable to "lumping"—that is, if later studies do not show important differences in the natural history of lesions classified in two adjacent categories of the system, the data in these two categories can be "lumped" together without difficulty. On the other hand, if lesions with different natural histories had initially been put into the same class, later separation and evaluation of such cases would be impossible.

TABLE 3. Hyperplasia (M0)

Description	Thickened urothelium without dysplastic changes
Mandatory features	
Polarization	Normal
Superficial cells	Present
Nuclear size	Normal
Nuclear crowding	None
Nuclear irregularity	None
Chromatin	Normal
Noncritical features	
Mitoses	Absent or very rare
Connective tissue	Inflammation may or may not be present.

Evaluation by the "Delphi" Technique

The Delphi survey approach was developed as a forecasting technique at the Rand Corporation,[2,3] and has been used in the medical field for the same purpose several times.[1,5] It is a way of maximizing the possibility of group consensus by lessening the opportunity for confrontational member interaction. Recognizing that group opinions tend to be influenced by their most eloquent, authoritative, and/or in-

TABLE 4. Mild Atypia/Dysplasia (M1)

Description	Urothelium with slight nuclear irregularities, not more pronounced than the features acceptable in "Grade 1 Transitional Cell Carcinoma" (WHO). Lesions may or may not be full thickness. In the past, this lesion has often been interpreted as normal.
Mandatory features	
Polarization	Slight and/or focal alteration
Superficial cells	Usually present and normal
Nuclear size	Slight variation from normal
Nuclear crowding	Slight
Nuclear irregularity	Slight
Chromatin	Finely granular and evenly distributed
Noncritical features	
Mitoses	Rare
Cytoplasm	Diminished glycogen
Connective tissue	Same as in M0

TABLE 5. Moderate Atypia/Dysplasia (M2)

Description	Urothelium with unequivocal nuclear irregularities, corresponding to changes in "Grade 2 Transitional Cell Carcinoma" (WHO). Lesions involve most or all of intermediate cell layers.
Mandatory features	
Polarization	Altered
Superficial cells	Usually present and normal
Nuclear size	More variation than in M1
Nuclear crowding	Present and more prominent than in M1
Nuclear irregularity	Prominent
Chromatin	Predominantly finely granular and evenly distributed. Some nuclei with coarsely granular chromatin may occur.
Noncritical features	
Mitoses	Not unusual
Nucleoli	May be prominent
Cytoplasm	Same as in M1
Connective tissue	Same as in M0

TABLE 6. Severe Atypia/Dysplasia (M3)

Description	Urothelium with severe cellular irregularities, corresponding to changes in a "Grade 3 Transitional Cell Carcinoma" (WHO). The lesion involves basal and intermediate cells but tends to spare the superficial layer. These changes are very similar to those of carcinoma in situ and may represent only a slight variation of the latter. The differentiation is particularly difficult if there is extensive denudation of the superficial layers.
Mandatory features	
Polarization	Markedly altered
Superficial cells	Present but may be abnormal
Nuclear size	Variable. Bizarre nuclei may occur
Nuclear crowding	Present
Nuclear irregularity	Present. Indentations and angularities of the nuclear borders are prominent.
Chromatin	Coarsely granular and irregularly distributed
Noncritical features	
Mitoses	Common
Nucleoli	Often prominent
Cytoplasm	Same as in M1
Connective tissue	Same as in M0

TABLE 7. Carcinoma In-Situ (M4)

Description	Urothelium with nuclear irregularities corresponding to changes in "Grade 3 Transitional Cell Carcinoma" (WHO). The lesions extend from the basal layer to the surface and include the superficial layer. Lesions need not be hyperplastic.
Mandatory features	
Polarization	Lost
Superficial cells	Absent
Nuclear size	Same as in M3
Nuclear crowding	Same as in M3
Nuclear irregularity	Same as in M3
Chromatin	Same as in M3
Noncritical features	
Mitoses	Common
Nucleoli	Same as in M3
Cytoplasm	Same as in M1
Connective tissue	Significant hyperemia is usual. Inflammation may be marked.
Denudation	Common

timidating members, the Delphi technique requires that each expert review the subject in question privately, and submit his or her opinion anonymously after examining several times the changes in the positions of other participants. In summary, the elements of the Delphi technique are:

1. Anonymity of the experts.
2. Repeated feedback with the possibility for adjustment of opinions.
3. Statistical analysis of results.

In our study, the set of photomicrographs was circulated four times among the 10 participating pathologists. Two of the coauthors (K.H. and R.S.W.) took part in the designing of the study but not in the evaluation of the set. Between the Delphi "rounds," the group repeatedly met and discussed the alternative approaches without identifying the individual sources of opinions. The participants were encouraged not to change their decision after they had concluded they could accept the majority opinion. This was, however, not enforced, and there was a relatively high frequency of switching opinions back and forth during the entire study. For technical reasons, the freedom to change an opinion had to be preserved; if a participant does not have the option to shift his or her decision after temporarily agreeing with the majority consensus, the results become bound and predictable whenever at least half of the participants reach an agreement.

Statistical Methods

Every numerical code value assigned to the answers was tabulated for each round and the means and standard deviations for each individual photomicrograph were computed. As an illustration, Table 8 is an excerpt from the summary diagnoses of photomicrographs. The arithmetic means of the numerical code values were considered to be the best approximations of the opinion of the group (e.g., a mean of 3.1 indicated that the opinions clustered near the code value 3, i.e., the diagnostic consensus of the group was "severe atypia/dysplasia, M3"). The standard deviation was considered to be only an indicator of the spread of opinions, and in no way was it implied that the code values of opinions followed a normal (Gaussian) distribution.

Since the distribution pattern of code values was unknown, a nonparametric statistical test—the Friedman two-way analysis of variance by ranks[11]—was used for comparison of the spread of opinions among the individual Delphi rounds. Since it appeared that the spread of opinions did not change between the third and fourth rounds, the t-test for nonindependent samples[12] was used for comparison of these data.

RESULTS

The changes in the spread of opinions are displayed in Table 9. According to the Friedman test, the spread of opinions, as expressed by the standard deviations of code values, significantly decreased during the study ($p < 0.001$). There was, however, no significant decrease of the spread of opinions between the third and

TABLE 8. Evaluation of 26 Transparencies by 10 Pathologists, 2nd Delphi Round. Excerpt

	Pathologists											
Transparencies	1	2	3	4	5	6	7	8	9	10	Mean	SD*
•												
•												
14	1	0.5	1	2	1	1	0.5	1	1	1	1.0	0.41
15	2	4	3	4	3	1	3	1	3	4	2.8	1.14
16	0	0	0	0	0	0	0	0	0	0	0.0	0.00
17	3	4	3	0.5	4	3	4	4	2	2	3.0	1.17
18	2	3	3	3	3	3	3	2	3	3	2.8	0.42
•												
•												

* SD: Standard deviation

TABLE 9. Standard Deviations (SD) of Code Values; Four Delphi Rounds

Number of Transparency	SD 1st Round	SD 2nd Round	SD 3rd Round	SD 4th Round
1	1.25	0.72	0.47	0.33
2	1.72	0.82	0.67	0.50
3	0.99	0.95	0.70	0.52
4	1.01	1.30	0.57	0.67
5	1.18	0.54	0.32	0.33
6	0.86	0.88	0.42	0.44
7	1.73	1.31	1.07	1.07
8	0.53	0.32	0.00	0.44
9	1.06	0.76	0.58	0.70
10	1.11	0.95	0.32	0.55
11		Deleted from study		
12	1.06	0.73	0.67	0.52
13	1.44	0.91	0.82	1.01
14	0.67	0.41	0.32	0.33
15	1.43	1.14	0.52	0.67
16	0.00	0.00	0.00	0.00
17	1.23	1.17	0.67	1.10
18	0.57	0.42	0.60	0.66
19	0.63	0.32	0.00	0.33
20		Deleted from study		
21	1.14	1.50	0.76	0.44
22	0.69	0.42	0.37	0.14
23	1.26	1.20	1.05	1.27
24	0.71	0.56	0.42	0.33
25	1.10	1.10	0.83	0.33
26	0.79	0.42	0.52	0.00

fourth rounds according to the t-test. Essentially, a relatively high level of agreement was reached after three "rounds," after which further improvement was not achieved.

Analysis of Individual Cases

After three rounds of the study, 19 of 24 cases were bracketed within one degree of morphologic severity by at least 9 of the 10 participating pathologists (Table 10). Of these cases, carcinoma in situ/severe dysplasia was recognized in six photomicrographs, moderate to severe dysplasia in six, and mild to moderate dysplasia in three; two cases were diagnosed as benign conditions and two cases as hyperplasia, mild atypia/dysplasia. All reviewers agreed about the photomicrographs illustrating

TABLE 10. Consensus of 10 Pathologists After Three Rounds of Delphi Study

	Code						
Transparency	B	M0	M0.5	M1	M2	M3	M4
1	–	–	–	–	2	8	–
2	–	1	1	5	3	–	–
3	–	–	–	–	5	4	1
4	–	–	–	–	1	7	2
5	–	–	–	9	1	–	–
6	–	–	–	–	8	2	–
7	–	1	–	–	4	4	1
8	–	–	–	–	–	–	10
9	–	–	1	2	7	–	–
10	–	–	–	–	–	1	9
11	Deleted from study						
12	–	–	–	–	1	4	5
13	–	2	–	3	5	–	–
14	–	–	–	9	1	–	–
15	–	–	–	–	–	4	6
16	10	–	–	–	–	–	–
17	–	–	–	1	5	4	–
18	–	–	–	–	1	8	1
19	10	–	–	–	–	–	–
20	Deleted from study						
21	–	–	1	5	3	1	–
22	–	2	5	3	–	–	–
23	–	1	–	1	6	1	1
24	–	–	–	–	2	8	–
25	–	–	1	–	3	6	–
26	–	4	–	6	–	–	–

normal urothelium and squamous metaplasia (Fig. 1, No. 16). In addition to the agreement on these two conditions, there was unanimous agreement for one other lesion (carcinoma in situ, Fig. 2, No. 8), and near unanimous agreement in four other lesions. Two other representative photomicrographs are shown: No. 4 (Fig. 3, majority opinion: severe atypia/dysplasia), and No. 6 (Fig. 4, majority opinion: moderate atypia/dysplasia). One other picture may represent an area of overgrowth of normal epithelium by slightly dysplastic epithelium (Fig. 5, No. 22). An illustration that could have been unequivocally recognized as hyperplasia was evidently not included in the study set.

A consensus could not be achieved in five instances. Interestingly, three of these photomicrographs (Nos. 7, 13, and 23) were from the same patient and illustrated cellular changes in von Brunn's nests (Fig. 6, No. 7), and in two of these three cases the opinions spread from benign lesion to carcinoma in situ, even after the third Delphi round.

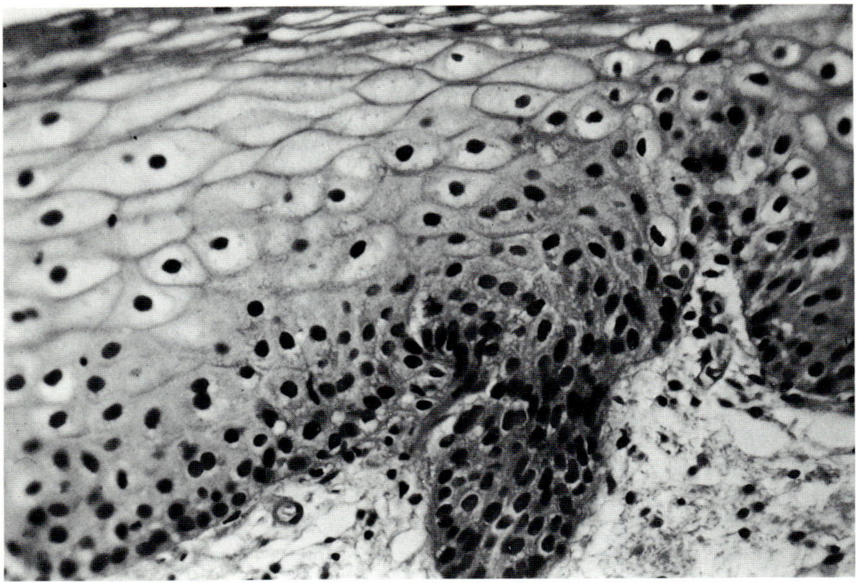

FIG. 1. Case No. 16. Squamous change ("squamous metaplasia") of urothelium. Complete consensus among ten pathologists. H&E. ×250.

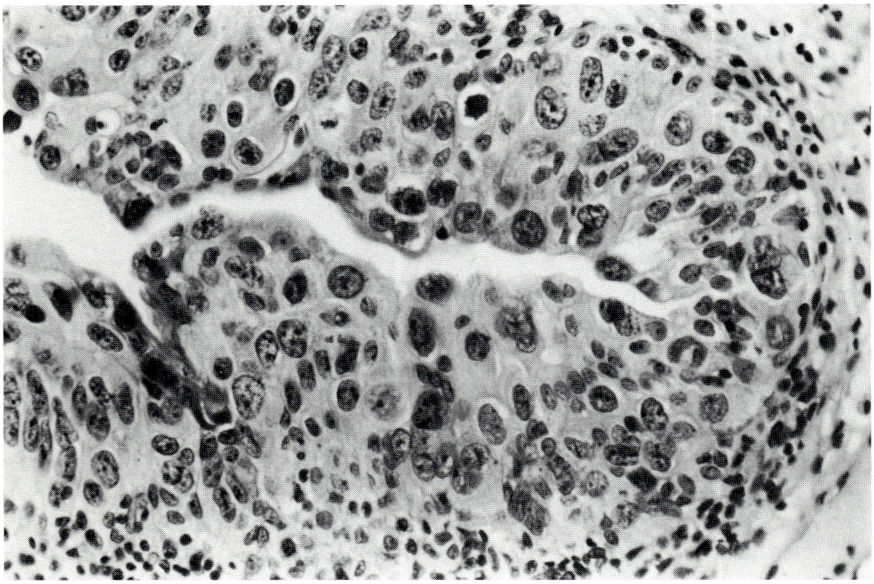

FIG. 2. Case No. 8. Carcinoma in situ of urothelium. Complete consensus in the third Delphi round. H&E. ×300.

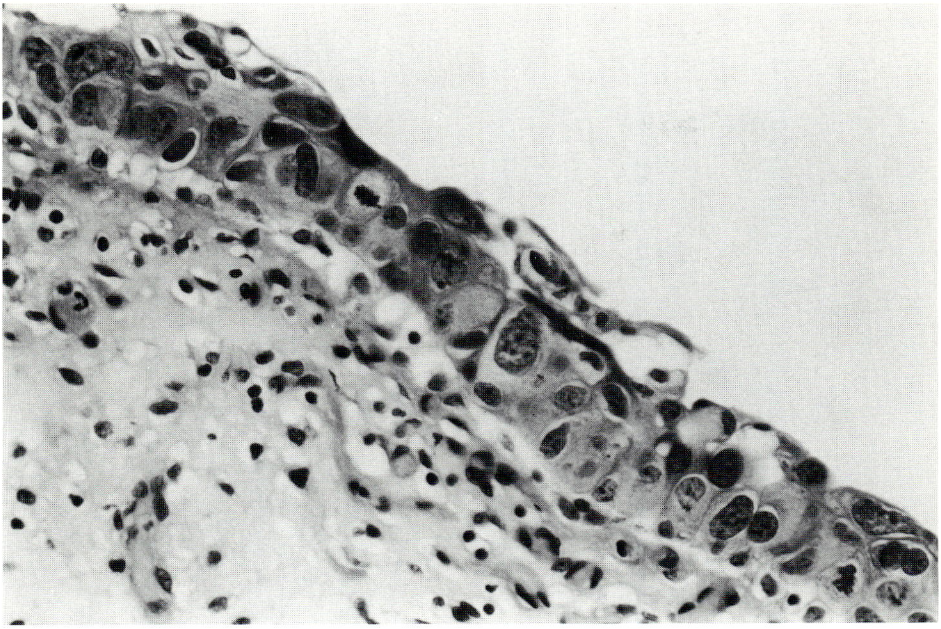

FIG. 3. Case No. 4. In the third Delphi round, seven participants classified this lesion as severe atypia/dysplasia of urothelium, two as carcinoma in situ, and one as moderate atypia/dysplasia. H&E. ×380.

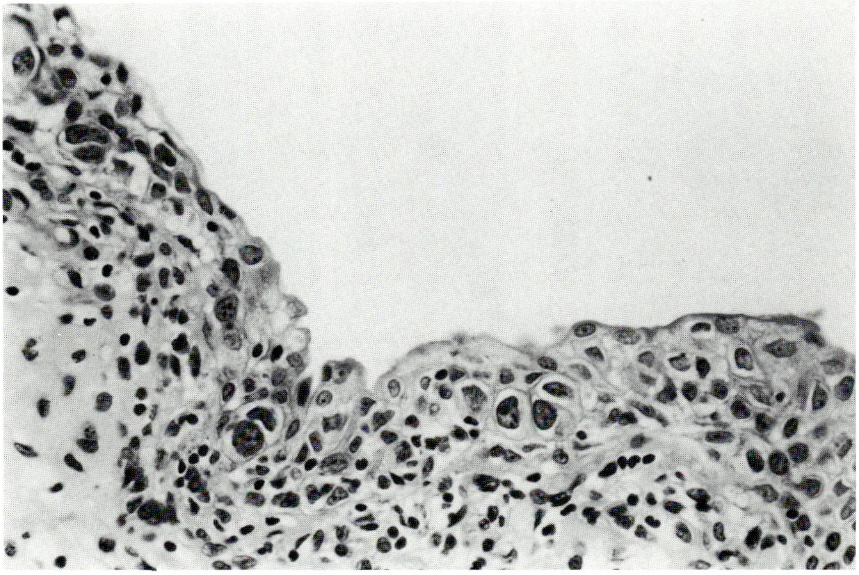

FIG. 4. Case No. 6. In the third round, eight reviewers classified this lesion as moderate atypia/dysplasia of urothelium, and two as severe atypia/dysplasia. H&E. ×250.

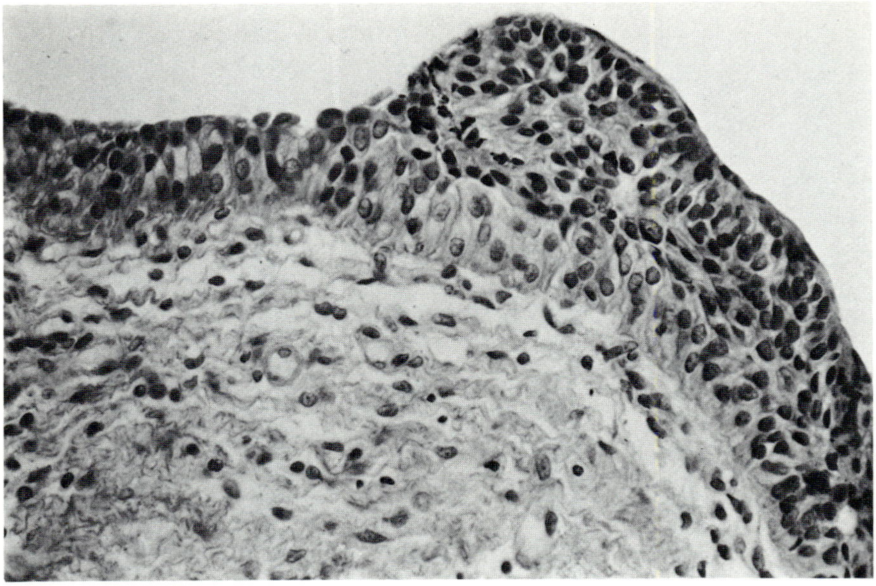

FIG. 5. Case No. 22. This lesion was difficult to classify. The majority of participants thought it was nonneoplastic but atypical epithelium ("M0.5") overgrowing normal urothelium. H&E. ×250.

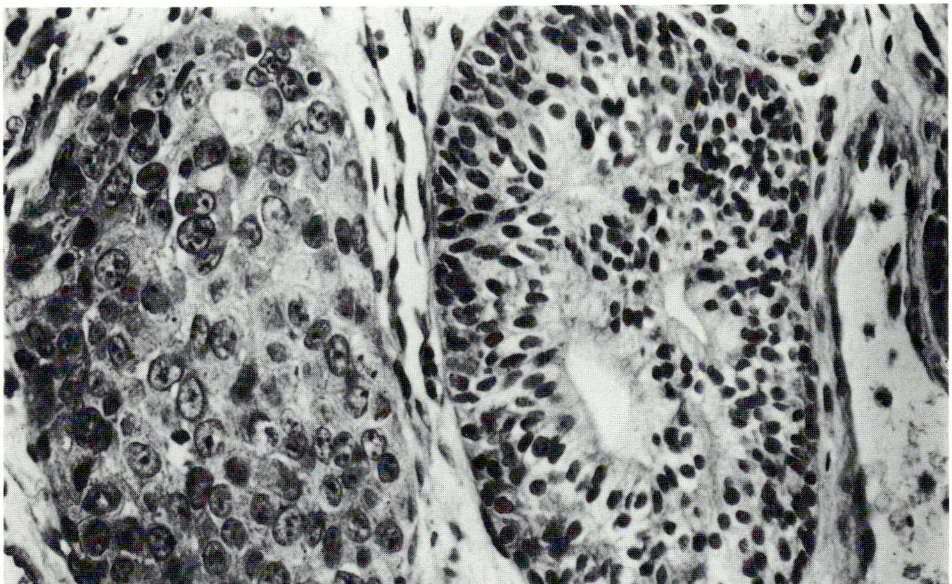

FIG. 6. Case No. 7. No consensus diagnosis for the abnormal epithelium in a von Brunn's nest. Opinions ranged from "benign" to carcinoma in situ. H&E. ×250.

DISCUSSION

The most important conclusion of this study is that a relatively high degree of diagnostic consensus can be reached by pathologists evaluating a spectrum of subtle histologic changes of urothelium. In this study, the urothelial alterations were chronologically or topically related to urothelial neoplasias, and probably represented morphologic expressions of a "field change." The method of study was the so-called Delphi technique, which provides pooling of opinions with anonymous appraisal and a feedback with adjustment of opinions.

The histologic definitions of urothelial abnormalities in this system were determined in such a way that they show parallelism to the definitions of the WHO system of grading.[8] For example, the cellular changes seen in the category "mild atypia/dysplasia, M1" roughly correspond to the cellular changes in grade 1 (WHO) papillary transitional cell carcinoma, and so forth. The WHO grading system is widely used in everyday practice, and its features are therefore usable as a baseline for our definitions of epithelial abnormalities.

The degree of consensus reached in this study was quite remarkable, considering the subjective nature of the analysis, the diverse background of the pathologists involved, and the rather arbitrary nature of the definitions and illustrations provided. During the first three Delphi "rounds," the indicators for the spread of opinions demonstrated a statistically significant improvement, i.e., the agreement grew at every round. There was no statistically significant improvement of consensus between the third and fourth rounds, a fact that reflects the limitations of the Delphi approach; after two reconsiderations, the diagnoses of individual pathologists are apparently settled, and nothing is to be gained by further review. Another limitation of this study is that, for technical reasons, the diagnosis in each case had to be based on the evaluation of one transparency, which might give only a narrow representation of diagnostic histologic and cellular changes.

The final results show that complete agreement occurred in cases illustrating normal urothelium and squamous change ("squamous metaplasia") as well as in one case of carcinoma in situ. Nine of 10 participants agreed with respect to the diagnosis of one carcinoma in situ and two mild atypias/dysplasias. Of the remaining 18 illustrations, 11 could be classified within one degree of morphologic severity by at least nine reviewers. Overall, 9 of 10 pathologists reached a consensus for 75 percent of lesions covering all morphologic stages of developing urothelial carcinoma. Among the seven photomicrographs for which no consensus was achieved, 8 of 10 reviewers classified five of these illustrations within one degree of severity. Failure to reach closer agreement in these instances may have been due to ambiguities of photographic reproduction in two cases, and to illustration of a nonhomogeneous pattern in one instance. The remaining photomicrographs were taken from the same specimen and depicted changes in von Brunn's nests. Obviously, the interpretation of these lesions remained highly individual.

On the basis of the results of this study, it can be stated that the morphologic features of potentially premalignant changes of urothelium can be defined and classified. When a genuine effort is made to minimize individuality and to reduce variation due to terminology, a consensus on the characteristics of hyperplasia, atypia/dysplasia, and carcinoma in situ can be reached. In this study, unanimity of opinion was achieved only for obviously benign and malignant lesions representing changes at the two extremes of the morphologic spectrum. Although further characterization of the diagnostic features of atypia/dysplasia would be helpful, we have to accept minor variations in the interpretation of developing urothelial carcinoma even among pathologists who have experience with these lesions. We hope that additional studies will lead to the recognition of morphologic patterns that will correlate relatively well with the biologic potential and clinical behavior of premalignant urothelial lesions.

ACKNOWLEDGMENTS

The authors are very grateful for help in the statistical analysis by L. Lipworth, M.B., B.Ch., Department of Family and Community Medicine, University of Massachusetts Medical Center, Worcester, Massachusetts; and E. Goldwater, M.S., Computing Center, University of Massachusetts, Amherst, Massachusetts. Participating pathologists for this chapter, from the Departments of Pathology, are: James J. Daly, M.D., Massachusetts General Hospital, Boston, Massachusetts; C. Lenore S. Englander, M.D., Roswell Park Memorial Institute, Buffalo, New York; Alexander W. Miller, M.D., and Ronald S. Weinstein, M.D., Rush-Presbyterian, St. Luke's Medical Center, Chicago, Illinois; George D. Penick, M.D., University of Iowa Hospitals, Iowa City, Iowa; Roger F. Wheelis, M.D., Virginia Mason Medical Center, Seattle, Washington; Gilbert H. Friedell, M.D., Kazuya Hirao, M.D., and Enrique A. Soto, M.D., Central Pathology Laboratory, National Bladder Cancer Collaborative Group A, St. Vincent Hospital, Worcester, Massachusetts.

REFERENCES

1. Goodale F, Gander GW: The future of pathology: A Delphi study by pathology department chairmen. J Med Educ 51:897–903, 1976
2. Gordon TJ, Helmer O: Report on a long-range forecasting study (P-2982). Santa Monica, California. The Rand Corporation, 1964
3. Hellriegel D, Slocum JW: Management: A contingency approach. Reading, Massachusetts, Addison-Wesley, 1974
4. Ito N, Matayoshi K, Arai M, et al.: Effect of various factors on induction of urinary bladder tumors in animals by N-butyl-N-(4-hydroxybutyl) nitrosamine. Gann 64:151–159, 1973
5. Keyes JA, Wilson MP, Becker J: The future of medical education: Forecast of the Council of Deans. J Med Educ 50:319–327, 1975
6. Koss LG, Tiamson EM, Robbins MA: Mapping cancerous and pre-cancerous bladder changes. JAMA 227:281–286, 1974
7. Melicow MM: Histological study of vesical urothelium intervening between gross neoplasms in total cystectomy. J Urol 68:261–279, 1952
8. Mostofi FK, Sobin LH, Torloni H (eds): Histological typing of urinary bladder tumours. International Histological Classification of Tumours, No. 10. Geneva, World Health Organization, 1973

9. National Bladder Cancer Collaborative Group A: Development of a strategy for a longitudinal study of patients with bladder cancer. Cancer Res 37:2898–2906, 1977
10. National Bladder Cancer Collaborative Group A: Surveillance, initial assessment, and subsequent progress of patients with superficial bladder cancer in a prospective longitudinal study. Cancer Res 37:2907–2910, 1977
11. Siegel S: Nonparametric Statistics for the Behavioral Sciences. New York, McGraw-Hill, 1956, pp 166–172
12. Steel RGD, Torrie JH: Principles and Procedures of Statistics, a Biometrical Approach, ed 2. New York, McGraw-Hill, 1980, pp 102–103

THE ULTRASTRUCTURE OF MALIGNANT EPITHELIAL NEOPLASMS OF THE LUNG

GURDIP S. SIDHU

The quest for the increasingly accurate morphologic diagnosis of tumors presupposes a predictable relationship between their appearance and behavior. Structural variations in tumors may reflect consistent qualitative or quantitative differences in metabolism, with the implication that such differences could be exploited to enhance therapeutic specificity and effectiveness. With tumors demonstrating readily observable differential characteristics, light-microscopic classifications have been eminently successful, but there has necessarily been a tendency to relegate highly anaplastic tumors to wastebasket categories, such as "undifferentiated" carcinoma. In the case of the lung, the "undifferentiated" carcinoma group constitutes a significant proportion of malignant tumors and, to this extent, introduces an element of doubt into studies evaluating prognosis and therapeutic regimens.

The most widely accepted classification of lung tumors, and that around which most other classifications are structured, is the WHO classification.[33,37] Diagnostic problems exist in several tumor categories, including poorly differentiated adenocarcinoma, poorly differentiated epidermoid carcinoma, and large-cell carcinoma. The distinction of these from one another, and their pathogenetic relationship to giant-cell carcinoma, are often unclear. The histogenesis of small-cell carcinoma and carcinoid tumors, and their relationship to squamous cell carcinoma, adenocarcinoma, and large-cell carcinoma has also been unclear. Electron microscopy has helped unravel many of these problems. It has also demonstrated that mesothelioma is a genuine entity that can be readily distinguished from adenocarcinoma of pulmonary origin, and that bronchioloalveolar carcinoma is composed of histogenetically overlapping cell types. Finally, the nature of tumorlets, benign clear-cell (sugar) tumors, and the so-called "chemodectomas" has been greatly clarified by electron microscopy.

This paper discusses the ultrastructure of the major categories of lung carcinoma and pleural mesothelioma on the basis of material examined at the New

TABLE 1. Tumor Types and Number of Cases Examined

Neoplasm	No. Cases
Small-cell carcinoma	43
Carcinoids and tumorlets	3, 1
Squamous cell carcinoma	71
Adenocarcinoma	63
Large-cell undifferentiated carcinoma	11
Bronchioloalveolar carcinoma	31
Mesothelioma	6
Total	229

York Veterans Administration Hospital (Table 1). In each instance, the morphology of the normal cell type(s) is presented briefly before that of the tumor category which is related to or resembles it. Finally, a histogenetic classification of lung carcinoma based on this discussion is presented.

THE NORMAL TRACHEOBRONCHIAL EPITHELIUM

The normal tracheobronchial epithelium[5] is composed of basal cells, intermediate cells, ciliated cells, and mucous cells. Other rare cells are Kultschitzky-like cells (K cells, small granule cells), brush cells, and ''special type'' cells. Of these cell types, the basal, intermediate, and mucous cells are capable of division.[27]

Present evidence suggests that all of these cell types differentiate from the basal cell, which may be viewed as an undifferentiated stem cell representing the endoderm from which the respiratory epithelium arises. The basal cell is small, wedge-shaped, and lies along the basal lamina, with no access to the lumen. The cytoplasm of the basal cell reflects its primitive nature, being small in amount and containing free ribosomes, glycogen, and a few tonofibrils. The intercellular space is wide and irregular, being crossed by intercellular cytoplasmic bridges that are joined by desmosomal junctions. Many microvillous-like cytoplasmic processes also project into this space. The nucleus of the basal cell is large and indented. The ''special type'' cell is a basal-cell variant seen in smokers. It has a prominent Golgi complex and numerous, pleomorphic, cytoplasmic granules.

The intermediate (indifferent) cell lies on the pathway to ciliated or mucous cell differentiation. It has more cytoplasm, mitochondria, and granular endoplasmic reticulum than the basal cell. The apex reaches the lumen. The cell surface is less complex, and desmosomal junctions and tonofibrils are fewer. Ciliogenesis is accompanied by increasing cytoplasmic pallor and mucinous differentiation is accompanied by increasing cytoplasmic density.

The ciliated cell has numerous apical cilia and microvilli, numerous mitochondria in the apical cytoplasm, a prominent Golgi complex, a scanty granular endoplasmic reticulum, and some smooth-surfaced vesicles, multivesicular bodies, lysosomes, and tonofibrils.

The mucous (goblet) cell has an abundant granular endoplasmic reticulum, a prominent Golgi apparatus, and mucin droplets in the apical cytoplasm. In mature goblet cells, these droplets are large and distend the apical cytoplasm. They often have a discontinuous limiting membrane due to coalescence with neighboring granules. Discharge of the granules is frequently within an intact granule membrane, and portions of cytoplasm may accompany the granules. This results in the presence of small, bead-like vesicles in the neighborhood of the cell surface, and a scalloped, luminal profile. A few apical microvilli with a characteristic spiked surface[28,41] are present; they are more numerous in discharged goblet cells. Often, the cells have only a few small, noncoalescing mucin granules. These are "small mucous granule cells" which incorporate thymidine whereas goblet cells do not. It has been suggested that goblet cells reflect a stimulated epithelium and may be rare normally.[27]

The brush cell is rare in humans but common in rats. It is distinguished by a prominent tuft of tall, thick, straight microvilli on the apical surface, which have filamentous cores extending down into and filling up most of the supranuclear cytoplasm. Brush cells may represent immature ciliated cells or discharged goblet cells.[3]

K cells[3,21] are rare in adults but more frequent in fetuses[16-18,21,22] and newborns. They are argyrophilic but not argentaffinic, wedge-shaped, and have a broad base on the basal lamina. The apex may or may not reach the lumen.[16,26] The cytoplasm of the K cell is pale and the smooth endoplasmic reticulum is prominent. Microtubules are prominent and many 10-nm-diameter filament bundles are present. A few lipofuscin granules are usually seen. The most characteristic feature is the presence of 80- to 170-nm-diameter, round, membrane-bound granules in the basal cytoplasm. These have a dense, finely granular matrix.

On the basis of granule morphology, Hage[17] has described three cell types. Type 1 cells have small granules (110-nm diameter) with a dense or filamentous core and a narrow, submembranous, lucent zone. Occasionally, these granules are larger, with an eccentric accumulation of dense or filamentous material giving the appearance of bubbles. Type 2 cells have larger (140-nm diameter) granules with a dense core and a narrow, lucent zone. Type 3 cells have large (190-nm diameter), uniformly dense granules without a lucent zone. Dense core granules similar to those in K cells may occur in bronchial goblet cells in disease states.

SMALL-CELL CARCINOMA

By light-microscopy, the tumor cells in small-cell carcinoma are small, but in different neoplasms may vary in size from that of a small lymphocyte to two or three times as large. They may be round, but are more frequently oval and are sometimes spindled. The cytoplasm is generally scanty, particularly in the small round-cell type (Fig. 1 Left). The nuclei are very hyperchromatic and nuclear detail is usually difficult to discern. Tumors with more abundant cytoplasm have been designated "intermediate cell type" in the revised WHO classification.

Necrosis in small-cell carcinoma is extensive and is an important diagnostic clue in endoscopic biopsy material. The stroma is so scanty as to be virtually nonex-

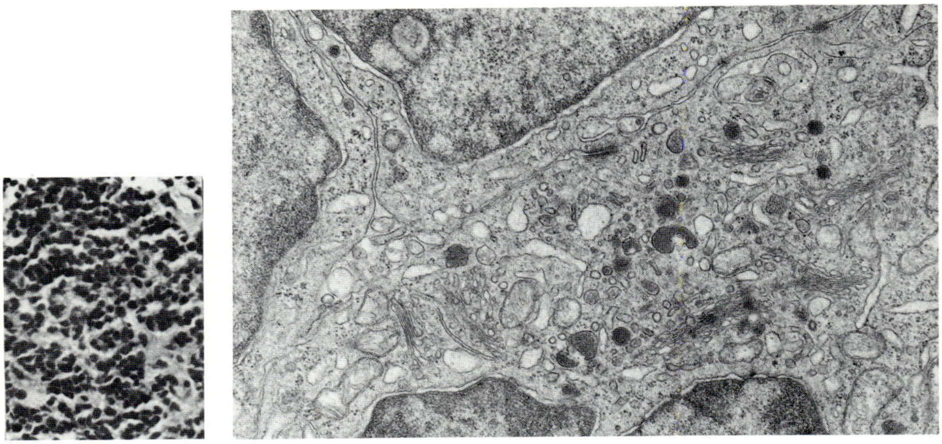

FIG. 1. Small-cell carcinoma, oat-cell type. **Left.** Small, round cells with dark nuclei and scanty cytoplasm. ×360. **Right.** Several neurosecretory-type granules are seen. ×13,050.

istent. This is probably the reason for the so-called crush artifact that is seen almost invariably in endoscopic biopsy material. This crush artifact is present even in material directly processed for electron microscopy, suggesting that it is not a result of paraffin embedding and sectioning. A similar artifact occurs in other pathologic infiltrates with scanty stroma, such as dense inflammatory lymphocytic infiltrates and lymphomas in the bronchial lamina propria. Lymphocytic inflammation and small-cell lymphomas can be confused with small-cell carcinoma; however, they lack necrosis. Large-cell lymphomas do not resemble small-cell carcinoma.

By electron microscopy, the cell preservation in small-cell tumors is often poor. In areas with good cell viability, the tumor-cell nuclei have multiple small foci of chromatin condensation corresponding to the light-microscopic hyperchromasia, giving a leopard-skin-like appearance. In some cells, the chromatin may be finely dispersed. Nuclear irregularities are present, but are obscured on light-microscopy by the chromatin density. Nucleoli are not prominent.

Cytoplasmic organelles are few. There may be numerous polyribosomes, but mitochondria, granular endoplasmic reticulum, and Golgi complexes are not prominent. In about 30 percent of the tumors, a variable number of small, cytoplasmic, membrane-bound, dense-core granules may be present (Fig. 1 Right). These are nearly always scanty and may or may not have a submembranous halo. Their scarcity may be one explanation for the absence of light-microscopically visible cytoplasmic argyrophilia. The granules are more frequently found in tumors with a relatively more abundant cytoplasm and more organelles, suggesting that their presence correlates with the degree of cellular differentiation. The intermediate-cell-type carcinoma[33] has more regular borders, better developed junctions, and neurosecretory-type granules in a higher percentage of cases (Fig. 2).

Other signs of differentiation may be present in a small percentage of neoplasms. These include well-developed desmosomal junctions, in contrast to the poorly formed ones usually seen in these neoplasms, cytoplasmic tonofibrils, and lumen formation (Fig. 3). In some cases, obvious squamous differentiation, in-

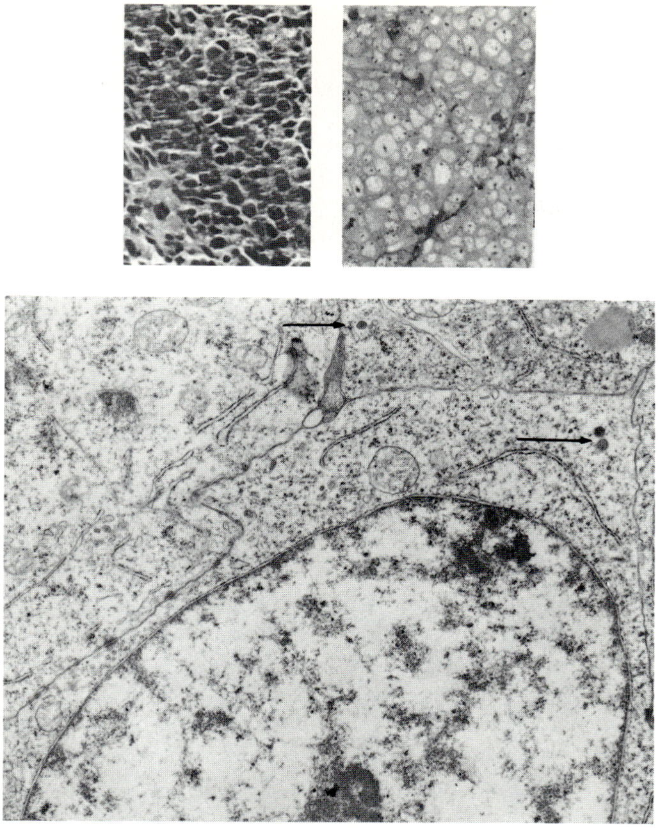

FIG. 2. Small-cell carcinoma, intermediate-cell type. **Top left.** The cells are oval and larger than oat cells. ×360. **Top right.** Epon-embedded, 1-μ-thick section. ×360. **Bottom.** The cells have a more regular cell surface and better developed junctions than in the oat-cell type. A few neurosecretory-type granules are present (arrows). ×8,000.

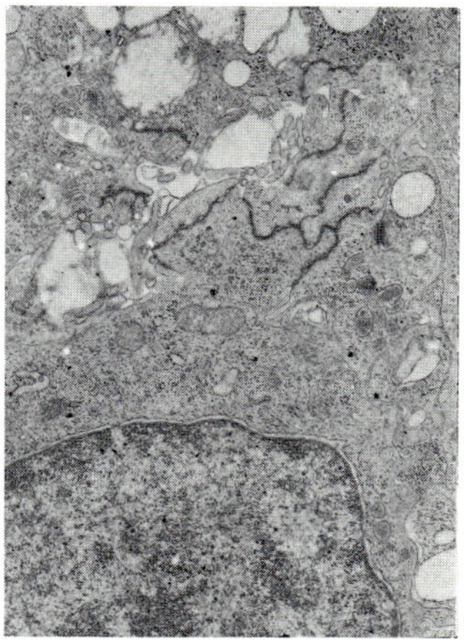

FIG. 3. Small-cell carcinoma, metastatic, in mediastinal lymph node. Several junctional complexes converge toward a poorly formed lumen in which lie a few irregular microvilli. ×5,500.

cluding intercellular bridges, is seen. The lumens are associated with the presence of delimiting tight junctions or junctional complexes incorporating a tight junction. These signs of differentiation correspond to the occasional presence of squamous differentiation or mucin on light-microscopy.[35] Such tumors have been placed in the combined oat-cell carcinoma category of the revised WHO classification.

Another morphologic feature unique to small-cell carcinomas is the frequent deposition of hematoxyphilic material in the walls of blood vessels or on collagen within the neoplasm (Fig. 4 Top left). This phenomenon is associated with extensive tumor necrosis. Ultrastructurally, the earliest lesion shows the deposition of irregular, very dense, finely granular material in the basal lamina of endothelial cells and pericytes (Fig. 4 Top right) and in the adjacent stromal matrix. A fine filamentous structure can be discerned in this material at high magnification (Fig. 4 Bottom left). In later stages, the deposition of granular material is too heavy for any localization to be evident, and similar material is found encrusting collagen fibrils (Fig. 4 Bottom right).

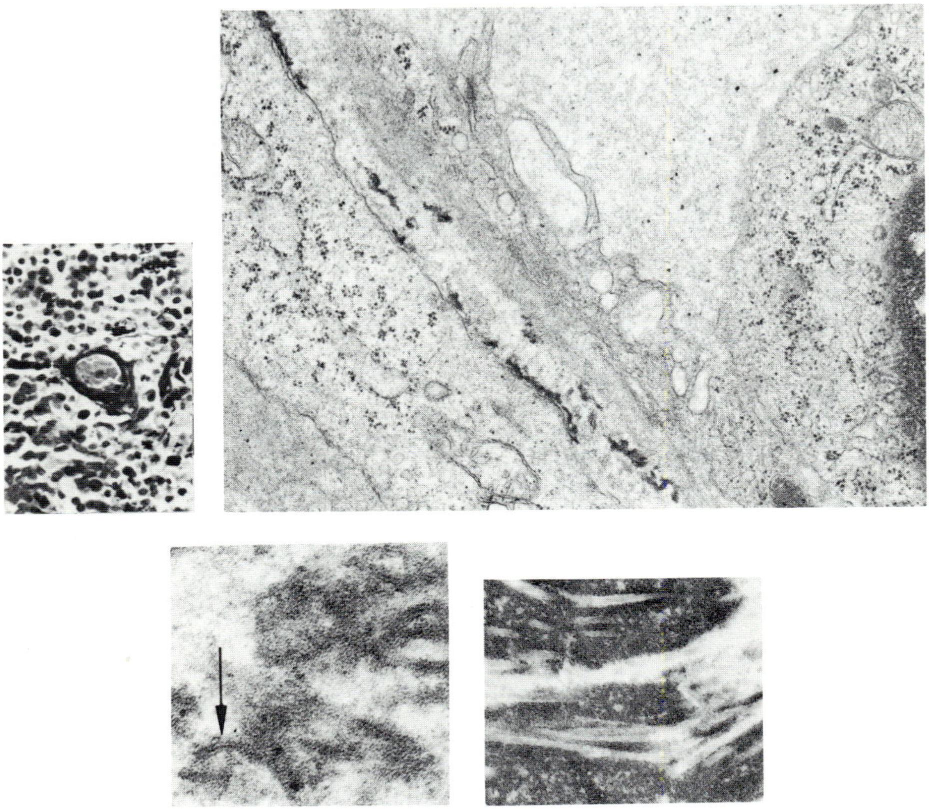

FIG. 4. Small-cell carcinoma with hematoxyphilic (blue) blood vessels. **Top left.** Basophilic material in wall of small blood vessel. ×360. **Top right.** Dense, granular material is deposited in and between pericytic and endothelial cell basal laminae. ×18,620. **Bottom left.** A filamentous substructure is seen (arrow). ×86,213. **Bottom right.** Dense material encrusting collagen fibrils. ×13,063.

This hematoxyphil material is derived from the degeneration and breakdown of tumor-cell nuclei. A sequence of progressive morphologic changes in the nuclear chromatin, progressing all the way to this extracellular material, can be demonstrated. The basophilic material is Feulgen-positive but is negative with stains for calcium and iron.[1]

Several factors can be implicated in the pathogenesis of the "blue blood vessels" in small-cell carcinoma. First, the poorly supported, fragile vascular network readily breaks down, leading to massive tumor necrosis. Second, the tumor cells, due to a sparsity of organelles, lack the lysosomal enzymes necessary to digest the necrotic nuclear material. Finally, because of a lack of vascular access to the tumor or because of an absence of chemotactic material, there is almost no inflammatory response to the necrosis, thus excluding any external source of digestive enzymes. Because of these factors, the nucleoprotein from the breakdown of tumor-cell nuclei accumulates locally in whatever structures are on the exit route for fluid, such as blood vessels and their stromal supports.

CARCINOID TUMORS

Carcinoid tumors of the lung are generally composed of uniform small cells with finely granular cytoplasm and round, uniform nuclei. Mitoses are rare. The cells are generally arranged in clusters or trabeculae in a very vascular, sometimes hyalinized stroma (Fig. 5 Left). Occasionally, acinus formation is seen. An oncocytic subtype

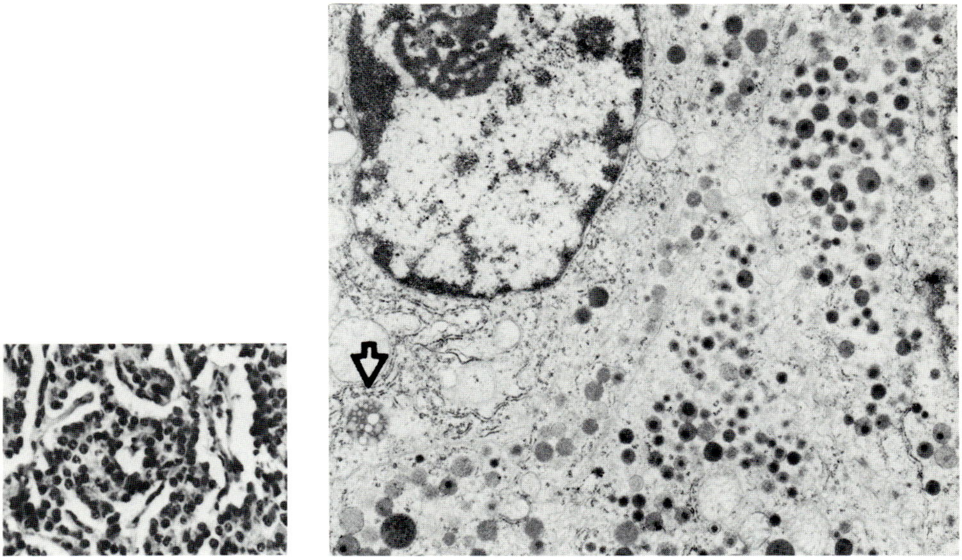

FIG. 5. Carcinoid of the bronchus. **Left.** The cells are uniform and have a trabecular pattern and a very vascular stroma. ×360. **Right.** Numerous round granules of varying size and staining intensity are seen. Some granules have a focus of increased density within their matrix. A lipofuscin granule is present (arrow). ×8,000.

also occurs in which the cytoplasm is eosinophilic, abundant, and more obviously granular (Fig. 6 Left).

Ultrastructurally, as opposed to the case in small-cell carcinoma, the cell preservation in carcinoid tumors is good. The cell surface is more regular and a few, poorly developed desmosomal junctions are present. The cells adhere better to each other, and clusters of cells are surrounded by a basal lamina investment. Small-cell carcinomas generally lack a basal lamina.

Mitochondria are more numerous than in small-cell carcinomas. The nuclei are round and regular, although the chromatin condensation is similar to that seen in small-cell carcinoma. Nucleoli are inconspicuous. Polyribosomes and a granular endoplasmic reticulum are moderately developed. The cytoplasm is generally filled with numerous, round, membrane-bound granules (see Fig. 8). These are larger than the secretory granules of small-cell carcinomas; their content is finely granular and of moderate to extreme density. A few large and small granules are scattered among the other granules. Submembranous halos may or may not be seen. Some granules may have an area of increased density within the matrix. A few lipofuscin granules are generally present.

The oncocytic variety of carcinoid-tumor cell is distinguished by the presence of secretory granules that resemble membrane-bound vacuoles (Fig. 6 Right). However, dense cores of variable size are present within these vacuoles and occasional granules have no vacuole. These granules resemble those of Hage's type 1 bronchial K cells. Recently, an oncocytic carcinoid having a cytoplasm packed with mitochondria, as in oncocytomas of other organs, has been reported.[32] Secretory granules in this tumor were fewer than in ordinary carcinoids.

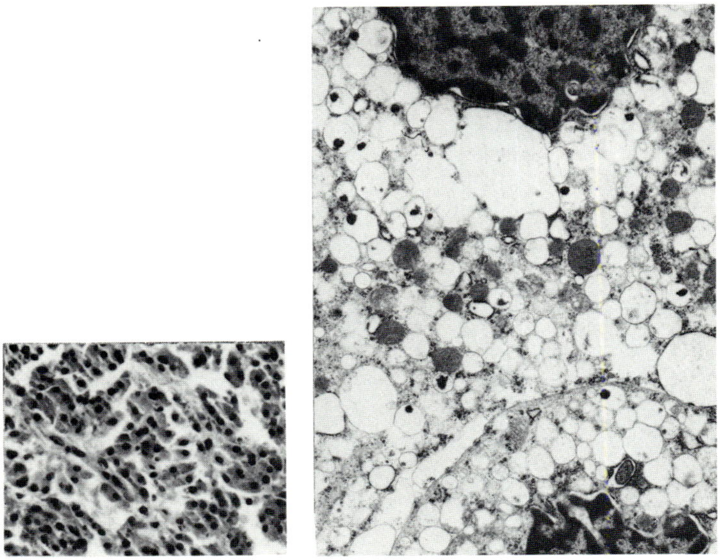

FIG. 6. Oncocytic carcinoid of bronchus. **Left.** The cells have more abundant, granular, acidophilic cytoplasm. ×360. **Right.** Markedly vacuolated granules fill the cytoplasm. ×6,270.

The granules of bronchial carcinoids are argyrophilic, although they may rarely be argentaffinic.

Spindle cell carcinoids occur peripherally in the lung, probably arising from bronchioles. The cells are elongated, may form fascicles, and are argyrophilic. Small groups of similar cells may be found associated with the epithelium of bronchioles or small bronchi in these or otherwise normal lungs. These tumorlets vary from microscopic to a few millimeters in size. On electron microscopy, the secretory granules in cells of spindle-cell carcinoids and tumorlets are much smaller than those in other lung carcinoids. A submembranous halo may be present.

In occasional carcinoid tumors, bundles of 10-nm-diameter cytoplasmic filaments may be present. These may occur in large whorls entrapping secretory granules and mitochondria or displacing them to the cell periphery.[2]

RELATIONSHIP OF SMALL-CELL CARCINOMA AND CARCINOID

The cells of carcinoids resemble the K cells of the bronchus. Small-cell carcinomas are poorly differentiated with some features of K cells, but more often resemble bronchial basal cells.

It is likely that the cell of origin of small-cell carcinoma is the basal cell; normal K cells are now believed to arise from the bronchial basal cells.[35] It is possible that carcinoids arise from cells already on the pathway of differentiation toward K cells. This hypothesis may explain the epidemiologic divergence of small-cell carcinoma and carcinoid of the lung.[15] Perhaps only the basal cell is susceptible to the influences that result in an increased incidence of small-cell carcinomas; cells more differentiated toward K cells may be less susceptible, explaining why carcinoids have not increased with the rising incidence of small-cell carcinoma.

SQUAMOUS CELL CARCINOMA

The term ''squamous'' is used here in preference to ''epidermoid'' because: (1) the epidermis is not the only squamous epithelium in the body; and (2) the word epidermoid refers to an organized arrangement of cells forming a structure, and not to a particular cell type. Tumors are best named after the cell type into which they differentiate. The word squamous expresses this much better than epidermoid.

Squamous cell carcinomas are composed of polygonal or elongated epithelial cells arranged in sheets and anastomosing clusters of varying size. The cytoplasm is abundant and eosinophilic. Intercellular bridges and keratinization may be present and are considered important diagnostic criteria. On the basis of the facility with which these features can be demonstrated, squamous cell carcinomas can be divided into well-differentiated, moderately differentiated, and poorly differentiated types. In the last category, there may be considerable uncertainty as to the squamous nature of the neoplasm.

Ultrastructurally, well-differentiated tumor cells (Fig. 7 Top and Bottom) have an abundant cytoplasm which is covered on all surfaces by numerous microvillous

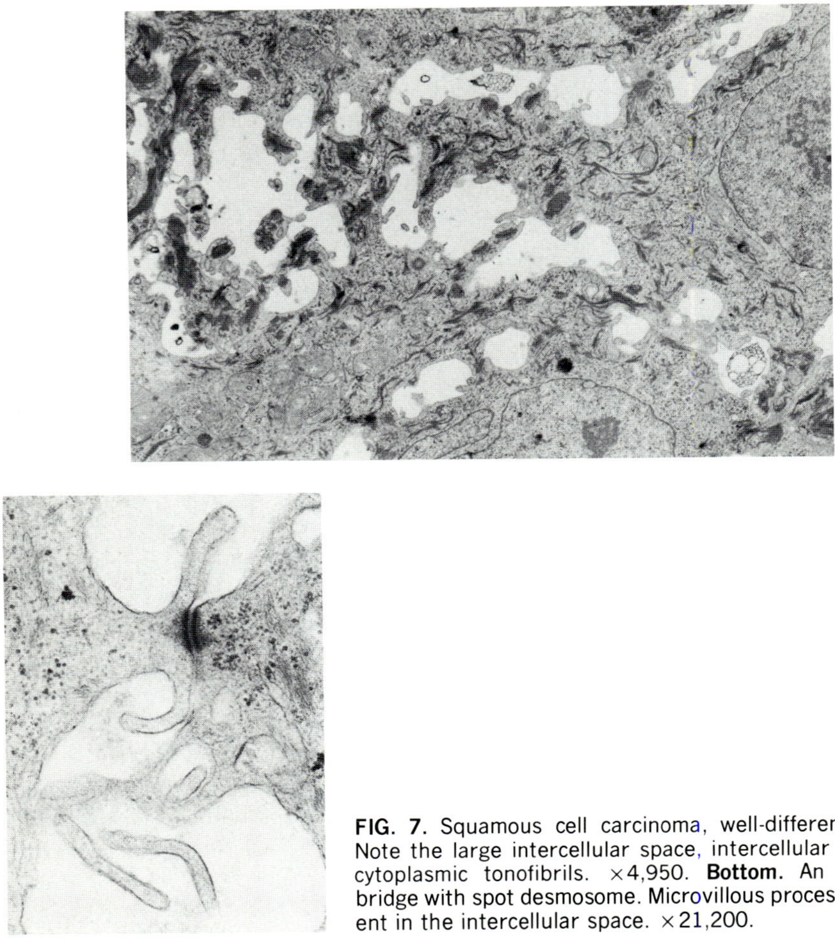

FIG. 7. Squamous cell carcinoma, well-differentiated. **Top.** Note the large intercellular space, intercellular bridges and cytoplasmic tonofibrils. ×4,950. **Bottom.** An intercellular bridge with spot desmosome. Microvillous processes are present in the intercellular space. ×21,200.

processes. These differ from the microvilli on the luminal surface of ductal or glandular structures by the fact that they are bent to a varying degree, suggesting lesser rigidity. Fine filaments similar to those in glandular microvilli may be present in the core of these structures, but there is no cytoplasmic filamentous web into which they merge. The intercellular space is wide. Cell processes broader than the microvilli but lesser in number also arise from the cell surface. They are joined to similar processes of adjoining cells by well-developed spot desmosomes; the complex of two cell processes and a desmosome corresponds to the intercellular bridge of light-microscopy. Sometimes, the complex is comprised of a cytoplasmic process of one cell joined to the cell body rather than to a cytoplasmic process of the neighboring cell.

The cytoplasm has a relative sparsity of organelles such as the granular endoplasmic reticulum and Golgi apparatus, in contrast to the cytoplasm of secretory cells, such as those of adenocarcinomas. Free ribosomes are generally abundant and glycogen, often in the form of large clusters, is usually present. An important feature is the presence of numerous cytoplasmic tonofibrils. The tonofibrils are composed of tonofilaments that are grouped together into dense, curving, compact bundles with frayed ends. They lie free in the cytoplasm or attach to desmosomal junctions. In spindled squamous cells, long, broad processes of cytoplasm may be interposed between other cells, and the tonofibrils tend to be concentrated in these processes.

Squamous epithelium is typically stratified. In such circumstances, cells toward the centers of clusters, as in tumors, or toward the free surface, as in normal skin and mucosa, must obtain their nutrition by diffusion across a multilayered barrier of cells. This is facilitated by the large intercellular space. However, squamous epithelia also have to withstand considerable shearing and other stresses. Large intercellular spaces tend to compromise the structural integrity of squamous tissue; this is counteracted by the structural rigidity imparted by the intercellular bridges and by the cytoplasmic tonofibrils in much the same manner as the steel skeleton imparts rigidity to a modern skyscraper. The microvillous processes increase the absorptive surface.

Occasionally, membrane-bound structures with transverse lamellae resembling keratinosomes (surface-coating granules) are seen in the cytoplasm. In some cells, clusters of membrane-bound glycogen granules are seen. This probably represents autophagic digestion of glycogen.

In keratinized areas, a homogeneous material (keratin) is deposited on the tonofibrils. Ultimately, the entire cytoplasm is replaced by a diffuse mass of closely packed parallel filaments without evidence of aggregation into tonofibrils. During the process of keratinization, the intercellular space disappears and a layer of dense material derived from keratinosomes is deposited on the surface, making the membrane appear thicker (Fig. 8).

With decreasing differentiation, the intercellular space shrinks and the number of cytoplasmic tonofibrils decreases. Polyribosomes become more abundant and the granular endoplasmic reticulum increases. Myofilaments may be visible in the peripheral cytoplasm (Fig. 9). In some tumors, well-developed desmosomal junc-

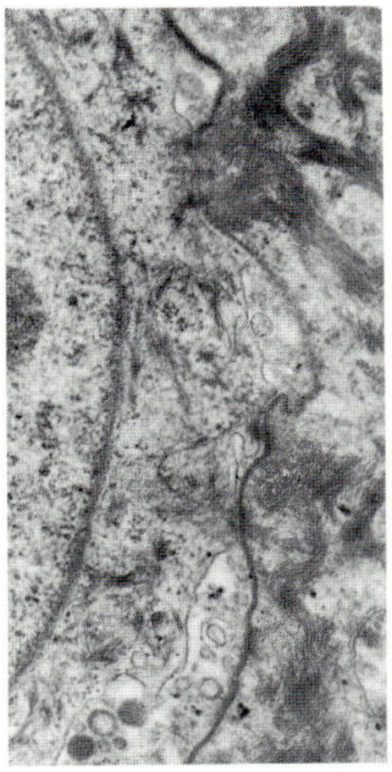

FIG. 8. Squamous cell carcinoma, well-differentiated. A fully keratinized cell is seen on the right with marked thickening of its plasma membrane. ×13,860.

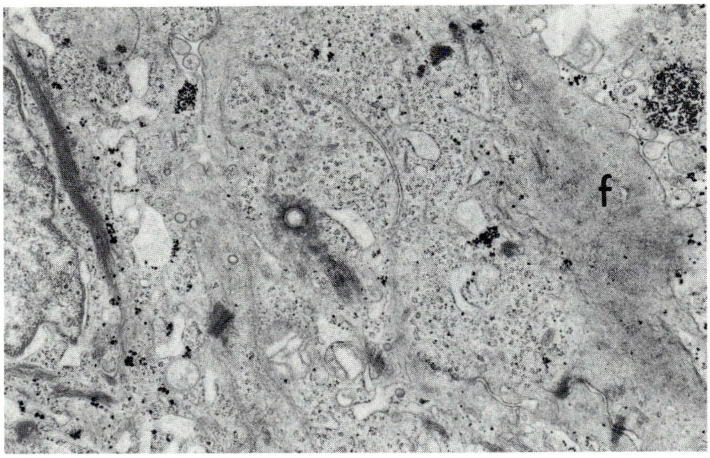

FIG. 9. Squamous cell carcinoma, poorly differentiated. The intercellular space is narrow. Myofilaments (f) are seen in the peripheral cytoplasm. ×9,300.

tions with some slight suggestion of intercellular-bridge formation may be the only evidence of differentiation. In such instances, whether the neoplasm is placed in the poorly differentiated squamous cell carcinoma or the large-cell undifferentiated carcinoma category becomes a matter of personal preference, since the presence of desmosomal junctions alone is not a sufficient criterion for the designation "squamous." Examination of additional tissue samples may demonstrate cytoplasmic tonofibrils.

Sometimes, necrosis and lysis of single tumor cells can lead to a pseudoglandular appearance (Fig. 10 Top). The cells lining the spaces formed in this manner have surface microvilli like other squamous cells, but tight junctions or junctional complexes of the type seen with true lumens are not present (Fig. 10 Bottom).

Occasionally, a squamous cell carcinoma may present with the light-microscopic appearance of a spindle-cell sarcoma (Fig. 11 Left). On electron microscopy, however, desmosomal junctions and cytoplasmic tonofibrils can be readily demonstrated. The granular endoplasmic reticulum may be prominent so that single cells may resemble fibroblasts, but tonofibrils are frequent enough that the distinction is not difficult (Fig. 11 Right).

ADENOCARCINOMA

This category includes the acinar-adenocarcinoma and solid-carcinoma-with-mucus-formation categories of the revised WHO classification. These categories represent well-differentiated and poorly differentiated tumors, respectively. In the revised WHO classification, papillary carcinomas are listed as a separate adenocarcinoma category from the bronchioloalveolar carcinoma group. For histogenetic reasons explained later, papillary carcinomas are included here among the bronchioloalveolar carcinomas.

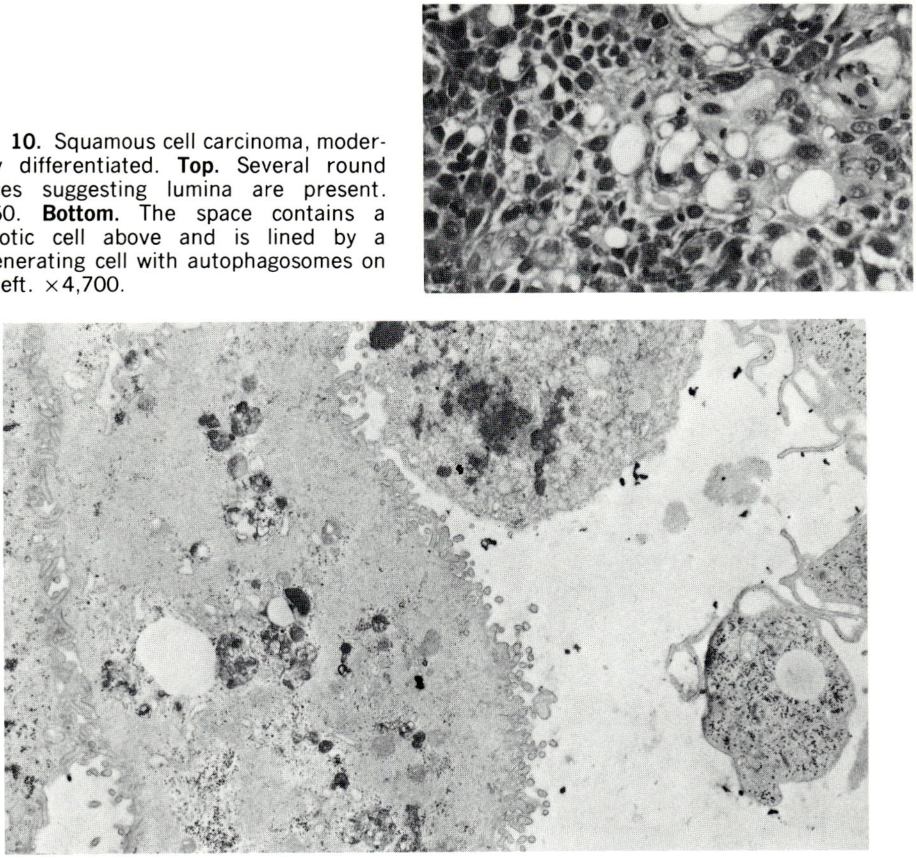

FIG. 10. Squamous cell carcinoma, moderately differentiated. **Top.** Several round spaces suggesting lumina are present. ×360. **Bottom.** The space contains a necrotic cell above and is lined by a degenerating cell with autophagosomes on the left. ×4,700.

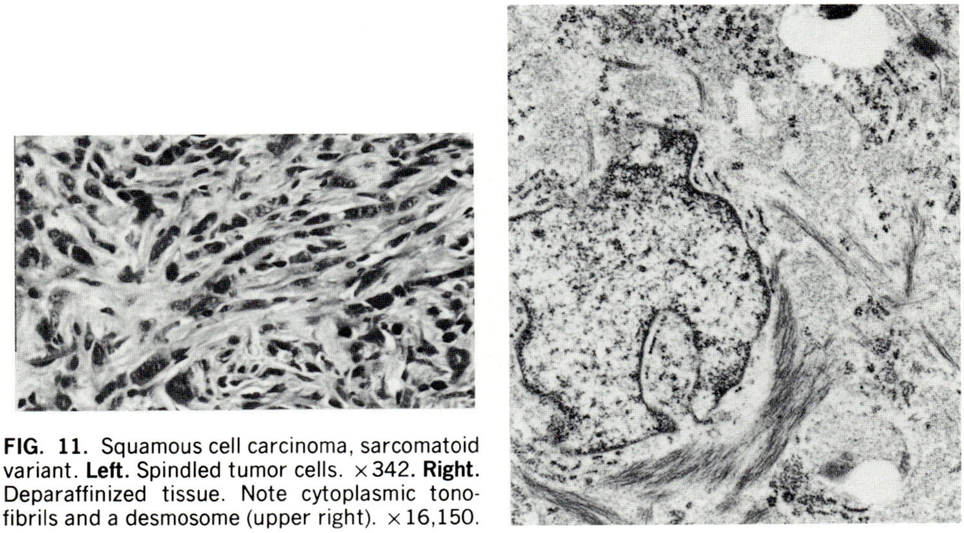

FIG. 11. Squamous cell carcinoma, sarcomatoid variant. **Left.** Spindled tumor cells. ×342. **Right.** Deparaffinized tissue. Note cytoplasmic tonofibrils and a desmosome (upper right). ×16,150.

An adenocarcinoma is a tumor whose cells form tubules, ducts, acini, or glands. The cells of these structures separate two extracellular compartments of different chemical composition—the intraluminal and stromal compartments. This separation is accomplished by the presence of an impermeable intercellular junction—the tight junction—between the adjoining lateral aspects of the tumor cells near the lumen. The tight junction is present as a ring that encircles the cell. It may be present alone or accompanied by an intermediate junction, which is also circumferential, and by a spot desmosome, in that order, from the cell apex toward the base. This combination is a junctional complex. Seven-nanometer-diameter, actin-type filaments form a web-like structure in the apical cytoplasm and insert into the cytoplasmic dense material associated with the tight and intermediate junctions. Tonofibrils insert into the desmosome. Other desmosomes not associated with the junctional complex may be present along the lateral aspect of the cells.

The luminal surface of the cells is covered by a varying number of microvilli. These are most numerous and well developed in well-differentiated tumors. Fine filaments are present in the cores of the microvilli and extend down into the apical cytoplasm to mingle with the apical web.

In keeping with their secretory function, adenocarcinoma cells have a prominent Golgi apparatus and granular endoplasmic reticulum. Mucin granules may be present in the cytoplasm. In well-differentiated tumors, these granules may be similar to those seen in goblet cells—that is, large and coalescing (Fig. 12); in most tumors, however, they are of the small mucus granule variety (Fig. 13). Here the granule content is less evenly distributed and often has an eccentric density.

In the lumina, the mucin consists partly of dense aggregates of finely granular or reticular material and partly of microvesicles which are much smaller than cross-

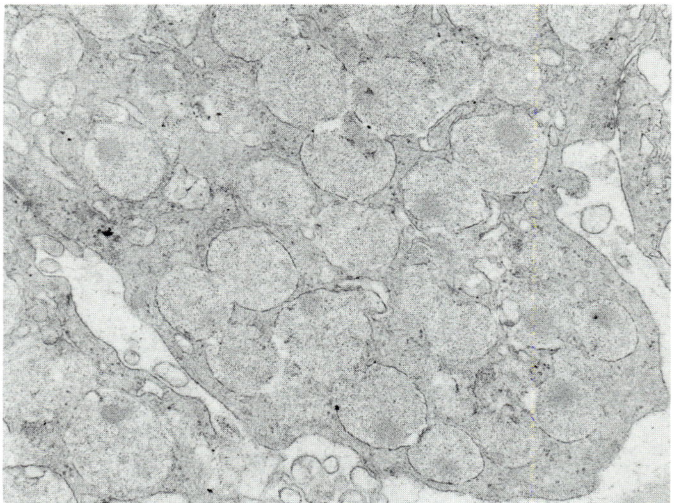

FIG. 12. Adenocarcinoma. A mucous cell containing large, coalescent mucus granules is seen. ×21,350.

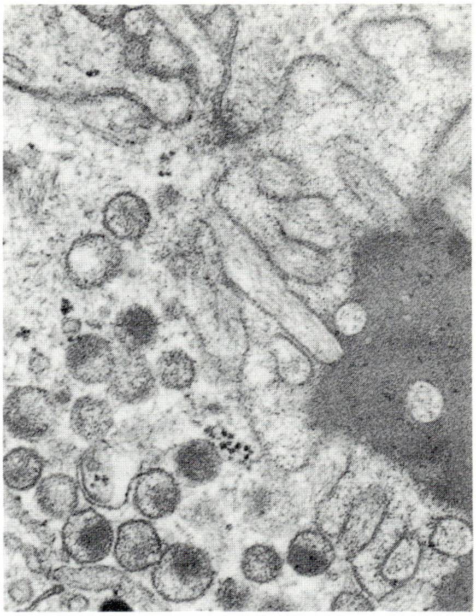

FIG. 13. Adenocarcinoma. Cytoplasmic small mucus granules, a gland lumen, microvilli, and dense luminal content are seen. ×30,550.

sections of microvilli (Fig. 14). With the alcian blue-PAS stain, one part of the luminal mucin stains only with PAS, while the other part stains with both stains.

In some cells, the lumens appear to be completely enclosed by cytoplasm. They may be invaginations from the apical surface or truly intracytoplasmic lumina (Fig. 15).

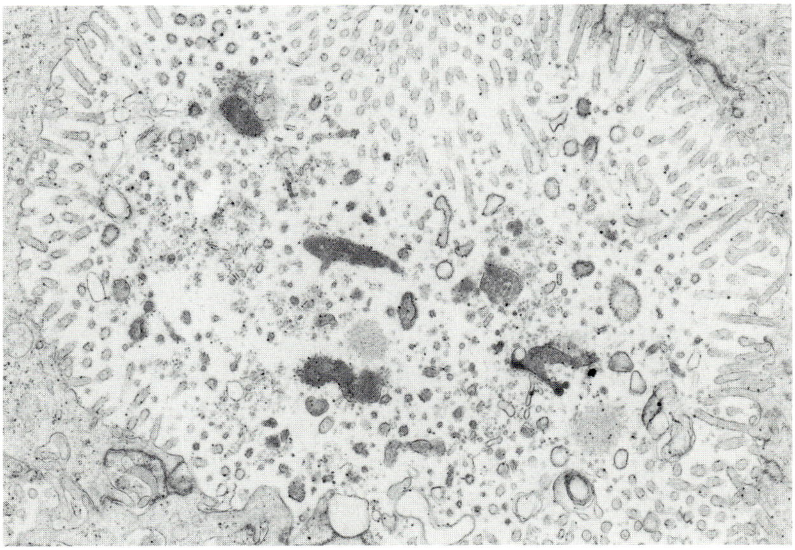

FIG. 14. Adenocarcinoma. Gland lumen containing mucin composed of granular and microvesicular material. Apical junctional complexes and luminal microvilli are seen. ×9,075.

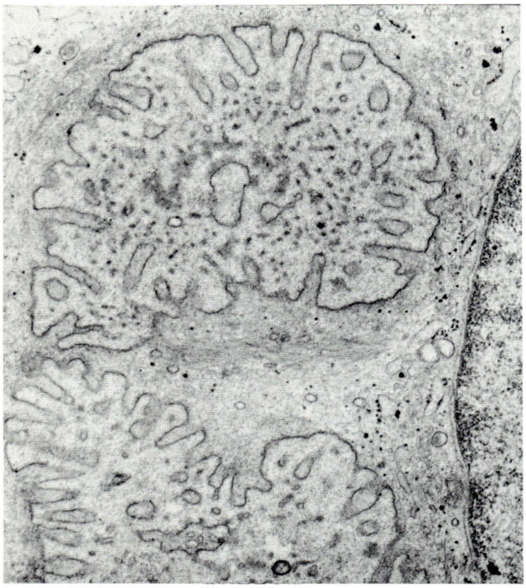

FIG. 15. Adenocarcinoma. Two intracytoplasmic lumens containing granulovesicular mucin are seen in a tumor cell. ×12,500.

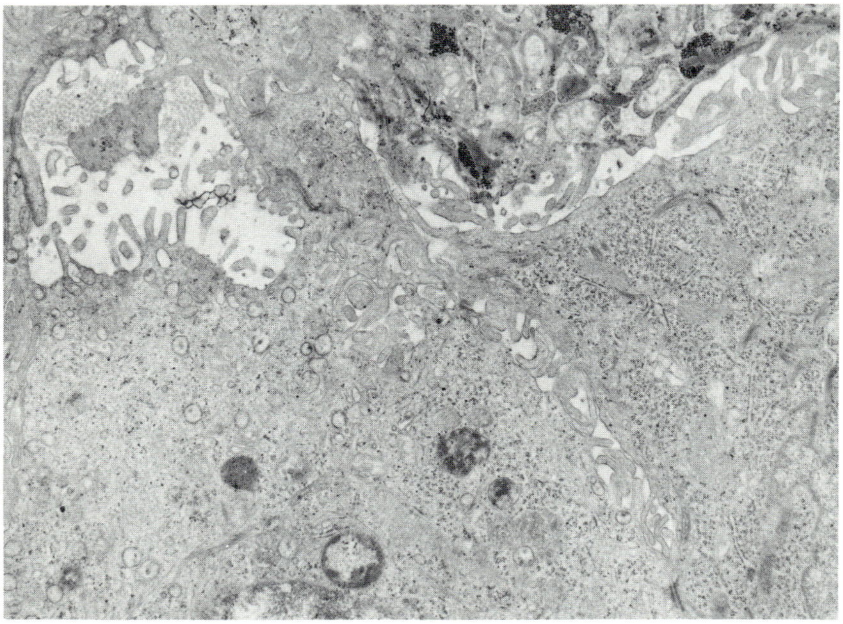

FIG. 16. Adenosquamous carcinoma. A cell with several tonofibrils is seen on the right. A gland lumen is seen on the upper left. The cell below it contains several small mucus granules. ×6,500.

In a small percentage of adenocarcinomas, cells with squamous differentiation, in the form of many cytoplasmic tonofibrils and intercellular bridges, may be present, in addition to cells forming lumens and containing mucin granules (Fig. 16). These tumors have been termed adenosquamous carcinomas in the revised WHO classification. A few isolated tonofibrils in the cytoplasm are common in adenocarcinomas of endodermal origin and should not be considered as evidence of squamous differentiation.

LARGE-CELL UNDIFFERENTIATED CARCINOMA

This name is applied to tumors that, by light-microscopy, do not show any obvious signs of differentiation other than enough cellular cohesiveness to suggest a carcinoma. The cells are larger and have more abundant cytoplasm than the cells of small-cell carcinoma (Fig. 17 Top). In some cases, multinucleated tumor cells may

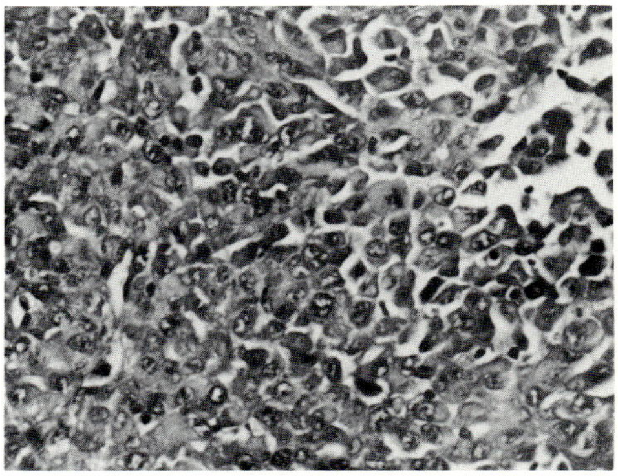

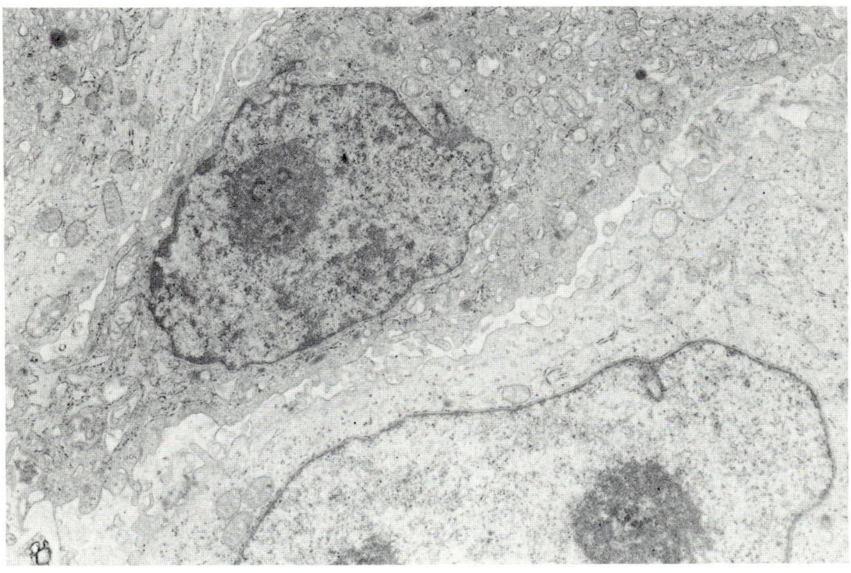

FIG. 17. Large-cell undifferentiated carcinoma. **Top.** Large pleomorphic tumor cells showing no differentiation. ×360. **Bottom.** The cytoplasm has a filamentous matrix and lacks distinctive features such as tonofibrils, secretory granules, or lumen formation. ×5,500.

be present in varying numbers. If these cells are numerous, the designation "giant-cell carcinoma" may be applied. The adjective "undifferentiated" is not included in the WHO classification. I prefer to use it to avoid confusion with other large-cell neoplasms, such as squamous cell carcinoma and adenocarcinoma.

Ultrastructurally, there may be no evidence of squamous or adenocarcinomatous differentiation in large-cell undifferentiated carcinoma. A few intercellular junctions as well as the absence of stromal components in the intercellular space attest to the epithelial nature of these tumors. Cytoplasmic, 10-nm-diameter filaments may be abundant, and a granular endoplasmic reticulum may be prominent, but no evidence of mucin granules is seen (Fig. 17 Bottom). In other cases, minimal evidence of squamous differentiation in the form of tonofibrils (Fig. 18), or minimal evidence of glandular differentiation in the form of lumina (Fig. 19) with or without mucin, may be seen.[10] In one case, neurosecretory-type granules were present in many of the tumor cells (Fig. 20 Top and Bottom). This case also had extensive areas of necrosis with "blue blood vessels" like those observed in small-cell carcinoma.

One case of large-cell undifferentiated carcinoma with minimal glandular differentiation had peculiar large, membrane-bound, intracytoplasmic granules composed of closely packed cylindrical structures with a hexagonal cross-section (Fig. 21 Left and Right). A stain for mucin was negative.

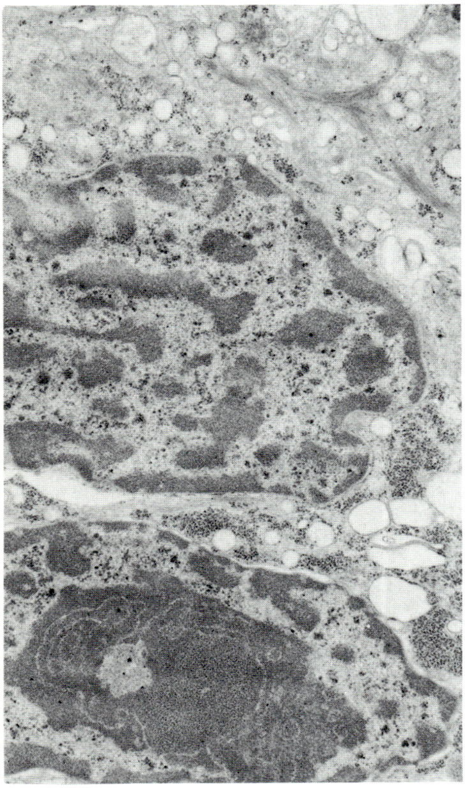

FIG. 18. Large-cell undifferentiated carcinoma. Note cytoplasmic tonofibrils. ×9,500.

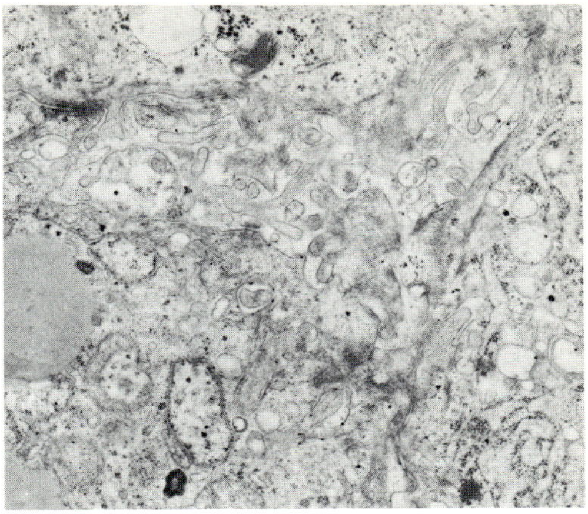

FIG. 19. Large-cell undifferentiated carcinoma. A poorly formed lumen and cytoplasmic lipid droplets are seen. ×9,075.

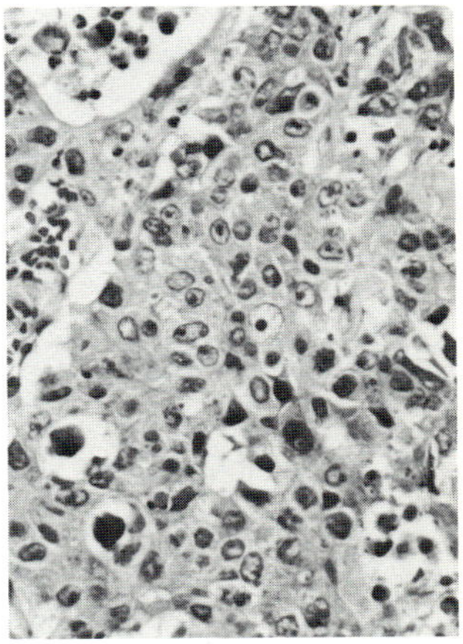

FIG. 20. Large-cell undifferentiated carcinoma. **Top.** Pleomorphic epithelial cells with abundant cytoplasm. ×360. **Bottom.** Neurosecretory-type cytoplasmic granules are present. ×11,600.

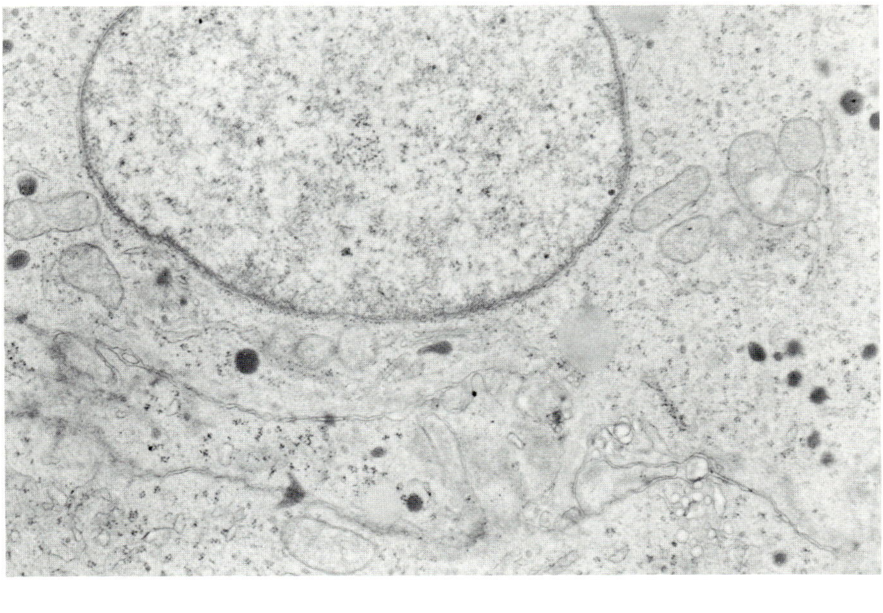

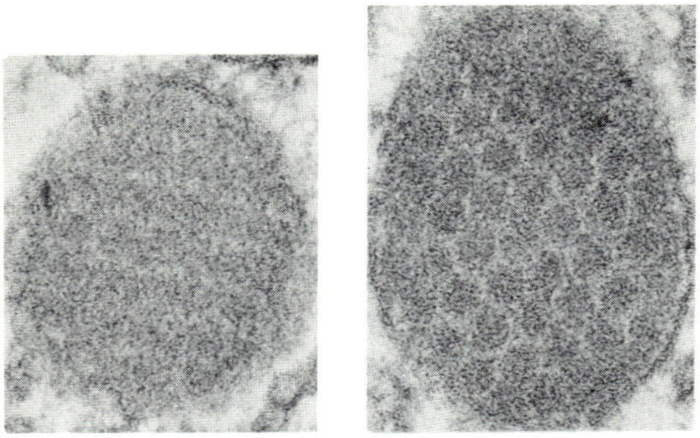

FIG. 21. Large-cell undifferentiated carcinoma. Membrane-bound cytoplasmic granules containing cylindrical structures **(Left)** are arranged in a hexagonal pattern **Right.** ×21,500.

THE EPITHELIAL LINING OF BRONCHIOLES AND ALVEOLI

Two types of epithelial cells line the bronchiole—the ciliated and the Clara cell (nonciliated, bronchiolar, secretory cell). Mucous cells develop following injurious stimuli. There are no basal cells. The Clara cell acts as the reserve cell by virtue of its ability to divide and differentiate into ciliated and mucous cells.[14] In the larger bronchioles, there is an admixture of ciliated and Clara cells, but the latter are predominant distally, being virtually exclusive in the smallest bronchioles.

The Clara cell is columnar and protrudes into the lumen in a dome-shaped manner beyond the level of the adjacent ciliated cells. It has a well-developed Golgi apparatus and abundant granular endoplasmic reticulum and mitochondria. Specific, membrane-bound, large round-to-oval secretory granules are present in the apical cytoplasm. In humans, the content of these granules is uniformly electron-dense and homogeneous. A large amount of glycogen may be present in the supranuclear cytoplasm. The luminal surface of Clara cells is covered with microvilli. Present evidence suggests that the Clara cells are responsible for producing the bronchiolar extracellular lining layer and perhaps for the hypophase or supporting portion, but not the tensio-active portion of the alveolar surfactant film. In the rat, the granules of the Clara cells in chlorphentermine-induced hyperplasia have a compact lamellar pattern that is lacking in the normal granules.

The alveoli and alveolar ducts are lined by type I and II pneumocytes. The type I cell is squamoid and covers most of the alveolar surface. The attenuated cytoplasm of this cell is part of the air–blood barrier across which gas exchange occurs. This cell type is not capable of division.

The type II pneumocyte (granular pneumocyte) can divide and is the precursor of the type I cell; it is cuboidal and present as rows of two or three cells in niches at alveolar septal junctions. The most conspicuous cytoplasmic feature of the type II pneumocyte is the presence of round, osmiophilic, lamellar bodies, 0.5 to 1.0 μ in diameter, that are seen as vacuoles on light-microscopy and as a structure composed of loosely arranged, concentric, membranous lamellae ultrastructurally. There is a prominent Golgi zone associated with numerous multivesicular bodies. Transitions from the latter to lamellar bodies are readily demonstrable. The surface is covered by apical microvilli, and the lamellar body content is released by exocytosis. This secretion, which consists largely of a dipalmityl lecithin, forms the tensio-active superficial layer of the extracellular alveolar lining material.

BRONCHIOLOALVEOLAR CARCINOMA

This entity was isolated on a clinicopathologic basis from other pulmonary neoplasms by Liebow[24] in 1960. He defined it as a peripheral adenocarcinoma whose cells tend to line the walls of distal air spaces without destroying them, and spread via aerogenous and lymphatic routes. The tumor is generally well differentiated, being composed of tall columnar cells that often have a papillary growth pattern. It may be composed entirely of mucus-producing cells or may be largely devoid of them. The papillary-adenocarcinoma category of the WHO classification is here included with the bronchioloalveolar carcinomas.

Thirty-one peripheral adenocarcinomas of the lung have been examined ultrastructurally at the New York Veterans Administration Hospital. The primary tumor was available for study in 27 cases. Twenty-four of these had varying amounts of a bronchioloalveolar growth pattern. A purely or predominantly Clara-cell-type differentiation was seen in 17 of these 24 neoplasms. In another Clara-cell tumor, not enough tissue was available to assess the pattern. Purely mucous-cell differentiation was seen in five cases, and a substantially mixed Clara cell–mucous cell pattern in seven cases. One case showed type II pneumocyte differentiation ultrastructurally, and by light-microscopy, a moderate number of cells also showed mucus production. Two of the neoplasms in the mixed category had a solid growth pattern. The following discussion is based on the findings of this study and published reports in the literature.

The vast majority of nonmucus-producing tumors (Fig. 22 Top left) show Clara-cell differentiation (Fig. 22 Bottom). These cells have the features of secretory cells—a prominent Golgi complex, an abundant granular endoplasmic reticulum, and many mitochondria with well-developed cristae. The most important feature of the cells is the presence of numerous, large (250- to 1000-nm diameter), round or oval, membrane-bound granules with a dense amorphous content (Fig. 22 Top right and Bottom). Some of the granules, however, may show a fingerprint-like or concentric, paracrystalline internal structure.[34] The concentric pattern is sometimes due to compact, membranous lamellae. In two Clara-cell neoplasms seen by the author, the majority of the secretory granules had a complex internal pattern. This may consist of dense material with an irregular or whorled morphology, parallel membranous lamellae, and even glycogen granules. The lack of accompanying degenerative changes suggests that these structures are not autophagosomes. Similar granules have been reported by Montes et al.[29] The secretory granules of Clara cells show a varying PAS-positivity.

Large quantities of cytoplasmic glycogen are usually present. Occasionally, this accumulation may be massive enough to present a clear-cell appearance on light-microscopy[34] (Fig. 22 Top left). In some cells, the glycogen may also be present in membrane-bound granules. Cytoplasmic annulate lamellae are not infrequent.

In mucus-secreting bronchioloalveolar carcinomas, virtually all of the cells produce mucus. This may be so abundant as to fill the alveoli and bronchioles lined by the tumor cells and to spill over into the adjoining air spaces. Ultrastructurally, the supranuclear cytoplasm of the majority of tumor cells is packed with mature mucus granules that show membrane fusion to each other and have a reticulated content that is paler than that of Clara-cell granules. Some of the cells may have

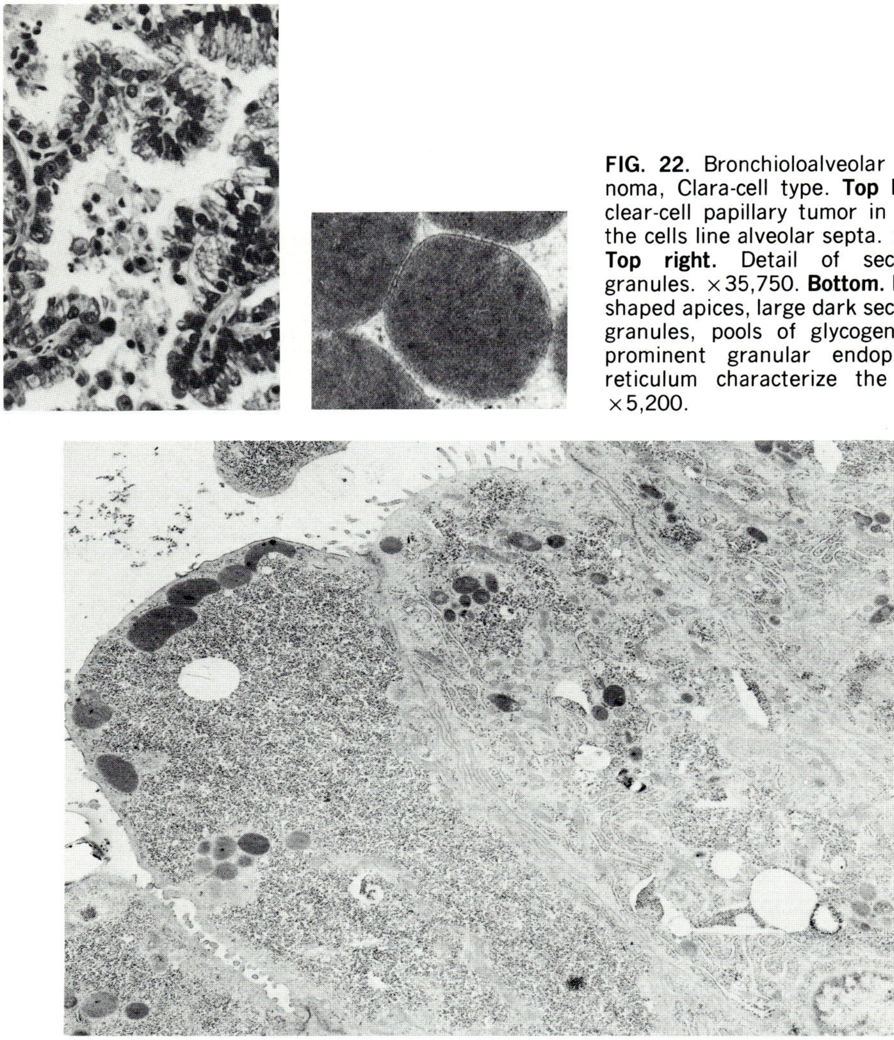

FIG. 22. Bronchioloalveolar carcinoma, Clara-cell type. **Top left.** A clear-cell papillary tumor in which the cells line alveolar septa. ×360. **Top right.** Detail of secretory granules. ×35,750. **Bottom.** Dome-shaped apices, large dark secretory granules, pools of glycogen, and prominent granular endoplasmic reticulum characterize the cells. ×5,200.

small or intermediate-sized discrete mucus granules in addition to or exclusive of the mature granules. Microvesicular and granular material representing extracellular mucus is seen on the luminal surface.

The Golgi complex and granular endoplasmic reticulum are prominent, particularly in cells that have discharged their secretion. In the latter cells, the luminal border may have a scalloped outline. The cytoplasmic glycogen content of the mucus-secreting cells in bronchioalveolar carcinomas is significantly lower than in Clara-cell tumors and, in about half the neoplasms, it may be nil.

In the mixed category of tumors (Fig. 23 Top left and right), most cells show one or the other type of differentiation, but individual cells with both Clara-cell-type secretory granules and small mucus granules are not infrequent (Fig. 23 Bot-

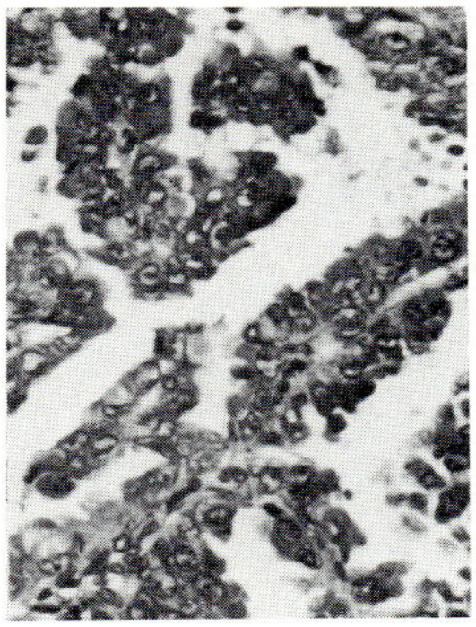
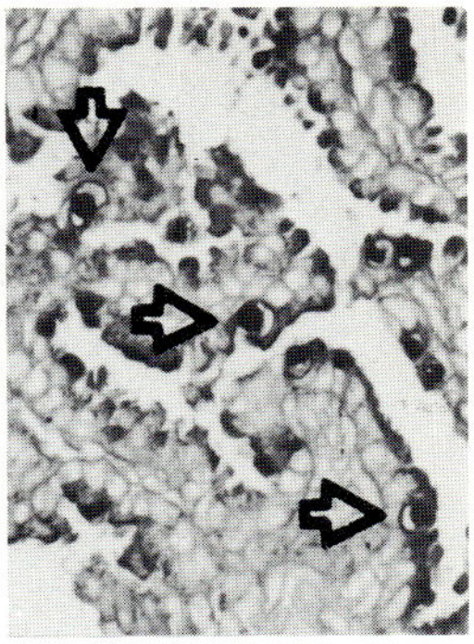

FIG. 23. Bronchioloalveolar carcinoma with mixed differentiation. **Top left.** Papillary pattern of cells lining alveoli. ×360. **Top right.** Alcian blue–PAS stain. Several mucin-containing cells are seen (arrows). The apical, PAS-positive material in other cells represents mostly glycogen. ×360. **Bottom.** The cell on the lower left and center contains both Clara-cell granules and small mucus granules. The cell on the right has three lamellar bodies and a Clara-cell granule. ×10,000.

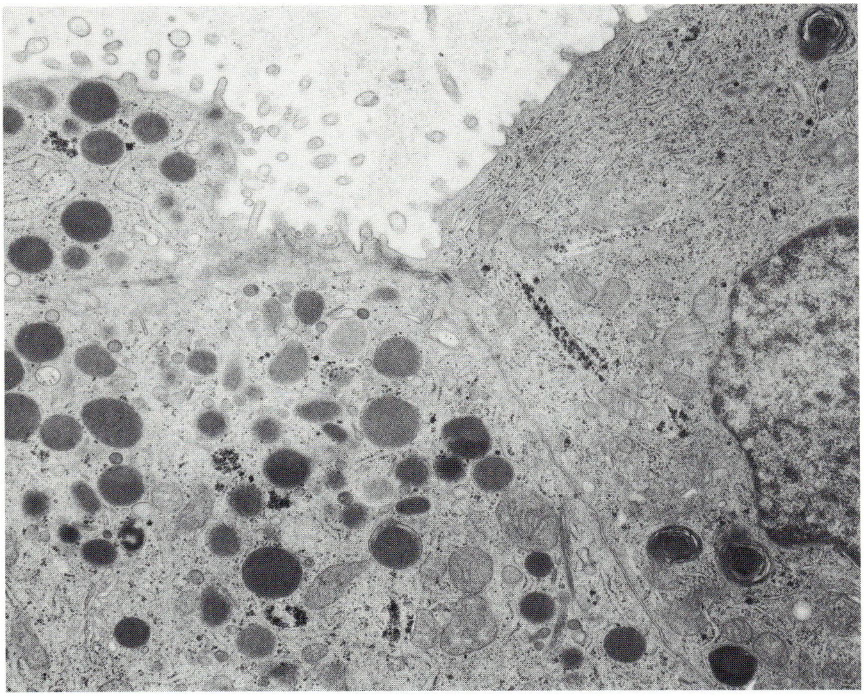

tom). The glycogen content is intermediate between that of the pure mucus and Clara-cell-type tumors.

The one tumor with extensive type II pneumocyte differentiation ultrastructurally had a radiologically visible peripheral mass in one lung and a metastatic tumor nodule in the brain. Only the metastatic nodule was available for examination. It was composed of well-differentiated papillary adenocarcinomatous areas (Fig. 24 Top) and poorly differentiated, more solid adenocarcinomatous areas. Type II pneumocyte differentiation, in the form of numerous mature lamellar bodies in the cell cytoplasm, was seen in both areas (Fig. 24 Bottom). A few mucus-producing cells were present in the solid area on light-microscopic examination. Other examples of tumors with type II pneumocyte differentiation have been described by Bonikos et al.[4] and Morningstar and Hassan.[30]

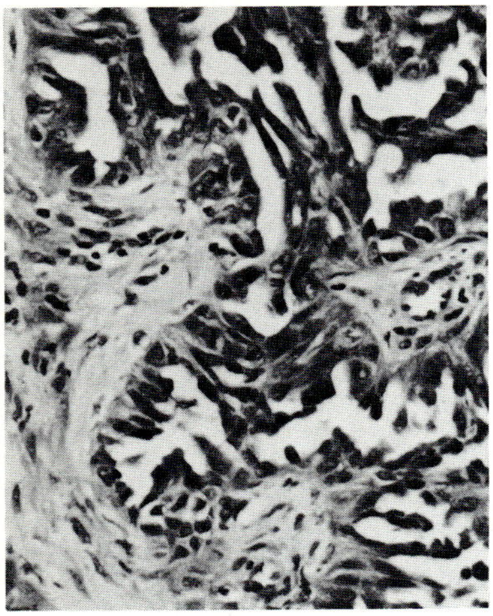

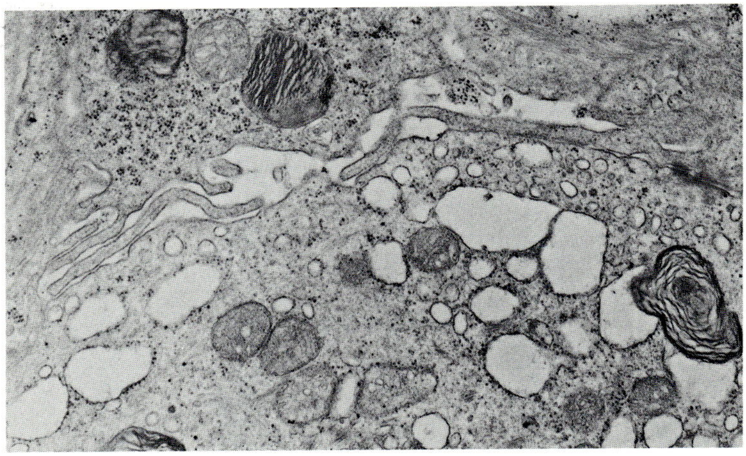

FIG. 24. Bronchioloalveolar carcinoma, type II pneumocyte type, metastatic in the brain. **Top.** The tumor has a papillary pattern. ×360. **Bottom.** Evidence of type II pneumocyte differentiation in the form of three lamellar bodies is seen. ×14,850.

In four of the neoplasms with only Clara-cell-type differentiation, granules morphologically intermediate between Clara-cell granules and lamellar bodies were present. Rare typical lamellar bodies were also seen. Similar intermediate granules and occasional lamellar bodies were seen in some of the Clara cells of the majority of tumors of mixed Clara-cell–mucous cell type. Examples of typical Clara-cell granules, lamellar bodies, and small mucus granules in the same tumor were also seen (Fig. 23 Bottom).

On the basis of these ultrastructural findings, it seems obvious that the classification of bronchioloalveolar carcinomas into separate, entirely independent subtypes is not feasible. Most of the tumors that appeared to be solely of the Clara-cell type ultrastructurally showed at least some mucus production on light-microscopic examination. Purely mucus-producing tumors did occur but were less common than those of mixed mucus cell–Clara-cell type. The one tumor with extensive type II pneumocyte differentiation also had some mucus production. Individual cells with mixed differentiation features were not infrequent.

Two possible histogenetic explanations exist for these findings. First, the tumors may arise from Clara cells. These cells act as stem cells in the bronchiole and can differentiate into mucous and ciliated cells.

The problem with this explanation is that it is not known if Clara cells can develop into type II pneumocytes. In human fetuses, prior to the development of Clara cells and type II pneumocytes, the distal airways are lined by cuboidal epithelial cells with abundant cytoplasmic glycogen.[6,17,18,40] Clara cells and type II pneumocytes differentiate from these cells. Also, in postnatal lung, undifferentiated cuboidal epithelial cells lacking the features of either Clara cells or type II pneumocytes have been described in the respiratory bronchioles of subhuman primates[7,8] and in human bronchioles.[3] An origin from these undifferentiated cells would explain all of the morphologic admixtures of cell types encountered in human bronchioloalveolar carcinomas.

Whether a subclassification of bronchioloalveolar carcinomas based on the predominant cell type is of value or not will have to await the results of future clinical studies of the behavior of these tumors. A light-microscopic subdivision of the tumors into mucous-cell (those in which almost every cell produces mucus), non-mucous-(Clara) cell, and mixed-cell varieties seems entirely reasonable. Because only a rare non-mucus-producing tumor is of the type II pneumocyte variety, such tumors would not significantly interfere with the value of the classification. This minor compromise eliminates the need for electron microscopy in clinical studies of bronchioloalveolar carcinoma. The presence of mucin should preferably be determined with the alcian blue–PAS stain rather than with mucicarmine. The former is more sensitive, gives better tinctorial visibility, and has the added advantage of being able to reveal the presence of cytoplasmic glycogen.

NORMAL MESOTHELIUM

The surface of the pleura is lined by a single layer of large, flattened cells that lie on a basal lamina and have a moderate number of microvilli and many pinocytotic vesicles on all of the cell surfaces. Junctional complexes incorporating apical tight junctions connect adjoining cells, giving them the properties of glandular cells. Gap junctions are also present. Cell organelles are scanty in unstimulated cells. The underlying connective tissue contains fibroblasts, smooth-muscle cells, collagen, and elastic fibers.

Clarke[11] has shown that regeneration of the mesothelial lining after experimental wounds of mesothelial surfaces occurs largely from subjacent mesenchyme rather than by the lateral spread of adjacent mesothelial cells over the wound, suggesting that the precursor cells of the mesothelial lining cells lie in this mesenchyme. Lewis,[23] using tissue cultures of embryonic cardiac mesenchyme, demonstrated its transformation into endothelium and mesothelium. Endothelial differentiation ceases at some time during embryonic life, with the result that endothelial cells can thereafter only be formed from preexisting endothelial cells. In contrast, mesothelium can continue to be formed from mesenchyme throughout life.

Maximow[25] showed that outgrowths from cultures of mesothelial cells could adopt a spindle-cell, fibroblastic pattern, demonstrating the biphasic potential of these cells.

PLEURAL MESOTHELIOMA

Since neoplasms arise by transformation of precursor cells, mesotheliomas can be expected to consist of mesenchymal and/or epithelial cells. In the experimental induction of peritoneal mesotheliomas in rats and mice, Davis[12] has shown that the neoplasms develop from spindle cells beneath the surface lining, and that the preexisting surface layer of epithelium does not take any part in the formation of the tumors. It does not even show evidence of hyperplasia.

In human malignant mesotheliomas of the pleura, the neoplasm may be epithelial, mixed epithelial and mesenchymal, or sarcomatoid. The epithelial neoplasms are adenocarcinomas, often well differentiated, with tubular, cystic, or cystopapillary formations (Fig. 25 Top). The stroma may be scanty or desmoplastic. The alcian blue–PAS stain is very helpful in distinguishing epithelial mesotheliomas from metastatic adenocarcinomas of pulmonary or other origin. Mesotheliomas lack epithelial mucin. They may, however, produce connective-tissue mucin (proteoglycan). This is seen as a thin layer of sky-blue-staining material on the surface of the cells. In contrast, epithelial mucins stain deep blue, purple, or magenta, and are frequently intracellular in addition to being extracellular. This distinction can be confirmed by showing that the blue staining can be abolished in mesotheliomas, but not in other adenocarcinomas, by pretreatment of the tissue sections with hyaluronidase. This technique is usually not necessary. Mucicarmine and PAS staining alone are not helpful. The light-microscopic distinction from tumors not producing mucin, such as Clara-cell- or type II-pneumocyte-type bronchioloalveolar carcinomas with pleural extension, can be difficult, particularly when only a small biopsy is available. Electron microscopy is very helpful in such instances.

Ultrastructurally, the tumor cells in pleural mesotheliomas form ductal structures. The luminal and intercellular surfaces are covered by a profusion of long, often interlocking, microvilli (Fig. 25 Bottom). Some of these may arise from short, pseudopod-like cytoplasmic processes. Reactive mesothelial cells have more microvilli than unstimulated mesothelial cells, but these are neither as profuse nor as elongated as those in tumors. The microvilli in benign mesotheliomas[36] are similar to those in the malignant variety. Apical junctional complexes and desmosomal junctions are present. Intercellular spaces are distended and can produce a vacuolated appearance on light-microscopy. The cytoplasm has a fibrillar matrix and is abundant. Tonofibrils may be present. The granular endoplasmic reticulum is prominent. Mitochondria may be numerous, are elongated, and have a dense matrix and prominent cristae. Lysosomal dense bodies and multivesicular bodies may be seen. Cytoplasmic aggregates of glycogen granules are frequently present. A basal lamina invests groups of tumor cells.

In mixed-type mesotheliomas, the neoplasm is composed of anastomosing cords of cells in a desmoplastic stroma. Slit-like structures lined by low cuboidal or

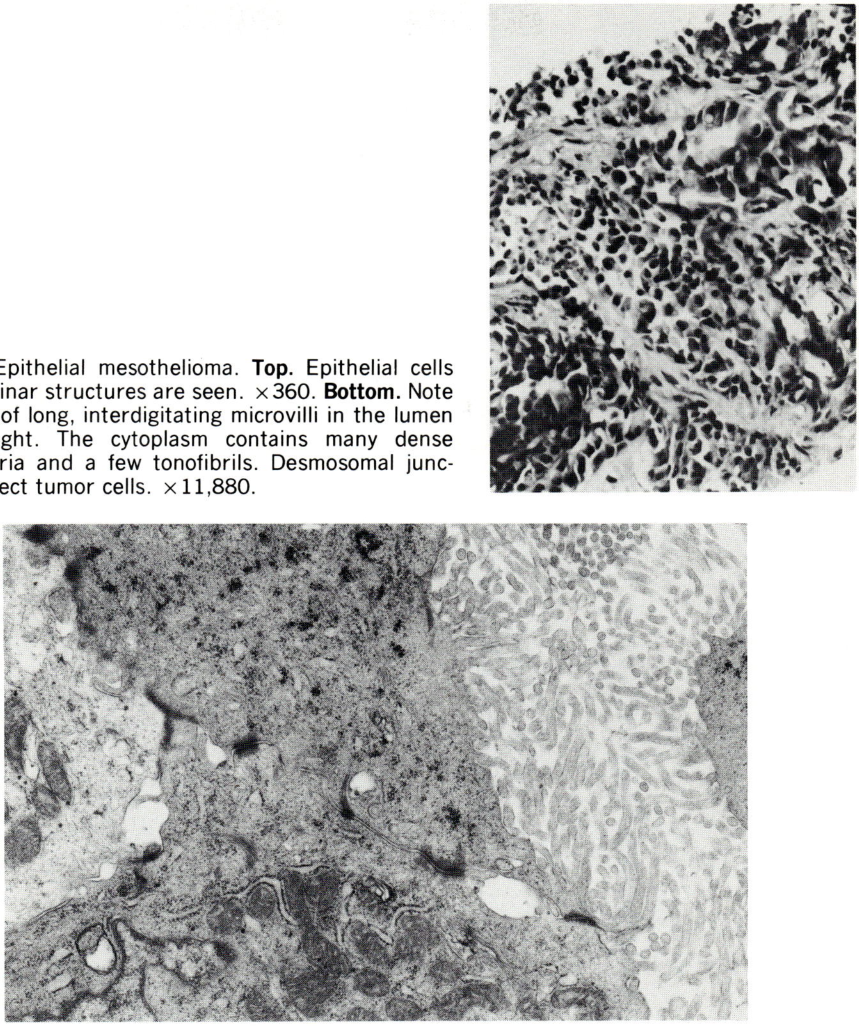

FIG. 25. Epithelial mesothelioma. **Top.** Epithelial cells forming acinar structures are seen. ×360. **Bottom.** Note the forest of long, interdigitating microvilli in the lumen on the right. The cytoplasm contains many dense mitochondria and a few tonofibrils. Desmosomal junctions connect tumor cells. ×11,880.

flattened epithelial cells may be seen. Ultrastructurally, the features of mixed-type mesothelioma cells are similar to those of cells in the epithelial type of tumor. However, the cells are arranged in a more disorganized manner, intercellular junctions are less well developed, and a basal lamina is present only focally. Irregular microvillous processes and pseudopodia are present at the stromal–cellular interface. Poorly differentiated and well-differentiated cells often coexist.

The sarcomatoid variant of pleural mesothelioma resembles a fibrosarcoma on light-microscopy (Fig. 26 Top). There is, however, some clustering of cells, and the cytoplasm may be more abundant than expected in a fibrosarcoma. Ultrastructurally, the clustering is seen to be due to extensive areas of continuous side-to-side contact of the cell membranes of adjoining cells (Fig. 26 Middle). Occasional in-

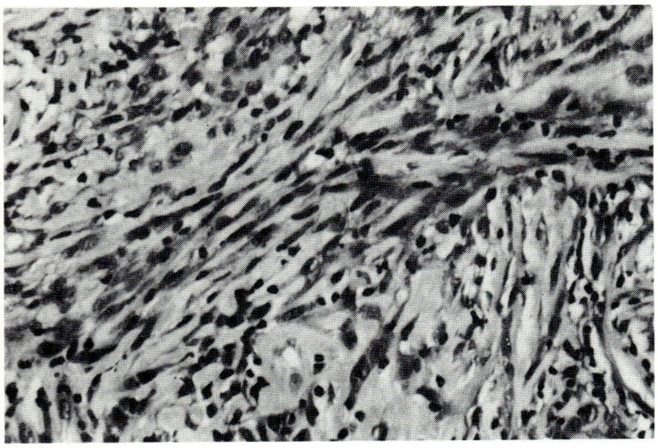

FIG. 26. Biphasic mesothelioma. **Top.** The spindled cells resemble a sarcoma. ×360. **Middle.** Elongated cells with extensive, continuous areas of membrane contact and a few cytoplasmic glycogen granules are seen. ×5,800. **Bottom.** A junctional complex is seen at the upper left along with some microvilli. Other junctions, resembling intermediate junctions with attached myofilaments, are also seen. ×10,890.

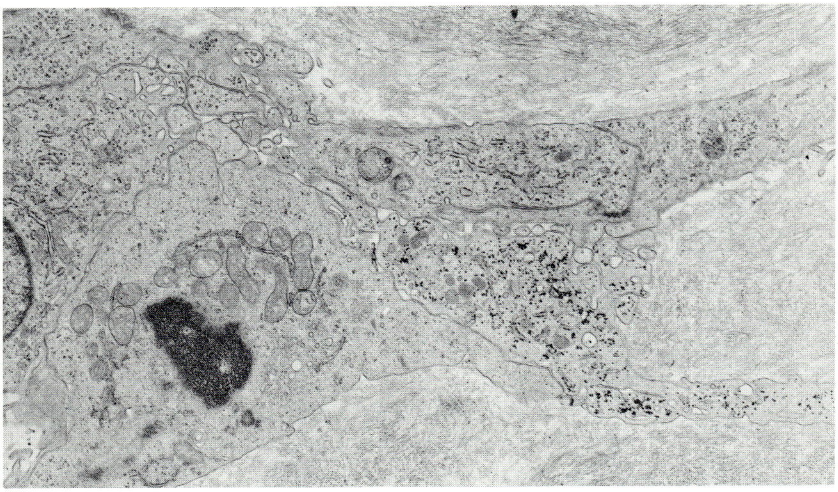

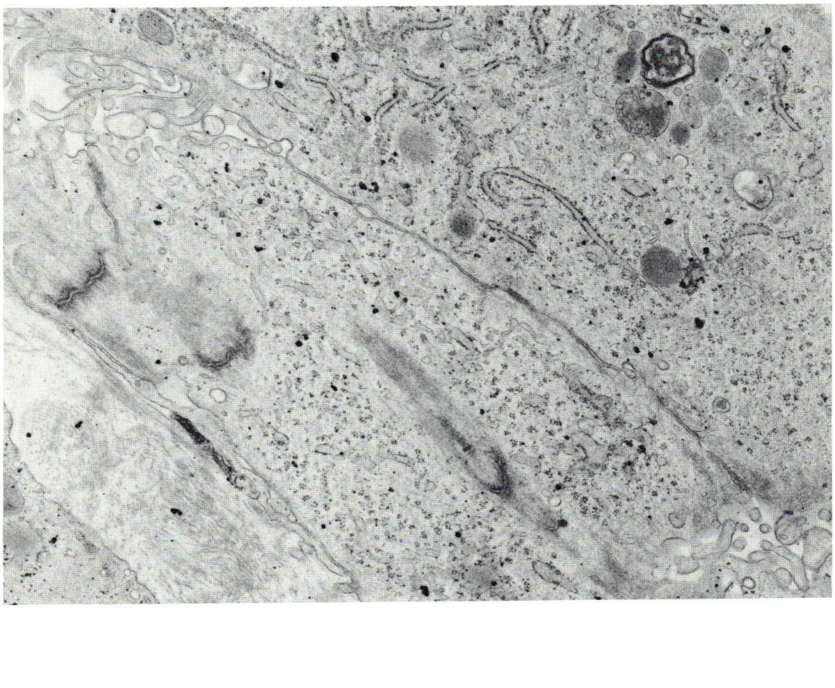

tercellular junctions are also seen (Fig. 26 Bottom); these may consist of poorly formed desmosomes, tight junctions, junctional complexes, or gap junctions. Occasional areas of microvillous formations in association with abortive lumina are seen. Cytoplasmic myofilaments may be present. Elongated cells with fibroblastic features are present, but usually show extensive areas of membrane contact with neighboring cells. Basal lamina may be absent or present only focally. The cytoplasmic matrix is very filamentous and varying quantities of cytoplasmic glycogen are usually present.

It appears that malignant mesotheliomas are epithelial or biphasic.[13,19,20,39] In tissue culture, they produce hyaluronic acid and extracellular collagen,[9] and sarcomatoid or "fibrous" forms of the tumor grow as terraced sheets of squamous-like cells.[31,38]

CONCLUSION

On the basis of the data presented above, a histogenetic classification of the major categories of lung carcinoma and pleural mesothelioma is proposed (Table 2).

Carcinoma in the bronchi can arise from one of two primary cells of origin—the basal and the mucous cells. Of the tumors that arise from basal cells, some may show no further differentiation. These are small-cell carcinomas that are totally undifferentiated ultrastructurally. Other tumors may show varying, but never marked, degrees of endocrine (K cell-type) differentiation. These form about one-third of small-cell carcinomas. A third group shows differentiation into larger (intermediate) cells that may also have evidence of endocrine differentiation. The relationship to the intermediate cells of normal bronchial epithelium should not be taken literally because the similarity is essentially only one of size. Nevertheless, it may be useful to retain this separate category until clinical studies can vindicate or nullify the value of such a separation.

Carcinoids can be viewed as tumors of basal-cell origin showing well differentiated K cell features. In most of these tumors, the granules resemble those of Hage's type 2 and 3 K cells. The oncocytic variant may be a tumor with granules resembling those of Hage's type 1 K cells or it may be any variety of carcinoid with marked mitochondrial proliferation. Spindle-cell carcinoids and tumorlets are peripheral carcinoids with granules resembling the smaller granules of Hage's type 1 K cells.

Squamous carcinoma may arise from basal cells. Adenocarcinomas arise from basal and/or mucous cells. Adenosquamous carcinomas may also arise from basal and/or mucous cells, since metaplastic squamous cells can develop from mucous cells.[28]

Large-cell undifferentiated carcinomas are tumors of basal- and/or mucous-cell origin that have developed beyond the basal-cell stage but lack sufficient adenocarcinomatous or squamous differentiation to permit classifying them into these categories. A giant-cell carcinoma is probably just a very pleomorphic large-cell carcinoma. A separate category of clear-cell carcinoma is probably not warranted, since tumors with extensive areas of clear cells often occur in Clara-cell car-

TABLE 2. Histogenetic Classification of Carcinomas of the Lung

Tumors from basal and/or mucous cells of bronchi
- Small-cell carcinoma
  - Oat-and spindle-cell carcinoma
  - Intermediate-cell carcinoma
- Carcinoids
  - Variants:
  - Oncocytic type
  - Spindle-cell type and tumorlets
- Squamous cell carcinoma
  - Well-differentiated
  - Moderately differentiated
  - Poorly differentiated
- Adenocarcinoma
  - Well-differentiated
  - Poorly differentiated
- Adenosquamous carcinoma
- Large-cell undifferentiated carcinoma
  - Variant:
  - Giant-cell carcinoma

Tumors from undifferentiated bronchiolar cells, Clara cells, type II pneumocytes, or bronchiolar mucous cells
- Bronchioloalveolar carcinoma
  - Mucous cell
  - Non-mucous-cell (Clara or type II pneumocyte)
  - Mixed cell

Tumors from pluripotent pleural mesenchymal cells
- Mesothelioma
  - Epithelial
  - Biphasic

cinoma and squamous cell carcinoma, most often due to cytoplasmic aggregates of glycogen but occasionally due to cytoplasmic lipid accumulation. Large-cell tumors with endocrine differentiation are too rare to warrant separate classification.

A bronchioloalveolar carcinoma in the histogenetic sense implies a carcinoma that arises from cells of the bronchiolar or alveolar epithelium, irrespective of the histologic pattern adopted by the neoplastic cells. Fortunately, the vast majority of these neoplasms have what Liebow described as a bronchioloalveolar growth pattern, but a small percentage are solid. The tumors could arise from Clara cells, type II pneumocytes, or mucous cells that have developed from Clara cells. However, since the neoplasms more often than not show a mixture of these cell types, an origin from undifferentiated bronchiolar epithelial cells is probably more frequent.

By light microscopy, the most reasonable subdivision would be into mucinous, nonmucinous, and mixed bronchioloalveolar carcinomas, with the understanding that although the nonmucinous group would be comprised mostly of Clara cell tumors, a small percentage would be type II pneumocyte tumors.

Mesotheliomas appear to arise from multipotential mesenchymal stem cells present in the stroma supporting the mesothelium. These tumors may be purely epithelial or mixed mesenchymal and epithelial (biphasic). The latter resemble fibrosarcomas upon light-microscopy. A tumor that was purely mesenchymal ultrastructurally could be called mesothelial if an epithelial potential were demonstrated by other means such as tissue culture. Such a neoplasm has not yet been described.

ACKNOWLEDGMENTS

The author is grateful to Eulee Forrester, Nicholas Cassai, and Sarah Gourley for expert technical assistance.

REFERENCES

1. Ahmed A: Some ultrastructural observations of haematoxyphil vascular change in oat cell carcinoma. J Pathol 112:1-3, 1974
2. An T: Cytoplasmic inclusions in bronchial carcinoid. Hum Pathol 9:241-242, 1978
3. Basset F, Poirier J, Le Crom M, Turiaf J: Étude ultrastructurale de l'epithelium bronchiolaire humain. Z Zellforsch 116:425-442, 1971
4. Bonikos DS, Hendrickson M, Bensch KG: Pulmonary alveolar cell carcinoma. Fine structure and in vitro study of a case and critical review of this entity. Am J Surg Pathol 1:93-108, 1977
5. Breeze RG, Wheeldon EB: The cells of the pulmonary airways. Am Rev Resp Dis 116:705-777, 1977
6. Campiche MA, Gautier A, Hernandez EI, Reymond A: An electron microscope study of the fetal development of human lung. Pediatrics 32:976-994, 1963
7. Castleman WL, Dungworth DL, Tyler WS: Intrapulmonary airway morphology in three species of monkeys: a correlated scanning and transmission electron microscopic study. Am J Anat 142:107-122, 1975
8. Castleman WL, Dungworth DL, Schwartz W, Tyler WS: Acute respiratory bronchiolitis. An ultrastructural and autoradiographic study of epithelial cell injury and renewal in rhesus monkeys exposed to ozone. Am J Pathol 98:811-840, 1980
9. Castor CW, Naylor B: Characteristics of normal and malignant human mesothelial cells studied in vitro. Lab Invest 20:437-443, 1969
10. Churg A: The fine structure of large cell undifferentiated carcinoma of the lung. Evidence for its relation to squamous cell carcinomas and adenocarcinomas. Hum Pathol 9:143-156, 1978
11. Clarke WC: Experimental mesothelium. Anat Rec 10:301-316, 1915-1916
12. Davis JMG: Histogenesis and fine structure of peritoneal tumors produced in animals by injections of asbestos. J Natl Cancer Inst 52:1823-1837, 1974a
13. Davis JMG: Ultrastructure of human mesotheliomas. J Natl Cancer Inst 52:1715-1725, 1974b
14. Evans MJ, Johnson LV, Stephens RJ, Freeman G: Renewal of the terminal bronchiolar epithelium in the rat following exposure to NO_2 or O_3. Lab Invest 35:246-257, 1976
15. Godwin JD, Brown CC: Comparative epidemiology of carcinoid and oat-cell tumors of the lung. Cancer 40:1671-1673, 1977
16. Hage E: Endocrine cells in the bronchial mucosa of human fetuses. Acta Pathol Microbiol Scand 80A:225-234, 1972
17. Hage E: Electron microscopic identification of several types of endocrine cells in the bronchial epithelium of human fetuses. Z Zellforsch 141:401-412, 1973a

18. Hage E: The morphological development of the pulmonary epithelium of human fetuses studied by light and electron microscopy. Z Anat Entw Gesch 140:271–279, 1973b
19. Kay S, Silverberg SG: Ultrastructural studies of a malignant fibrous mesothelioma of the pleura. Arch Pathol 92:449–455, 1971
20. Klima M, Spjut HJ, Seybold WD: Diffuse malignant mesothelioma. Am J Clin Pathol 65:583–600, 1976
21. Lauweryns JM, Peuskens JC: Argyrophil (kinin and amine producing?) cells in human infant airway epithelium. Life Sci 8(Part I):577–585, 1969
22. Lauweryns JM, Peuskens JC, Cokelaere M: Argyrophil, fluorescent and granulated (peptide and amine producing?) AFG cells in human infant bronchial epithelium. Light and electron microscopic studies. Life Sci 9(Part I):1417–1429, 1970
23. Lewis WH: Mesenchyme and mesothelium. J Exp Med 38:257–262, 1923
24. Liebow AA: Bronchiolo-alveolar cell carcinoma. Adv Intern Med 10:329–358, 1960
25. Maximow A: Uber das Mesothel (Deckzellen der serosen Haute) und die Zellen der serosen Exsudate. Untersuchungen an entzundetem Gewebe und an Gewebskulturen. Arch Exp Zellforsch 4:1–36, 1927
26. McDowell EM, Barrett LA, Trump BF: Observations on small granules cells in adult human bronchial epithelium and in carcinoid and oat cell tumors. Lab Invest 34:202–206, 1976
27. McDowell EM, Barrett LA, Glavin F, et al: The respiratory epithelium. I. Human bronchus. J Natl Cancer Inst 61:539–549, 1978a
28. McDowell EM, McLaughlin JS, Merenyi DK, et al.: The respiratory epithelium. V. Histogenesis of lung carcinomas in the human. J Natl Cancer Inst 61:587–606, 1978b
29. Montes M, Binette JP, Chaudhry AP, et al.: Clara cell adenocarcinoma. Light and electron microscopic studies. Am J Surg Pathol 1:245–253, 1977
30. Morningstar WA, Hassan MO: Bronchiolo-alveolar carcinoma with nodal metastases. An ultrastructural study. Am J Surg Pathol 3:273–278, 1979
31. Sano ME, Weiss E, Gault ES: Pleural mesothelioma; further evidence of its histogenesis. J Thorac Surg 19:783–788, 1950
32. Scharifker D, Marchevsky A: Oncocytic carcinoid of lung: an ultrastructural analysis. Cancer 47:530–532, 1981
33. Shimosato Y: Pathology of lung cancer. In Hansen HH, Rorth M (eds): Lung Cancer, 1980. Postgraduate Course, II World Congress on Lung Cancer, Copenhagen, June 9–13, 1980. Amsterdam-Oxford-Princeton, Excerpta Medica, 1980, pp 27–48
34. Sidhu GS, Forrester EM: Glycogen-rich Clara cell-type bronchiolo-alveolar carcinoma. Light and electron microscopic study. Cancer 40:2209–2215, 1977
35. Sidhu GS: The endodermal origin of digestive and respiratory tract APUD cells. Histopathologic evidence and a review of the literature. Am J Pathol 96:5–20, 1979
36. Sidhu GS, Fresko O: Adenomatoid tumor of the epididymis: ultrastructural evidence of its biphasic nature. Ultrastruct Pathol 1:39–47, 1980
37. Sobin LH: The WHO Classification of Lung Tumors, Revised Edition. XII Congress Internacional del Cancer; Buenos Aires, October 5–11, 1978, pp 105–106 (Abstract)
38. Stout AP, Murray MR: Localized pleural mesothelioma. Investigation of its characteristics and histogenesis by the method of tissue culture. Arch Pathol 34:951–964, 1942
39. Suzuki Y, Churg J, Kannerstein M: Ultrastructure of human malignant diffuse mesothelioma. Am J Pathol 85:241–262, 1976
40. Thurlbeck WM: Postnatal growth and development of the lung. Am Rev Resp Dis 111:803–844, 1975
41. Watson JHL, Brinkhous GL: Electron microscopy of the epithelial cells of normal and bronchitic human bronchus. Am Rev Resp Dis 90:851–866, 1964

CROHN'S COLITIS

ROBERT ROWLAND AND DERRICK J. POUNDER

Published accounts of nontuberculous granulomatous inflammation of the large and small bowel have appeared intermittently since the turn of the century.[1] In a landmark paper[2] in 1932, Crohn, Ginzberg, and Oppenheimer drew attention to the importance of the entity which they called "regional ileitis." At first it was thought that Crohn's disease only affected the terminal ileum, but over the years it has become apparent that any part of the gastrointestinal tract, from the mouth to the anus, may become involved. Today, Crohn's colitis is a well-established entity, and its differentiation from ulcerative colitis has emerged as a challenging problem for both clinician and pathologist.

Large-intestinal involvement in Crohn's disease occurs in approximately 40 percent of cases, and in one-half of these the disease is confined to the large bowel.[3] Large-bowel involvement is second in incidence only to terminal ileal disease, and is more common than upper small-bowel, duodenal, or gastric disease.[4] Although Crohn's disease of the large bowel may occur at any age, the age incidence is bimodal,[5] with the main peak being in the third decade and a second, smaller peak occurring in the elderly; the overall increase in the incidence of the disease has been largely attributed[6] to increasing numbers of persons in the older age group. These elderly patients often have localized left-sided colonic involvement,[5] which sometimes coexists with diverticular disease.[7] A recent epidemiologic study suggests that this rising incidence of Crohn's disease has not been maintained.[8]

In the absence of any known etiologic factors, the diagnosis of Crohn's disease is of necessity based upon anatomic features which may be assessed clinically, radiologically, or histopathologically. The pathology of Crohn's colitis is not fundamentally different from that of ileal disease, but in the histopathologic interpretation of material from the large bowel there is an important distinction of Crohn's disease from ulcerative colitis. In biopsy material, this distinction has implications for both medical and surgical management. In colectomy specimens, the distinction is of prognostic importance as recurrent ileal disease may occur following proctocolectomy for Crohn's colitis[9] while by contrast proctocolectomy effectively cures ulcerative colitis.

MACROSCOPIC APPEARANCE

Crohn's disease affects the right side of the colon more often than the left,[10] and in only half of the cases is the rectum involved.[11] The disease can be diffuse, segmental with strictures, or mainly confined to the rectum.[12] These differing patterns contrast with the manner in which ulcerative colitis invariably affects the rectum and spreads proximally in continuity.[3]

At laparotomy[13] in active Crohn's disease, a small amount of free peritoneal fluid is usually present, and adhesions are frequently seen. The affected areas may be "fat wrapped" and the mesentery is often indurated. The diseased segments can be readily identified since they are edematous and thickened. The serosa is congested, a fibrinous exudate is present, and numerous tiny serosal tubercles (granulomata) may occasionally be apparent. Draining lymph nodes are usually enlarged. When examined from the serosal aspect, the presence of diseased bowel is more obvious in Crohn's disease than in ulcerative colitis. This is because the inflammatory process in Crohn's disease is transmural, whereas in ulcerative colitis it is confined to the mucosa. At laparotomy in Crohn's disease, althought the proximal margins of the disease segments appear well demarcated, this can be deceptive, since mucosal involvement is often more extensive.

When the bowel is opened in the typical case of Crohn's colitis, two features are present that distinguish this condition from ulcerative colitis. Firstly, the disease is segmental, and second, the inflammation is transmural. Mucosal ulceration is usually present, but the pattern of the ulceration is variable. Some ulcers remain shallow despite becoming quite large, while others are deeply penetrating fissures. The smallest lesions are tiny aphthoid ulcers (Fig. 1), which have been so termed because of their resemblance to the common aphthous ulcers of the mouth. These aphthoid ulcers develop over lymphoid aggregates[14] and vary in appearance from hemorrhagic spots to small, clearly defined, shallow and white-floored ulcers (Fig. 2). It is particularly important to note their presence at the lines of resection, for if they are present the patient has an increased risk of developing recurrent disease. The shallow aphthoid ulcers may enlarge to become extensive, shallow serpiginous ulcers.

Fissures are narrow ulcers which may penetrate deeply into the bowel wall. They appear radiologically as spiculations of barium aligned at right angles to the lumen. These fissures give rise to abscesses and fistulae, which often complicate Crohn's disease. The characteristic cobblestone mucosal pattern observed in small-bowel disease is less commonly seen in colonic disease. This cobblestone appearance is created by numerous raised islands of edematous mucosa surrounded by intercommunicating and fissuring ulceration.

Longitudinal guttering ulceration,[4] with intact normal or near normal surrounding muscosa, is another well-recognized pattern of ulceration, and this heals to leave parallel "rail-track" scars (Fig. 3). Pseudopolyps produced by undermining

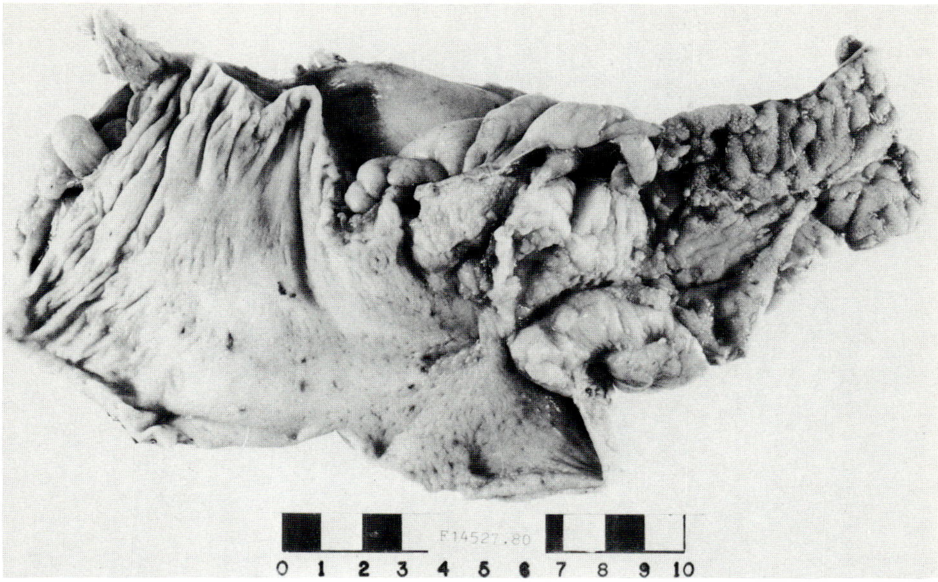

FIG. 1. Terminal ileum and ascending colon. Ileal ulceration is extensive, while the colon has many small hemorrhagic aphthoid ulcers.

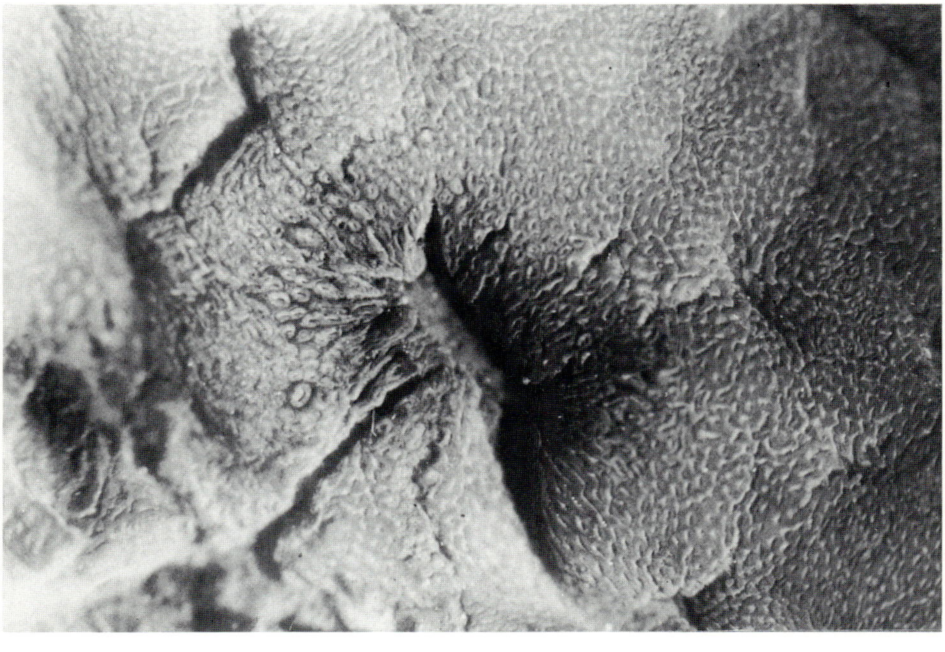

FIG. 2. An aphthoid ulcer as seen under the dissecting microscope. The margin of the ulcer is congested and a single inflamed crypt is present nearby.

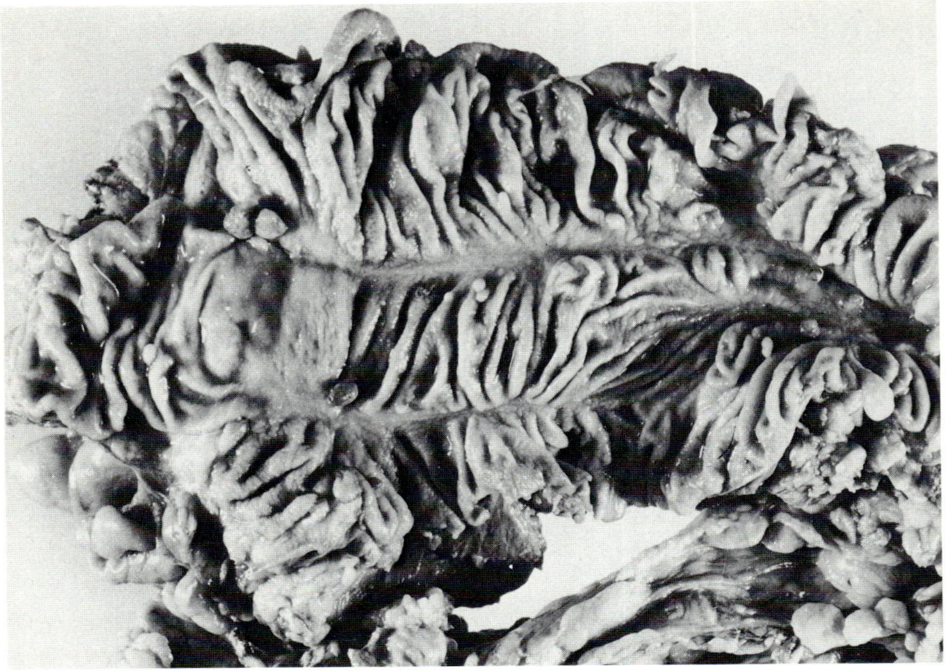

FIG. 3. Rail-track scarring and pseudopolyp formation in the ascending colon.

ulceration may be found in Crohn's disease as well as in ulcerative colitis. When present, strictures may be single or multiple and have a similar appearance to those seen in the small bowel (Fig. 4). The wall of the bowel is asymmetrically thickened and feels rubbery. The lumen is reduced and the mucosa is usually ulcerated or atrophic.

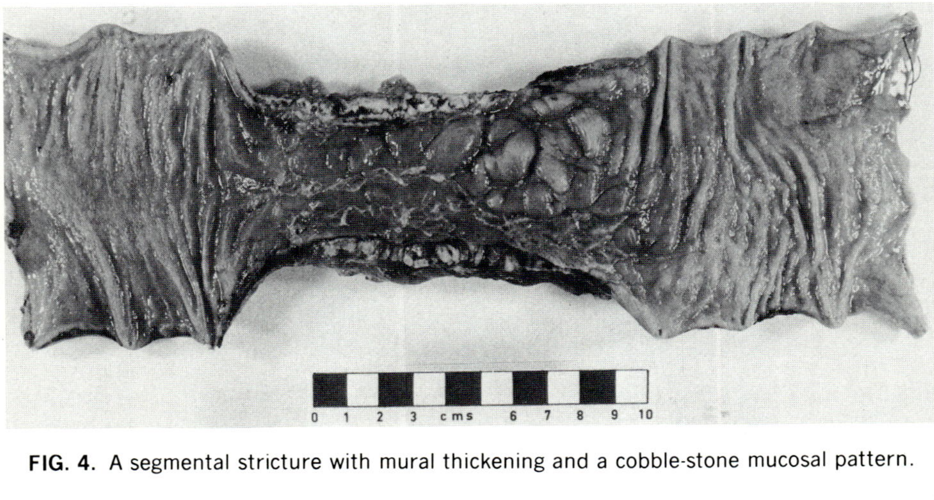

FIG. 4. A segmental stricture with mural thickening and a cobble-stone mucosal pattern.

Two macroscopic patterns of disease seen in ulcerative colitis may be confused with Crohn's colitis. In some cases of ulcerative colitis, there is apparent anomalous rectal sparing. This may be misinterpreted on sigmoidoscopy as segmental disease, favoring a diagnosis of Crohn's colitis. However, in ulcerative colitis, although the rectum may appear normal on sigmoidoscopy, the mucosa is always microscopically abnormal. This pattern of anomalous rectal sparing is seen particularly in fulminant disease and following local steroid therapy. Another difficulty that may be encountered is in distinguishing ulcerative colitis with "backwash ileitis" from Crohn's colitis with associated disease of the terminal ileum. "Backwash ileitis" always occurs in continuity with diseased colon, and the inflammation is primarily mucosal and involves only 5 to 25 cm of the terminal ileum. By contrast, terminal ileal Crohn's disease may be separated from disease in the colon by a segment of normal mucosa. In addition, Crohn's disease is transmural and the affected segment may be longer than 25 cm.

MICROSCOPIC APPEARANCE

In order to correlate the microscopic with the macroscopic appearance of the bowel in Crohn's disease, it is important to display the mucosa properly by pinning out the specimen, fixing it well, and making a photographic as well as a descriptive record. Tissue taken for histologic examination should include the lines of resection, apparently normal mucosa, diseased areas, lymph nodes, and vessels.

Crohn's disease is a transmural inflammation which is characteristically aggregated and principally lymphocytic in type. The presence of granulomata is the single most helpful diagnostic feature and also provides the basis for an absolute distinction from ulcerative colitis. However, granulomata are only present in 50 to 70 percent of cases.[15] The granulomata may be sparse, necessitating the careful examination of many tissue sections. They are usually located in the submucosa and serosa, but may be found in any layer of the bowel wall (Fig. 5). Granulomata occur less commonly in lymph nodes, and when these are present they are always associated with granulomata in the bowel wall. There is a poor correlation between lymph node size and the presence of granulomata.[11]

Small, poorly formed microgranulomata[16] should be noted, for they provide valuable suggestive evidence of Crohn's disease. These microgranulomata comprise small collections of a few histiocytes intermingled with lymphocytes (Fig. 6). When well-formed, the granulomata in Crohn's disease consist of clusters of epithelioid histiocytes with or without giant cells, and with only a few surrounding lymphocytes being present. Although some necrosis may be found in the granulomata of Crohn's disease, the presence of caseation should arouse suspicion of tuberculosis.

Typically in Crohn's disease the basic mucosal architecture is only mildly disturbed. The mucosa is edematous and there is an increase in lamina propria round cells, particularly lymphocytes. Crypt abscesses are usually present but few in number. Goblet-cell mucin is not depleted and cannot be used as a guide to the activity of the disease, as it can in ulcerative colitis. Edema and lymphatic dilatation

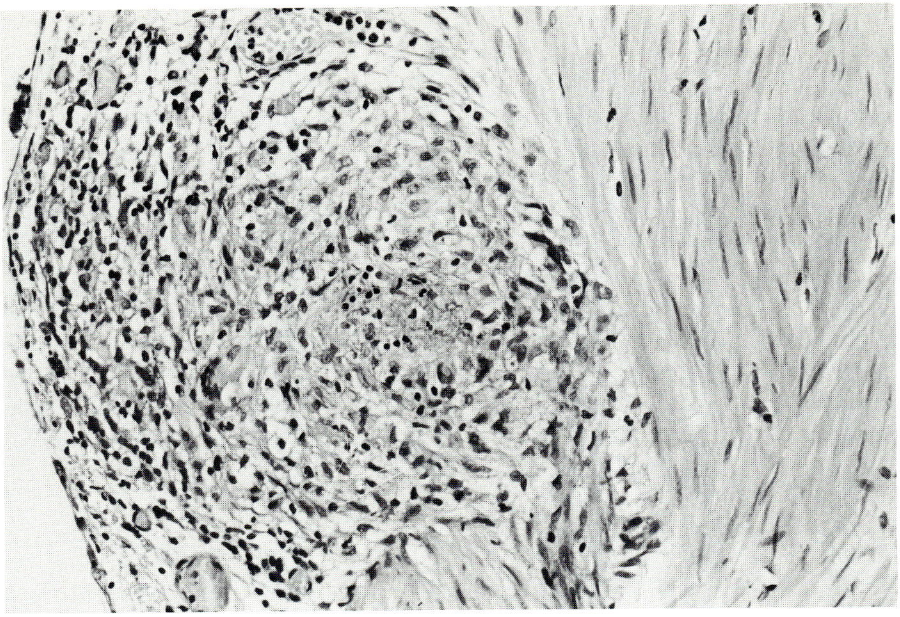

FIG. 5. A subserosal granuloma containing a small focus of necrosis. ×221.

are dominant features and involve the full thickness of the bowel wall. The pronounced vascular component to the inflammatory process that is seen in the mucosa in ulcerative colitis is missing in Crohn's disease. When present, fissuring ulceration is a distinctive feature of Crohn's disease but must be distinguished from the broader-based ulcers found in fulminant colitis of all etiologies.[17] The submucosa is edematous and fibrotic, and this submucosal fibrosis contributes substantially to stricture formation.

The granulomatous and lymphocytic inflammations in Crohn's disease often develop in close proximity to blood vessels and lymphatics, and this may reflect a pathogenetic relationship (Fig. 7). Several patterns of vascular change are observed,[18] at least some of which are secondary to adjacent inflammation. The vein walls commonly show irregular thickening and the arteries typically display concentric fibroelastic subintimal proliferation with variable medial hypertrophy. These changes may progress to vascular obliteration. Less common is segmental necrosis of the vessel walls with a granulomatous reaction surrounding a vessel or involving its wall or lumen. This appearance may reflect entrapment of the vessel by an adjacent granulomatous reaction. A more classical, giant-cell type of arteritis, with fragmentation of the internal elastic lamina and a giant-cell reaction at the intima-media interface, has also been described (Fig. 8).[19] Takayasu's arteritis, which may involve larger mesenteric vessels, has only rarely been reported in association with inflammatory bowel disease.[20]

There are several other histologic features which, although adding to the overall picture, are of little diagnostic importance in Crohn's disease.[21] Eccentric thickening of the main muscle coat and neuromatous hyperplasia of the nerve

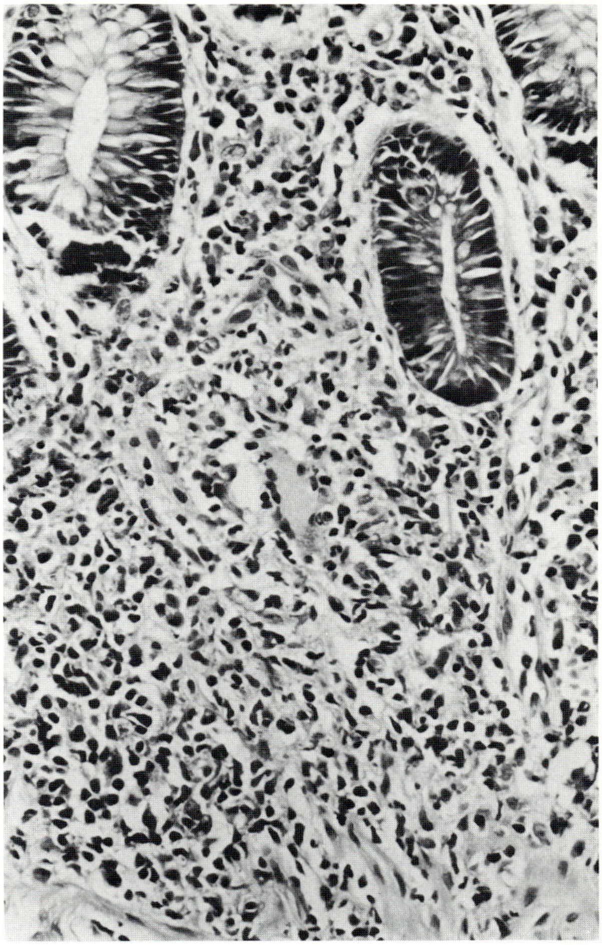

FIG. 6. A microgranuloma in the lamina propria. A giant cell is surrounded by lymphocytes and admixed histiocytes which have little cytoplasm. ×350.

fascicles of the intermyenteric and submucosal regions may be observed. Pseudopyloric gland metaplasia, Paneth cell metaplasia, and lipocytes in the lamina propria are other nonspecific changes which may be seen. Healed areas of ulceration may show mucosal atrophy with branching and loss of parallelism of crypts, but the architectural disturbance is generally less than that seen in ulcerative colitis. Absence of the muscularis mucosae provides evidence of previous ulceration even if the overlying mucosa is intact.[22]

BIOPSY APPEARANCE

Rectal biopsy is a safe, simple, and painless procedure of value both in the diagnosis of Crohn's colitis[23,24] and in the distinction of this condition from ulcerative colitis.[25-27] The recent development of fiberoptic colonoscopy has made it possible to biopsy the entire length of the colon. Biopsies should be taken from nor-

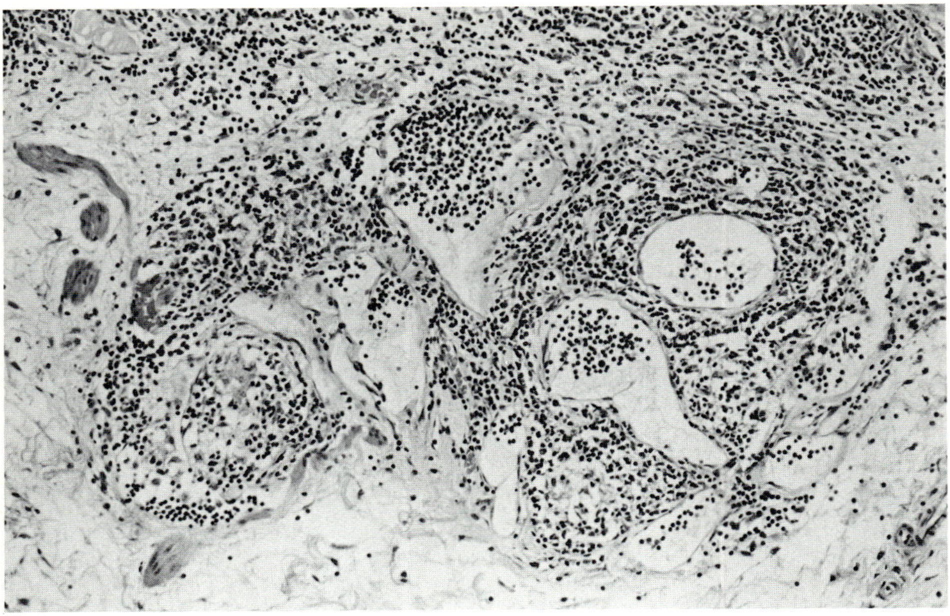

FIG. 7. Dilated submucosal lymphatics with surrounding aggregates of lymphocytes. Two small, poorly formed granulomata are present. ×140.

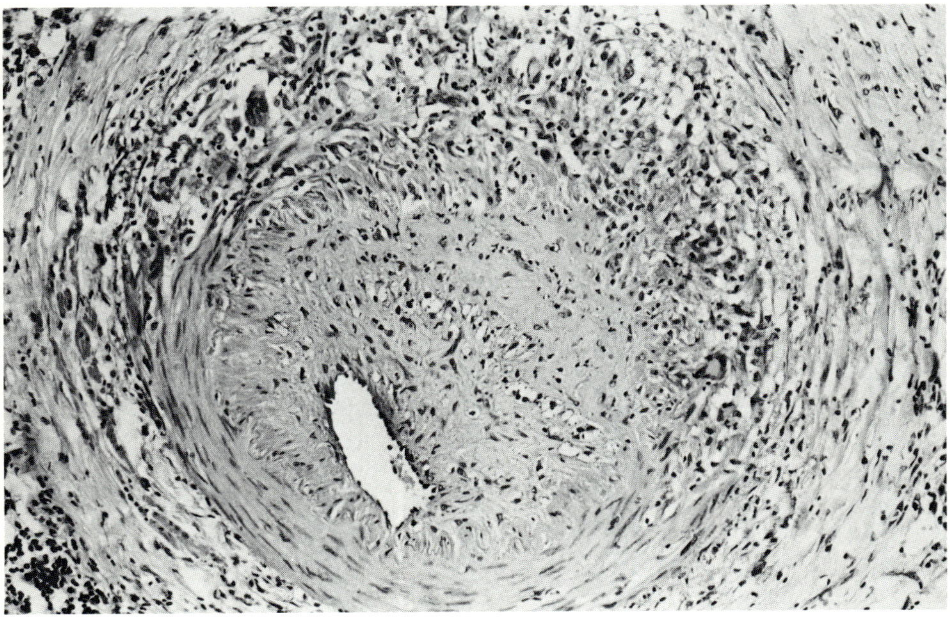

FIG. 8. A small muscular artery with a giant cell and granulomatous reaction within the media. There is prominent intimal proliferation. ×140.

mal and abnormal areas of the colonic mucosa, and the sigmoidoscopist should attempt to include submucosa in the specimen. Nodular areas, reflecting submucosal involvement, and the edges of ulcers should always be biopsied because they are most productive of granulomata.[11] When present, granulomata are the single most valuable diagnostic feature of Crohn's colitis (Fig. 9). Well-formed granulomata are not found in ulcerative colitis, although occasional giant cells may be seen. In ulcerative colitis, and to a lesser extent in Crohn's disease, rectal mucosa that sigmoidoscopically appears normal may be microscopically abnormal and harbor valuable diagnostic information. Approximately one-half of all cases of Crohn's colitis have rectal involvement. In the remainder, the confirmation of lack of rectal involvement effectively excludes a diagnosis of ulcerative colitis, which invariably shows such involvement.

In the typical case of Crohn's colitis, the various biopsy fragments show evidence of the patchy nature of the disease, with only some fragments being involved by the inflammatory process. Small foci of inflammation flanked by relatively normal mucosa may be seen in a single fragment. These inflammatory foci typically comprise a lymphocytic infiltrate surrounding a degenerating crypt that shows goblet-cell depletion (Fig. 10).

The mucosal architecture of the inflamed fragments of the colon is usually well preserved, and the muscularis mucosae is not thickened. The lamina propria of the inflamed areas contains increased numbers of round cells, many of which are lymphocytes. Crypt abscesses are usually seen but are not numerous, and the melting away of crypts seen in ulcerative colitis is not a feature. Prominent lymphoid aggregates in an otherwise normal mucosa are suggestive of Crohn's colitis,

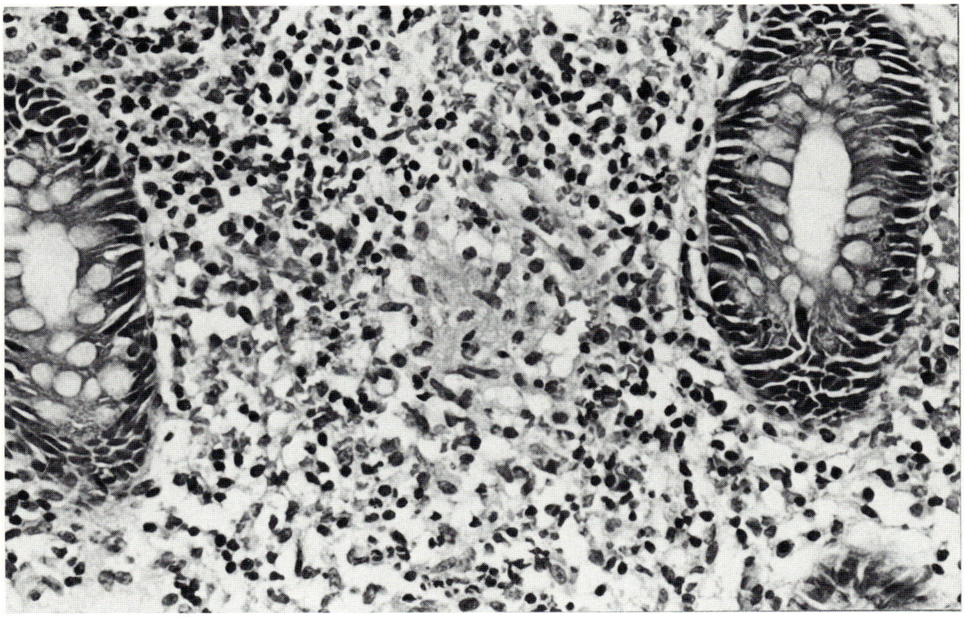

FIG. 9. A poorly formed granuloma within the lamina propria of a colonic biopsy. ×350.

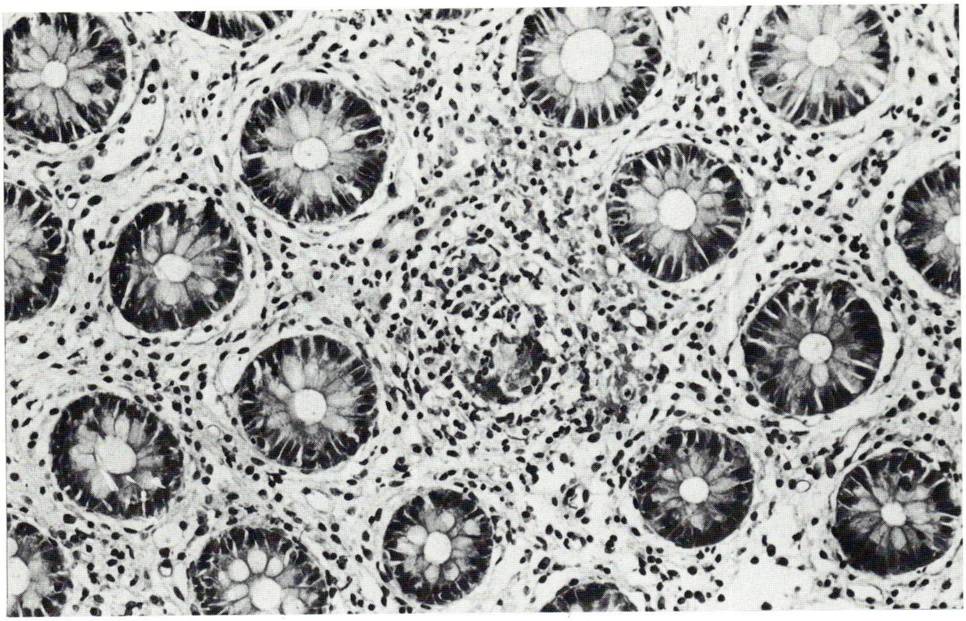

FIG. 10. A single crypt is partly destroyed and surrounded by mononuclear cells. The goblet-cell population of the adjacent crypts is preserved. ×221.

but must be distinguished from the excessive lymphoid tissue seen in chronic ulcerative colitis. In the latter there is always other evidence of mucosal damage, in the form of crypt irregularity. By comparison with ulcerative colitis, the goblet-cell population in Crohn's colitis is well preserved, and the histochemical assessment of epithelial mucosubstances[28] can be helpful in differentiating Crohn's disease from ulcerative colitis.

Normally in the rectal mucosa, the goblet cells of the lower two-thirds of the crypts contain predominantly sulfated mucosubstances, which may be stained with a high iron diamine technique or with alcian blue at pH 1.0. The goblet cells of the surface and upper third of the crypts contain a mixture of sulfated and nonsulfated mucosubstances, the latter staining with alcian blue at pH 2.5, together with a variable amount of neutral mucosubstances, staining brightly with the periodic acid-Schiff (PAS) reagent. Generally in cases of Crohn's disease, the mucin-secretion pattern remains remarkably normal. By contrast, in ulcerative colitis there is a marked diminution in mucin secretion and the remaining mucin is predominantly acid nonsulfated mucin.

With a sufficiently deep biopsy, submucosal inflammation unrelated to mucosal ulceration may be seen. The inflammatory infiltrate may comprise only focal aggregates of lymphocytes in an edematous submucosa, although granulomata may also be present.

In Crohn's disease, when the mucosa appears normal sigmoidoscopically, microscopy of biopsy material may reveal minor early changes, such as mucosal or submucosal edema and lymphatic dilatation (Fig. 11). Lamina propria edema may

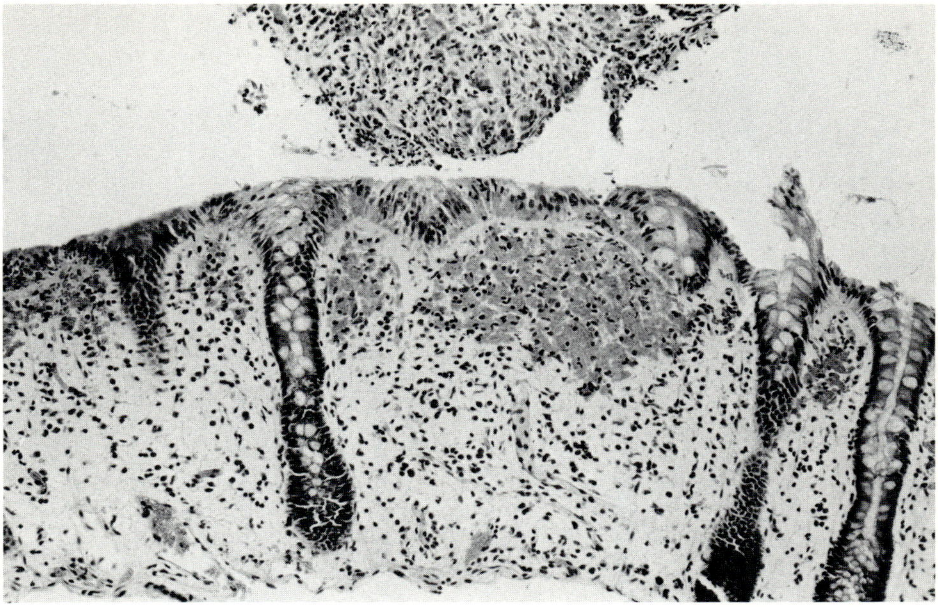

FIG. 11. Mucosal edema and areas of superficial hemorrhage. The smaller biopsy fragment contains a granuloma. ×140.

separate the base of the crypts from the muscularis mucosae, causing apparent crypt shortening. This must be distinguished from the mucosal atrophy with irregular shortening and branching of crypts seen in chronic ulcerative colitis.

A significant number of cases of Crohn's disease mimic ulcerative colitis when first seen because on sigmoidoscopy the disease is diffuse and biopsy reveals a "nonspecific" proctitis without the diagnostic features of Crohn's disease. The correct diagnosis will be established in due course provided that the case is reevaluated clinically, radiologically, and pathologically on a regular basis. Thus, it must be accepted that some cases which initially appear to be ulcerative colitis turn out later to be Crohn's disease.

Once the diagnosis of Crohn's colitis is established—in contrast to the situation obtaining in ulcerative colitis—further biopsy is not very helpful in assessing disease severity or monitoring the response to therapy.

COMPLICATIONS

Toxic Megacolon

Toxic megacolon[29] describes a syndrome in which a severe attack of a colitis is associated with dilatation of part or the whole of the colon (Fig. 12). The dilatation affects the transverse and sigmoid colon more often than the retroperitoneal segments.

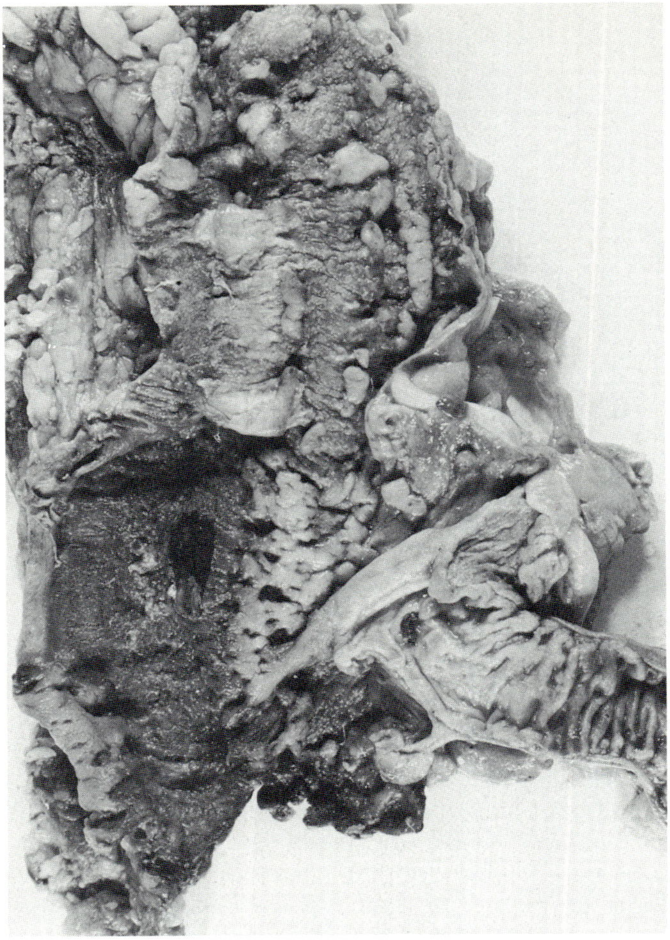

FIG. 12. Terminal ileum and ascending colon from a case of fulminant colitis with perforation. Extensive mucosal sloughing has exposed the main muscle coat of the cecum.

Although it is more common in ulcerative colitis, toxic megacolon also occurs in Crohn's colitis with sufficient frequency to prevent it from being a useful point of distinction. It is approximately twice as common in total Crohn's colitis than in segmental disease, and occurs in both recent-onset and long-standing disease.

At surgery,[30] the serosal surface of the affected colon is red and the vessels are congested. A fibrinous exudate with straw-colored, slightly turbid ascitic fluid is present in established cases. The adjacent omentum is edematous, thickened, and inflamed, and the bowel wall is so friable that it has been compared with wet blotting paper. Adhesions of omentum to the colon usually indicate the presence of a sealed colonic perforation. Free perforation increases the mortality rate to 80 percent compared with an overall mortality rate of 30 percent for toxic dilatation alone.

The colectomy specimen[17] shows intense transmural congestion, and there is usually extensive sloughing of the mucosa and submucosa, exposing a thin and edematous, often partly necrotic, muscularis propria. The lumen contains gas and a little seropurulent or sanguinous exudate. A variable intensity of the inflammatory process, with intermittent ulceration, is seen in both ulcerative and Crohn's colitis. Fissuring ulcers are typically seen in fulminant colitis but differ from those characteristic of Crohn's colitis in being more numerous, broad and V-shaped, and in having only a sparse lining of inflammatory cells (Fig. 13). Myocytolysis is a prominent feature of toxic megacolon and is associated with capillary engorgement (Fig. 14). It has been suggested that this deep ulceration and myocytolysis produce paralysis of the smooth muscle of the muscularis propria, resulting in colonic dilatation.

Transmural inflammation is common in fulminant colitis. The inflammation is nonaggregated, has a mixed cell population, and is always related to areas of deep ulceration. In fulminant colitis, the surviving islands of mucosa are usually surpris-

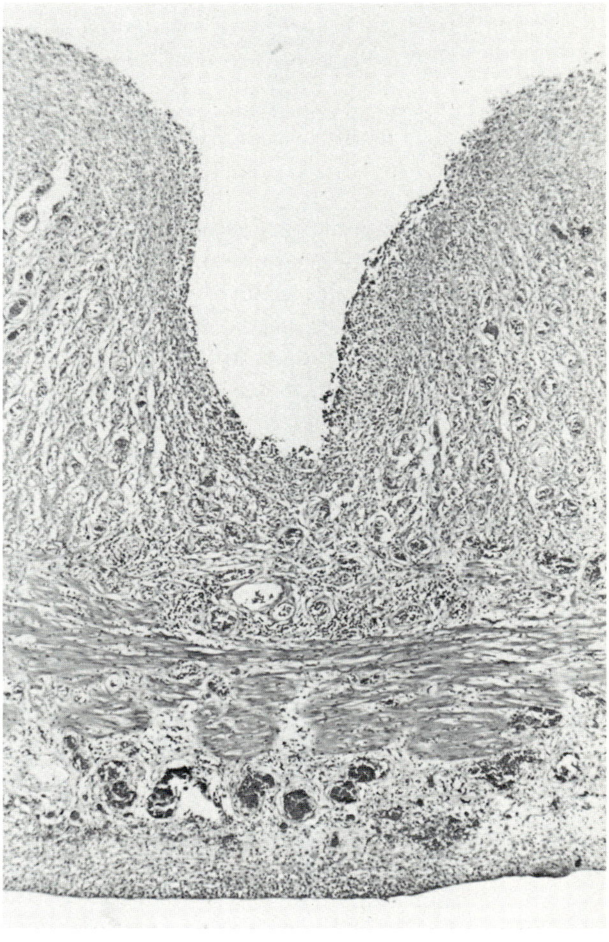

FIG. 13. Fulminant colitis with a broad V-shaped fissure. Vascular dilatation is marked but inflammatory cells are relatively few in number. ×63.

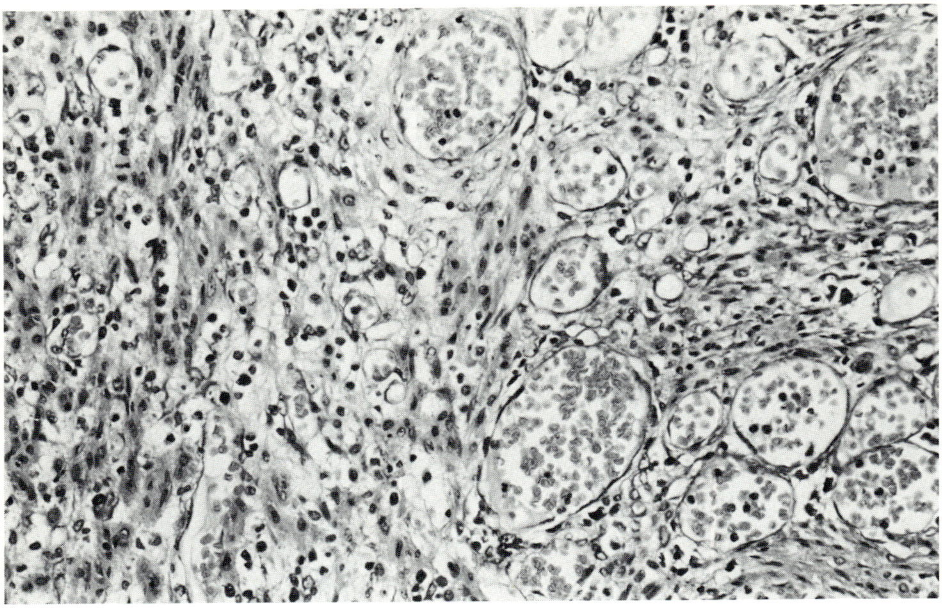

FIG. 14. Fulminant Crohn's colitis with myocytolysis of the muscularis propria. Degenerating muscle cells are present between dilated vessels. ×221.

ingly normal. Granulomas are said to be less frequent in fulminant Crohn's colitis.

Thus, the most discriminating diagnostic features of Crohn's colitis—segmental disease, granulomata, fissures, transmural inflammation, and focal mucosal inflammation with preservation of the goblet-cell population, are of less value in colectomy specimens removed for fulminant acute disease. Many of the 15 percent of cases of colitis in which it is not possible to distinguish Crohn's disease from ulcerative colitis are instances of fulminant disease (Fig. 15).

Anal Disease

Anal lesions[31-33] are a common complication of Crohn's disease of the large bowel, and may occur synchronously with the intestinal disease or antedate it by many years. The high incidence of anal involvement may be a reflection of the tendency of the disease to affect areas of gut where large amounts of lymphoid tissue are normally present.

When the anal disease occurs in continuity with rectal disease, it is usually ulcerative in type. Other anal lesions seen in Crohn's disease include fissures, fistulae, and edematous skin tags. The fissures are often multiple and are typically relatively painless and indolent. They represent longitudinal ulcers in the anal canal and characteristically have undermined edges.

Ulceration may involve the perineum and the groins, and may even extend onto the anterior abdominal wall. Anterior abdominal-wall ulceration may also occur around an ileostomy or colostomy site, usually in continuity with recurrent

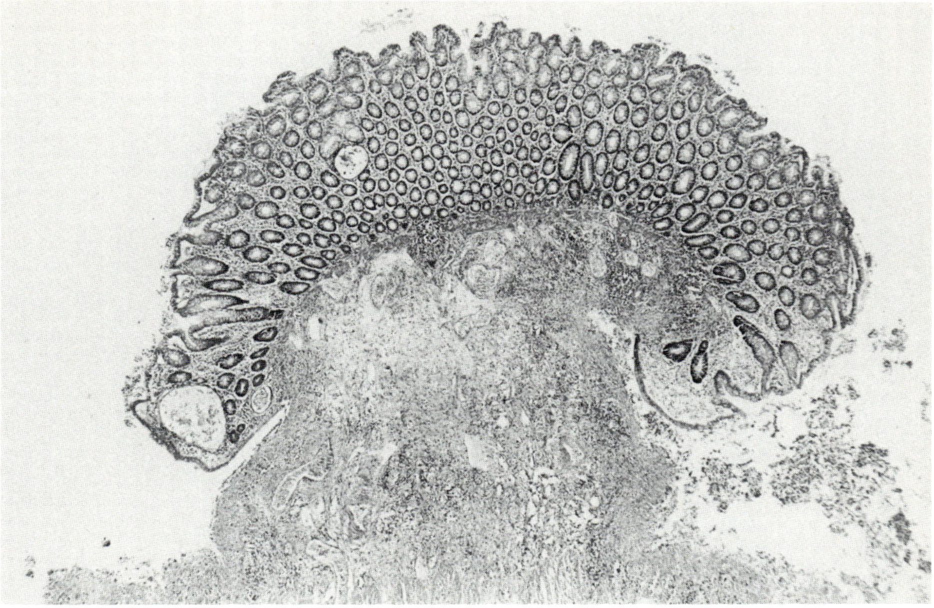

FIG. 15. Fulminant colitis with a mucosal pseudopolyp formed as a result of undermining ulceration. The mucosal architecture and goblet-cell population are well preserved, features which in other circumstances would suggest Crohn's colitis. ×25.

disease in the bowel. "Metastatic" granulomatous ulceration of the skin, completely remote from the gastrointestinal tract, is rare in Crohn's disease but has been reported to affect the penis, vulva, submammary skin fold, and skin folds of the lower abdomen.[34,35]

The only useful histologic feature in the diagnosis of anal Crohn's disease is the presence of noncaseating granulomata (Fig. 16). However, these are found in only two-thirds of cases. Even when granulomata are present, they may be sparse and in some cases are poorly-formed. They must be distinguished from foreign-body-type granulomata, which are commonly found in tissue from anal ulcers. Tuberculosis, syphilis, bilharziasis, and lymphogranuloma inguinale must be considered in the differential diagnosis.

Since anal Crohn's disease may antedate detectable intestinal disease, its significance can pass unrecognized unless a histologic diagnosis is possible at the time of surgery. Consequently, all tissue removed from anal lesions should be submitted for histologic examination.

Granulomatous Appendicitis

In colectomy specimens removed for known Crohn's disease, granulomata may be found in the appendix in about one-quarter of cases, and are more common when there is cecal disease.[36] The symptoms of Crohn's disease can mimic acute appendicitis, and the diagnosis of Crohn's disease is initially suggested on occasions by

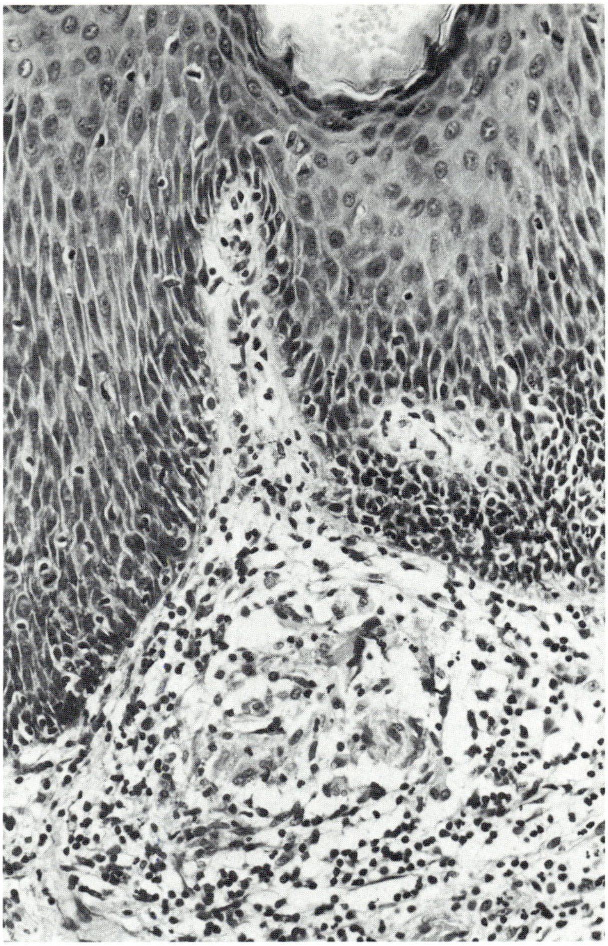

FIG. 16. Anal skin with a noncaseating granuloma in the upper dermis. ×350.

the presence of granulomata in the appendectomy specimen. Other causes of a granulomatous appendicitis, particularly infection by *Yersinia pseudotuberculosis* and *Mycobacterium tuberculosis,* must be excluded. Rarely, Crohn's disease is initially confined to the appendix and only later manifests itself elsewhere in the bowel.[37]

Carcinoma

The development of carcinomas of the small and large bowel in patients with Crohn's disease is being increasingly recognized, and this association may be significant.[38,39] The majority of carcinomas complicating Crohn's disease of the large bowel occur in the more frequently diseased proximal or transverse colon. However, the risk of malignancy complicating Crohn's disease is very low when compared with this risk in ulcerative colitis.

DIFFERENTIAL DIAGNOSIS

Ulcerative Colitis

Distinguishing Crohn's disease from ulcerative colitis is a major diagnostic problem, and may prove difficult in up to 25 percent of cases.[3,12,17,21] Consequently, the diagnosis should be based upon the combined clinical, radiologic, and pathologic features. Points of pathologic distinction have already been referred to in the text. In some cases, repeated evaluations over a period of time may be necessary before the correct diagnosis becomes apparent.[40] It is important to arrive at the correct diagnosis because the two diseases differ in their prognosis, response to therapy, complications, and surgical management.

Ischemic Colitis

Ischemic colitis[22,41,42] displays a wide spectrum of clinical and pathologic appearances commensurate with its varied etiology and complex pathogenesis. A colitis-like clinical picture, segmental involvement of the bowel, and stricture formation are three facets of ischemic colitis which may cause confusion with Crohn's disease.

The splenic flexure is particularly susceptible to ischemia, since it represents the watershed area between the superior and inferior mesenteric vessels. The descending colon and sigmoid colon are also commonly affected by ischemia. Rectal involvement, which was previously considered rare, is being increasingly recognized in ischemic colitis.

In the acute phase, ischemic colitis may mimic Crohn's disease radiologically and sigmoidoscopically. However, the histologic features are characteristic and quite different from those seen in inflammatory bowel disease. The mucosa shows hemorrhagic necrosis, and any inflammation present is secondary to necrosis or ulceration. The submucosa is typically congested and edematous with foci of hemorrhage, and these changes may occur in the presence of an intact mucosa. In the later, reparative phase, there is exuberant granulation tissue which contains hemosiderin-laden macrophages. Foreign-body-type giant cells may be seen.

Ischemic strictures are typically fusiform or tubular. Sacculations may be present and rarely occur other than in ischemic strictures and systemic sclerosis. There is usually patchy mucosal ulceration, and the submucosa is widened by characteristically dense, hyalinized, and poorly vascularized connective tissue which is relatively free of inflammation. A useful diagnostic feature is fibrosis affecting the middle third of the circular layer of the main muscle coat.

Late gastrointestinal complications in patients who have received pelvic irradiation are generally considered to be the result of obliterative vascular changes, and most frequently involve the rectosigmoid area. In addition to the histologic features common to all types of ischemic colitis, characteristic findings which indicate previous irradiation are brightly eosinophilic fibrinoid material at the base of ulcers, prominent hyalinization of blood vessels, and fibroblasts with bizarre nuclei and prominent nucleoli.

In some cases of ischemic colitis not associated with major vessel obstruction, microthrombi are apparent in the small vessels of the affected areas. Any part or the whole of the large bowel may be involved by the small-vessel type of ischemic colitis, and the prognosis is usually poor, with the diagnosis often being made at autopsy.

Pseudomembranous plaques are seen in cases of small-vessel ischemic colitis but are more typical of cases of antibiotic-associated pseudomembranous colitis[43,44] from which toxin-producing *Clostridium difficile* may be cultured. The adherent yellow-green plaques are scattered diffusely over the hyperemic mucosa. Microscopically, the plaques consist of an explosive, mushroom-like exudate of mucus, epithelial cells, fibrin, red cells, and polymorphs which overlie foci of mucosal ulceration and necrosis. The adjacent mucosa is surprisingly normal. This pseudomembranous-type of inflammatory response is not seen in uncomplicated Crohn's colitis.

Diverticular Disease

Although Crohn's disease localized to the sigmoid colon may be clinically misdiagnosed as diverticular disease, the pathologist usually has no difficulty in distinguishing between the two. The principal problem for the pathologist lies in recognizing when the two diseases coexist, particularly in elderly patients.[7,45] In cases of diverticular disease, the presence of coexistent Crohn's disease may be suspected if the diseased segment of colon is unusually long or if there is other evidence of Crohn's disease, such as rectal involvement or anal lesions. By contrast with Crohn's disease, the abscess cavities in diverticulitis are centered outside the bowel wall, and the associated inflammation tends to spare the main muscle coat and submucosa. In diverticular disease, lymphoid hyperplasia tends to be restricted to the neck regions of the diverticula, as is mucosal inflammation, and the giant cells and granulomata observed are of the foreign body-type.

Granulomatous Colitis

It is important to differentiate Crohn's disease of the large bowel from other causes of granulomatous colitis, especially tuberculosis.[46] The presence of fistulae, serosal tubercles, a thickened mesentery, superficial ulceration, and fissures are common to both Crohn's colitis and tuberculosis. However, strictures in tuberculosis are usually multiple and the ulceration tends to be circumferential and undermining, and not linear or serpiginous as is seen in Crohn's disease. In tuberculosis, unlike Crohn's disease, the submucosa is not widened, and there may be fibrosis of the main muscle coat. Compared with Crohn's disease, the granulomatous reaction in tuberculosis typically is more florid, with frequent confluence of granulomata, which may show fibrosis or hyalinization. In contrast to Crohn's disease, tuberculous granulomata may be found in the regional lymph nodes when they are not present in the bowel wall itself. A histologic distinction based upon the presence of caseous necrosis and acid-fast bacilli is possible in most cases.

Although sarcoidosis is occasionally associated with asymptomatic gastric granulomata,[47] involvement of the large bowel has not been convincingly demonstrated as far as we are aware.

Histoplasma capsulatum is a yeast that varies from 2 to 4 μ in diameter and stains positively with the periodic acid-Schiff (PAS), Gridley, and Gomori's methenamine silver methods. The colonic lesions found in histoplasmosis[48] typically consist of multiple ulcerated nodules measuring from a few millimeters to a few centimeters in diameter. Histologically, there is a dense lymphocytic and histiocytic infiltrate of the mucosa and submucosa, with numerous yeast forms within the histiocytes. Noncaseating granulomata may be seen in the mesenteric lymph nodes.

Necrotizing granulomata are seen in intestinal infections due to *Yersinia pseudotuberculosis,* a small, Gram-negative coccobacillus, and a histopathologically similar picture is produced by the closely related organism *Yersinia enterocolitica.*[49] Typically, there is an ileocecal lymphadenopathy which may be associated with ileal inflammation. The appendix and cecum are less commonly affected. Since the clinical diagnosis in such cases is often one of acute appendicitis, the appendix is frequently resected. Histologically, it typically shows submucosal lymphoid hyperplasia with prominent germinal centers, together with granulomata which are frequently sited within the germinal centers. By contrast with Crohn's disease, central coagulative necrosis of the granulomata is characteristic, and is associated with a polymorph infiltrate that leads to the formation of irregular or stellate microabscesses which can progress to mucosal ulceration. An identical necrotizing granulomatous reaction is seen in the paracortical zone of the draining mesenteric lymph nodes. The histologic suspicion of *Yersinia* infection can be confirmed serologically.

The Dysenteries

On a worldwide basis, dysenteries are the commonest cause of colitis. Since the treatment of the various enteric infections is so different from that of inflammatory bowel disease, it is important to exclude infectious agents by use of the appropriate bacteriologic tests.

Salmonellosis usually presents as an acute, self-limiting enteric infection which may clinically simulate chronic inflammatory bowel disease. Rectal biopsy[50] reveals the histologic pattern of an infectious colitis. This pattern may also be observed in bacillary dysentery, amoebiasis, gonorrheal proctitis, and *Campylobacter fetus* infection. In mild cases, edema and congestion alone are present. In more severely affected cases, the lamina propria contains increased numbers of inflammatory cells, which are mainly neutrophils. Crypt abscesses may be present, but the basic architecture of the mucosa and the goblet-cell population are generally well preserved. In chronic cases, the lamina propria may also contain increased numbers of mononuclear cells, including plasma cells, histiocytes, and lymphocytes. In those cases in which salmonellosis and inflammatory bowel disease coexist, it is generally not possible to identify the infective element from rectal biopsy examination alone.

Sporadic cases of bacillary dysentery[51] are more often confused with ulcerative colitis than with Crohn's disease. Sigmoidoscopically, the mucosa is congested, edematous, and granular. Serpiginous ulceration may be seen but is uncommon. Rectal biopsy reveals an infectious-colitis pattern. In severe cases, considerable architectural disturbance may occur and persist to leave an atrophic mucosa with a disturbed crypt pattern. It should be noted that some cases of ulcerative colitis present following an attack of dysentery.

Campylobacter fetus has been recognized recently as a cause of diarrheal illness in humans. Sigmoidoscopically, there may be diffuse mucosal inflammation resembling ulcerative colitis[52] or patchy involvement with ulceration mimicking Crohn's colitis.[53] Histologically, there is a mixed inflammatory infiltrate of the lamina propria, with crypt abscess formation, mucosal atrophy, and mucus depletion producing a picture which may be confused with ulcerative colitis rather than with Crohn's colitis.[52,53]

Amoebic dysentery[54] may simulate chronic inflammatory bowel disease clinically and sigmoidoscopically. Characteristically, isolated ulcers of 5 to 15 mm diameter are usually seen in the rectum or the cecum, but sometimes affect the entire bowel. The ulcers have undermined edges, and amoebae, which are distinctive in having ingested red blood corpuscles, are most commonly found in the tissue of the ulcer edge. The amoebic trophozoites may also be seen on the bowel surface or in fecal debris. A periodic acid-Schiff (PAS) stain is helpful in locating the organisms since they contain glycogen. Occasionally, the rectal mucosa has the appearance of a nonspecific colitis, both on sigmoidoscopy and on biopsy. Amoebae may not be found in the rectal biopsy of some of these cases.

An infrequent complication of amoebiasis is the development of an amoeboma[55] which presents as a localized mass, usually in the cecum or rectum. The macroscopic appearance of these inflammatory masses has given rise to the term ''amoebic granuloma.'' The histologic appearance of the amoeboma is that of a localized exaggeration of the inflammatory process seen in colonic amoebiasis, with secondary infection and much fibrosis.

Intestinal schistosomiasis[56,57] is usually caused by *Schistosoma mansoni* or *S. japonicum,* but may also be caused by *S. haematobium*. In the early stages, there is an acute proctitis. Chronic disease is associated with ulceration, stricture formation, mucosal polyposis, and the development of pericolic abscesses. Microscopically, the basic lesion is an inflammatory response to the presence of the ova in the tissues. The ova can be observed in the center of a granulomatous reaction, and numerous eosinophils are present in the surrounding tissues.

Actinomycosis[58] involving the ileocecal region, the appendix, or the rectum may be complicated by abscess or fistula formation similar to that in Crohn's disease. On histology, the Gram-positive colonies of filamentous fungi can be seen within abscess cavities.

Venereal Infections

Lymphogranuloma venereum[59,60] is a venereally transmitted chlamydial infection characterised by inguinal lymphadenopathy. A proctocolitis with mucosal ulceration may occur, and this is more common in females. The inflammation is usually confined to the rectum, but left-sided colitis and pancolitis are described. Rectal stricture is a characteristic late sequel, and lymphogranuloma venereum is said to be the most common cause of benign stricture of the rectum. Multiple localized areas of stricturing may also occur on the left side of the colon. The inflammatory reaction tends to be centered in the submucosa and, although intense, is nonspecific. The diagnosis of lymphogranuloma venereum may be confirmed by the Frei test and a complement fixation (CF) test.

Gonorrhea[61] may also present as an acute proctitis, but the symptoms and the sigmoidoscopic findings are suggestive of ulcerative proctitis rather than of Crohn's disease. The abnormalities are confined to the rectum, and biopsy reveals a severe, acute infectious type of colitis showing epithelial destruction, submucosal inflammation, and crypt abscess formation. Gram-negative intracellular diplococci are seen in only half the cases, but bacteriologic studies should lead to the correct diagnosis.

Primary syphilitic proctitis[62] is usually found in male homosexuals and may imitate Crohn's colitis, ulcerative colitis, or carcinoma. The diagnosis is usually made serologically as a result of clinical suspicion. The inflammation is confined to the rectum and anus, and proctoscopically the mucosa may be ulcerated or appear granular. Biopsy discloses an intense lymphohistiocytic infiltrate of the mucosa and submucosa, with a prominent perivascular distribution. Crypt abscesses and mucosal ulceration may be seen. Spirochetes may be identified using the Warthin-Starry silver stain. The spirochetes of syphilis must be distinguished from those seen in intestinal spirochetosis. In the latter, the spirochetes lie on the epithelial cell surface, parallel to the microvilli, creating a blue haze in sections stained with H&E. The associated intense inflammation of syphilis is absent, and the condition is probably of no significance.

Most important in the diagnosis of all of these venereal infections is a forthright enquiry regarding the sexual habits of patients presenting with an acute proctitis.[63]

Miscellaneous Disorders

A miscellany of other disorders may occasionally be confused clinically with Crohn's disease of the large bowel.

Solitary ulcer of the rectum[54] is characterized by an area of proctitis with or without mucosal ulceration, and is ascribed to prolapse, often due to excessive straining at stool. Rectal biopsy is distinctive, and the principal features are fibrosis of the lamina propria and bundles of smooth-muscle cells streaming up from the muscularis mucosae between the crypts. In about 10 percent of cases, cystic glands are displaced beneath the muscularis mucosae, giving a false impression of invasion. The histologic appearances of rectal prolapse are similar to those which occur in solitary ulcer of the rectum.

Rarely, rectal and colonic irritation from enemas can cause bloody diarrhea and leave an inflamed mucosa which has a histologic pattern similar to that of an infectious colitis[50] but is associated with severe mucin depletion.

Secondary amyloidosis may involve the colon and rectum, with resultant mucosal ulceration and hemorrhage. Even in the absence of gastrointestinal symptoms, rectal biopsy is a valuable means of diagnosing amyloidosis,[54] which may itself complicate Crohn's disease.[64]

Collagenous colitis[65] is a rare disorder characterized by a diarrheal illness. Histologically, there is a continuous, collagenous zone up to 50 μ thick beneath the surface epithelium of the large-bowel mucosa. This appearance has not been described in Crohn's disease but resembles that seen in the small bowel in collagenous sprue.

Crohn's disease and lymphoma of the small bowel may have similar clinical and radiologic features and pose a diagnostic dilemma. In such cases, rectal-biopsy evidence of an associated Crohn's colitis may prevent an unnecessary diagnostic laparotomy.[66]

REFERENCES

1. Fielding JF: The history of granulomatous colitis. Gastroenterology 64:510, 1973
2. Crohn BB, Ginzburg L, Oppenheimer GD: Regional ileitis: a pathologic and clinical entity. JAMA 99:1323, 1932
3. Price AB, Morson BC: Inflammatory bowel disease. The surgical pathology of Crohn's disease and ulcerative colitis. Hum Pathol 6:7, 1975
4. Goldberg HI, Caruthers SB, Nelson JA, Singleton JW: Radiographic findings of the National Co-operative Crohn's Disease Study. Gastroenterology 77:925, 1979
5. Editorial: Crohn's disease in the elderly: A diagnostic problem. Br Med J 2:188, 1973
6. Kyle J: An epidemiological study of Crohn's disease in northeast Scotland. Gastroenterology 61:826, 1971
7. Schmidt GT, Lennard-Jones JE, Morson BC, Young AC: Crohn's disease of the colon and its distinction from diverticulitis. Gut 9:7, 1968
8. Kyle J, Stark G: Fall in the incidence of Crohn's disease. Gut 21:340, 1980
9. Editorial: Crohn's disease of the large bowel. Br Med J 1:125, 1972
10. Allan R, Steinberg DM, Alexander-Williams J, Cooke WT: Crohn's disease involving the colon: An audit of clinical management. Gastroenterology 73:723, 1977
11. Lockhart-Mummery HE, Morson BC: Crohn's disease of the large intestine. Gut 5:493, 1964
12. Lockhart-Mummery HE, Morson BC: Crohn's disease (regional enteritis) of the large intestine and its distinction from ulcerative colitis. Gut 1:87, 1960
13. Mottet NF: Histopathologic spectrum of regional enteritis and ulcerative colitis. In Bennington JL (ed): Major Problems in Pathology, Vol 2. Philadelphia, W.B. Saunders, 1971
14. McGovern VJ, Goulston SJM: Crohn's disease of the colon. Gut 9:164, 1968
15. Morson BC: Histopathology 15–33. In Engel A, Larsson T (eds): Regional Enteritis (Crohn's Disease). Skandia International Symposia. Stockholm, Nordiska Bokhandelns Förlag, 1977
16. Rotterdam H, Korelitz BI, Sommers SC: Microgranulomas in grossly normal rectal mucosa in Crohn's disease. Am J Clin Pathol 67:550, 1977

17. Price AB: Overlap in the spectrum of non-specific inflammatory bowel disease - "Colitis indeterminate." J Clin Pathol 31:567, 1978
18. Knutson H, Lunderquist L, Lunderquist A: Vascular changes in Crohn's disease. Am J Roentgenol 103:380, 1968
19. Teja K, Crum CP, Friedman C: Giant cell arteritis and Crohn's disease. An unreported association. Gastroenterology 78:796, 1980
20. Owyang C, Miller LJ, Lie JT, Fleming CR: Takayasu's arteritis in Crohn's disease. Gastroenterology 76:825, 1979
21. Cook MG, Dixon MF: An analysis of the reliability of detection and diagnostic value of various pathological features in Crohn's disease and ulcerative colitis. Gut 14:255, 1973
22. Whitehead R: The pathology of ischaemia of the intestines. Pathol Annu 11:1, 1976
23. Crucioli V: Rectal biopsy in Crohn's disease. Rendic Gastroenterol 4:73, 1972
24. Dyer NH, Stansfeld AG, Dawson AM: The value of rectal biopsy in the diagnosis of Crohn's disease. Scand J Gastroenterol 5:491, 1970
25. Morson BC: Rectal biopsy in inflammatory bowel disease. N Engl J Med 287:1337, 1972
26. Goulston SJM, McGovern VJ: The value of rectal biopsies. Med J Aust 1:1234, 1972
27. McGovern VJ: Rectal biopsy in the differential diagnosis of colitis. Rendic Gastroenterol 4:94, 1972
28. Dawson IMP: The histochemistry of Crohn's disease. Clin Gastroenterol 1:309, 1972
29. Editorial: Toxic megacolon. Lancet 1:480, 1979
30. Fazio VW: Toxic megacolon in ulcerative colitis and Crohn's colitis. Clin Gastroenterol 9(2):389, 1980
31. Morson BC, Lockhart-Mummery HE: Anal lesions in Crohn's disease. Lancet 2:1122, 1959
32. Gray BK, Lockhart-Mummery HE, Morson BC: Crohn's disease of the anal region. Gut 6:515, 1965
33. Buchmann P, Alexander-Williams J: Classification of peri-anal Crohn's disease. Clin Gastroenterol 9(2):323, 1980
34. Mountain JC: Cutaneous ulceration in Crohn's disease. Gut 11:18, 1970
35. Devroede G, Schlaeder G, Sanchez G, Haddad H: Crohn's disease of the vulva. Am J Clin Pathol 63:348, 1975
36. Larsen E, Axelsson C, Johansen A: The pathology of the appendix in morbus Crohn and ulcerative colitis. Acta Pathol Microbiol Scand 212:161, 1970
37. Ewen SWB, Anderson J, Galloway JMD, et al.: Crohn's disease initially confined to the appendix. Gastroenterology 60:853, 1971
38. Weedon DD, Shorter RG, Ilstrup DM, et al.: Crohn's disease and cancer. N Engl J Med 289:1099, 1973
39. Lightdale CJ, Sternberg SS, Posner G, et al.: Carcinoma complicating Crohn's disease. Am J Med 59:262, 1975
40. Kirsner JB: Problems in the differentiation of ulcerative colitis and Crohn's disease of the colon: The need for repeated diagnostic evaluation. Gastroenterology 68:187, 1975
41. McGovern VJ, Goulston SJM: Ischaemic enterocolitis. Gut 6:213, 1965
42. Alschibaja T, Morson BC: Ischaemic bowel disease. J Clin Pathol (Suppl 11) 30:68, 1977
43. Medline A, Shin DH, Medline NM: Pseudomembranous colitis associated with antibiotics. Hum Pathol 7:693, 1976
44. Editorial: Antibiotic associated colitis - A bacterial disease. Br Med J 2:349, 1979
45. Editorial: Is malignant diverticulitis a true bill? Br Med J 1:1156, 1980
46. Tandon HD, Prakash A: Pathology of intestinal tuberculosis and its distinction from Crohn's disease. Gut 13:260, 1972
47. Present DH, Lindner AE, Janowitz HD: Granulomatous diseases of the gastrointestinal tract. Annu Rev Med 17:243, 1966
48. Shull HJ: Human histoplasmosis: a disease with protean manifestations often with digestive system involvement. Gastroenterology 25:582, 1953

49. El-Maraghi NRH, Mair NS: The histopathology of enteric infection with Yersinia pseudotuberculosis. Am J Clin Pathol 71:631, 1979
50. Day DW, Mandal BK, Morson BC: The rectal biopsy appearances in Salmonella colitis. Histopathology 2:117, 1978
51. Morson BC, Dawson IMP: Gastrointestinal Pathology, ed 2. Oxford, Blackwell, 1979
52. Lambert ME, Schofield PF, Ironside AG, Mandal BK: Campylobacter colitis. Br Med J 1:857, 1979
53. Loss RW, Mangla JC, Pereira M: Campylobacter colitis presenting as inflammatory bowel disease with segmental colonic ulcerations. Gastroenterology 79:138, 1980
54. Whitehead R: Mucosal Biopsy of the Gastrointestinal Tract. London, W.B. Saunders, 1973
55. Ruiz-Moreno F: Amoebic granuloma of the colon and rectum. Dis Colon Rectum 6:201, 1963
56. Diaz-Rivera RS, Ramos-Morales F, Sotomayor ZR, et al.: The pathogenesis of Manson's schistosomiasis. Ann Intern Med 47:1082, 1957
57. Binford CH, Connor DH (eds): Pathology of Tropical and Extraordinary Diseases. Washington, D.C., Armed Forces Institute of Pathology, 1976
58. Wilson E: Abdominal actinomycosis with special reference to the stomach. Br J Surg 48:266, 1961
59. Miles RP: Rectal lymphogranuloma venereum. Br J Surg 45:180, 1957
60. Levine JS, Smith PD, Brugge WR: Chronic proctitis in male homosexuals due to lymphogranuloma venereum. Gastroenterology 79:563, 1980
61. Zellner SR, Trudeau WL: Anorectal gonorrhea presenting as ulcerative proctitis. South Med J 66:706, 1973
62. Akdamar K, Martin RJ, Ichinose H: Syphilitic proctitis. Digest Dis 22:701, 1977
63. Babb RR: Evaluation of acute proctitis. JAMA 244:358, 1980
64. Fitchen JH: Amyloidosis and granulomatous ileo-colitis. Regression after surgical removal of the involved bowel. N Engl J Med 292:352, 1975
65. Nielsen VT, Vetner M, Harslof E: Collagenous colitis. Histopathology 4:83, 1980
66. Hyams JS, Goldman H, Katz AJ: Differentiating small bowel Crohn's disease from lymphoma. Role of rectal biopsy. Gastroenterology 79:340, 1980

THE KIDNEY IN LYMPHOPLASMACYTIC DISORDERS

GLORIA R. GALLO, HELEN D. FEINER, AND JOEL N. BUXBAUM

A wide spectrum of kidney diseases resulting from different pathogenetic mechanisms may occur in the course of lymphoplasmacytic neoplasms and dyscrasias. In those neoplasms characterized by proliferation of a single clone of B cells that secrete a homogeneous monoclonal (M) protein, the renal disease may be functionally related to the plasma concentration, physicochemical properties, or specific nephrotoxic effects of the M protein. In the same group of neoplasms renal dysfunction may be structurally related to the deposition of M proteins, their fragments, or immune complexes.[1] In the predominantly nonsecretory monoclonal B-cell disorders, and in the T-cell lymphoproliferative disorders, renal damage may occur secondary to the deposition of immune complexes or by unknown mechanisms.

Some of the glomerular functional abnormalities in lymphoplasmacytic disorders have not been associated with structural changes, and may be related to the actions of humoral permeability factors produced by the proliferating cells.[2] The application of immunohistologic and electron microscopic techniques to the study of the renal tissue in these disorders has allowed better detection of subtle changes in kidney morphology. One can specifically identify the deposits of M proteins in a way that is not possible with conventional light- or electron microscopy. The integration of observations that have been made using the new technology with the analysis of the well-defined clinical syndromes manifest in the lymphoplasmacytic disorders has led to the characterization of a group of renal diseases associated with the gammopathies.

The renal biopsy is often useful in distinguishing the different mechanisms of renal damage. In some patients who present with the nephrotic syndrome or azotemia as the first clinical manifestation of a lymphoplasmacytic disorder, the biopsy may provide the diagnostic clue that initiates the search for an overt or occult myeloma or dyscrasia.[3-6] Through the routine use of fluoresceinated antisera—each one monospecific for the individual heavy- or light-chain determinants of the Ig molecule—it is possible to determine if Ig deposits are present, if they are monoclonal and contain both heavy- and light-chain antigenic determinants of a single class (G, A, M, D or E, kappa, or lambda), if they are comprised solely of monoclonal heavy or light chains, or if they are polyclonal and contain light-chain determinants of both the kappa and lambda classes. The staining patterns with fluoresceinated antisera thus offer useful clues concerning the pathogenesis of the renal disease in a lymphoplasmacytic disorder by providing evidence for the deposition of material synthesized by a single plasma-cell clone or the polyclonal deposition more typical of immune-complex disease.[5] The application of now standard immunochemical techniques, plus more analytically sensitive biosynthetic studies, allows the comparison between those molecules synthesized and those deposited.

We will briefly survey the spectrum of renal lesions that has been observed in association with the lymphoplasmacytic disorders. The major part of the discussion will focus on those diseases that result from the deposition of the M protein or its subunits in the kidney.

It is evident from the foregoing discussion that renal diseases associated with lymphoplasmacytic disorders may be divided into several broad categories.

1. Dysfunctions associated with neoplastic cellular infiltration which either disrupts or compresses the renal parenchyma.
2. Functional disorders in which no anatomic lesion of the renal parenchyma has yet been detected.
3. Monoclonal deposition states in which a single-component protein, its subunits, or fragments thereof are deposited in renal tissue and produce dysfunction with: (1) fibril formation (amyloidosis); (2) clustered, granular, nonfibrillar deposits; or (3) fibrillar-crystalline deposits frequently associated with cryoprecipitation properties.
4. Polyclonal deposition states in which immune-complexes are deposited and cause renal dysfunction with: (1) granular deposits; or (2) with fibrillar-crystalline deposits frequently associated with cryoprecipitation properties.

There are substantial data available concerning mechanism number 1, and the reader is referred to other reviews.[7-9]

Knowledge concerning the purely functional abnormalities is somewhat limited. It has been known for many years that tubular dysfunction may be associated with either polyclonal or monoclonal hyperglobulinemic states, not all of which exhibit excess monoclonal light-chain excretion.[10] The characteristic functional abnormality in these hyperglobulinemic states appears to be a defect in acidification (vide infra).

The deposition diseases, which will be discussed at length, can be subdivided into those characterized by a monoclonal Ig deposit, and those characterized by polyclonal Ig deposits of immune complexes. The monoclonal diseases can be classified according to the nature of the protein, i.e., whether it contains a single-component Ig with antigenic determinants of both heavy and light chains, or only a single light chain, and their respective classes. These diseases can also be classified by the ultrastructural appearance of the deposits, i.e., whether they are fibrillar or nonfibrillar. The AL type of amyloid, which is composed of light chains or their variable (V)-region fragments, represents the major form of renal fibrillar deposition associated with lymphoplasmacytic disease. Immune-complex renal disease has been described accompanying a large number of malignant tumors, including lymphoplasmacytic neoplasms.[11]

DISORDERS OF IMMUNOGLOBULIN SYNTHESIS AND RENAL DISEASE

The morphologic spectrum of B-cell dyscrasias associated with overt or cryptogenic monoclonal gammopathy includes benign, malignant, and transitional forms of plasma-cell dyscrasias (multiple myeloma, extraosseous plasmacytomas, plasma-cell leukemia, and amyloidosis), lymphoplasmacytic dyscrasias (Waldenström's macroglobulinemia, heavy-chain diseases, lymphocytic lymphoma, chronic lymphocytic leukemia), and monoclonal gammopathies of undetermined significance.[12,13] These disorders, all of which may be associated with kidney disease, are currently classified on the basis of their clinical features as well as the functional and morphological properties of the lymphoplasmacytic cells. It must be noted, however, that there is overlap among some of the B-cell disorders and that there is no absolute correlation between the cell type, the M protein produced, and the clinical manifestations. Thus, myeloma and the various related syndromes, such as heavy-chain and light-chain diseases and macroglobulinemia, are identified by the precise definition of the secretory products.

The biosynthetic processes of normal plasma cells are approximately balanced, i.e., the cells synthesize and secrete intact Ig (H_2L_2) and a small excess of light chains of a single class.[14,15] The disorders of Ig synthesis and the associated clinical syndromes have been previously reviewed.[12,13] The synthesis and secretion of intact (H_2L_2) molecules and excess light chains occur in most patients with myeloma.[16] Monoclonal IgM's with or without excess light chains are produced in Waldenström's macroglobulinemia and occasionally in chronic lymphocytic leukemia, lymphocytic lymphoma, and histiocytic lymphoma.[13] The production of monoclonal proteins of other classes has also been described in the latter four disorders.[13]

In about 25 percent of patients with myeloma, who have what is termed "light-chain disease,"[17,18] and in rare patients with monoclonal gammopathies of undetermined significance,[19] only kappa or lambda light chains are synthesized. Portions of heavy chains corresponding to the Fc fragments of IgG, IgA, and IgM are synthesized and secreted in the disorders known as heavy-chain diseases.[20] More recently, other qualitative disorders of Ig synthesis have been defined, in which abnormal heavy and light chains are synthesized.[21,22] In the last group of syndromes, the determination of the precise defect requires the study of cellular Ig biosynthesis, since the abnormal proteins may be rapidly degraded or deposited in the tissues. Some of the latter patients appear to characterize a subset of individuals in whom a proliferative disorder of plasma cells is identified but in whom no monoclonal serum or urinary protein can be found—patients with the so-called nonsecretory myelomas.[23,24] However, while such nonsecretory myelomas clearly exist, the cells from many of these patients, when they have been analyzed by either immunofluorescence or biosynthetic labeling techniques, or both, have been found to synthesize and secrete small amounts of normal and apparently abnormal polypeptides even though the products are not detected in the patient's serum or urine. Hence, these myelomas are not truly nonsecretory.[25-27]

The M protein may have purely functional effects on the kidney. These effects may be related to the high Ig concentration in the serum, the intrinsic properties of the M proteins that affect polymerization and aggregation, or protein–protein interactions that may increase plasma viscosity[28] and thereby reduce the glomerular filtration rate (GFR). These elements may be found in patients with polyclonal hyperglobulinemia not associated with malignancy[10] as well as in patients with Waldenström's macroglobulinemia and those with myeloma.[13] The nephrotoxic effects of light chains on the renal tubular epithelium are believed to give rise to the proximal and/or distal tubular dysfunction in patients with light-chain proteinuria.[29-31] These clinical observations are supported by in vitro studies that have shown defects in the tubular transport mechanisms in kidney slices incubated with Bence Jones proteins.[32] It is not yet clear whether in vivo functional tubular disorders are associated with deposits of light chains in tubular basement membranes, or whether dysfunction can occur in the absence of deposits. The absence of light-chain deposits in the kidney biopsy, examined by immunofluorescence, of one patient with tubular dysfunction suggests that the functional abnormalities may occur without in vivo tissue deposition.[30]

Little is known concerning the mechanisms responsible for the tissue deposition of monoclonal proteins. Such deposition may be due to the intrinsic properties of the M protein, such as the altered solubility or cryoprecipitability that is sometimes found in patients with Waldenström's macroglobulinemia, myeloma, monoclonal gammopathy of undetermined significance, lymphoma, and chronic lymphocytic leukemia. The glomerular deposits that occur in some patients with cryoglobulinemia often have a crystalline ultrastructure.[33-40] It is likely that pH, tissue osmolality, and ionic concentration affect the protein deposition; however, the details of the process have not been elucidated. In other instances, specific antibody activity of the M proteins for other Igs or other unknown antigens may produce circulating immune complexes that are deposited in the glomeruli, as in other forms of immune-complex disease.[34,40-42] Thus, renal deposits are believed to occur by two mechanisms: (1) the direct deposition of the M protein; or (2) the deposition of immune complexes containing a monoclonal antibody.

RENAL DISEASE IN MULTIPLE MYELOMA AND MONOCLONAL GAMMOPATHY OF UNDETERMINED SIGNIFICANCE (PLASMA CELL DYSCRASIAS)

Renal damage in myeloma was recognized in the early 1900s.[43] The histologic finding of tubular protein casts surrounded by syncytial giant cells, with tubular atrophy and nephrocalcinosis, has been called "myeloma kidney" or "myeloma nephrosis.''[44] The renal failure that occurs in about half of the patients with myeloma correlates best with the severity of the tubular atrophy and degeneration, and the presence and magnitude of the Bence Jones proteinuria.[31] While obstruction of the tubules by Bence Jones casts has been thought to be a cause of renal failure in myeloma, recent observations suggest that cast formation is a late event.[31] However, virtually all clinical studies have found that the occurrence of renal insufficiency in myeloma is best correlated with excess light-chain production. Hypercalcemia may be a major contributory factor[45] to the acute renal failure of myeloma.

Other patterns of renal involvement in myeloma have long been recognized,[3] so that the term ''myeloma kidney,'' as often used to designate the lesion of tubulointerstitial disease and Bence Jones cast nephropathy, requires further qualification for precise use. Renal tubular transport defects are observed in patients with light-chain proteinuria, usually in association with overt or occult myeloma. Renal amyloidosis complicates from 6 to 15 percent of myeloma[46] and has been the subject of previous reviews.[47,48]

Primary amyloid in the absence of overt myeloma is now considered to be a monoclonal plasma-cell dyscrasia, because most patients with primary amyloid can be demonstrated to have free monoclonal light chains in their serum and/or urine.[49] Furthermore, it has been demonstrated in at least one patient that the primary amino acid sequence of the deposited amyloid protein corresponds to that of the light chain isolated from the serum or urine.[50,51]

While amyloid deposition in the glomeruli was recognized as one of the types of renal involvement in myeloma, other glomerular disease was not emphasized until the late 1950s and in 1960, when mesangial nodules lacking the staining characteristics of amyloid were described in patients with myeloma.[3,52] A review of the reported cases[5] and data from more recent series indicate that, of the nonamyloidotic glomerular diseases, lobular or nodular glomerulopathy has been the most frequently reported condition in albuminuric patients with myeloma or lymphoplasmacytic dycrasias.[3-5,27,33,35,52-71] The nature of the nodular glomerulopathy only became apparent following the demonstration of monoclonal light-chain antigenic determinants in the glomeruli and tubular basement membranes in two patients with similar nodular lesions, one of whom had myeloma.[59] An identical nonamyloidotic nodular glomerulopathy (Fig. 1a), with deposits containing monoclonal kappa light-chain determinants (Fig. 1b), was demonstrated in another patient without myeloma or light chains in the serum or urine, in whom biosynthetic studies of bone marrow cells demonstrated excess kappa light-chain synthesis.[4,5] The evidence suggested that the observed glomerulopathy resulted from the deposition of the monoclonal kappa light chains produced by the bone marrow cells, and provided a conceptual link between the renal disease of overt myeloma and that in occult dyscrasias.

In most of the reported cases of glomerulopathy associated with the dyscrasias which have been studied by immunofluorescence, monoclonal kappa light-chain determinants have been detected in both the glomeruli and tubular basement membranes[4,5,59,61,62,67-72]. However, there are exceptions. In one patient with myeloma who had electron-dense deposits in the glomeruli and tubular basement membranes,

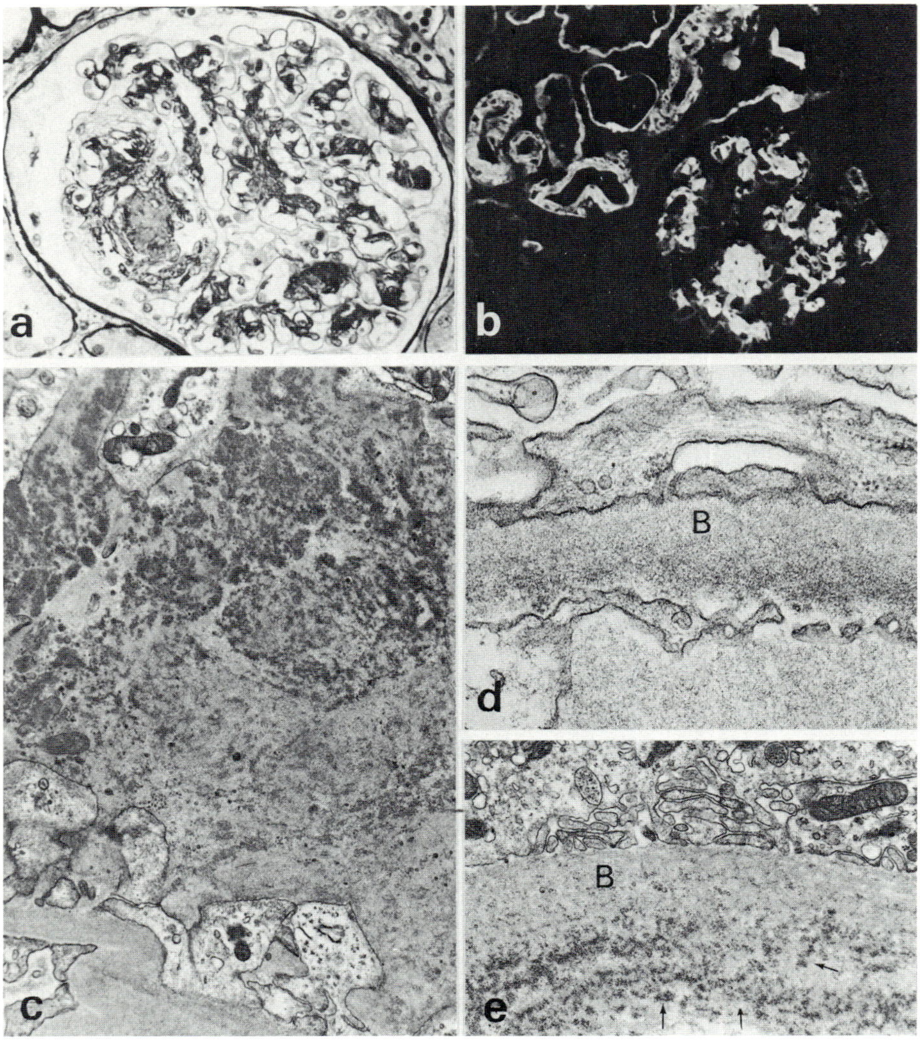

FIG. 1. Renal biopsy from a 56-year-old male without myeloma or M protein in the serum or urine. Biosynthetic studies of the patient's bone marrow cells demonstrated an excess production of kappa light chains.[5] **a.** A light-micrograph of a glomerulus demonstrates mesangial widening and a mesangial nodule containing non-silver-staining amorphous deposits. Periodic acid silver-methenamine, counterstained with H&E. ×409. **b.** A frozen section of the kidney incubated with fluorescein-conjugated goat anti-human kappa antiserum (light-chain specific) is shown. The glomerulus in the lower right corner shows nodular mesangial deposits. There is also diffuse staining of tubular basement membranes and walls of arterioles. No other Ig's nor C_3 were detected. ×219. **c–f.** Electron micrographs of the kidney biopsy double-stained with uranyl acetate and lead citrate are shown. **c.** A portion of a mesangial nodule contains clusters of dense deposits in the matrix. ×7,125. **d.** The glomerular basement membrane (B) shows a layer of dense material within the lamina rara interna. ×24,320. **e.** Electron-dense deposits are present in clusters (arrows) in the outer aspect of the tubular basement membrane (B) and adjacent interstitium. ×7,125. (Continued)

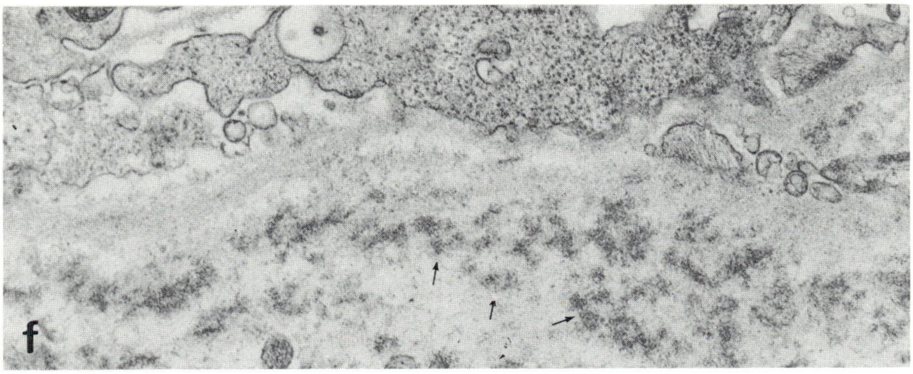

FIG. 1. (cont.) f. Clustered deposits (arrows) are demonstrated in a capillary basement membrane and adjacent tissue. ×24,320. (Reproduced with permission from Gallo et al.: Am J Pathol 99:621, 1980.)

no light-chain determinants were detected by immunofluorescence.[65] This observation suggests either that the deposits were not kappa light chains or that the antigenic determinants of the light chains deposited in situ were not recognized by the antisera used, most of which detect constant (C)-region determinants. Hence, V-region-fragment deposits would not be detectable with C-region antisera. In other cases, deposits were demonstrated in the tubular basement membranes but not in the glomeruli,[22,63,68,71,73] suggesting that in situ alterations could render the deposits in some sites unrecognizable or that the deposits in the tubular basement membranes differed from those in the glomeruli.

The electron-dense deposits seen ultrastructurally in the kidney generally correspond to the sites of specific immunofluorescence. They have a rather characteristic granular appearance that clearly differs from that of the fibrils of amyloid. Deposits present in the lamina rara interna and the mesangial matrix of the glomeruli, and in the tubular basement membrane and the vessel walls, are dense and often distributed in small clusters (Fig. 1c, d, e, and f). When these ultrastructural features are found in renal biopsies obtained from undiagnosed patients with proteinuria, it should suggest the possibility of a monoclonal light-chain deposition disease, and appropriate immunohistologic analysis should be performed.

It is now apparent that immunohistologic variants of glomerular disease other than kappa light-chain nodular glomerulopathy occur in association with the disorders of Ig synthesis. Intra- and extracapillary cell proliferation in the glomeruli, associated with clustered electron-dense deposits in the glomerular and tubular basement membranes and in the mesangium, has been observed in a patient with myeloma who had kappa light-chain determinants in the tubular basement membranes but not in the glomeruli.[73] Segmental proliferation, mild mesangial widening, or minimal changes, all associated with granular dense deposits containing kappa light-chain determinants as demonstrated by electron microscopy and immunofluorescence, have been observed in patients with myeloma or other plasmacytic dyscrasias.[68-72] We have seen biopsies from two patients with minimal

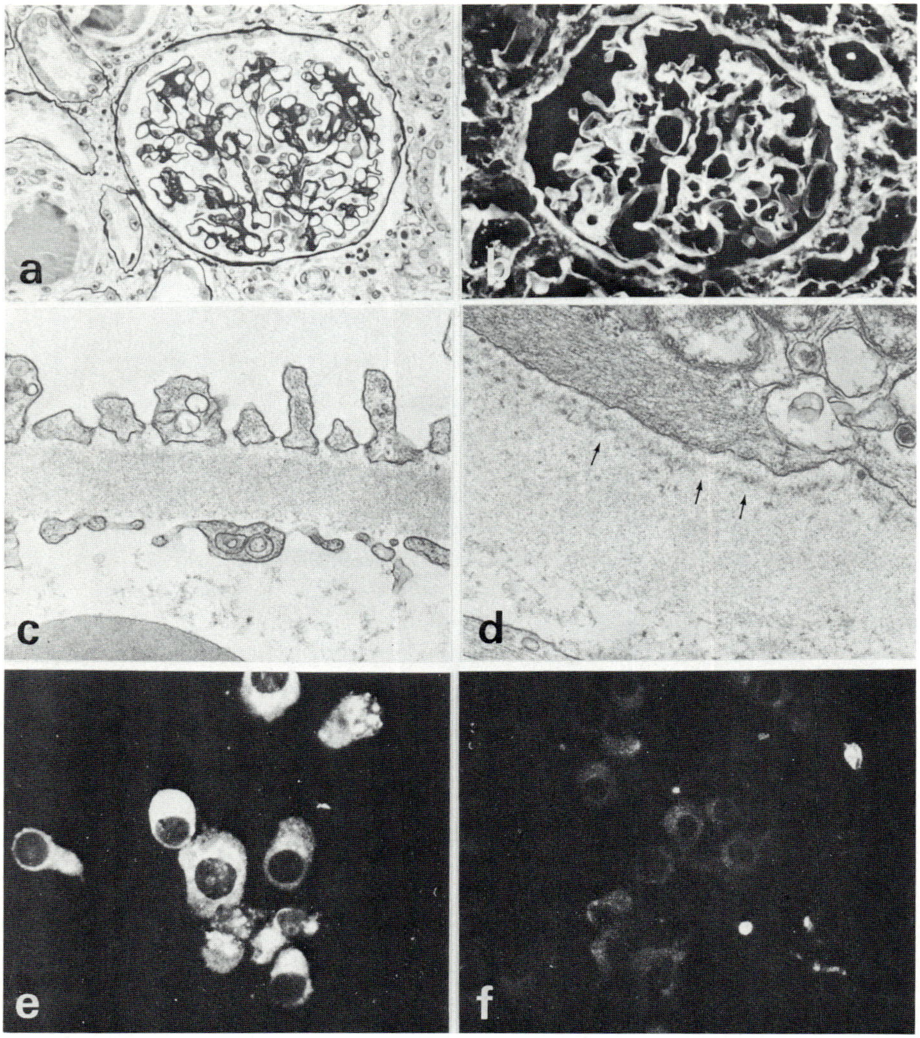

FIG. 2. Renal biopsy and bone marrow smear from a 59-year-old male with myeloma. The patient had monoclonal IgG-kappa in his serum and kappa light chains in the urine. **a.** A light-micrograph of a glomerulus demonstrates only mild mesangial widening. No mesangial nodules were present in any glomeruli. Tubules with casts are seen on the left side of the glomerulus. Periodic acid silver-methenamine, H&E. ×352. **b.** A frozen section of the kidney incubated with fluorescein-conjugated anti-human kappa antiserum (light-chain specific) demonstrates outlining of glomerular, capsular, and tubular basement membranes. No other Ig's were found. ×380. **c, d.** Electron micrographs of glomerular and tubular basement membranes double-stained with uranyl acetate and lead citrate are shown. No electron-dense deposits are visible in the glomerular basement membrane (**c**), but are demonstrated (arrows) in the tubular basement membrane (**d**). **c.** ×23,750; **d.** ×23,750. **e,f.** Bone marrow smears from the same patient, stained with fluoresceinated monospecific anti-kappa light chain (**e**) and lambda light chain (**f**) antisera are shown. The cytoplasm of the plasma cells stains brightly for kappa, but not for lambda light chains. Gamma heavy-chain determinants were not detected in the cells of smears double-stained with rhodaminated anti-gamma (heavy-chain specific) and fluoresceinated anti-kappa light-chain antisera. **e.** ×1,330; **f.** ×665.

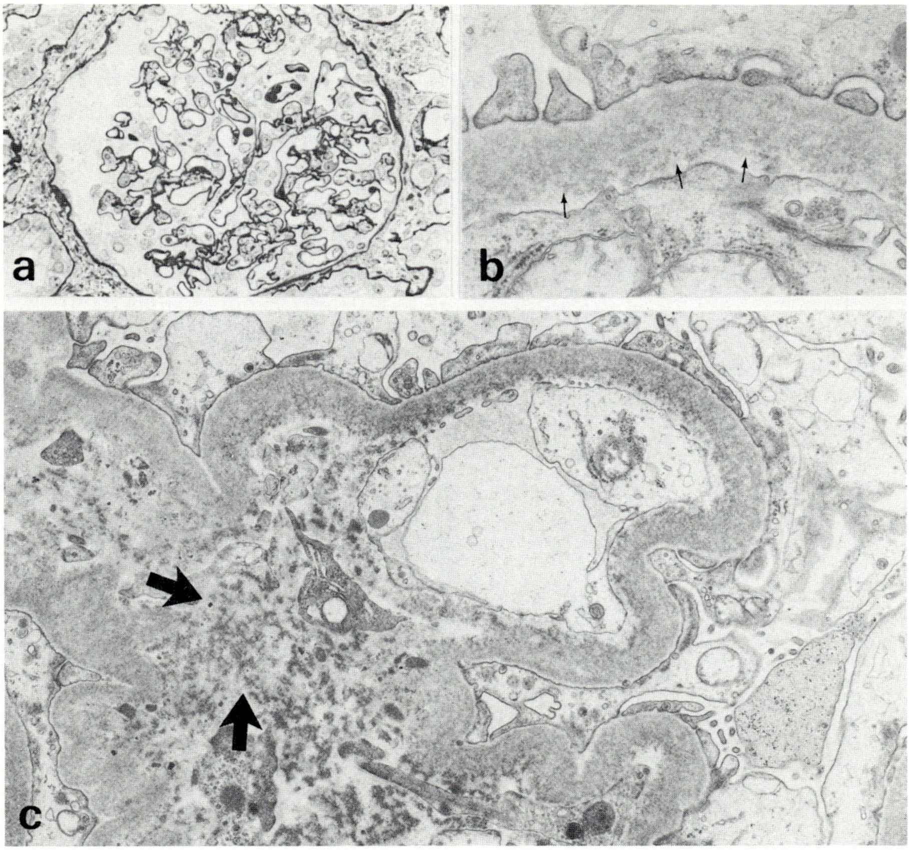

FIG. 3. This is a renal biopsy from a 63-year-old male with myeloma and oliguric renal failure. There were Bence Jones casts with giant-cell reactions in the tubules (not shown). **a.** A light-micrograph of the thick section of Epon-embedded tissue shows a glomerulus in which no detectable abnormalities are seen. Periodic acid silver-methenamine, H&E. ×380. **b, c.** Electron micrographs of the same glomerulus depict clustered deposits (arrows) in the lamina rara interna (**b**) and in the mesangium (**c**) (arrows). **b.** ×19,000; **c.** ×11,400.

changes seen upon light microscopy (Figs. 2a and 3a) that exhibited kappa light-chain deposits in the glomeruli and tubular basement membranes by immunofluorescence microscopy. (Fig. 2b). Only one of these had detectable corresponding electron-dense deposits in the glomerular basement membrane and mesangial matrix (Fig. 3b, c); the other had no visible deposits in either the glomerular basement membrane (Fig. 2c) or mesangial matrix, but deposits were demonstrated in the tubular basement membranes (Fig. 2d). Thus, light-chain deposits, although detected by immunofluorescence, may not always be visualized as ultrastructurally dense. Serial histologic examinations in some patients with minimal or mild mesangial light microscopic changes on initial observation have shown progression to a lobular or nodular glomerulopathy.[59,68,69] These findings suggest that the different morphologic forms of glomerular lesions may represent stages in the evolution of disease.

Deposits of monoclonal Ig's other than solely kappa light-chain type also have been observed in the kidney in some glomerulopathies with light microscopic minimal changes or with mesangial nodules. Monoclonal lambda light-chain determinants with corresponding ultrastructural deposits have been detected in the glomeruli and in tubular basement membranes in a few cases.[6,70,71] In a single case with dense granular ultrastructural deposits, staining for IgG of the lambda type was found, but the specificity of the reagents used was not given.[66] We have observed mild mesangial widening and focal segmental proliferation without nodules in a biopsy from one patient (Fig. 4a), in whose glomerular and tubular basement membranes only antigenic determinants of monoclonal lambda light chain were detected by immunofluorescence (Fig. 4b). Only a few small, electron-dense deposits were visualized in the glomerular basement membrane (Fig. 4c), and none were seen in tubular basement membranes. Other nodular glomerulopathies have

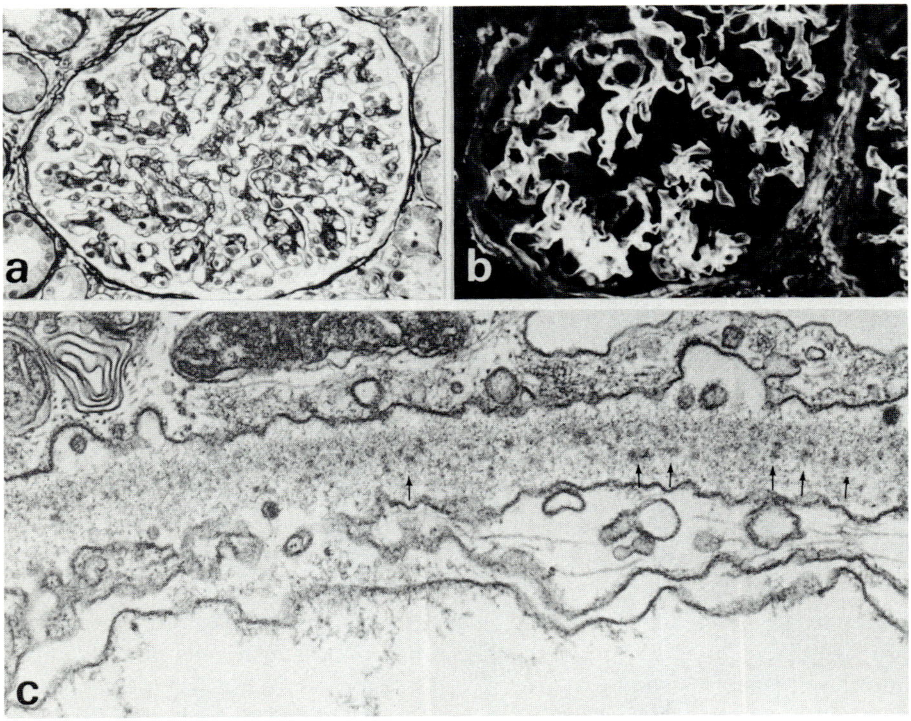

FIG. 4. Renal biopsy from a 75-year-old woman without myeloma. Free lambda light chains were found in the serum and urine. Biosynthesis studies of the bone marrow cells demonstrated excess production of normal light chains as well as short polypeptides. **a.** A light-micrograph of a glomerulus shows only mild mesangial widening. No mesangial nodules were present in any of the glomeruli. Periodic acid silver-methenamine, H&E. ×380. **b.** A frozen section of kidney incubated with fluoresceinated anti-human lambda antiserum (light-chain specific) demonstrates localization in the glomerular basement membrane. There was also diffuse staining of the tubular basement membranes (not shown). ×380. **c.** An electron micrograph of the glomerular basement membrane double-stained with uranyl acetate and lead citrate demonstrates scattered electron-dense material in the lamina densa (arrows). ×19,000.

been associated with monoclonal deposits containing both alpha heavy- and kappa light-chain determinants.[21] We have observed one nodular glomerulopathy with deposits (Fig. 5a) in which both gamma heavy- and lambda light-chain determinants (Fig. 5b) were the only ones found. Only equivocal corresponding electron-dense deposits were detectable ultrastructurally (Fig. 5c).

Thus, it is clear that similar lesions can occur in overt myeloma, occult myeloma presenting with a glomerulopathy, and monoclonal gammopathies of undetermined significance. A variety of immunopathologic features can be seen, ranging from minimal glomerular changes to nodular glomerulopathy associated with the deposition of either a monoclonal single-component heavy and light chain, its subunit light chain, or fragments thereof. The most characteristic and frequent immunohistologic lesion found thus far has been a nodular glomerulopathy with deposits containing only monoclonal kappa light-chain antigenic determinants. In other instances, glomeruli appeared normal by light- and sometimes by electron microscopy, but have shown deposits of monoclonal light chains upon immunofluorescence microscopy. Therefore, immunofluorescence examination was essential for detection of the lesion, particularly in those patients who had no other evidence of a lymphoplasmacytic disease nor a monoclonal gammopathy by serum or urine electrophoresis (Table 1). We believe that antisera, each monospecific for heavy-or light-chain determinants, should be used routinely to examine all renal biopsies. This permits the detection of unsuspected disease having minimal glomerular light microscopic changes. The specific nature of the glomerular disease can only be completely characterized by immunologic methods.

The immunofluorescence analysis of renal biopsy specimens obtained from patients with lymphoplasmacytic disease is straightforward, assuming that the appropriate monospecific antisera are available. However, knowledge concerning the mechanisms responsible for the Ig deposition is far from complete. It is evident from several of the well-studied cases that the phenomenon of deposition was not merely a reflection of mass action, since in many of the cases it was difficult to find any monoclonal light-chain in either serum or concentrated urine. The lack of substantial amounts of serum or urine light chains also suggested that the light chains in question must have had a predisposition for tissue deposition, either because they had a specific affinity for tissue sites or because they tended to become insoluble under the physiologic conditions present in certain tissues, most notably the kidney. Hence, the newly synthesized chains rapidly disappeared from the serum and did not appear in the urine. In the past when large numbers of plasma cells have been found in the marrow of such patients, it is likely that they would have been given the diagnosis of nonsecretory myeloma.[74]

Biosynthetic experiments designed to examine the nature of the proteins secreted and ultimately deposited resulted in a series of observations which indicated that in at least four patients the deposited light chains were abnormal in size, with two being larger and two smaller than normal.[21,22] In addition, some of the molecules were assembled into higher-molecular-weight polymers at the time of synthesis. The investigators also noted molecules, precipitable with anti-light chain antisera, that had molecular weights in the 12,000- to 14,000-dalton range. In one of the patients, a short alpha heavy-chain was also synthesized and detected in the

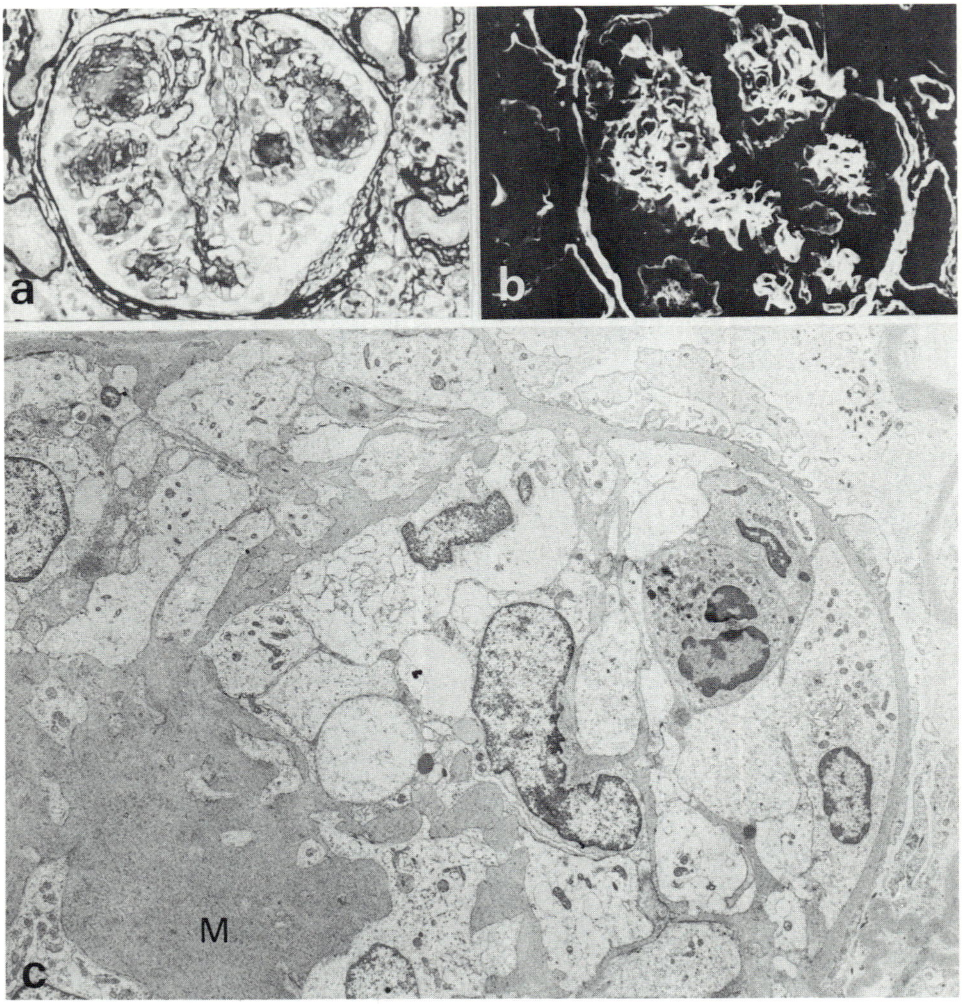

FIG. 5. Renal biopsy from a 75-year-old female with increased plasma cells in the bone marrow. An IgG-lambda M protein was found in the serum and lambda light chains in the urine. **a.** The glomerulus shown in the light-micrograph displays prominent mesangial nodules which contained eosinophilic, amorphous deposits. Periodic acid silver-methenamine, H&E. ×400. **b.** A frozen section double-stained with fluorescein-conjugated anti-lambda and rhodamine-conjugated anti-gamma heavy chain antisera (each monospecific) demonstrated both of these determinants in the same locations in the same section. There is staining within mesangial nodules and glomerular, capsular, and tubular basement membranes (lambda light chain shown). Kappa light-chain and other heavy-chain determinants were not detected. ×400. **c.** In the electron micrograph, a portion of a glomerular lobule demonstrates a mesangial nodule (M) in the lower left corner. Only equivocal electron-dense deposits could be demonstrated in the mesangium despite the evident bright staining by immunofluorescence. ×3,850.

renal deposits. These results led the investigators to hypothesize that structural abnormalities in the Ig polypeptides predisposed these molecules to tissue deposition.

Our own biosynthetic studies of three patients with monoclonal renal light-chain deposition (Table 1) indicated that normal-sized light chains were synthesized in all. In one of the patients, only normal light chains were found.[5] In the other two, normal-sized light chains were the major species synthesized, but other, shorter polypeptides, bearing light-chain antigenic determinants, were also detected (Buxbaum, unpublished observations). In one of the two patients an abnormal, small gamma heavy-chain was also produced, and the renal biopsy showed gamma heavy-chain and monoclonal lambda light-chain deposition (Fig. 5b).

These studies tend to support the hypothesis that abnormal Ig chains are predisposed to tissue deposition, but also amply document that chains that are normal in size at the time of their synthesis may be susceptible to renal parenchymal deposition. It should be noted that in cases of heavy-chain disease in which the abnormal chains have been studied in detail, clinical renal disease suggesting a deposition state has not been described. Hence, the type of polypeptide abnormality may be crucial to tissue deposition.

The known data clearly call for some comparison of the deposition seen in AL amyloid renal disease[75] with that seen in nonamyloidotic light-chain glomerulopathy. Both are characterized by excess light-chain synthesis and deposition. It has been well documented that the amyloid deposits consist of intact light chains or V-region fragments.[48] Additionally, analyses of tissue amyloid and urinary light chains from the same patient have shown that they share the same amino acid sequence.[50,51] Less is known concerning the chemical nature of the deposits of nonamyloidotic light-chain nephropathy, since the only characterization to date has been the limited antigenic analysis carried out by immunofluorescence microscopy on tissues in this condition. Hence, while it is clear that in AL amyloid renal disease and nonamyloidotic light-chain glomerulopathy, the synthetic products and the deposits share antigenic determinants, it has not yet been determined if the cell products and the deposited molecules are identical or if the primary synthetic product must undergo processing prior to deposition. From the available synthetic studies in both conditions, it appears that polymerization may occur but does not appear to be obligatory in the genesis of the deposits.

At present, it is our view that similar processes are involved in the synthesis and deposition of both the fibrillar deposits of the AL type of amyloid and the granular deposits of nonamyloidotic light-chain glomerulopathy. In the case of the AL proteins, their primary amino acid sequence leads them to fold into beta-pleated sheets, to become insoluble, and to form fibrils that have the characteristics of amyloid. The light chains found in the nonfibrillar type of deposits apparently have different primary structures which do not result in fibril formation. The first steps involved in the synthesis and secretion of both the soluble and insoluble forms of light chains appear to be similar.

The chemical nature of the proteins in the AL fibrillar deposits has been defined in detail.[48] This has not yet been achieved for the nonamyloidotic light-chain deposits. In neither case have the steps between synthesis and deposition been elucidated. It appears that both substances are the synthetic products of single

TABLE 1. Correlation of Lymphoplasmacytic Disorder and Glomerular Disease With Presence of M Protein in Serum, Urine, and Kidney

Group A	References	Case No.	M Protein		
			SERUM	URINE	BIOSYNTHESIS
Myeloma (or plasmacytosis of bone marrow)	Antonovych[72]	1	Klch		
	Randall[59]	1	Klch	Klch	
	Noël[61]	1	IgAK	Klch	
	Noël	2	IgAK	Klch	
	Silva[73]	1	Klch	Klch	
	King[65]	1	–	Klch	
	Colvin[69]		–	–	
	Seymour[68]	1	–	Klch	
	Seymour	2	IgGK	Klch	
	Seymour	3	–	Klch	
	Seymour	4	–	Klch	
	Seymour	5	IgGK	Klch	
	Seymour	6	–	Klch	
	Seymour	8	IgAL	Llch	
	Tubbs[71]	1	–	Klch	
	Tubbs	2	–	–	
	Tubbs	4	IgGK	Klch	
	Tubbs	7	–		
	Elfenbein[63]	1	–	–	
	Elfenbein	2	–	–	
	Rao[62]	1	–		
	Preud'homme[22]	1	Klch	Klch	Large Klch (28,000D)
	Preud'homme[22]	3*	–	–	Short Klch (12,000D)
	†	Fig. 2	IgGK	Klch	
	†	Fig. 3	Klch	Klch	
	Preud'homme[21]		IgAK	–	Short alpha Hch Normal lch Short free lch
	†	Fig. 5	IgGL	Llch	Normal Llch Short polypeptides Small gamma Hch
	Tange[66]		IgGL	–	
	Tubbs[71]	9	Llch	Llch	
	Tubbs	10*	Llch	Llch	
	Tubbs	11	Llch	Llch	
	Tubbs	3	–	–	

*This patient had a diagnosis of lymphoma.

TABLE 1 (cont.)

Deposits (IF)			Deposits (EM)			
GLOMERULI	TBM	VES	GLOMERULI	TBM	VES	**Glomerular Lesion**
Klch	Klch	Klch	+	+	+	Minimal
Klch	Klch	Klch	+	+	+	Minimal→nodular
Klch	Klch		+	+		Nodular
Klch	Klch		+	+		Nodular
–	Klch		+	+		Proliferative GN; crescents
–	–	Klch	+	+		Mes. widening
Klch	Klch		+	+	+	Mes. widening→ nodular
Klch	Klch	Klch	+	+	+	Enlarged→nodular
Klch	Klch	Klch	+	+	+	Nodular
Klch	Klch	Klch	+	+	+	Seg. proliferation
Klch	Klch	Klch	+	+	+	Enlarged
–	–	–	+	+	+	Enlarged
Klch	Klch	Klch	+	–	–	Proliferation
Klch	–	–	+	+	+	Mes. widening
Klch	Klch	–	+	+		
Klch	Klch	–	+	+		
Klch	Klch	Klch	+	+		
Klch	Klch	–	+	+		
Klch	Klch	–	+	+	+	
–	Klch		+	+		Nodular
–	–		+	+		Nodular
Klch	Klch		+	+		Nodular
–	Klch					Nodular
Klch	Klch					Mes. widening
Klch	Klch		–	+		Minimal
Klch	Klch		+	+		Minimal
alpha Hch	alpha Hch					Nodular
Klch	Klch					
gamma Hch	gamma Hch		–	–		Nodular
Llch	Llch					
IgGL	IgGL		+			Minimal
Llch	Llch	–	+	–		
Llch	Llch	–	+	–		
Llch	Llch	+	+	–		

(Continued)

TABLE 1. (Continued)

Group B	Reference	Case No.	M Protein		
			SERUM	URINE	BIOSYNTHESIS
Without myeloma (or data not stated)	Randall[59]	2	–	–	
	Herf[67]	1			
	Tubbs[71]	5			
	Tubbs	6	Klch	Klch	
	Tubbs	8			
	Gallo[5]	Fig. 1	–	–	Excess normal Klch
	Blaustein[5]		–	–	
	Preud'homme[22]	2	–	+	
	†	Fig. 4	Llch	Llch	Normal Llch Short polypeptides

†Unpublished observations.

clones of plasma cells, that both are processed in similar ways, and that both are deposited in normal tissues, with resulting compromised function. There is some suggestion that lambda light chains may be more predisposed to amyloid fibril formation, while to date the nonamyloidotic monoclonal Ig's have more frequently been associated with excess kappa-chain synthesis. However, these are generalizations drawn from a few observations, and await more data to test their validity.

Previous immunofluorescence studies of the kidneys, from many patients with myeloma and a gammopathy, have not detected light-chain determinants in the glomeruli or tubular basement membranes.[76,77] Hence, not all monoclonal Ig's localize in the glomeruli or tubular basement membranes. The reason why some but not all monoclonal Ig's are pathogenic remains unclear; antibody specificity for kidney antigens seems an unlikely cause for localization in view of the widespread distribution of deposits previously observed.[21,22,59,68,69] Furthermore, monoclonal light chains in serum or urine from patients with nonamyloidotic light-chain glomerulopathy have not demonstrated in vitro binding to renal substrates.[70,71] The same question has been raised regarding the differences in tissue deposition between amyloid-related light chains versus nonamyloid light chains.[49] A comparison of tissue-binding affinities was investigated utilizing immunofluorescence analysis of tissue sections incubated with the different fluorescein-conjugated light chains. Quantitative but not qualitative differences were observed between the binding of amyloid-related light chains and that of nonamyloid light chains.[48] These results must be viewed with reservation, since with the methods used, quantification is difficult at best. Thus, the reasons for deposition of amyloid-related light chains or nonfibrillar light chains remain unclear.

Other recent observations suggest an alternative mechanism to account for the tissue deposition of amyloid-related light chains and nonamyloid light chains —namely, electrostatic interactions. The distribution of the deposits in clusters in

TABLE 1. (Continued)

Desposits (IF)			Deposits (EM)			
GLOMERULI	TBM	VES	GLOMERULI	TBM	VES	**Glomerular Lesion**
Klch	Klch	Klch	+	+	+	Nodular
Klch	Klch					Nodular
–	Klch	–	+	+		
Klch	Klch		+	+		
–	Klch	–	+	+		
Klch	Klch	Klch	+	+	+	Nodular
Klch	Klch		+	+		Nodular
–	Klch					Mes. widening
Llch	Llch	Llch	+	–		Mild mesangial widening

IF: immunofluorescence; EM: electron microscopy; TBM: tubular basement membranes; Ves: vessels MES: mesangial; Seg: segmental; Klch: kappa light chain; Llch: lambda light chain; Hch: heavy chain; +: present; –: absent; no entry: data not stated.

the glomerular and tubular basement membrane and the mesangium is reminiscent of the binding of cationic probes to anionic sites in glomeruli, as previously described in experimental animals.[78,79] Additionally, studies in experimental passive serum sickness, using immune complexes formed with bovine gamma globulin antigen and rabbit antibovine gamma globulin antibody, have shown that cationic but not anionic antigen or antigen–antibody complexes bind electrostatically to the anionic sites in the glomerular and tubular basement membranes in a manner similar to the binding of cationic probes.[80] The electrophoretic heterogeneity of Ig's allows for this possibility and may explain why some M proteins do bind to kidney structures, while others do not. This hypothesis remains to be tested.

RENAL DISEASE IN CRYOGLOBULINEMIA

Monoclonal Ig's may have cryoprecipitable properties, and have been detected in patients with myeloma, lymphoma, monoclonal gammopathy of undetermined significance, and Waldenström's macroglobulinemia.[81,82] Several types of cryoglobulins have been described: Type I, monoclonal, comprising a single Ig component; Type II, mixed polyclonal, comprising a monoclonal antibody against a polyclonal Ig; and Type III, mixed polyclonal, comprising two or more polyclonal components.

Renal disease occurs in approximately 20 percent of patients with cryoglobulinemia, and is most common in patients with type II cryo-Ig's, representing a type of immune-complex glomerulonephritis.[82] The Ig's in the glomerular deposits have generally corresponded to those comprising the serum cryoprecipitate.[33,37] A fibrillar-crystalline ultrastructure of the renal deposits and serum cryoprecipitate has been described in patients with types I and II cryoglobulins.[36-38,83] However, although repeatedly observed in patients with cryoglobulinemia, these ultrastructural features do not appear to be unique to the cryoprecipitable property of the Ig, since crystalline deposits have been found in the kidneys of patients who have dysproteinemia but not cryoglobulinemia[84] (Fig. 6c).

RENAL DISEASE IN MACROGLOBULINEMIA

Glomerular thrombi, the hallmark lesion first described in light-microscopic studies,[85] are now recognized as a feature of renal involvement in macroglobulinemia (Fig. 6a). In the largest series of patients with macroglobulinemia whose kidneys have been examined by light- and immunofluorescence microscopy, 8 of the 19 patients had capillary "thrombi" or endomembranous deposits.[34,86] Of those examined by immunofluorescence, all the deposits stained for IgM but not for other Igs. The IgM deposited in the glomeruli was shown to be monoclonal in those patients examined with antisera monospecific for light chains. It was proposed that the deposits and thrombi resulted from the direct deposition of the M protein, and that their mechanism of deposition thus differed from that of immune complexes. This hypothesis is consistent with what is known of the properties of macroglobulins and the local glomerular factors that can promote precipitation. The presence of hyperviscosity with slow perfusion, high protein concentration, low osmotic pressure, and low ionic strength all predispose to decreased solubility. In other studies, there is evidence to suggest an immune-complex pathogenesis of renal disease in macroglobulinemia. In one patient, glomerular deposits were polyclonal and contained, by immunofluorescence examination, both IgG and IgM, as well as C_3.[87] In two other patients with macroglobulinemia and cryoglobulinemia, one had a monoclonal IgM-kappa type and the other a mixed IgM-kappa and polyclonal IgG type of glomerular deposit.[39]

Thus, is some patients with macroglobulinemia, the glomerular deposits may contain only a single-component Ig, suggestive of a monoclonal Ig deposition state. In others, with polyclonal Ig deposits, an immune complex mechanism is implicated in which a monoclonal antibody is complexed with other polyclonal Ig's. It is also possible that the two types of deposition may co-exist.

Ultrastructurally, the deposits may be granular[87] or fibrillar-crystalline[39]; the latter was observed in a patient with cryo-Ig's. We have examined a biopsy from one patient with an IgM macroglobulinemia who had massive luminal and capillary wall polyclonal deposits which stained for IgM and IgG heavy-chain determinants and both kappa and lambda light-chain determinants, as well as C_3. Ultrastructurally the deposits present in the mesangium and in expanded subendothelial masses had a crystalline substructure (Fig. 6c). No serum cryoglobulins could be demonstrated.

Other glomerular lesions have been described in macroglobulinemia. Renal amyloid has been well documented.[86] Nodular nonamyloidotic glomerulopathy has also been reported in two patients.[57,88] These cases were not characterized by immunohistologic methods.

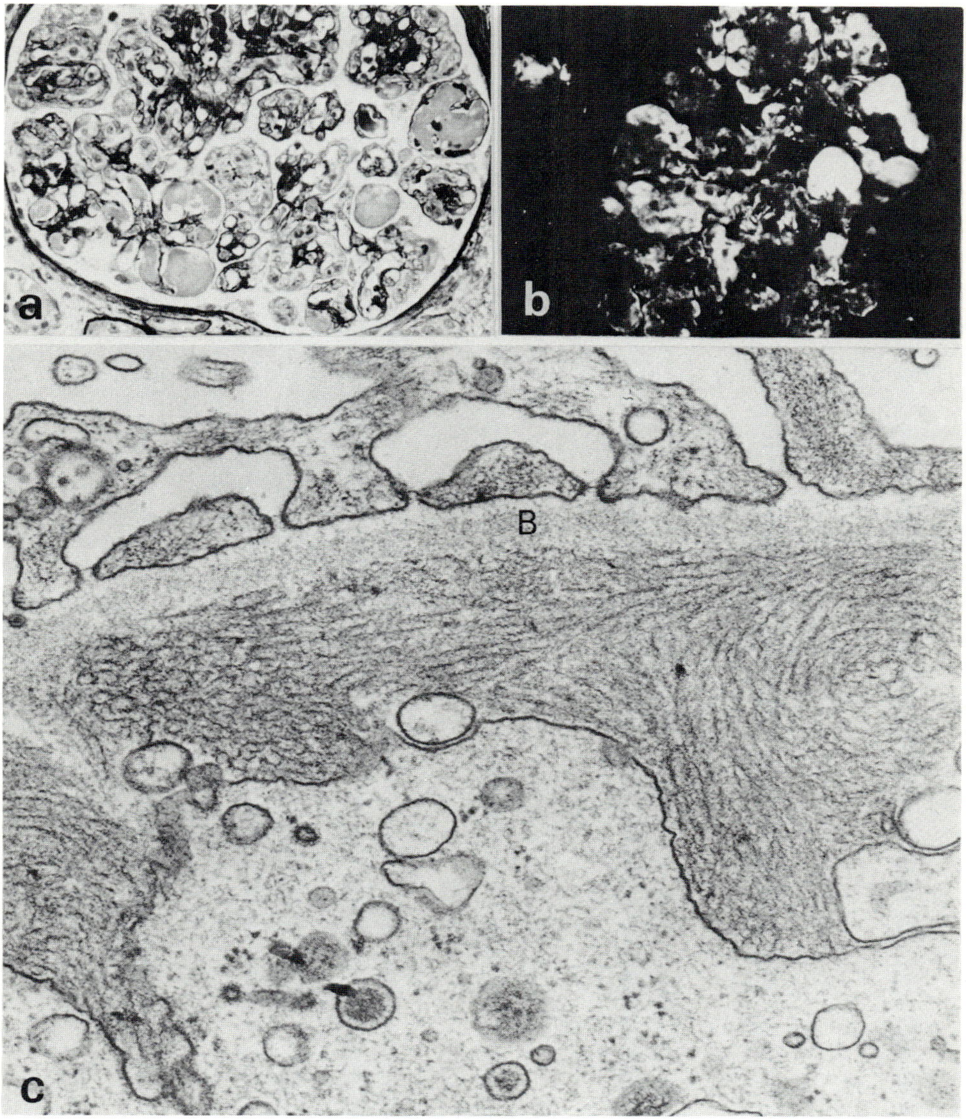

FIG. 6. Renal biopsy from a patient with IgM-kappa macroglobulinemia. **a.** A light-micrograph demonstrates a glomerulus with conspicuous capillary lumen "thrombi." Periodic acid silver-methenamine and H&E. ×430. **b.** Immunofluorescence examination of the frozen section shows a glomerulus stained with the fluoresceinated anti-IgM antiserum (heavy-chain specific). Large masses are seen in the capillary lumens (arrows). ×400. **c.** An electron micrograph of a glomerulus double-stained with uranyl acetate and lead citrate is shown. The deposits present in the inner zone of the glomerular basement membrane (B) have a fibrillar-crystalline substructure which does not resemble amyloid. ×50,000.

RENAL DISEASE IN HODGKIN'S LYMPHOMA, NON-HODGKIN'S LYMPHOMA, AND LEUKEMIA

Glomerular diseases in the lymphoproliferative disorders, excluding those associated with dysproteinemia, have been thoroughly reviewed,[11] and these data are only briefly discussed in the context of this review.

The glomerular diseases—often manifested as the nephrotic syndrome—that occur in association with Hodgkin's lymphoma, non-Hodgkin's lymphoma, chronic lymphocytic leukemia, and angioimmunoblastic lymphadenopathy are shown in Table 2.[2,7,9,22,40,89-140] Amyloidosis was the most frequently reported cause of the nephrotic syndrome in association with Hodgkin's lymphoma in the period from 1930 to 1962, whereas it was less frequent in the period from 1962 to 1976, when minimal change disease, membranous nephropathy, and proliferative glomerulonephritis were the most common causes. These differences may not reflect the true incidences of disease types, since the renal biopsy and the techniques necessary to accurately classify the glomerular lesions have only been routinely employed during the latter period.

Information regarding the pathogenesis of renal disease in these lymphoproliferative disorders is limited. The type of amyloid (AA or AL), that is deposited though not defined in earlier studies of Hodgkin's lymphoma,[105,106] has

TABLE 2. Association of Glomerulopathy With Lymphoproliferative Disorders

Lymphoproliferative Disorder	Glomerular Lesion	No. Cases	References
Hodgkin's lymphoma	Amyloidosis	30	7, 9, 89–106
	Minimal change nephrotic syndrome	25	2, 102, 108–120, 140
	Proliferative GN	6	106, 111, 120, 121, 125
	Renal vein or inferior vena cava occlusion	4	102, 122, 123
	Membranous nephropathy	3	124–126
	Anti-GBM disease	1	127
Non-Hodgkin's lymphoma	Proliferative GN	4	128–130
	Minimal change nephrotic syndrome	2	110, 131
	Membranous nephropathy	2	132, 133
	Membranoproliferative GN	1	120
	Diffuse GBM and TBM thickening	2	22, 134
Chronic lymphocytic leukemia	Proliferative GN	5	109, 135–137
	Membranoproliferative GN	3	40, 138
	Amyloidosis	2	100, 135
	Membranous nephropathy	1	136
Angioimmunoblastic lymphadenopathy	Minimal changes and mesangial Ig deposits	2	139

GN: glomerulonephritis; GBM: glomerular basement membrane; TBM: tubular basement membrane since been determined to be the AA type.[107] The mechanism of glomerular dysfunction in the minimal change glomerular disease associated with these disorders is not understood. As in the other neoplastic diseases, the evidence for an immune-complex mechanism of glomerular disease in the lymphoproliferative disorders is derived from several observations: (1) Ig's and C_3 have been detected in the glomeruli of patients with lymphoproliferative disorders;[11] (2) elevated levels of circulating immune complexes have been detected in the serum of 50 percent of untreated patients with Hodgkin's disease as compared with the normal levels detected posttreatment and the normal levels of control subjects;[141] and (3) specific antigen and antibodies have been demonstrated in the glomerular deposits.[11] Information about the antigen–antibody systems involved is based upon the detection of specific antigen or antibody in the deposits as determined by immunofluorescence microscopy, or by their detection in acid eluates of kidneys containing Ig deposits. Viral antigens, either tumor-related or due to intercurrent infections, have been implicated;[11] these include herpes zoster viral antigens in Hodgkin's disease,[120] Oncornavirus antigens in leukemia and lymphoma,[142] and Epstein-Barr virus antigens in African Burkitt's lymphoma and Hodgkin's disease.[143,144]

ACKNOWLEDGMENTS

We gratefully acknowledge the assistance of Virginia Meyer, who prepared the figure illustrations, and Gwynne Nemcek, who typed the manuscript. Studies in Dr. Buxbaum's laboratory were supported by VA research funds and the Rheumatic Diseases Study Group Program Grant AM 01431.

REFERENCES

1. Beaufils M, Morel-Maroger L: Pathogenesis of renal disease in monoclonal gammopathies: Current concepts. Nephron 20:125–131, 1978
2. Moorthy AV, Zimmerman SW, Burkholder PM: Nephrotic syndrome in Hodgkin's disease. Evidence for pathogenesis alternative to immune complex deposition. Am J Med 61:471–477, 1976
3. Sanchez LM, Domz CA: Renal patterns in myeloma. Ann Intern Med 52:44–54, 1960
4. Gallo GR, Feiner HD, Katz LA, Buxbaum JN: Nonamyloidotic light chain glomerulopathy associated with unbalanced immunoglobulins synthesis. Kidney Int 16:929, 1979 (Abstract)
5. Gallo GR, Feiner HD, Katz LA, et al.: Nodular glomerulopathy associated with nonamyloidotic kappa light chain deposits and excess immunoglobulin light chain synthesis. Am J Pathol 99:621–644, 1980
6. Silva F, Mesa-Tejada R, Williams GS, et al.: Light chain glomerulonephropathy (GN) as the first manifestation of plasma cell dyscrasia (PCD). Lab Invest 42:151, 1980 (Abstract)
7. Richmond J, Sherman RS, Diamond HD, Craver LF: Renal lesions associated with malignant lymphomas. Am J Med 32:184–207, 1962
8. Martinez-Maldonado M, Ramirez-Arellano GA: Renal involvement in malignant lymphomas: A survey of 49 cases. J Urol 95:485–488, 1966
9. Kiely JM, Wagoner RD, Holley KE: Renal complications of lymphoma. Ann Intern Med 71:1159–1175, 1969

10. Morris RC, Fudenberg HH: Impaired renal acidification in patients with hypergammaglobulinemia. Medicine 46:57–69, 1967
11. Eagen JW, Lewis EJ: Glomerulopathies of neoplasia. Kidney Int 11:297–306, 1977
12. Kyle RA, Greipp PR: Laboratory medicine-series on clinical testing. 3. The laboratory investigation of monoclonal gammopathies. Mayo Clin Proc 53:719–739, 1978
13. Fudenberg HH, Virella G: Multiple myeloma and Waldenström macroglobulinemia: Unusual presentations. Semin Hematol 17:63–79, 1980
14. Baumal R, Scharff MD: Synthesis, assembly and secretion of mouse immunoglobulins. Transpl Rev 14:163–183, 1973
15. Buxbaum JN: The biosythesis, assembly, and secretion of immunoglobulins. Semin Hematol 10:33–52, 1973
16. Zola S, Buxbaum JN, Franklin EC, Scharff MD: Synthesis and assembly of immunoglobulins by malignant plasmacytes. I. Myelomas producing γ chains and light chains. J Exp Med 132:148–162, 1970
17. Williams RC, Brunning RD, Wollheim FA: Light-chain disease. An abortive variant of multiple myeloma. Ann Intern Med 65:471–486, 1966
18. Stone MJ, Frenkel EP: The clinical spectrum of light chain myeloma: A study of 35 patients with special reference to the occurence of amyloidosis. Am J Med 58:601–619, 1975
19. Kyle RA: Monoclonal gammopathy of undetermined significance. Natural history in 241 cases. Am J Med 64:814–826, 1978
20. Buxbaum JN: Heavy chain diseases in man. Ric Clin Lab 6:301–317, 1976
21. Preud'homme JL, Morel-Maroger L, Brouet JC, et al.: Synthesis of abnormal heavy and light chains in multiple myeloma with visceral deposition of monoclonal immunoglobulins. Clin Exp Immunol 42:545–553, 1980
22. Preud'homme JL, Morel-Maroger L, Brouet JC, et al.: Synthesis of abnormal immunoglobulins in lymphoplasmacytic disorders with visceral light chain deposition. Am J Med 69:703–710, 1980
23. Azar HA, Zaino EC, Pham TD, Yannopoulos K: "Nonsecretory" plasma cell myeloma: Observations on seven cases with electron microscope studies. Am J Clin Pathol 58:618–629, 1972
24. River GL, Tewksbury DA, Fudenberg HH: "Nonsecretory" multiple myeloma. Blood 40:204–206, 1972
25. Hurez D, Preud'homme JL, Seligmann H: Intracellular "monoclonal" immunoglobulin in nonsecretory human myeloma. J Immunol 104:263–264, 1970
26. Preud'homme JL, Hurez D, Danon F, et al.: Intracytoplasmic and surface-bound immunoglobulins in "nonsecretory" and Bence Jones myeloma. Clin Exp Immunol 25:428–436, 1976
27. Arend WP, Adamson JW: Nonsecretory myeloma. Immunofluorescent demonstration of paraprotein within bone marrow plasma cells. Cancer 33:721–728, 1974
28. Capra JD, Kunkel HG: Aggregation of G3 proteins: Relevance to the hyperviscosity syndrome. J Clin Invest 49:610–621, 1970
29. Maldonado JE, Velosa JA, Kyle RA, et al.: Fanconi syndrome in adults: A manifestation of a latent form of myeloma. Am J Med 58:354–364, 1975
30. Smithline N, Kassirer JP, Cohen JJ: Light-chain nephropathy. Renal tubular dysfunction associated with light-chain proteinuria. N Engl J Med 294:71–74, 1976
31. DeFronza RA, Cooke CR, Wright JR, Humphrey RL: Renal function in patients with multiple myeloma. Medicine 57:151–166, 1978
32. Preuss HG, Weiss FR, Iammarino RM, et al.: Effects on rat kidney slice function *in vitro* of proteins from the urines of patients with myelomatosis and nephrosis. Clin Sci Mol Med 46:283–294, 1974
33. Verroust P, Mery J-P, Morel-Maroger L, et al: Glomerular lesions in monoclonal gammopathies and mixed essential cryoglobulinemia IgG-IgM. Adv Nephrol 1:161–194, 1974
34. Morel-Maroger L, Verroust P: Glomerular lesions in dysproteinemias. Kidney Int 5:249–252, 1974

35. Schuurman S, Stekhoven JH, Van Haelst UJ: Unusual findings in the human renal glomerulus in multiple myeloma: A light and electron microscopic study. Virchows Arch [Cell Pathol] 9:311–321, 1971
36. Bengtsson U, Larsson O, Lindstedt G, Svalander C: Monoclonal IgG cryoglobulinemia with secondary development of glomerulonephritis and nephrotic syndrome. QJ Med 44:491–503, 1975
37. Feiner H, Gallo GR: Ultrastructure in glomerulonephritis associated with cryoglobulinemia. A report of six cases and review of the literature. Am J Pathol 88:145–162, 1977
38. Gallo GR, Feiner H: Ultrastructure in glomerulonephritis associated with cryoglobulinemia. In Chenais F (ed): Colloque Cryoproteines. Villars-de-Lans, France, Inserm, 1978, pp 139–156
39. Faraggiana T, Parolini C, Previato G, Lupo A: Light and electron microscopic findings in five cases of cryoglobulinemic glomerulonephritis. Virchows Arch [Pathol Anat] 384:29–44, 1979
40. Gilboa N, Durante D, Guggenheim S, et al.: Immune deposit nephritis and single-component cryoglobulinemia associated with chronic lymphocytic leukemia. Nephron 24:223–231, 1979
41. Kaplan NG, Kaplan KC: Monoclonal gammopathy, glomerulonephritis and the nephrotic syndrome. Arch Intern Med 125:696–700, 1970
42. Avashti PS, Erickson DG, Williams RC, Tung KSK: Benign monoclonal gammaglobulinemia and glomerulonephritis. Am J Med 62:324–329, 1977
43. von Decastello A: Beiträge zur Kenntnis der Bence Jonesschen Albuminurie. Ztschr F klin Med 67:319–343, 1908–1909
44. Allen AC: The Kidney. Medical and Surgical Diseases, ed 2. New York, Grune and Stratton, 1962
45. DeFronza RA, Humphrey RL, Wright JR, Cooke CR: Acute renal failure in multiple myeloma. Medicine 54:209–223, 1975
46. Heptinstall R: Pathology of the Kidney, ed 2. Boston, Little, Brown, 1974
47. Limas C, Wright JR, Matsuzaki M, Calkins E: Amyloidosis and multiple myeloma: A reevaluation using a control population. Am J Med 54:166–173, 1973
48. Glenner GG: Amyloid deposits and amyloidosis. The β-fibrilloses. N Engl J Med 302:1283–1292, 1333–1343, 1980
49. Osserman EF, Takatsuki K, Talal N: The pathogenesis of "amyloidosis." Studies on the role of abnormal gammaglobulins and gammaglobulin fragments of the Bence Jones (L-Polypeptide) type in the pathogenesis of "primary" and "secondary amyloidosis" and the "amyloidosis" associated with plasma cell myeloma. Semin Hematol 1:3–85, 1964
50. Terry WD, Page DL, Kimura S, et al.: Structural identity of Bence Jones and amyloid fibril proteins in a patient with plasma cell dyscrasia and amyloidosis. J Clin Invest 52:1276–1281, 1973
51. Putnam FW, Whitley EJ Jr, Paul C, Davidson JN: Aminoacid sequence of a K Bence Jones protein from a case of primary amyloidosis. Biochemistry 12:3763–3780, 1973
52. Kobernick SD, Whiteside JH: Renal glomeruli in multiple myeloma. Lab Invest 6:478–485, 1957
53. Cauchie C, Kenis Y, Potvliege P, et al.: Les manifestations rénales du myéloma des dysglobulinemies: Rapports introductifs: Les manifestations rénales du myeloma. Societé du nephrologie. J Urol Nephrol (Paris) 68:41–56, 1962
54. Olsen S: Mesangial thickening and nodular sclerosis in diabetes mellitus and other diseases. Acta Pathol Microbiol Scand (A) (Suppl 233) 80:203–216, 1972
55. Solling K, Askjaer SA: Multiple myeloma with urinary excretion of heavy chain components of IgG and nodular glomerulosclerosis. Acta Med Scand 194:23–30, 1973
56. Schubert GE, Adam A: Glomerular nodules and long-spacing collagen in kidneys of patients with multiple myeloma. J Clin Pathol 27:800–805, 1974
57. Zlotnick A, Rosenmann E: Renal pathologic findings associated with monoclonal gammopathies. Arch Intern Med 135:40–45, 1975

58. Jensen H, Wiik A: Monoclonal immunoglobulinemia associated with glomerulopathy. Acta Med Scand 197:265–269, 1975
59. Randall RE, Williamson WC, Mullinax F, et al.: Manifestation of systemic light chain deposition. Am J Med 60:293–299, 1976
60. Vladutiu AO, Kohli RK, Prezyna AP: Monoclonal IgE with renal failure. Am J Med 61:957–962, 1976
61. Noël NH, Droz D, Ganeval D, Jungers P: Glomerulosclerose nodulaire du myeloma (Abstract). VII International Congress of Nephrology, Montreal, 1978 p L16.
62. Rao TKS, Nicastri AD, Chen CK, et al.: Membranoproliferative glomerulonephritis (MPGN), an unusual manifestation of multiple myeloma (MM). Kidney Int 14:659, 1978 (Abstr)
63. Elfenbein IB, Bastl CP, Guzzo JC, et al.: Nodular mesangial sclerosis lesions and nephrotic syndrome in multiple myeloma. Kidney Int 14:710, 1978 (Abstr)
64. Mallick NP, Dosa S, Acheson EJ, et al.: Detection, significance and treatment of paraprotein in patients presenting with 'idiopathic' proteinuria without myeloma. QJ Med 47:145–175, 1978
65. King JT, Valenzuela R, McCormack LJ, Osborne DG: Granular dense deposit disease. Lab Invest 39:591–596, 1978
66. Tange T, Kurumado K, Nakazawa M, et al.: Glomerular lesions in multiple myeloma. Acta Pathol Jpn 28:325–333, 1978
67. Herf S, Pohl SL, Sturgill B, Bolton WK: An evaluation of diabetic and pseudodiabetic glomerulosclerosis. Am J Med 66:1040–1045, 1979
68. Seymour AE, Thompson AJ, Smith PS, et al.: Kappa light chain glomerulosclerosis in multiple myeloma. Am J Pathol 101:557–580, 1980
69. Colvin R: Case records of the Massachusetts General Hospital. Case 1 - 1981. N Engl J Med 304:33–43, 1981
70. Tubbs RR, Gephardt GN, McMahon JT, et al.: Light chain nephropathy. Lab Invest 44:68A, 1981 (Abstr)
71. Tubbs RR, Gephardt GN, McMahon JT, et al.: Light chain nephropathy. Am J Med 71:263–269, 1981
72. Antonovych T, Linc C, Parrish E, Mostofi K: Light chain deposits in multiple myeloma (Abstract). Am. Soc. Nephrol. Seventh Annual Meeting, 1973
73. Silva FG, Meyrier A, Morel-Maroger L, Pirani CL: Proliferative glomerulonephropathy in multiple myeloma. J Pathol 130:229–236, 1980
74. Solling K, Solling J, Jacobsen NO, Thomsen OF: Nonsecretory myeloma associated with nodular glomerulosclerosis. Acta Med Scand 207:137–143, 1980
75. Buxbaum JN, Hurley ME, Chuba J, Spiro T: Amyloidosis of the AL type: Clinical, morphologic and biochemical aspects of the response to therapy with alkylating agents and prednisone. Am J Med 67:867–878, 1979
76. Levi DF, Williams RC, Lindstrom FD: Immunofluorescent studies of the myeloma kidney with special reference to light chain disease. Am J Med 44:922–933, 1968
77. Cohen AH, Border WA: Myeloma kidney: An immunomorphogenetic study of renal biopsies. Lab Invest 42:248–256, 1980
78. Caulfield JP, Farquhar MG: Distribution of anionic sites in the glomerular basement membranes: Their possible role in filtration and attachment. Proc Natl Acad Sci USA 73:1646–1650, 1976
79. Kanwar YS, Farquhar MG: Anionic sites in the glomerular basement membrane. In vivo and vitro localization to the laminae rarae by catonic probes. J Cell Biol 81:137–153, 1979
80. Gallo GR, Caulin-Glaser T, Lamm ME: Charge of circulating immune complexes as a factor in glomerular basement membrane localization in mice. J Clin Invest 67:1305–1313, 1981
81. Grey HM, Kohler PF: Cryoimmunoglobulins. Semin Hematol 10:87–112, 1973
82. Brouet J-C, Clauvel J-P, Danon F, et al.: Biologic and clinical significance of cryoglobulins. A report of 86 cases. Am J Med 57:775–788, 1974

83. Cordonnier D, Martin H, Groslambert P, et al.: Mixed IgG-IgM cryoglobulinemia with glomerulonephritis. Am J Med 59:867–872, 1975
84. Bogaars H: Personal communication.
85. Lamm ME: Macroglobulinemia: Report of two cases. Am J Clin Pathol 35:53–65, 1961
86. Morel-Maroger L, Basch A, Danon F, et al.: Pathology of the kidney in Waldenström's macroglobulinemia. N Engl J Med 283:123–129, 1970
87. Martelo OJ, Schultz DR, Pardo V, Perez-Stable E: Immunologically-mediated renal disease in Waldenström's macroglobulinemia. Am J Med 58:567–575, 1975
88. Lin JH, Orofino J, Sherlock J, et al.: Waldenström's macroglobulinemia, mesangiocapillary glomerulonephritis, angiitis and myositis. Nephron 10:262–270, 1973
89. Bannick EG, Barker NW: Diffuse amyloidosis of unknown etiology. Med Clin North Am 14:773–781, 1930
90. Lehman RG: Hodgkin's disease complicated by amyloidosis and a nephrotic syndrome: case report. Ohio State Med J 39:232–233, 1943
91. Jackson H: Hodgkin's Disease and Allied Disorders. New York, Oxford University Press, 1947
92. Short CL: Case records of the Massachusetts General Hospital Case #35391. N Engl J Med 241:497–500, 1949
93. Dahlin DC: Secondary amyloidosis. Ann Intern Med 31:105–119, 1949
94. Scott RB: The spleen and splenectomy. Br Med J 1:1063–1070, 1949
95. Wallace SC, Feldman DJ, Berlin I, et al.: Amyloidosis in Hodgkin's disease. Am J Med 8:552–557, 1950
96. Gledhill RC, Shillitoe AJ: Purpura and amyloidosis in Hodgkin's disease. Br Med J 1:1336–1337, 1952
97. Teilum G: Studies on pathogenesis of amyloidosis. II. Effect of nitrogen mustard on inducing amyloidosis. J Lab Clin Med 43:367–374, 1954
98. Sherman MJ, Morales JB, Bayrd ED, Schierman WD: Amyloid nephrosis secondary to Hodgkin's disease. Arch Intern Med 95:618–621, 1955
99. Spain DM: Rapid and extensive development of amyloidosis in association with nitrogen mustard therapy. Am J Clin Pathol 26:52–55, 1956
100. Leonard BJ: Chronic lymphatic leukemia and the nephrotic syndrome. Lancet 1:1356–1357, 1957
101. Winawer SJ, Feldman SM: Amyloid nephrosis in Hodgkin's disease. Arch Intern Med 104:793–796, 1959
102. Hamburger J: Nephrology, Vol 1. Philadelphia, W. B. Saunders, 1968
103. Clinico-pathologic conference. Hodgkin's disease complicated by thrombocytopenia and nephrotic syndrome. Am J Med 51:109–120, 1971
104. Wilks S: Cases of lardaceous disease and some allied affections. Guys Hosp Rep 52:103–132, 1856
105. Falkson G, Falkson HC: Amyloidosis in Hodgkin's disease. S Afr Med J 47:62–64, 1973
106. Yum MN, Edwards JL, Kleit S: Glomerular lesions in Hodgkin's disease. Arch Pathol Lab Med 99:645–649, 1975
107. Franklin EC, Gorevic PD: The amyloid diseases. In Fougereau M, Dausset J (eds): Immunology 80. Fourth International Congress of Immunology. Progress in Immunology IV. London, Academic, 1980, pp 1219–1230
108. Miller D: The association of immune disease and malignant lymphoma. Ann Intern Med 66:507–521, 1967
109. Brodovsky HS, Samuels ML, Migliore PJ, Howe CD: Chronic lymphocytic leukemia, Hodgkin's disease, and the nephrotic syndrome. Arch Intern Med 121:71–75, 1968
110. Ghosh LB, Muehrcke RC: The nephrotic syndrome: A prodrome to lymphoma. Ann Intern Med 72:379–382, 1970
111. Lowry WS, Munzenrider JE, Lynch GA: Nephrotic syndrome in Hodgkin's disease. Lancet 1:1127, 1971

112. Jackson RH, Oo M: Nephrotic syndrome with Hodgkin's disease. Lancet 2:821–822, 1971
113. Bichel J, Jensen KB: Nephrotic syndrome and Hodgkin's disease. Lancet 2:1425–1426, 1971
114. Plager J, Stutzman L: Acute nephrotic syndrome as a manifestation of active Hodgkin's disease. Am J Med 50:56–66, 1971
115. Sherman RL, Susin M, Weksler ME, Becker EL: Lipoid nephrosis in Hodgkin's disease. Am J Med 52:699–706, 1972
116. Hansen HE, Skov PE, Askjaer SA, Albertsen K: Hodgkin's disease associated with the nephrotic syndrome without kidney lesion. Acta Med Scand 191:307–313, 1972
117. Hayslett JP, Kashgarian M, Bensch KG, et al.: Clinicopathological correlations in the nephrotic syndrome due to primary renal disease. Medicine 52:93–120, 1973
118. Carpenter CB: Case records of the Massachusetts General Hospital. Case #49–1973. N Engl J Med 289:1241–1247, 1973
119. Routledge RC, Hann IM, Morris Jones PH: Hodgkin's disease complicated by the nephrotic syndrome. Cancer 38:1735–1740, 1976
120. Hyman LR, Burkholder PM, Joo PA, Segar WE: Malignant lymphoma and nephrotic syndrome. J Pediatr 82:207–217, 1973
121. Lockich J, Galvanek EG, Moloney WC: Nephrosis of Hodgkin's disease. Immune complex-induced lesion. Arch Intern Med 132:597–600, 1973
122. Foth R, Bader K: Development of the nephrotic syndrome secondary to renal vein thrombosis in a patient with bronchogenic carcinoma and Hodgkin's disease. IMJ 125:505–509, 1964
123. Piessens WF, Zeicher M: Hodgkin's disease causing a reversible nephrotic syndrome by compression of the inferior vena cava. Cancer 25:880–884, 1970
124. Hardin JG, Coker AS, Blanton JH: Medical grand rounds from the University of Alabama Medical Center. South Med J 1111–1118, 1969
125. Froom DW, Franklin WA, Hano JE, Potter EV: Immune deposits in Hodgkin's disease with nephrotic syndrome. Arch Pathol 94:547–553, 1972
126. Row PG, Cameron JS, Turner DR, et al.: Membranous nephropathy. Long term follow-up and association with neoplasia. QJ Med 44:207–239, 1975
127. Ma KW, Golbus SM, Kaufman R, et al.: Glomerulonephritis with Hodgkin's disease and herpes zoster. Arch Pathol Lab Med 102:527–529, 1978
128. Sagel J, Muller H, Logan E: Lymphoma and the nephrotic syndrome. S Afr Med J 45:79–80, 1971
129. Muggia FM, Ultmann JE: Glomerulonephritis or nephrotic syndrome in malignant lymphoma, reticulum cell type. Lancet 1:805, 1971
130. Petzel RA, Brown DC, Staley NA, et al.: Crescenteric glomerulonephritis and renal failure associated with malignant lymphoma. Am J Clin Patho 71:728–732, 1973
131. Gagliano RG, Costanzi JJ, Beathard GA, et al.: The nephrotic syndrome associated with neoplasia: An unusual paraneoplastic syndrome. Am J Med 60:1026–1031, 1976
132. Gluck MC, Gallo GR, Lowenstein J, Baldwin DS: Membranous glomerulonephritis. Evolution of clinical and pathologic features. Ann Intern Med 78:1–12, 1973
133. Rabkin R, Thatcher GN, Diamond LH, Eales L: The nephrotic syndrome, malignancy and immunosuppression. S Afr Med J 47:605–606, 1973
134. Berkel J, Granillo-Bodansky C, Kr v d Borne AEG: Acute renal failure associated with a malignant lymphoproliferative disorder with monoclonal light chain immunoglobulin production. Scand J Hematol 20:377–383, 1978
135. Scott RB: Leukemia. Lancet 1:1162–1167, 1957
136. Cameron S, Ogg CS: Nephrotic syndrome in chronic lymphatic leukemia. Br Med J 4:164, 1974
137. Dathan JRE, Heyworth MF, Maciver AG: Nephrotic syndrome in chronic lymphocytic leukemia. Br Med J 3:655–657, 1974
138. Mandalenakis N, Mendoza N, Pirani CL, Pollak VE: Lobular glomerulonephritis and membranoproliferative glomerulonephritis. Medicine 50:319–355, 1971

139. Wood WE, Harkins MH: Nephropathy in angioimmunoblastic lymphadenopathy. Am J Clin Pathol 71:58–63, 1979
140. Larson LS, Fritz RD: Nephrotic syndrome in association with Hodgkin's disease. Wis Med J 75:514–517, 1976
141. Brown CA, Hall CL, Long JC, et al.: Circulating immune complexes in Hodgkin's disease. Am J Med 64:289–294, 1978
142. Sutherland JC, Mardiney MR Jr: Immune complex disease in the kidneys of lymphoma-leukemia patients: The presence of an oncornavirus-related antigen. J Natl Cancer Inst 50:633–644, 1973
143. Oldstone MBA, Theofilopoulos AN, Gunven P, Klein G: Immune complexes associated with neoplasia: Presence of Epstein-Barr virus antigen-antibody complexes in Burkitt's lymphoma. Intervirology 4:292–302, 1974
144. Sutherland JC, Olweny CLM, Levine PH, Mardiney MR: Epstein-Barr virus-immune complexes in postmortem kidneys from African patients with Burkitt's lymphoma and American patients with and without lymphoma. J Natl Cancer Inst 60:941–946, 1978

"CLEAR-CELL" CHANGE WITHIN DUCT AND LOBULAR EPITHELIUM OF THE HUMAN BREAST

KENNETH W. BARWICK, MICHAEL KASHGARIAN, AND PAUL P. ROSEN

An infrequent microscopic finding, consisting of marked "clear-cell" change affecting the lobular and duct epithelium of the breast, has been noted during the examination of routine histologic sections. This study was undertaken to further characterize this finding by light and electron microscopy, and to seek possible causal factors.

MATERIALS AND METHODS

Occasional examples of epithelial clear-cell change in benign epithelium were noted by one of us (P.R.) during a review of breast carcinoma at the Memorial Sloan-Kettering Cancer Center. For the purposes of this study, other examples of the lesion were sought during the routine histologic evaluation of breast biopsies and mastectomies over a 9-month period. Neither the retrospective nor the prospective search involved consecutively performed surgical procedures.

The lesion to be described was identified in 31 patients (6 retrospectively and 25 prospectively). Clinical data were obtained from a review of hospital charts and were recorded when available.

Tissue was examined by electron microscopy in six cases. In each of these instances the tissues examined were removed from paraffin blocks and were deparaffinized in xylene prior to postfixation with osmium tetroxide. We were unable to find a single example of clear-cell change at the time of frozen section, in order to have fresh tissue for ultrastructural analysis.

RESULTS

Clinical Observations

The ages of the 31 patients at the time of biopsy or mastectomy ranged from 35 years to 82 years. The mean age was 56. Twenty-eight women were white, 1 was black, and 2 were of unknown race. Information regarding parity was available for 28 patients; 5 were nulliparous and the remainder had borne children. None had borne a child in the year preceding biopsy. Eight women had nursed at least one child and five had not; this information was not available for the other patients. Inquiry about the use of exogenous hormones had been made of 22 patients; 2 had previously used oral contraceptives and 6 had received conjugated estrogens for menopausal symptoms. Fourteen patients had never received any form of hormonal therapy. No patient was on any form of hormone therapy at the time of biopsy. Menstrual status was listed for 27 patients; 15 were postmenopausal, 9 were premenopausal, and 3 were perimenopausal (1 year or less from the time of menopause).

Associated diseases included hypertension in seven patients, cholecystitis in three, and anginal pain in two. One patient each had a history of rheumatic fever, breast abscess, tuberculosis, endometrial polyp, endometrial carcinoma, benign ovarian cyst, and epilepsy. No patient gave a history of diabetes mellitus.

On review of the tissue sections containing clear-cell changes in the benign epithelium, the following diagnoses were determined: intraductal and infiltrating duct carcinoma in 12 patients; intraductal and infiltrating duct carcinoma with foci of lobular carcinoma in situ in 6 patients; lobular carcinoma in situ and infiltrating lobular carcinoma in 2 patients; medullary carcinoma in 1 patient; intraductal carcinoma with foci of lobular carcinoma in situ in 1 patient; fibrocystic mastopathy in 6 patients; and fibroadenoma in 2 patients.

Light-Microscopic Observations

The histologic changes being considered in this study were most commonly seen in lobules, but often involved terminal ducts as well. They consisted of enlargement of the epithelial cells, with abundant pale cytoplasm marked by a fine granular or grainy appearance (Fig. 1). This graininess varied in texture, with some cells having coarse eosinophilic granules of differing size. The granules were irregularly distributed through the cytoplasm, and when prominent were invariably associated with a secretory product within the lumina of acini (Fig. 2). This luminal secretion and the granules were intensely PAS-positive and resisted diastase digestion. The nuclei were usually diminished in size, at times appearing pyknotic and dense. This characteristic was not consistent, however, and some nuclei were of normal size with pale, uniform chromatin distribution.

The involved lobules were usually enlarged, often to three to four times the size of uninvolved lobules. Within lobules the acini were expanded, with the ballooned, clear epithelial cells assuming a cuboidal shape about dilated lumina.

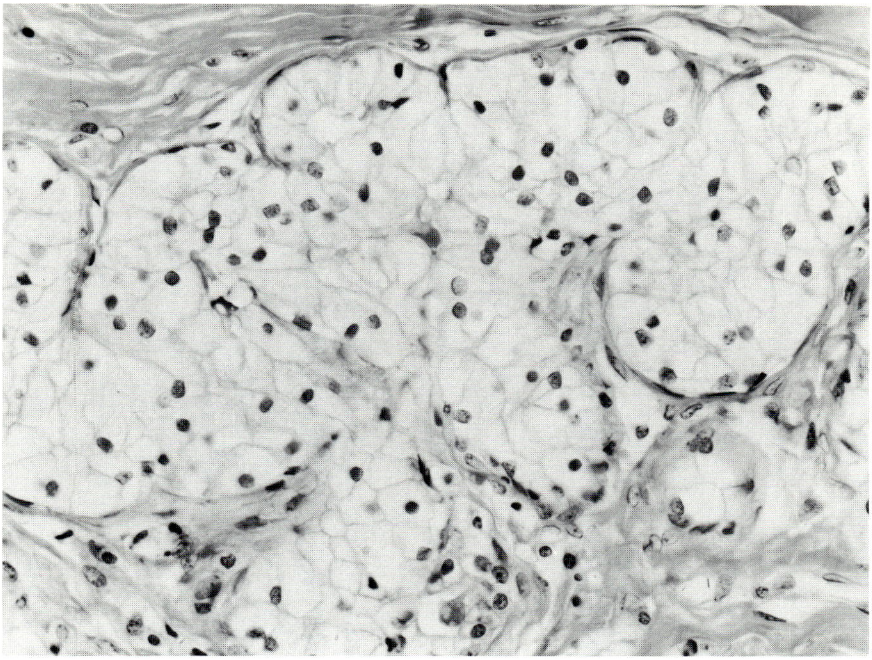

FIG. 1. Mammary lobule comprised of epithelial cells having abundant clear cytoplasm and bland nuclei. H&E. ×320.

Luminal dilatation of acini or terminal ducts was most marked when seen in association with prominent cytoplasmic granules (Fig. 3). Myoepithelial cells were often, although not invariably, evident beneath the epithelial lining cells.

A second pattern of clear-cell change was present within lobules and terminal ducts, and involved cells which lay beneath the epithelial lining cells (Fig. 4). The affected cells were assumed to be myoepithelial cells by virtue of their location. The cytoplasmic and nuclear changes seen were similar to those described above, but prominent cytoplasmic granules were not seen. The epithelial lining cells overlying the affected cells showed varying degrees of attenuation from field to field, and in some acini were not evident. The two patterns were usually found together in the same breast tissue, and intermediate areas were invariably present.

Two other types of benign breast epithelium showed unusual histologic changes in the patients under study. The first type was apocrine metaplasia. The apocrine cells of 10 patients exhibited cytoplasmic vacuolization. When marked, this resulted in a "clear-cell" appearance very similar to that present in lobular epithelial cells of the same tissue. Cytoplasmic granules of varying size and random location were also occasionally dispersed within the apocrine cells. These were distinct from the so-called apical bodies which are commonly seen in cells of apocrine metaplasia.

The second type of benign epithelium that demonstrated histologic alteration

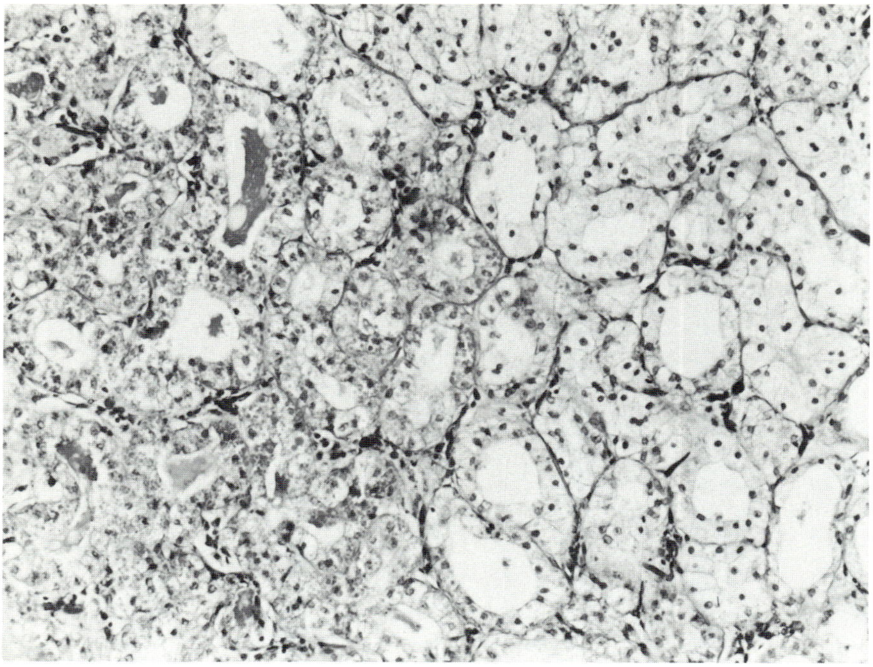

FIG. 2. Acini within an expanded lobule showing luminal dilatation. The epithelial cells on the left show prominent coarse cytoplasmic granules associated with eosinophilic material within lumina. H&E. ×160.

was sclerosing adenosis. Here cytoplasmic clearing and nuclear attenuation comparable to that seen in ordinary lobules were observed. Cytoplasmic granules were occasionally also seen within the cells, but never to a marked degree in sclerosing adenosis.

The distribution of the clear-cell changes varied widely within the tissue examined in each case. Occasionally only limited areas were affected, but more commonly the changes were widespread. The myoepithelial pattern of change particularly tended to be widespread and extensive. Of 13 cases in which bilateral breast tissue was available for examination, 11 showed the histologic changes in both breasts.

Twenty-three patients in this study had had a malignant primary tumor of the breast at some point in their course. Slides of these tumors were available for 22 of the patients and were studied for evidence of alterations similar to those observed in the benign epithelium. Cytoplasmic changes consisting of clearing or vacuolization were evident in 17 cases. In most cases these changes within the tumor were focal; they were more widespread in five cases. Both duct and lobular carcinomas showed the changes, but they were more pronounced in the latter neoplasm, and were of greater degree than the cytoplasmic pallor frequently seen in lobular carcinoma. All five tumors in which no cytoplasmic changes were present were infiltrating duct carcinomas.

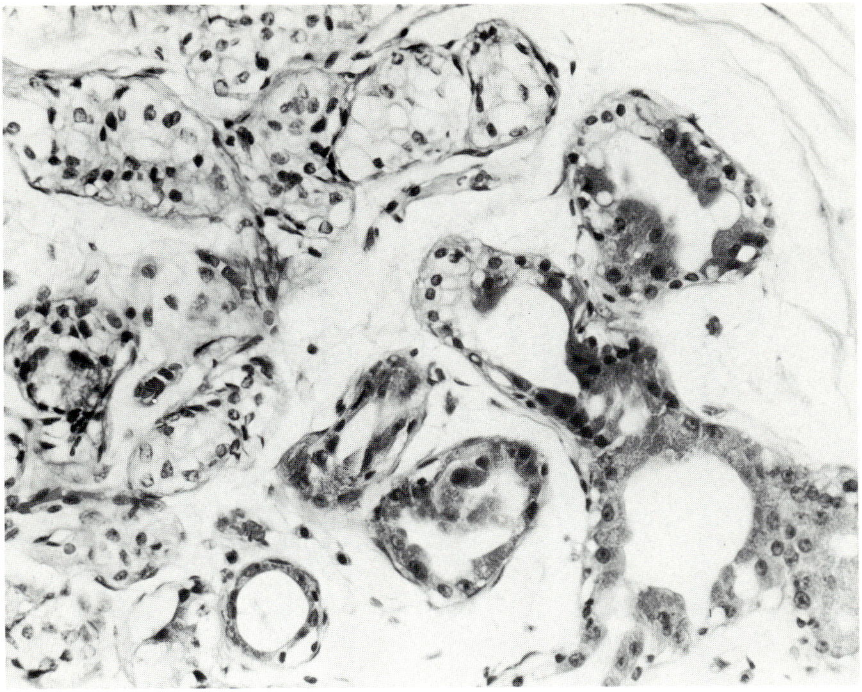

FIG. 3. Acini and terminal ducts, with the epithelium about the dilated lumina of the latter containing fine cytoplasmic granules. H&E. ×250.

Ultrastructural Observations

The most consistent finding by electron microscopy was the presence of cytoplasmic granules. These corresponded to the granules seen by light microscopy. But, whereas only two of the six cases selected for ultrastructural analysis showed these cytoplasmic granules by light-microscopy, all six contained granules upon electron microscopic examination. The granules were of two types which varied considerably in size and general configuration. The more common type was membrane delimited and contained internal, electron-dense beading (Fig. 5). These granules were generally round, but at times assumed an oblong or tear-shaped configuration. They varied in size from granules larger than a nucleus to others smaller than mitochondria. The second granule type was seen only occasionally. It was dense and amorphous with no internal structure, and when seen was invariably present with the membrane-delimited granules.

Within the acini containing the "clear cells," both epithelial and myoepithelial cells were identified. The latter were characterized by their oblong nuclear shape, by myofilaments, and by hemidesmosomes. Both cell types were noted to contain cytoplasmic granules, but these were more abundant in the epithelial-type cells. An occasional third type of cell was seen which demonstrated morphologic features intermediate between those of the myoepithelial and the epithelial cells.

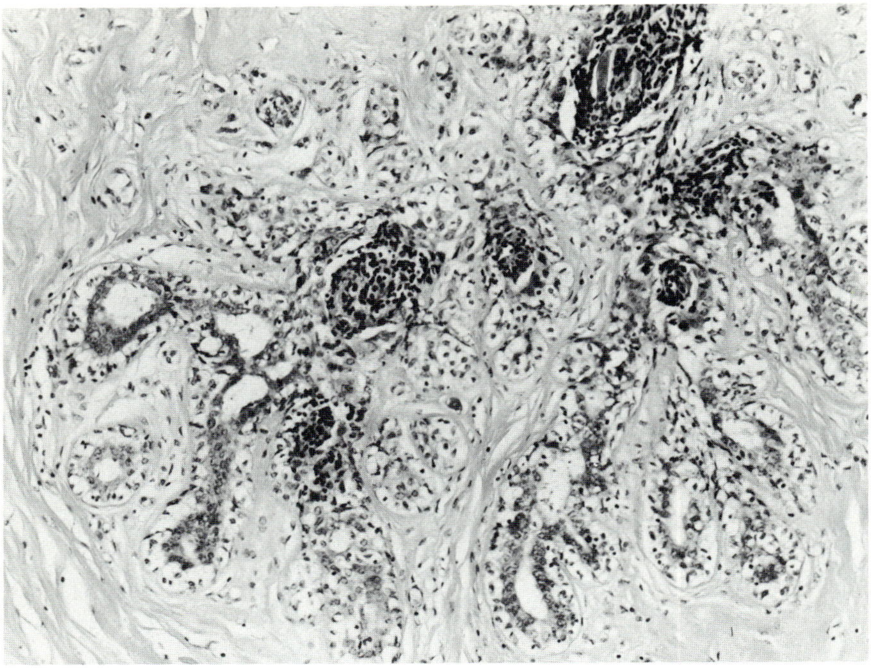

FIG. 4. Prominent cytoplasmic clearing of apparent myoepithelial cells of terminal ducts and lobular acini. H&E. ×128.

Granules within the cytoplasm of clear cells were often contained within vacuoles which appeared to be associated with the Golgi apparatus, although the preservation of the cells was not sufficient to confirm this. Much of the cytoplasm was rarefied and tenuous in most of the cells, but the exact nature of this change was not evident. Frequently it appeared that the rarefied texture of the cytoplasm might have resulted from the loss of some cytoplasmic substance during tissue fixation, or from retraction of the granule substance.

Several cells demonstrated a ballooning of the outer nuclear membrane, with consequent bleb formation resulting from an increase in size of the nuclear envelope cistern. Within these blebs were often encountered granules having the same morphology as those seen within the cytoplasm (Fig. 6).

Electron microscopy was undertaken on one duct carcinoma which showed "clear cell" change. The preservation of this tumor was poor, but it was evident that membrane-delimited cytoplasmic granules, with the same appearance as those in the benign tissues, were present.

DISCUSSION

We have studied a cellular change of lobular and duct epithelium consisting of marked clearing of the cytoplasm, with frequent attenuation or shrinkage of the nucleus. By light microscopy, this change was most often present in lobules, but

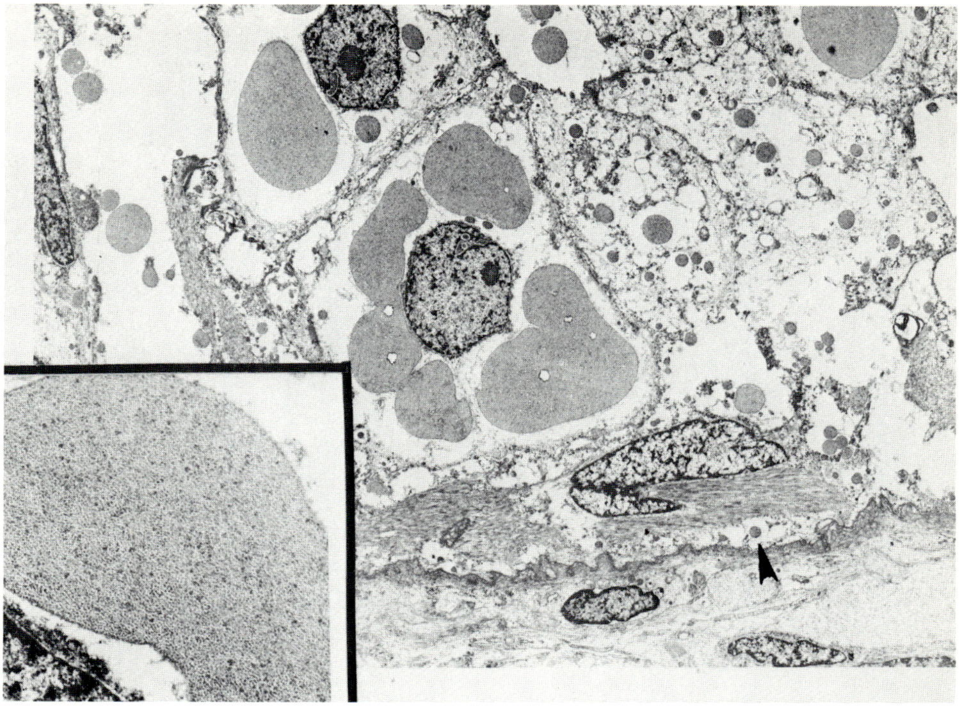

FIG. 5. Electron micrograph illustrating cytoplasmic granules of varying size. Granules are present within both epithelial and myoepithelial cells (arrow localizes a small granule in a myoepithelial cell). ×3,900. Inset: Fine detail of a cytoplasmic granule with internal beading and a delimiting membrane. ×10,350.

commonly involved terminal ducts as well. Eosinophilic cytoplasmic granules of varying size were frequently present in the cytoplasm, and this was associated with luminal secretion.

Ultrastructural studies demonstrated the presence of two types of cytoplasmic granules within epithelial cells and myoepithelial cells, as well as within cells having morphologic features intermediate to those of the former two cell types. The more frequent of these granule types had the same appearance as the secretory product demonstrated by Wellings et al.[1] in the mammary glands of pregnant and lactating rats. Similar granules have also been demonstrated in human breast tissue and have been interpreted as secretory product.[2,3] A second, less common granule identified in this study was characterized by an amorphous, electron-dense substance lacking internal structure. This substance is identical to a second secretory product seen by Wellings and associates[1] in lactating rats. In a companion study,[4] Wellings et al. established the chemical nature of the two granule types by appropriate digestion studies. The membrane-delimited granules were sensitive to tryptic digestion, and were therefore identified as comprising a protein product. The dense, amorphous granules were sensitive to methanol-ethyl ether dissolution and were thus identified as comprising a lipid substance. In the current study it is possible that most of the lipid moiety was dissolved by the formalin-fixation and paraffin-embedding pro-

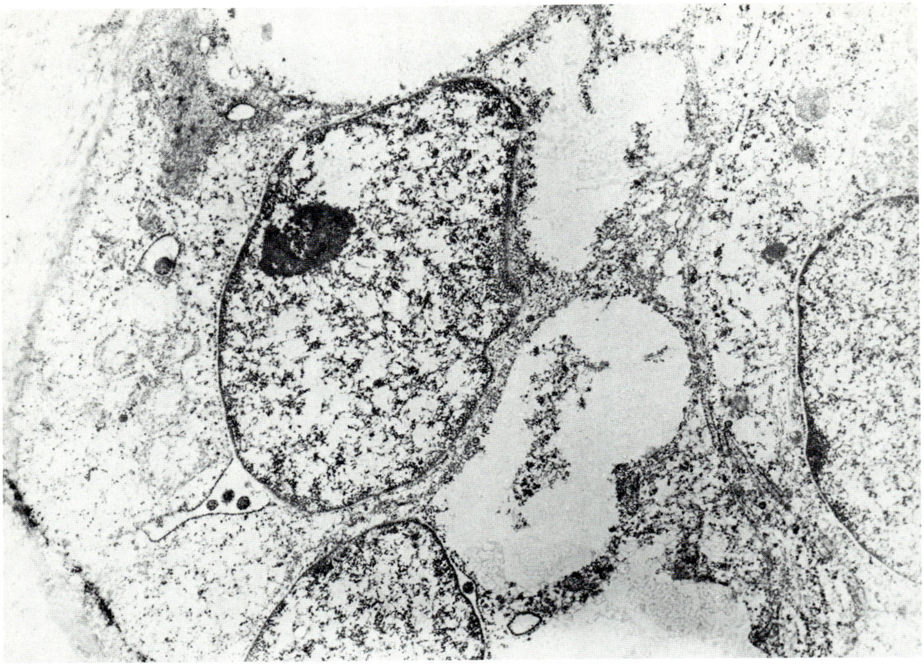

FIG. 6. Bleb, containing granules, formed by the outer nuclear membrane. ×10,350.

cesses. This would account for the relative paucity of this moiety as compared with the protein-granule type material. It is also possible that much of the "clear-cell" appearance of the lesion under study results from a residual cytoplasmic volume previously occupied by lipid substance.

The significance of the reduplication of the nuclear envelope as seen ultrastructurally in clear cells is not apparent. Such changes have been previously demonstrated, and have been attributed to a viral-induced alteration,[5-7] but viral particles were not seen in this study. Other investigators have assumed such nuclear-envelope changes to be normal and perhaps a mechanism of nucleocytoplasmic exchanges.[8,9]

Despite a similarity by light microscopic examination between some of the cells showing clear-cell change and the cells of apocrine metaplasia, the ultrastructural features did not confirm this. The increased numbers and size of mitochondria, and the dense homogeneous, apical granules characteristic of apocrine metaplasia[10-12] were not present in the clear cells we observed.

The apparent secretory activity within the cells we studied raised the question of either endogenous or exogenous hormonal activity in these patients. It seems unlikely that exogenous hormones are responsible for the activity, since only eight of the patients in the study had ever received such agents, and none were receiving them at the time of biopsy. Furthermore, we have observed clear-cell changes in biopsies obtained in the 1930s and 1940s, prior to the availability of exogenous hormones.

The question of an endogenous hormonal stimulus inducing the histopathologic changes described here is much more difficult to address, and would require extensive hormone analyses that were not done in our patients. It is possible, however, that the epithelium in some individuals is inordinately sensitive, and that slight amounts of hormone, not causing systemic effects, could produce these cytologic changes.

The association of primary breast carcinoma with the lesion being described must be interpreted cautiously. The patient population studied was treated because carcinoma was suspected clinically. The relationship of the lesion to breast neoplasia, or the incidence of the change in either benign or malignant lesions of the breast, cannot be absolutely determined by this study. Furthermore, the association of the lesion with any particular age group is biased by the age distribution of the patients treated. It is perhaps significant, however, that only 1 of the 31 women in this study was under 40 years of age, including those patients with benign disease.

Both cytoplasmic clearing and protein-secretory product were demonstrated in myoepithelial cells and epithelial cells in the cases we studied. The relationship between these cell types in the human breast and in other organs remains incompletely understood.[3,10,11] Many ultrastructural investigations of breast tissue have demonstrated cells with features intermediate to those of myoepithelial and epithelial cells, leading to the suggestion that the two cell types either have a common progenitor or have the capacity of undergoing transition from one to the other. Murad et al. have demonstrated a transition of myoepithelial cells to secretory epithelial cells in pregnant rats.[13] Such a transformation has also been illustrated in sweat glands.[14] Tannenbaum et al.[3] illustrated a number of structural and functional similarities between myoepithelial and epithelial cells, including the presence of structures resembling secretory granules. The present study further illustrates similarities between these two cell types, and demonstrates cytoplasmic structures which we interpret as comprising secretory product in both types. Cells with features intermediate between those of the myoepithelial and the epithelial cell were also identified. While the genesis of clear-cell change remains undetermined it does not appear to be directly related to breast neoplasia, nor does the change appear to represent a premalignant change.

ACKNOWLEDGMENTS

The authors wish to acknowledge Ms. Margaret Uibel and Mr. John Braslin for photography, Ms. Margaret Koonce and Ms. Michaele Kashgarian for their electron microscopy assistance, and Mrs. Susan Kekacs for typing the manuscript.

REFERENCES

1. Wellings SR, Deome KB, Pitelka DR: Electron microscopy of milk secretion in the mammary gland of the C3H/Crgl mouse. I. Cytomorphology of the prelactating and the lactating mouse. J Natl Cancer Inst 25:393, 1960

2. Waugh D, van der Hoeven E: Fine structure of the human female breast. Lab Invest 11:220, 1962
3. Tannenbaum M, Weiss M, Marx AJ: Ultrastructure of the human mammary ductule. Cancer 23:958, 1969
4. Wellings SR, Grunbaum BW, Deome KB: Electron microscopy of milk secretion in the mammary gland of the C3H/Crgl mouse. II. Identification of fat and protein particles in milk and in tissue. J Natl Cancer Inst 25:423, 1960
5. Gregg MB, Morgan C: Reduplication of nuclear membranes in HeLa cells infected with adenovirus. J Biophys Biochem Cytol 6:539, 1959
6. Patrizi G, Middelkamp JN, Reed CA: Reduplication of nuclear membranes in tissue culture cells infected with guinea pig cytomegalovirus. Am J Pathol 50:779, 1967
7. Shipkey FH, Erlandson RH, Bailey RB, et al.: Viral biographies. II. Growth of Herpes simplex virus in tissue culture. Exp Mol Pathol 6:39, 1967
8. Pomerat CM, Lefeber CG, Smith McD: Quantitative cine analysis of cell organoid activity. Ann NY Acad Sci 58:1311, 1954
9. Baud CA: Nuclear membrane and permeability. In Seno S, Cowdry EV (eds): In Intracellular Membrane Structure. Okayama, Okayama Press, 1963, p. 323
10. Fisher ER: Ultrastructure of the human breast and its disorders. Am J Clin Pathol 66:291, 1976
11. Ozzello L: Ultrastructure of the human mammary gland. Pathol Annu 6:1, 1971
12. Archer F, Omar M: Pink cell (oncocytic) metaplasia in a fibroadenoma of the human breast: Electron microscopic observations. J Pathol 99:119, 1969
13. Murad TM, von Hamm E: Ultrastructure of myoepithelial cells in human mammary gland tumors. Cancer 21:1137, 1968
14. Hibbs RG: The fine structure of human eccrine sweat glands. Am J Anat 103:201, 1958

PERIODIC DISK-LIKE STRUCTURES OF THE LOOP OF HENLE: DESCRIPTION OF A NEWLY RECOGNIZED ANATOMIC NETWORK

ROBERT R. BELLIVEAU

The following description concerns a heretofore unrecognized anatomic network located in the basement membrane of the loop of Henle. This network is not apparent with the H&E stain, but is clearly visualized with the periodic acid–Schiff (PAS) stain. The network has not been previously described by light-or electron microscopy with regard to its extent or components, but portions of the individual components of the network have been described in electron microscopic studies.

The basement membrane of the thin limbs of the loop of Henle has been described[1] as being "segmentally covered with multiple dense layers of ground substance." Referring to these multiple dense layers, a subsequent publication stated that "they rarely surround a tubule completely, but usually cover only one portion of the circumference,"[2] and that "such multilayering is not seen around collecting tubules." McDonald et al.,[3] studying the effects of experimental potassium deficiency, stated that "the most obvious lesion was in the basement membrane of the thin segment of the loop of Henle. This membrane was found to be thickened and fibrillar." "In some areas, thickening was very marked and the basilar membrane looked like a meshwork." Bulger et al.[4] stated that "The basement membrane generally consisted of one thick layer of moderately dense material. The thickness of this layer varied considerably even along the length seen in a given picture. In other regions, the basement membrane consisted of several thick layers." In a subsequent publication, Bulger[5] noted simply that "the basement membrane is of variable thickness."

Tisher[6] wrote that "the basement membrane of a thin limb segment varies greatly in thickness from species to species, and in many animals is multilayered. The possible physiological significance of the variations in basement membrane structure, if any, is presently unknown. The thin limb cells in the human kidney have . . . a thicker basement membrane." Chatelanant[7] stated that "the human basement membrane, thicker than that of the rat kidney, seems stratified.'' Bloom and Fawcett,[8] in their Textbook of Histology, simply noted that ''the epithelium (of the loop of Henle) rests upon a moderately thick basement lamina.'' Rhodin,[9] in his Textbook of Histology, made no mention of the basement membrane of the loop of Henle. Kaissling and Kriz[10] described the thin limbs of the short loops of Henle thus: ''Basically the epithelium is wrapped by a thin, single layered, uninterrupted basal lamina.'' Schwartz and Venketachalam,[11] in a detailed description of the thin limbs of Henle, made no reference to the basement membrane. The Mollendorf Handbuch der Mikroskopischen Anatomie des Menschen stated that ''The basement membrane is made of a homogeneous transparent membrane and this membrane on the very outside has a rough textured covering to strengthen it and connect it to the interstitium,''[12] but no mention was made of any focal thickenings of the basement membrane.

In summary, a review of the literature, including original articles as well as standard texts, indicates that investigators have determined that the basement membrane of the loop of Henle is variably thickened and focally multilayered, but there is no exact description of the size, shape, and extent of these thickened multilayered areas or of their interrelationship with each other. This report presents the light-microscopic findings of the size, shape, and interrelationship of these structures which have not previously been adequately described and are presently not generally understood.

MATERIALS AND METHODS

Thirty-five kidneys were selected from three different sources. Ten were from patients on whom autopsies were performed at Southern Nevada Memorial Hospital. The kidneys were taken from 8 male and 2 female cadavers of persons ranging from 10 to 83 years of age; these kidneys were selected from patients who did not have significant clinical or pathologic evidence of renal disease. Five other kidneys selected were removed at surgery for adenocarcinoma (four) or for a penetrating gunshot wound (one). These came from 3 males and 2 females, ranging from 25 to 51 years of age. Twenty kidneys came from patients autopsied by the local medical examiner. These individuals died as a result of accident or murder; there were 12 males and 8 females, ranging from 2 months to 40 years of age. The kidneys were stained with periodic acid–Schiff, phosphotungstic acid hematoxylin (PTAH), and H&E, and were examined microscopically, with special attention given to the basement membrane of the loop of Henle.

RESULTS

Figure 1 represents a longitudinal section through a loop of Henle, which demonstrates relatively regular periodic thickening of the basement membrane. This longitudinal section demonstrates the thickenings on opposite walls of the loop of Henle. Figures 2 and 3 represent more tangential sections of the loop, which give

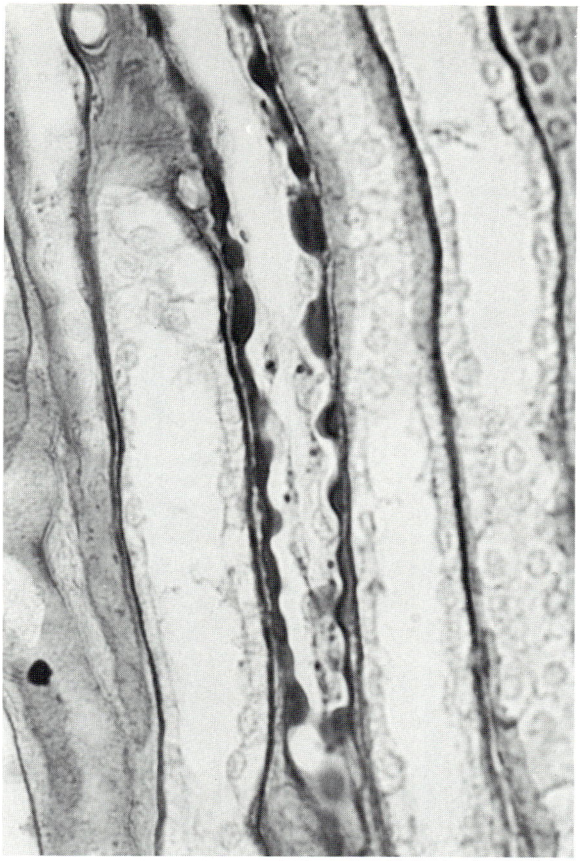

FIG. 1. Periodic nodular thickenings of the Henle-loop basement membranes are clearly seen. PAS. ×650.

the appearance of a three-dimensional view. These views clearly demonstrate that the thickenings of the basement membrane have a round-to-ovoid shape and comprise an extensive network involving the tubule. The essentially round-to-ovoid disks range from 10 to 15 μ in maximal diameter and are usually separated by nonthickened areas that range from 5 to 10 μ. The number of disks present circumferentially at different levels of the tubules is variable. Multiple sections taken perpendicular to the loops of Henle reveal tubules which usually had five to seven disks situated around the tubule (Fig. 4). The disks were never identified within the cortical portion of the kidneys, nor were they seen in the most distal portions of the collecting tubules. They were essentially limited to the outer-stripe and the inner-stripe regions of the medulla. Most of the disks were located on tubules having the flat epithelium which characterizes the loop of Henle. Occasionally the disks were present on portions of tubules having tall epithelium, consistent with either the distal (straight) portions of the proximal tubules or the thick portions of the ascending loop of Henle. However, utilizing the PAS stain and light microscopy, it could

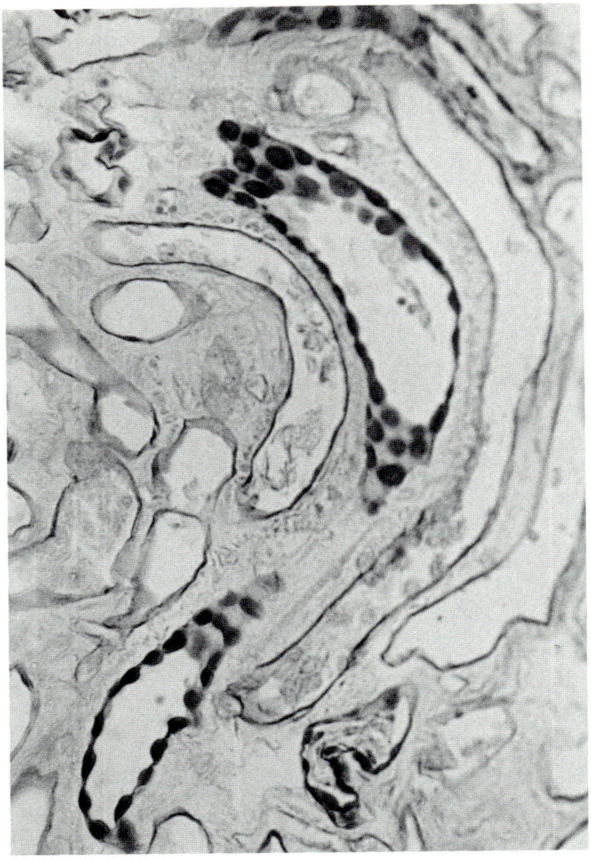

FIG. 2. Slightly tangential section of a tubule reveals that the basement membrane thickenings are disk-like structures. PAS. × 500.

not be definitely determined whether or not these cells with taller epithelium were the proximal portions of collecting tubules. All kidneys from the 35 patients, except that from the 2-month-old child, demonstrated these same disk-like structures in most Henle loops, although it sometimes required some searching to find sections of the kidney that gave the appearance of the three-dimensional view. In contrast, it was relatively simple to find longitudinal sections through the loops that demonstrated thickened disks on opposite walls of the loop. It should be emphasized that the disks were never seen on sections stained with H&E, and that they stained less strongly with PTAH than with PAS.

The electron microscopy on all kidney specimens was done on material reprocessed from the original paraffin blocks used to illustrate the light-microscopic findings. Two well-preserved disks are demonstrated in Figure 5. Their appearance is the same as that of basement membrane, with a faint cleavage line of less electron density between the disk and the tubular basement membrane.

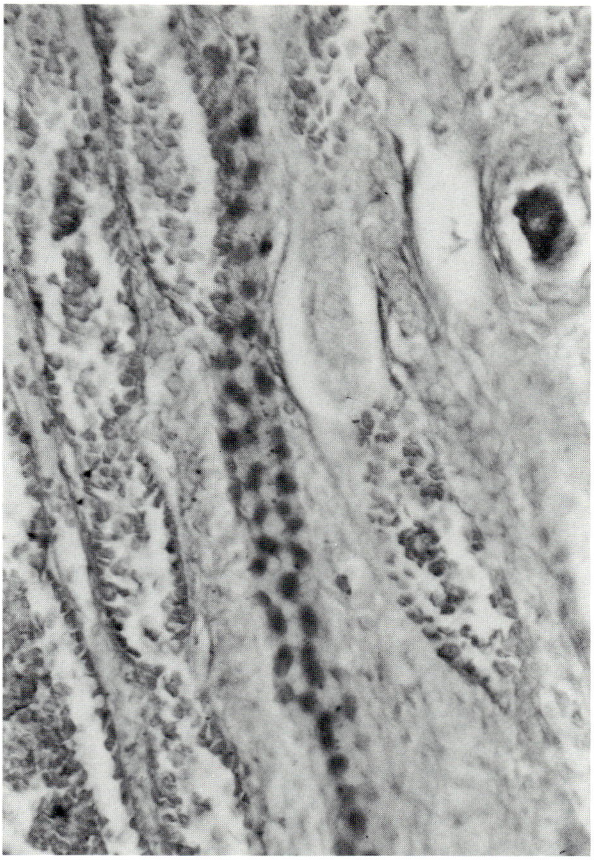

FIG. 3. Tangential section of another Henle-loop tubule shows arrangement of disk-like structures. ×500.

DISCUSSION

The usefulness of PAS and PTAH staining to bring out the hitherto undescribed thickened disks of the tubular basement membranes of the loop of Henle is evident. McManus,[13] in a report devoted entirely to the histologic evaluation of kidney tissue stained with periodic acid, stated simply that "the basement membranes of glomeruli and tubules are so well shown by this technique that it is proposed as a method of choice," but he made no reference to the disks. The electron microscopic recognition of the variable thickening of the basement membrane has not improved understanding the overall relationship of this network of disks.

Although these disks were not identified on basement membranes other than those of the loop of Henle, they are not necessarily specific for this segment of the nephron. If they are present elsewhere in significantly smaller numbers, an exhaustive search of a large number of kidney sections may be necessary before their

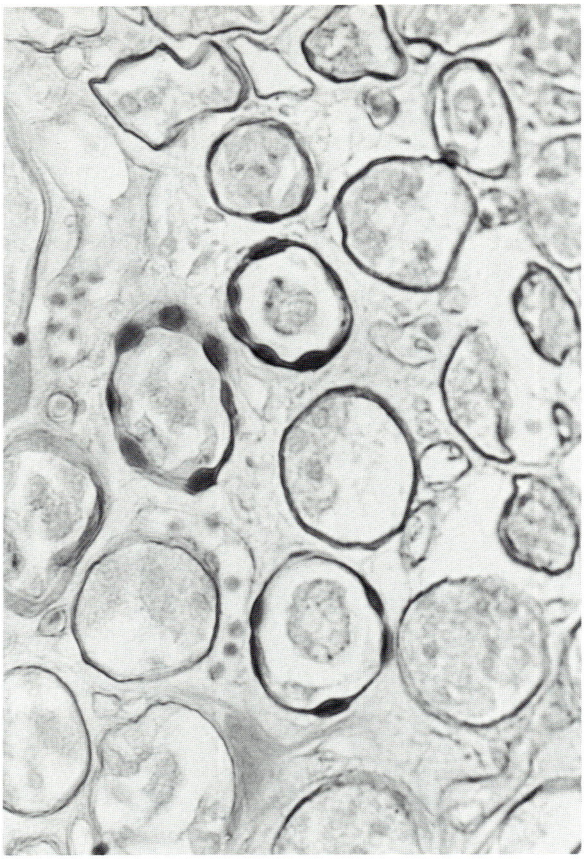

FIG. 4. Cross-section of tubules demonstrates five to seven disks around the circumference of each. ×500.

absence can be averred with any surety. The function of this network of disks—if any—must remain speculative. In view of current knowledge of this portion of the nephron, one is tempted to postulate that the thickened areas of the basement membrane might serve to slow fluid transport into and out of the loop of Henle. If the disks network does in fact have a function, one might expect hypertrophy, hyperplasia, atrophy, degeneration, or other pathologic processes to occur with different pathologic conditions. A study is presently underway to examine this possibility.

SUMMARY

A light-microscopic examination of sections of kidneys from 35 patients was performed utilizing the PAS stain. A previously unrecognized anatomic network of the basement membrane of the loop of Henle is described. The network consists of

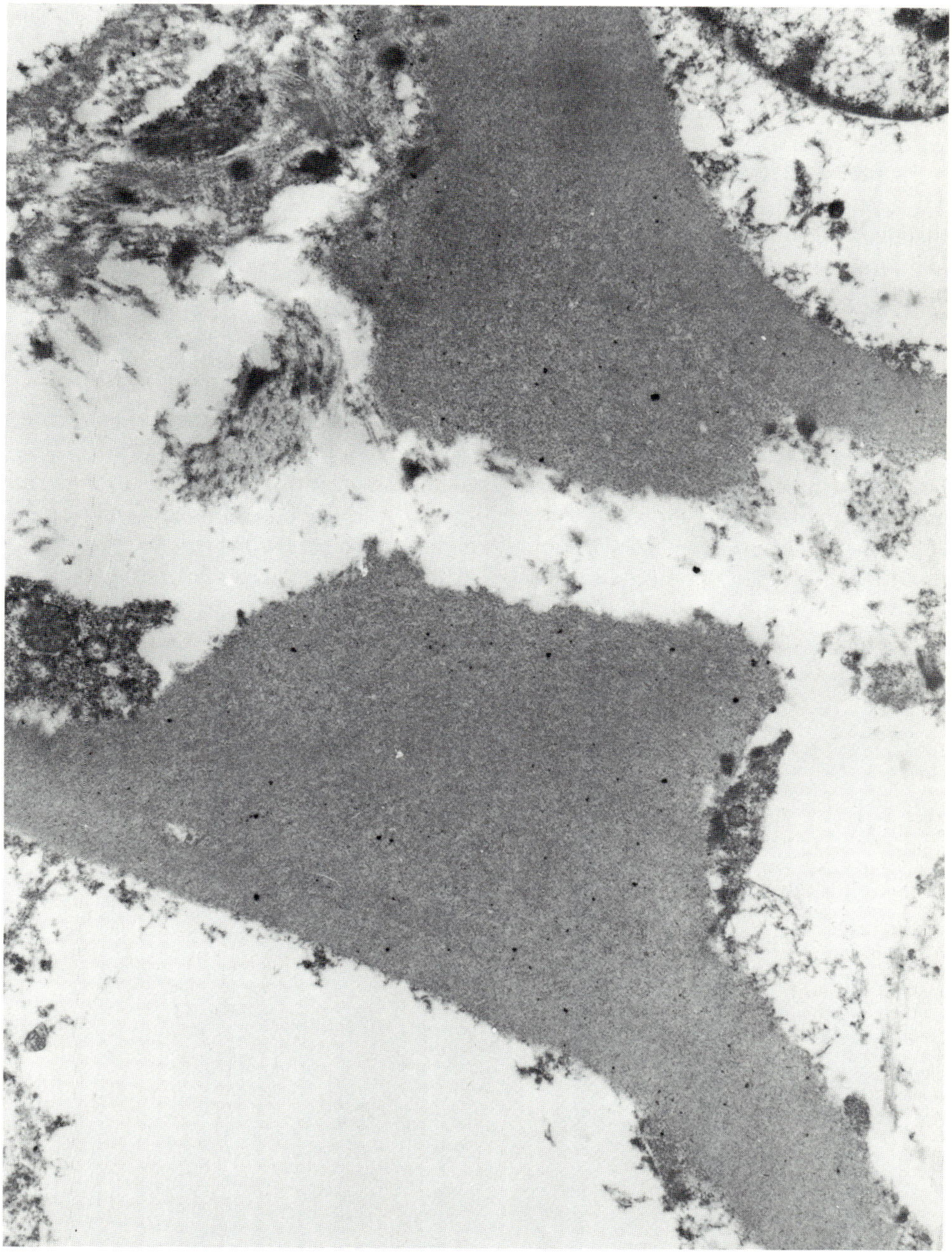

FIG. 5. Electron microscopy demonstrates the disks and a slight cleavage plane between them and the Henle-loop tubular basement membrane. ×12,250.

10-to 15-μ-diameter, round-to-ovoid, disk-like areas of thickening of the basement membrane occurring along most loops of Henle and appearing to be present on both thin and thick portions. These disks are present around the entire circumference of the tubule and are separated by areas of 5 to 10 μ of nonthickened basement membranes. Their function, if any, is not presently understood.

ACKNOWLEDGMENTS

Electron microscopy was performed by Dr. Claude Biava, Department of Pathology, University of California, San Francisco.

REFEREE'S COMMENT

To my best knowledge and belief the change described by Dr. Belliveau, that is, thickening of the basement membranes of Henle's loops, represents a new finding. Dr. Belliveau is to be commended for this acute observation. Review of his material and of our own cases shows that the tubules with thick basement membranes are found with varying frequency in individual cases, from few or none to many, and that they are focally distributed. Moreover, there is variation in thickness from nor-

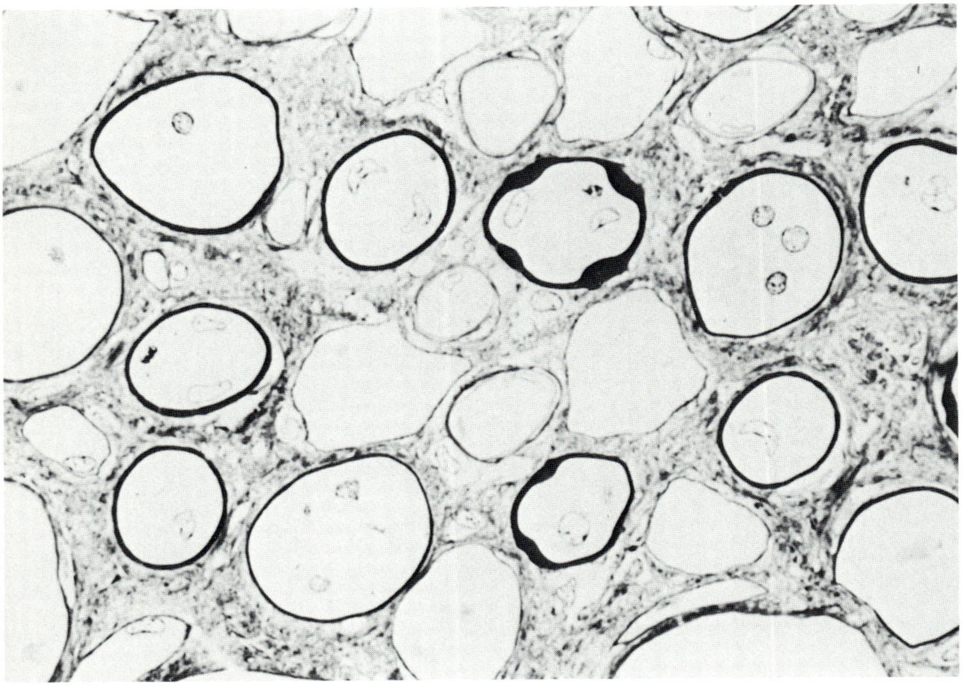

FIG. 6.

mal, to moderately, diffusely, or segmentally thickened, and finally, to projections described by Dr. Belliveau. This variation could very well represent progression of the basement membrane changes. It is best seen in thin sections (2μ) and is illustrated in Figure 6 from one of Dr. Belliveau's cases. The focal distribution and indications of progressive thickening suggest that this is not a normal finding but rather a pathologic change. The cause of this change is not presently apparent, but further studies might demonstrate its origin and its functional significance.

Jacob Churg

REFERENCES

1. Osvaldo L, Latta H: The thin limbs of the loop of Henle. J Ultrastruct Res 15:144–168, 1966
2. Osvaldo L, Latta H: Interstitial cells of the renal medulla. J Ultrastruct Res 15:589–613, 1966
3. MacDonald MK, Sabout MS, Lambie AT, Robson JS: The nephropathy of experimental potassium deficiency: An electron microscopic study. Q J Exp Physiol 47:262–272, 1962
4. Bulger RE, Tisher CC, Myers CH, Trump BF: Human renal ultrastructure II: The thin limb of Henle's loop and the interstitium in healthy individuals. Lab Invest 16:124–141, 1967
5. Bulger R: Kidney morphology. In Straus and Welt's Diseases of the Kidney, ed 3. Boston, Little, Brown, 1979, p 25
6. Tisher CC: Anatomy of the kidney. In Brenner B, Rector F (eds): The Kidney. Philadelphia, Saunders, 1976, p 37
7. Chatelanat F: Anatomy of the kidney. In Hamberger J, Crosnier J, Grünfeld J (eds): Nephrology. New York, Wiley, 1979, p 22
8. Bloom W, Fawcett DW: A Textbook of Histology, ed 9. Philadelphia, Saunders, 1968, p 662
9. Rhodin AGJ: Histology, a Textbook and Atlas. New York, Oxford University Press, 1974
10. Kaissling B, Kriz W: Advances in Anatomy, Embryology and Cell Biology: Structural Analysis of the Rabbit Kidney, volume 56. Berlin, Springer-Verlag, 1979
11. Schwartz MM, Venkatachalam MA: Structural differences in thin limbs of Henle: Physiological implications. Kidney Int 6:193–208, 1974
12. von Mollendorff W: Der Exkretionsapparat. In Handbuch der Mikroskopischen Anatomie des Menschen, Vol 7. Berlin, Springer, 1930, p 61
13. McManus JFA: The periodic acid routine applied to the kidney. Am J Pathol 24:643–653, 1948

THE PATHOLOGY OF TUBEROUS SCLEROSIS

BRUCE L. BENDER AND EDUARDO J. YUNIS

The first recognizable description of a case of tuberous sclerosis was published by von Recklinghausen in 1862.[1] He reported a neonate who died after taking a few breaths and was found to have multiple "myomata" of the heart and "a great number of scleroses" of the brain. Eighteen years later, Bourneville coined the name tuberous sclerosis, which refers to the potato-like thickenings of the cerebral cortex characteristic of this disease.[2] In papers that followed, Bourneville and Brissaud further defined the clinical and pathologic findings associated with tuberous sclerosis.[3,4]

During the same period, Balzer and Menetrier[5] redescribed some previously reported[6] cutaneous lesions of the face and scalp as "sebaceous adenoma".[5] In 1890, Pringle described adenoma sebaceum in a 25-year-old mildly mentally-disturbed woman and noted decreased intelligence in several other patients with this cutaneous finding.[7]

In 1905, Perusini[8] reported the association of the cerebral, renal, and cardiac lesions of tuberous sclerosis and "cutaneous adenomas." Finally, in 1908, Vogt[9] linked the finding of sebaceous adenomas, mental deficiency, and epilepsy into the classic triad that has been used to diagnose tuberous sclerosis for the last 70 years.

During this century, the protean pathologic manifestations of tuberous sclerosis have been catalogued. Ocular symptoms were first described by Campbell[10] in 1905. Marcus[11] demonstrated osseous lesions radiologically in 1924. By 1933, almost all of the lesions currently considered part of the tuberous sclerosis complex had been described in association with it; these were summarized in tabular form by Van der Hoeve[12] and included cortical tumefaction, ventricular tumors, heterotopias of the white matter, cysts of the central nervous system, cysts and tumors of the eye, intrathoracic tumors, cysts and tumors of bone including defects of the skull, deformity of the vertebral column, and multiple nevi and tumors of the skin. Diverse lesions of the endocrine glands, spina bifida, and ectopia of the testis had also been reported in patients with tuberous sclerosis.[12]

Although new lesions are occasionally reported,[13] the current outline of the tuberous sclerosis complex is not much longer than that compiled almost 50 years ago.[12] Most of the intervening reports have had new information about the nature of previously described lesions[13-28] or have addressed themselves to the question of the pathogenesis of the complex.[29-37] It is our purpose to review systematically the pathology of tuberous sclerosis and comment upon the various theories of pathogenesis that have been proposed.[29-37]

INCIDENCE AND GENETICS

Tuberous sclerosis is a rare disorder, with an incidence in the general population estimated at approximately 1 case per 50,000 to 150,000 persons. There is a familial history of the disease in about half of the patients,[38] with autosomal dominant behavior and variable expression.[38,39] Gunther and Penrose[38] proposed a modifier gene, the existence of which was supported by Marshall et al.[39]

The cases without a family history are assumed to be due to mutation. This theory is strengthened by the minimal reproduction of severely affected patients. Mutation rates of 8[38] and 10.5[40] per million have been calculated. The occurrence of the disorder is not related to advanced maternal age or consanguinity. The disease occurs in all races at approximately the same rate.[41,42]

LESIONS

The lesions included in the tuberous sclerosis complex are summarized in Table 1. Although every organ in the body has been reported involved, the brain, skin, eye, heart, and kidneys are the classic sites. Most symptoms are ascribable to central nervous system or cardiac lesions.

The lesions of tuberous sclerosis are hamartomas or collections of abnormal cells, the nature of which varies from organ to organ. Many of them, including angiomyolipoma of the kidney, facial angiofibromas, parungual fibroma, lymphangiomyomatosis, splenic hemangioma, and hepatic hamartoma are vascular and mesenchymal malformations. The central nervous system lesions, phakomata, cardiac rhabdomyomata, renal cysts, and focal histiocytoid cells of the spleen consist of collections of distinctly abnormal but relatively uniform cells. All of the lesions are either slow-growing or static.

Symptoms generally result from mass effects rather than from the invasion and destruction of surrounding tissue. Occasionally, one of the vascular lesions is the site of hemorrhage. Many of the malformations that have been reported intermittently in patients with tuberous sclerosis are probably either incidental findings or random expressions of general tissue dysplasia in these patients.

Brain

Central nervous system lesions are responsible for the epilepsy and mental retardation that comprise two-thirds of the classic diagnostic triad of tuberous sclerosis. These findings are spectacular, and have led to the common impression that all pa-

TABLE 1. The Tuberous Sclerosis Complex and Associated Lesions

- Central nervous system
  - Cortical tubers
  - Heterotopias in the white matter
  - Subependymal nodules
  - Malformations
  - Corpus callosum dysplasia*
  - Spina bifida*
  - Syringomyelia*
  - Decreased pituitary eosinophilic cells*
- Eyes
  - Retinal
    - Hamartomas
    - Pigmentary defects*
  - Nonretinal
    - Papilledema and optic nerve atrophy*
    - Disc anomaly*
    - Coloboma*
    - Megalocornea*
    - Keratoconus*
    - Iris sector depigmentation*
    - Enophthalmos*
  - Eyelids
    - Adenoma sebaceum
    - Vitiligo*
    - Poliosis*
    - Epicanthal folds*
- Skin
  - Facial angiofibroma
    - collagenous plaques, forehead
  - Hypopigmented areas
  - Shagreen patch
  - Parungual fibroma
  - Café-au-lait spots*
  - Cutaneous nodules*
- Kidneys
  - Cysts
  - Malformations*
- Heart
  - Rhabdomyoma
- Lungs
  - Lymphangiomyomatosis
- Reticuloendothelial
  - Spleen
    - Vascular hamartoma
    - Focal histiocytoid cells
  - Lymph Nodes
    - Lymphangiomyomatosis
- Skeleton
  - Pagetoid changes, skull
  - Cysts, phalanges
  - Periosteal new bone, metatarsals
- Liver
  - Hamartoma
- Oral Cavity
  - Fibromas*
  - Enamel defects*
- Other
  - Vascular hamartoma of intestines, genitals
  - Genital hypoplasia*
  - Pancreatic adenoma*
  - Adrenal fatty tumor*
  - Paraganglioma*

*Indicates presumably nonspecific or incidental associations.

tients with tuberous sclerosis have severe mental deficiency. However, it is likely that the disease is not diagnosed in mildly affected patients.[43,44] In addition, it has been demonstrated that at least one-third of patients have no mental retardation,[38,45,46] and that almost all of those who are mentally retarded have epileptic seizures,[40,47] with the implication that the mental retardation is usually a result of seizure activity and interruption of learning rather than a separate manifestation of central nervous system lesions. Conversely, patients with spontaneous or therapeutic cessation of seizures may have continued mental deterioration.[48] The brains of patients with tuberous sclerosis are usually within the normal weight range.

Cortical tubers are present in almost all cases of tuberous sclerosis. The external appearance of these may be spectacular, with a prominent white nodule in the cortical surface (Fig. 1), or very subtle, with a barely noticeable thickening of gyri. Cortical tubers are more easily felt than seen, and multiple areas of increased firmness can usually be palpated on the surface of the brain. These areas are moderately well circumscribed and rise slightly above the surrounding tissue. As stated by Bourneville,[3] their consistency is very much like that of a potato. On cross-section, expansion of the gyrus by white, apparently fibrotic, tissue is seen (Fig. 2). This tissue may proceed into the underlying white matter. There is no encapsulation. Foci of calcification may be present but are not common.

Histologically, the tubers have abnormal cells of somewhat variable appearance. They are 5 to 10 times as large as unaffected astrocytes. Many have astrocytic features, many resemble neurons, and there is a complete spectrum of cells of intermediate appearance.[23] The nuclei of these cells vary from small, without nucleoli, to large with marginated chromatin and a single prominent nucleolus, suggesting both astrocytes and neurons. The cytoplasm of the cells is abundant, and occasional cells have peripheral Nissl substance. The cells are separated by moderate amounts of stroma, and apparently normal cells are frequently interspersed with diseased ones. Cortical layering is frequently discernible, although abnormal. Most tubers have a predominance of abnormal cells in the deeper cortical layers and blend into the white matter. The overlying cortical surface may contain focal aggregates of small stellate cells (Fig. 3). It has been suggested that these aggregates represent persistence of the embryonal subpial germinal layer, which is also found in micropolygyria and mild cortical dysplasia.[49] The most cellular of the tubers have no residual normal architectural features, and the demarcation between cortex and white matter is obliterated.

The white matter is the least involved area of the brain in tuberous sclerosis. When lesions are present they consist of clusters of enlarged cells identical to those in the tubers. These clusters are poorly circumscribed, and the cells seem to stream along tracks (Fig. 4 Top). Occasionally the collections are large enough to approach tumefaction (Fig. 4 Bottom) and grossly visible lesions.

Subependymal lesions vary from microscopic collections of abnormal cells to large tumors, which may cause obstructive hydrocephalus. The larger lesions produce a candle-guttering effect on the ventricular surface, with multiple, firm white nodules protruding into the ventricles (Figs. 2 Bottom and 5). The tumors may attain large size without proceeding into the adjacent brain tissue. Subependymal le-

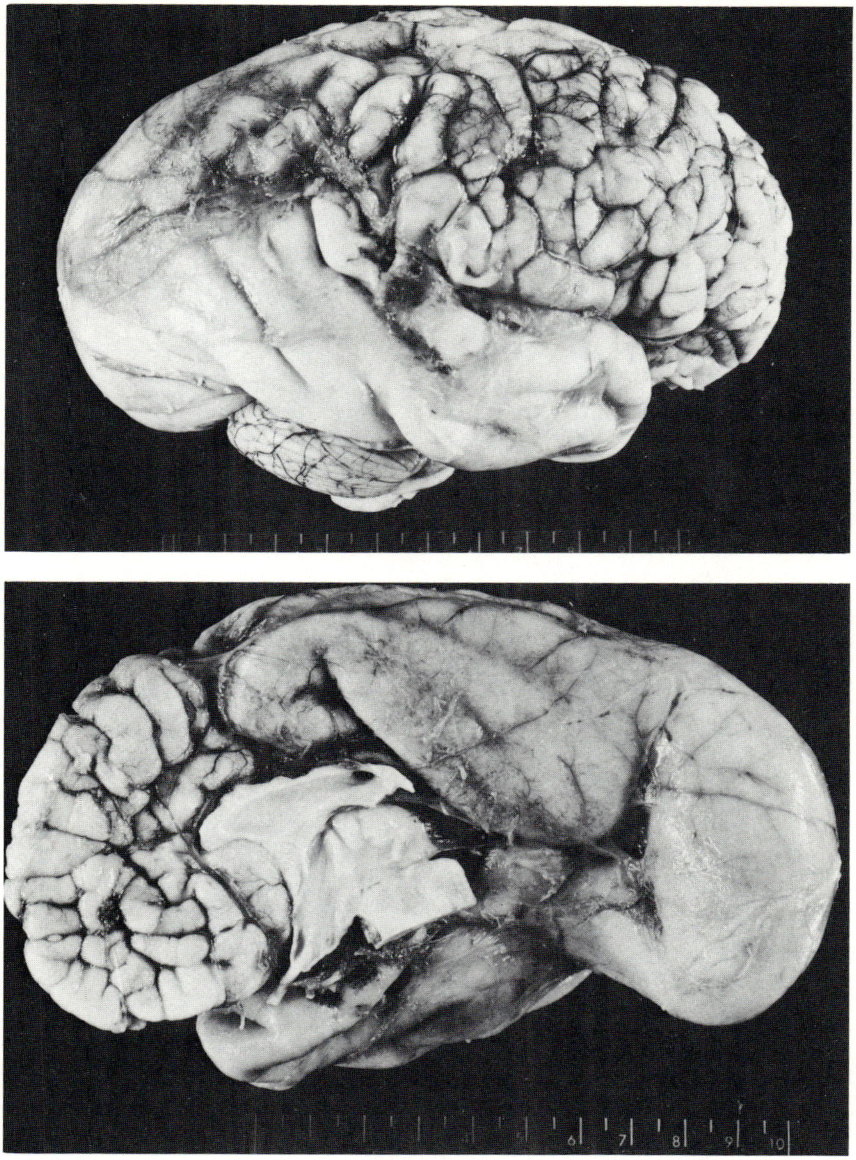

FIG. 1. Marked cortical abnormality including tubers and megagyrus: **Top.** External surface. **Bottom.** Medial surface.

sions are much more frequently hemorrhagic, focally necrotic, and calcified than tubers; in small children, their close relation to the subependymal germinal matrix layer is apparent. These lesions are usually better circumscribed grossly than the cortical tubers. The cerebellum and medulla also rarely contain similar sclerotic subependymal lesions.[50]

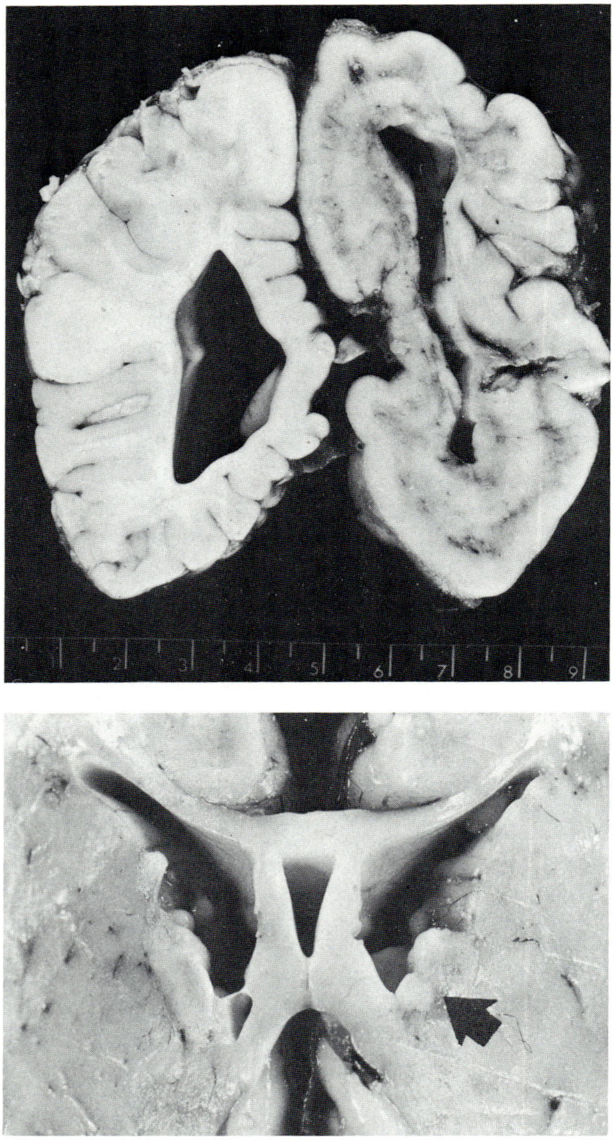

Fig. 2. Top. Cross-section of the same brain as in Figure 1. Cortical tubers and dilated ventricles. Only the lower portion of the right hemisphere is grossly unremarkable. **Bottom.** Small subependymal nodules (arrow). Such lesions may be easily overlooked.

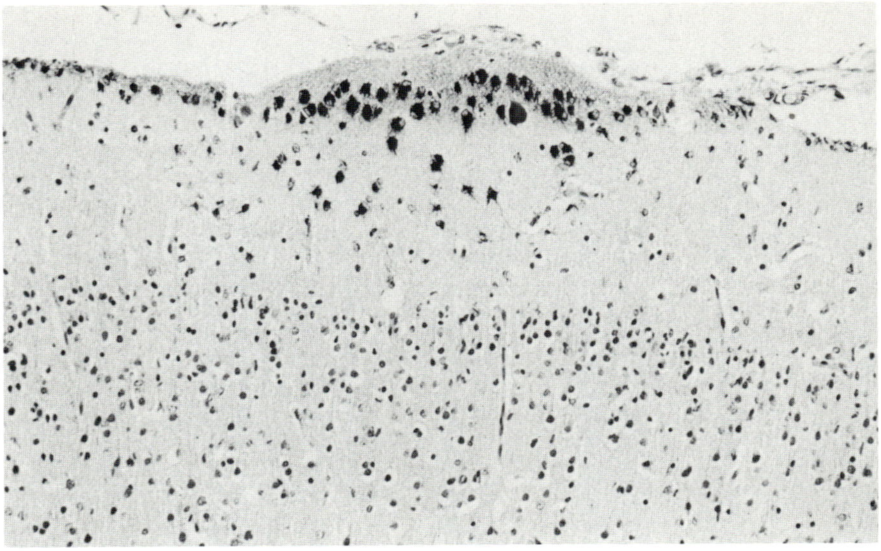

FIG. 3. Retention of the subpial germinal matrix is emphasized by immunostaining for GFAP, yielding deep brown staining. A small cortical nodule is also present and most of its cells are stained (immunoperoxidase counterstained with hematoxylin). ×135.

The distinction between nodules and tumors rests upon whether there is a symptomatic mass effect. Those lesions that have such an effect are designated tumors. Histologically, the nodules and tumors are indistinguishable. Both are overlain by intact ependyma. The majority consist of a simple sheet of large, uniform cells abutting against each other (Fig. 6A). In some areas the cells are elongated, with increased vascularity, occasional palisading around blood vessels, and frequent areas of necrosis (Fig. 6B), reminiscent of ependymoma. Both appearances are frequently present within a single tumor, with transitional areas of plump cells of varying size in a vascular fibrotic stroma (Fig. 6C). Focal calcification is common, but lumen formation or cilia are usually not found. Astrocytes that appear to be reactive and lack the changes suggestive of tuberous sclerosis are common within subependymal tumors.

In all lesions, Holzer's stain is positive in a small number of abnormal cell bodies, frequently staining a clump of apparent fibrils within a cleared area. Nissl staining is from faintly to strongly positive in approximately one-half of the cells, in a band of material at the periphery of the cell body. Immunostaining for glial fibrillary acidic protein (GFAP) demonstrates positivity in approximately one-third of the abnormal cells[23,51] (Fig. 7). Many of the GFAP-positive cells have neuronal features, and the stellate cells along the cortical surface stain strongly (Figs. 3 and 7).

Ultrastructurally, the abnormal cells in tuberous sclerosis have features of both astrocytes and neurons (Fig. 8). Many have an abundant rough endoplasmic reticulum (RER) and frequent dense bodies (Fig. 8 Top). In some cells, the rough endoplasmic reticulum is arranged in parallel stacks (Fig. 8 Top) with interdigitated

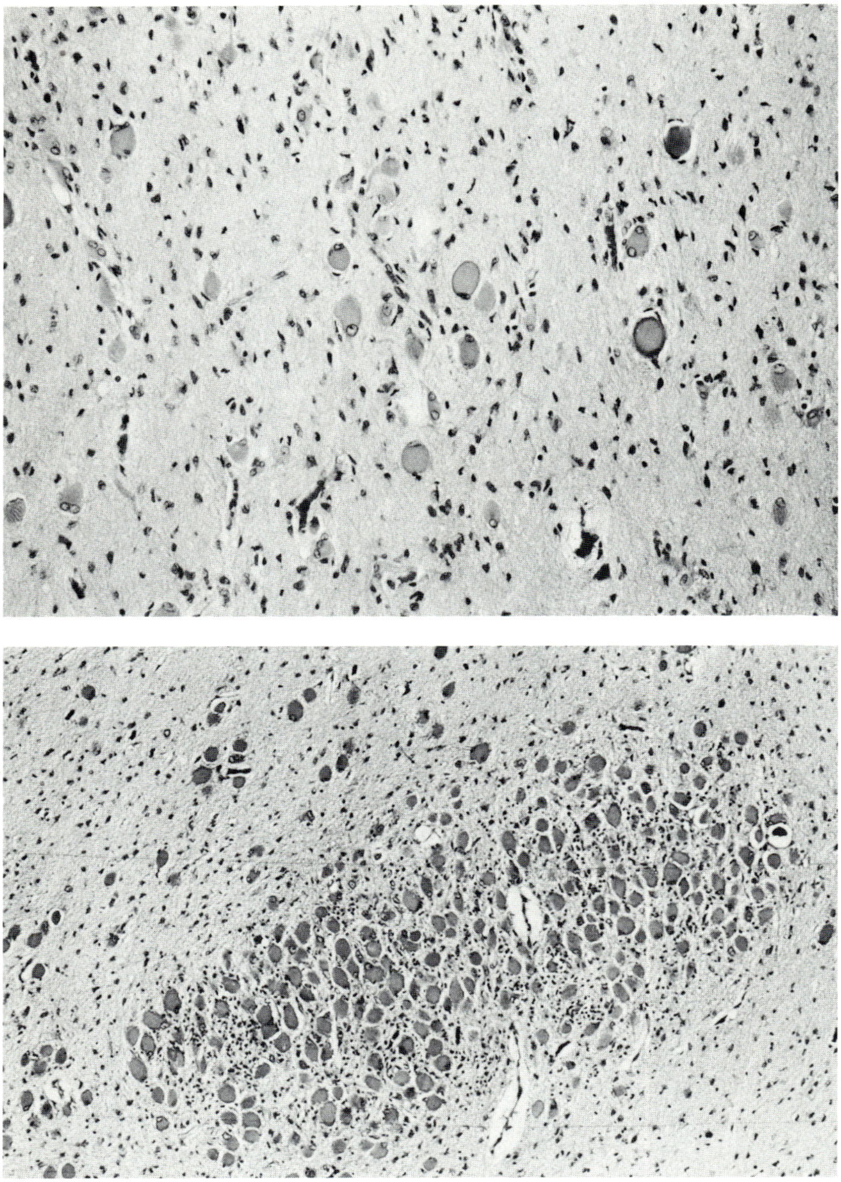

FIG. 4. White matter lesions: **Top.** Giant cells scattered loosely throughout otherwise unremarkable tissue. These cells have one or two nuclei, abundant eosinophilic cytoplasm, and occasionally a hematoxylin-stained periphery. H&E. ×135. **Bottom.** A poorly circumscribed aggregate of similar cells. H&E. ×65.

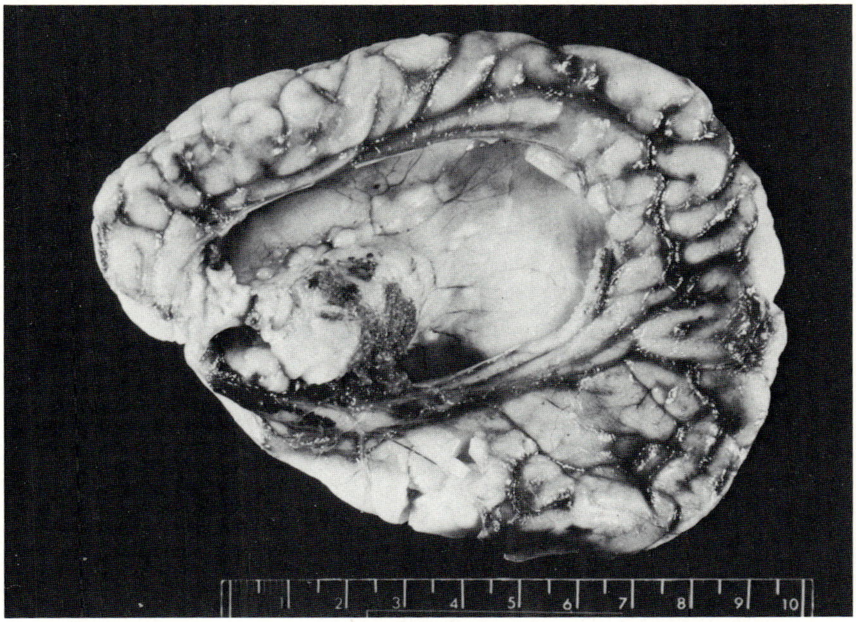

FIG. 5. Medial surface of a brain with tubers and subependymal tumors.

polyribosomes. Polyribosomes are not otherwise frequent. Dense bodies are very common[18,23] and usually have the appearance of lysosomes, with frequent internal crystalline formations.[23] Structures several hundred nanometers in length with a homogeneous crystalline structure having a 7-nm periodicity have been reported.[23] Mitochondria are frequent and vary in size. Glycogen is sparse or absent, although rare peripheral accumulations are present. The nuclear configuration is variable, with some small nuclei with dispersed chromatin and no nucleolus, and many large nuclei with marginated chromatin and a prominent, well-defined nucleolus (Fig. 8 Bottom). Most of the cells have abundant cytoplasm. They contain moderate to large numbers of 9–12 nm fibrils, most common in cytoplasmic processes but occasionally streaming around the nucleus (Fig. 8 Bottom). Only simple, apparently unspecialized, junctions are usually found, although junctional complexes have been reported.[17,20] A basal lamina is not present. Microvilli, abortive lumina, intracytoplasmic lumina, and basal lamina have all been reported by Chadarévian in a tumor which had an appearance suggestive of ependymoma.[20]

The light- and electron microscopic findings, including histochemistry and immunohistochemistry, in all of the central nervous system lesions of tuberous sclerosis reveal the cells in these lesions to be the same. These cells have a mixture of both astrocytic and neuronal features. Many appear to be one or the other type of cell, but individual cells may have the features of both (Figs. 6 to 8 and 23).

There is essentially no difference other than location between the subependymal nodules and tumors, the white matter lesions, and the cortical tubers in

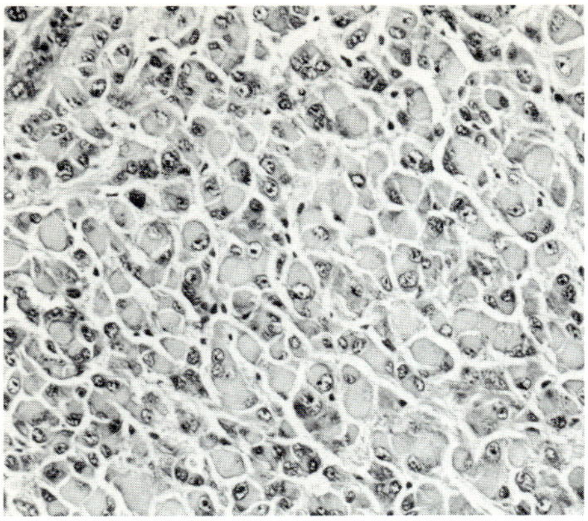

A.

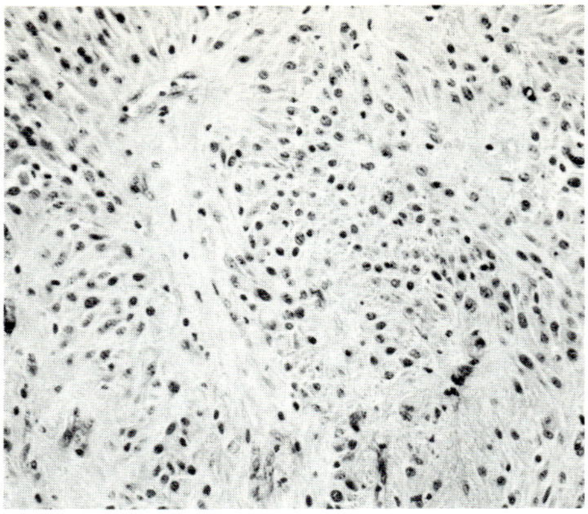

B.

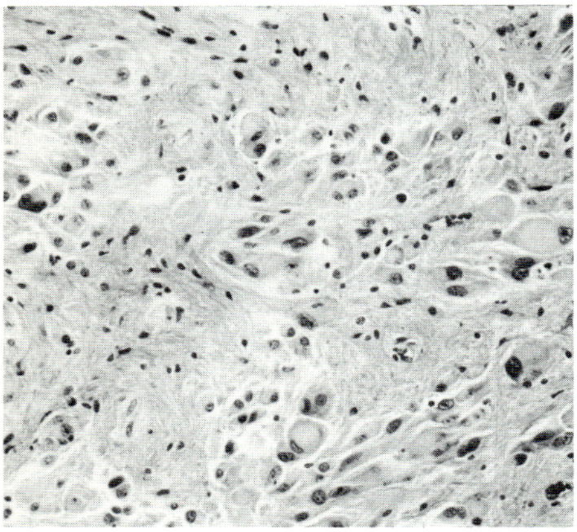

C.

FIG. 6. Subependymal tumor: **A.** A sheet of large cells identical to those in the white matter and cortex. H&E. ×128. **B.** Palisading elongated cells, resembling ependymoma. H&E. ×128. **C.** Intermediate appearance. H&E. ×128.

FIG. 7. A loose cortical tuber underlies subpial germinal matrix. Many cells are immunostained for GFAP (immunoperoxidase counterstained with hematoxylin). ×100.

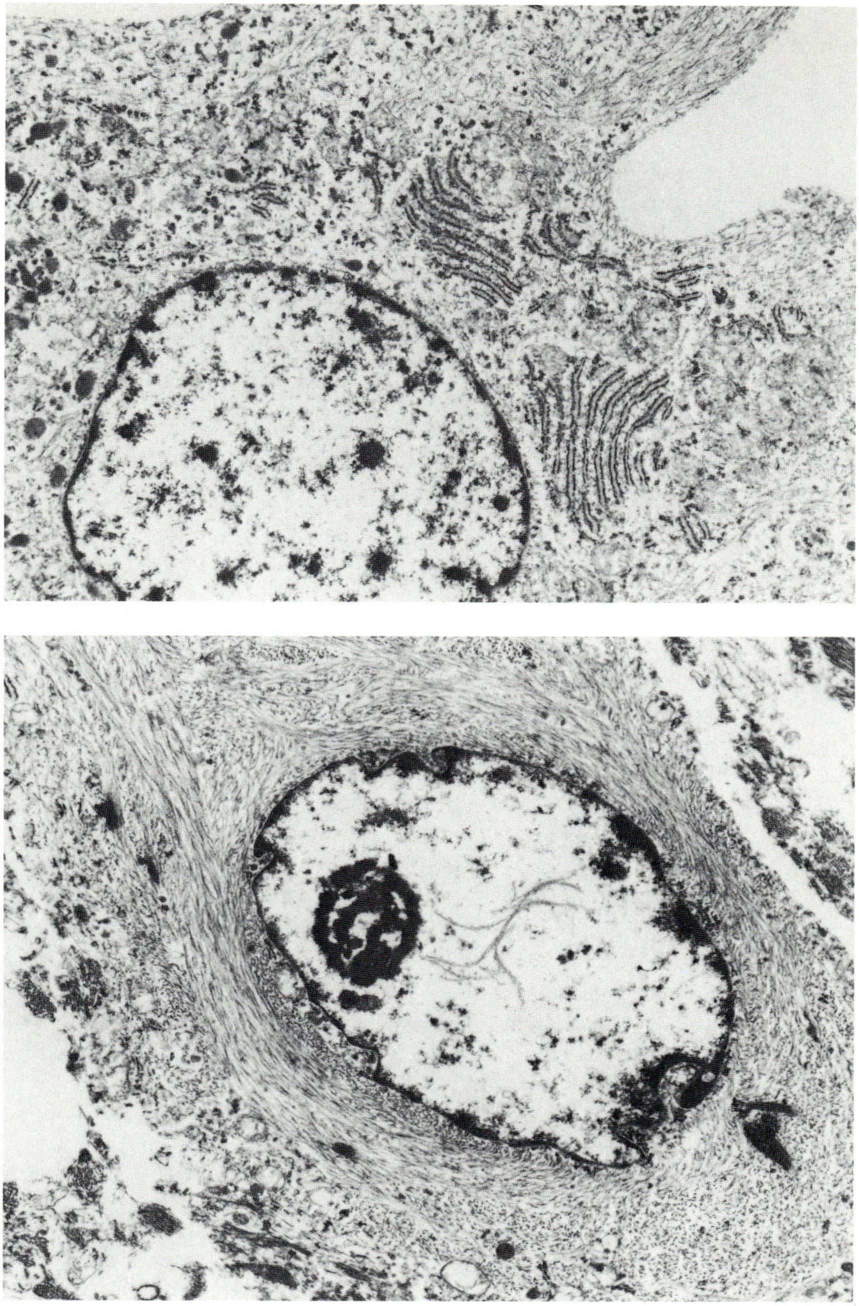

FIG. 8. Ultrastructural appearance of subependymal tumor cells: **Top.** Stacked rough endoplasmic reticulum, polyribosomes, dense bodies and scattered fibrils. ×10,000. **Bottom.** This cell has prominent streaming fibrils. ×10,000.

tuberous sclerosis. These lesions all seem to result from disordered migration and abnormal differentiation of embryonic cells.

It is likely that the diseased cells in tuberous sclerosis are affected early in their maturation; before differentiation as astrocytes or neurons, and that their subsequent development is altered to produce cells with features of both.[50] Thus the lesions are dysplasias or hamartomas which result from disordered cellular maturation. They do not appear to be true neoplasms.

Although other forms of glioma, including glioblastoma multiforme and ependymoma, have been described in patients with tuberous sclerosis,[53] most are probably actually variations of the above-described lesions. Convincing cases of glioblastoma multiforme or ependymoma associated with tuberous sclerosis are so rare[47] that they are probably coincidental.

Gross central nervous system malformations have also been reported in association with tuberous sclerosis. These include dysplasia of the corpus callosum,[21] syringo- and hydromyelia, and spina bifida.[52] It is likely that these are chance occurrences.

Eyes

Although many lesions have been reported in the eyes of patients with tuberous sclerosis, only retinal hamartomas are clearly a part of the syndrome. These were first described in detail by Van der Hoeve,[54] who termed them phakomas. The occurrence of similar lesions in patients with neurofibromatosis and Von Hippel-Lindau disease was the stimulus for grouping these diseases and varying numbers of others as the "phakomatoses," with some presumed common etiologic factor. Both the grouping and the name are still used occasionally,[55] despite the current belief that these diseases are not closely related.[47]

Once considered to be an uncommon aspect of the tuberous sclerosis complex,[44,56] retinal hamartomas have recently been demonstrated to be present in approximately one-half of all patients.[57] The low incidence of these reported in earlier series may have been the result of these lesions usually being asymptomatic or having caused stable changes since early life[55,58] which are not detected by the patient. Many patients have such severe central nervous system impairment that they can neither detect nor report visual deficiency. In addition, the lesions may be very difficult to detect by fundoscopic examination,[58] and the patients may be unable to cooperate, so that sedation and indirect ophthalmoscopy[57,59,60] may be required during examination for them.

The finding of retinal hamartomas has occasionally been the first indication of tuberous sclerosis, however.[61] This may result from a routine eye examination[62] or a hospital admission.[63,64] Thorough fundoscopic examination is a necessary part of the evaluation of a child with seizures and cutaneous lesions.[38] The retinal hamartomas have a variable fundoscopic appearance and are generally divided into a flat and an exophytic variety.[54] The flat tumors are most frequent. They are translucent and may be gray, yellow, or the same color as the surrounding eye. They are poorly circumscribed and may only be noticed because of a circular light reflex.[57] The tumors are slightly elevated and the underlying tissue, which usually includes a vessel, may be less visible than usual. The flat tumors usually occur in the posterior portion of the orbit, and may be single or multiple. Although some early authors emphasized the avascular appearance of these lesions,[65,66] fluorescein angiography has demonstrated that they are intensely vascular,[62] and has been used to locate otherwise undetectable lesions.[64] Some current authors suggest following a retinal vessel toward the periphery of the globe to find these lesions.[47]

The exophytic variety of retinal hamartoma is the more classic lesion. It is frequently likened to a mulberry in gross appearance, with clusters of opaque, cystic,[56] or calcified, variably colored nodules. Periodic filling of cystic areas and emptying into the vitreous humor has been recorded,[54] and vitreous hemorrhage may cause transient visual disturbance.[62] These lesions may be up to 4 disc diameters wide and protrude 7 diopters.[57] They characteristically occur at the disc margin,[56] but may occur as laterally as the midperiphery of the retina.[57]

Lesions of intermediate appearance between the flat and the mulberry type are seen in tuberous sclerosis, and transition from the former to the latter has been observed over a period of years.[57]

Although it has been suggested that the above lesions are diagnosable as tuberous sclerosis clinically,[65] and although a patient with only retinal hamartomas clinically has given birth to three children with fully developed tuberous sclerosis,[65] the lesions are indistinguishable from the ocular lesion of neurofibromatosis.[55] Only family studies allow differentiation.

The appearance of the mulberry-like lesions, particularly those in the periphery, may mimic that of retinoblastoma.[40,60,67–69] In most cases other findings of tuberous sclerosis will allow this differentiation. In those patients without any other signs, close follow-up for the size changes indicative of retinoblastoma is necessary.[70] Neither the honeycomb appearance of regressing retinoblastoma[71] nor a high aqueous-to-serum lactic acid dehydrogenase level should be present with retinal hamartoma. The mulberry-like lesions of retinal hamartoma may resemble drusen of the optic disc,[72] but have a greater tendency to obscure underlying vasculature.[57]

Histologically, the main component of the retinal hamartomas is a proliferation of large, highly variable cells which is limited to the nerve fiber and ganglion layers in small lesions (Fig. 9),[47] but which may involve the entire retina or optic papilla.[56,73] The cells usually have one oval nucleus, but may have as many as five, frequently with a single prominent nucleolus; their cytoplasm is abundant and has the range of appearances found in central nervous system tumors, resembling that of ganglion cells or glia. The cells may have processes which extend to envelop blood vessels,[74] or be rounded. The appearance of syncytium formation is frequently described.[47,57,73] Phosphotungstic acid staining has been used as evidence of glial differentiation,[73] and the Hortega stain has illustrated nerve fibers within a tumor.[74] The edges of the tumors may be abrupt or poorly circumscribed,[56] and microscopic collections of abnormal cells may be scattered throughout the retina.

The larger retinal hamartomas are frequently complicated by spaces filled with serous fluid or blood.[54,56,62] They may also have necrotic areas[74] with hyalinization and focal calcification.[47] Blood vessels are present in variable numbers, but are occasionally frequent enough to suggest that they are a part of the tumor.[75]

The origin of retinal hamartomas in tuberous sclerosis is probably identical to

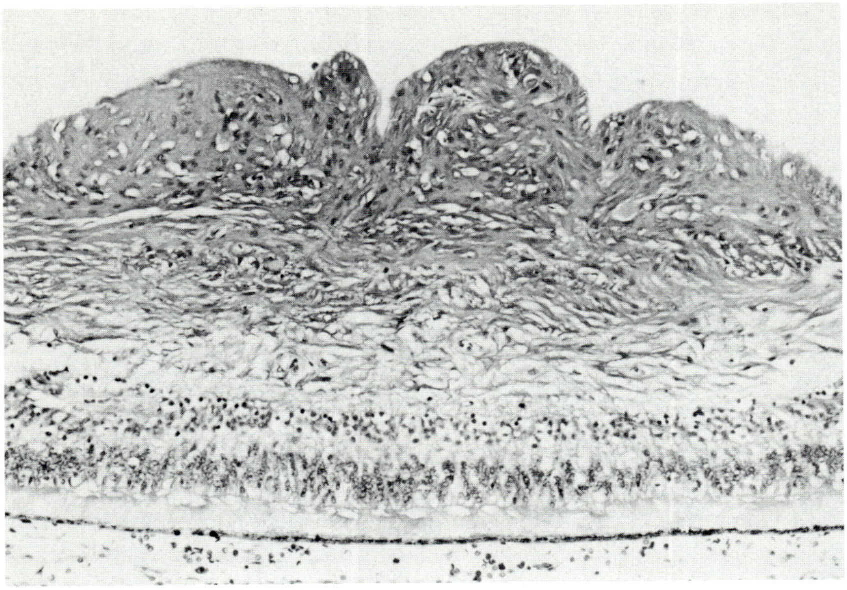

FIG. 9. Retinal hamartoma: Spindled glia-like cells in the superficial retinal layers. H&E. ×135.

that of the central nervous system lesions—a proliferation of undifferentiated "glioneurocytes" with development of variable neuronal or glial features, as proposed by Van de Hoeve[76] and suggested by Mann.[73] It is probable that the aberration occurs before the third month of gestation.[73]

Depigmented iris sector has been considered the ocular equivalent of hypopigmented skin lesions.[63] The presence of hypo-[40] and hyperpigmented[56,57] retinal lesions has also been reported, but their histologic correlate and frequency are unclear. The increased pigmentation may represent old hemorrhage within otherwise fundoscopically invisible lesions.

Adenoma sebaceum,[77] vitiligo, poliosis, ptosis, and epicanthal folds of the eyelids; conjunctival thickening;[78] glaucoma; rubeosis, iridocyclitis, and coloboma of the lens; and enopthalmos and phthisis of the globe[78] have all been seen in association with tuberous sclerosis,[47] but are likely to be incidental findings.

Secondary involvement of the eye occurs with intracranial hypertension. Such patients develop papilledema[35,44] and may have optic atrophy leading to visual disturbance.[47,66] Ocular nerve palsy may also occur.[79]

Skin

Almost all patients with tuberous sclerosis have cutaneous lesions.[40,80] Although these are not life-threatening, they are of great importance to the diagnosis of tuberous sclerosis, particularly in mild[81] and early cases.[82,83]

There are four cutaneous lesions that have been stated to be diagnostic of tuberous sclerosis; these are facial angiofibroma (adenoma sebaceum),[5,6,7,84] hypopigmented macules,[82,83] shagreen patch, and parungual fibromas.[80,85] Although all have some similarities, their differences are significant, and discussion of each is warranted.

Facial Angiofibroma. Facial angiofibromas were described by Rayer[6] in 1835 and again by Balzer and Menetrier in 1885.[5] Both Pringle[7] and Bourneville[2] described them in patients with probable tuberous sclerosis, but did not recognize their connection to that disease. Vogt[9] incorporated them into the tuberous sclerosis complex.

Occasional adult patients with tuberous sclerosis do not have facial angiofibromas,[44,81,86] but over 90 percent do.[80,81,84] Well-developed lesions are considered diagnostic of the disease. Most, if not all patients with facial angiofibroma have other manifestations of tuberous sclerosis,[84] and there is approximately a 50 percent incidence of tuberous sclerosis in their offspring.[81]

Facial angiofibroma may be present at birth,[47,66] but is usually diagnosed in patients between 2 and 6 years of age.[87] Only three of our eight pediatric patients for whom information about its presence at last follow-up was available had facial angiofibromas. Occasionally these lesions do not appear until adulthood. The only reported symptom is sensitivity to cold.[7,86] In some cases the lesions are noted by the patient or his family, but they are almost invariably ascribed to some other condition.[86] They are frequently diagnosed when the patient is evaluated for seizure or retardation.

The earliest visible abnormality usually appears in the first year of life, and consists of centrofacial flushing upon crying.[47] This is followed by the development of isolated, pale-pink flat or rounded papules.[87] These increase in number and size over several years. In many patients there is increased growth of the lesions at puberty[47] and the lesions are static after about age 20, although there is a tendency to recurrence if they are planed.

Involvement of the temporal region and forehead by angrofibroma is frequent in tuberous sclerosis patients.[84] There is sparing of the circumoral region which is both striking and useful in distinguishing facial angiofibromas from other lesions (Fig. 10). Papules are usually, but not always,[87] symmetrically distributed and do not extend below the clavicles.[88]

Individual papules evolve from near invisibility to the classic lesion, which averages about 4 mm in diameter and protudes up to 5 mm above the skin surface (Fig. 10). The papules frequently become pedunculated,[87] are variably brown, yellow, or red, and blanch incompletely under pressure, with the preservation of a central telangiectatic spot. Their firmness and surface texture are variable.[47] There are no comedones. Previous authors have subclassified these lesions into several categories,[86,87,89] but the current concensus is that this is unnecessary; all of the lesions are basically the same histologically and have the same prognostic implications. There is no correlation between the number of angiofibromas and the severity of other aspects of tuberous sclerosis.

Histologically, it is apparent that the designation adenoma sebaceum is a misnomer for the facial lesions in tuberous sclerosis. There is proliferation of the

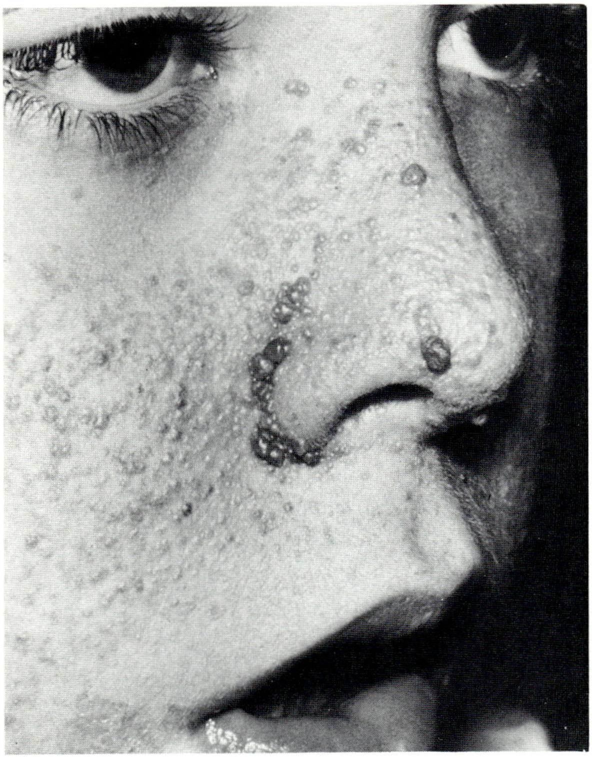

FIG. 10. Facial angiofibromas. The small papular lesions are distributed over the nose and cheeks, with sparing of the circumoral region. They are most prominent in the nasolabial fold and show a tendency to pedunculation.

dermal fibrous tissue and vasculature, with vascular dilatation (Fig. 11). There is diffusely increased cellularity with an increased size of fibroblasts. There may be stellate, frequently multinucleate, cells, lending a glial appearance to the tumor (Fig. 12)[32,84]; this has led to the suggestion that Schwann cells are involved,[32] but current methods demonstrate that these cells are more likely of fibroblastic origin.[27,84] Elastic tissue is essentially absent from the lesions. With increasing age there is an accumulation of collagen, with decreased cellularity and occasional formation of keloid-like bands around adnexal structures.[84]

These proliferated areas are poorly circumscribed. As the lesion enlarges, the sebaceous glands and hair follicles tend to remain at the base of the lesion, or to atrophy. The ducts and epidermis are stretched over the enlarging fibrous mass, giving them an elongated, thinned appearance.

A report of the ultrastructure of the facial lesions in tuberous sclerosis has illustrated dermal vessels lined by a single nonfenestrated layer of endothelial cells with luminal, poorly formed microvilli.[27] The stromal cells had a single large nucleus with a prominent nucleolus. The abundant cytoplasm contained rough endoplasmic reticulum. The cells frequently had a stellate appearance. No basement membrane or desmosomes were described. The intercellular space was filled by collagen (occasionally with a periodicity of 110 nm), electron-dense fibrillar material, and an amorphous ground substance.

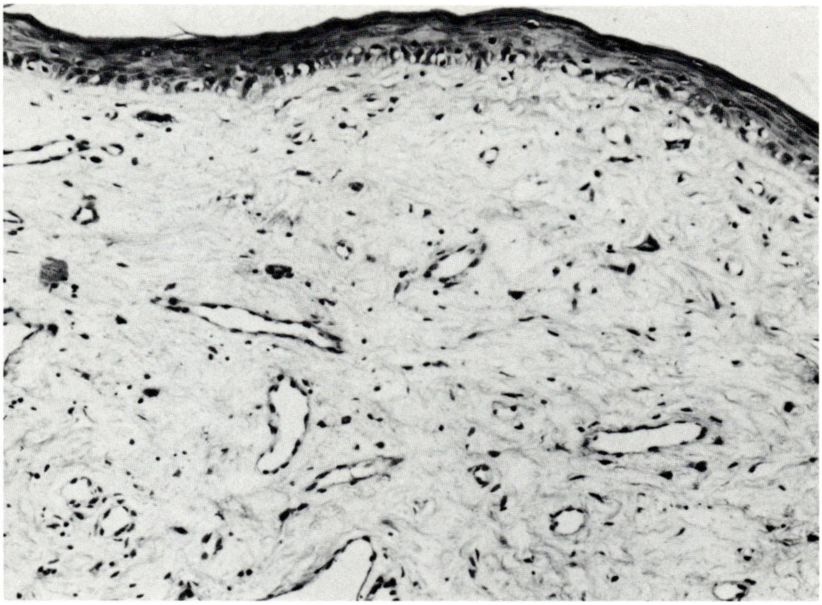

FIG. 11. Vascular dilatation and increased connective tissue in a facial angiofibroma. Sebaceous elements are decreased. H&E. ×135.

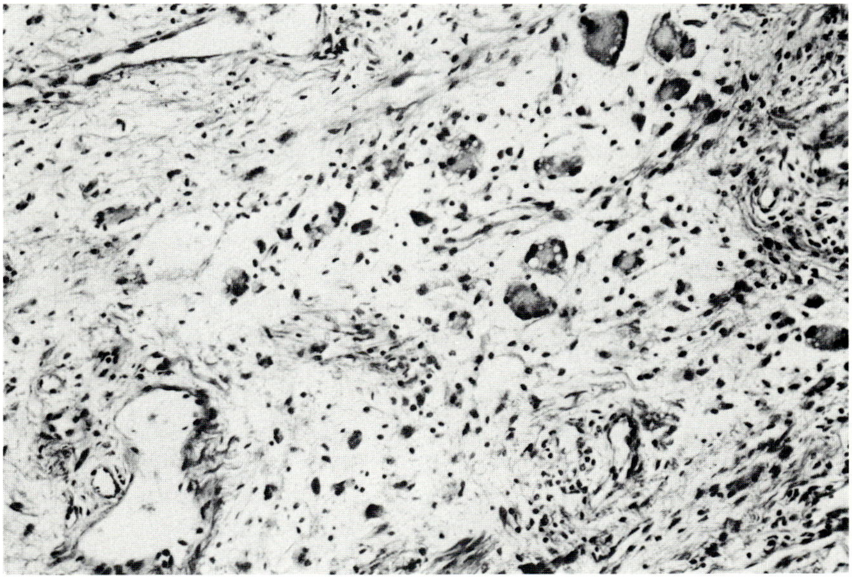

FIG. 12. Facial angiofibroma with giant cells and a "glial" appearance. H&E. ×135.

Hypopigmented Macules. Hypomelanotic macules (ash-leaf spots) are the most common lesions on the trunk of patients with tuberous sclerosis. Although distinguishing these macules from vitiligo and piebaldism may be difficult,[47] it is said to be possible. The macules are virtually pathognomonic of tuberous sclerosis.

These lesions have been reported in from 55 to 70 percent of patients with tuberous sclerosis,[47,84] with the recent suggestion that they are actually much more common.[47,83] They were present in six of our eight patients for whom the information was available. They are usually the earliest cutaneous sign of tuberous sclerosis, frequently being present at birth.[82,83]

The hypopigmented macules are scattered about the body, most frequently occurring on the trunk and buttocks,[47] differing from the sun-exposed-area location of vitiligo. There may be a few or as many as 100. They may increase in number for a few years after birth, although that is difficult to ascertain owing to the difficulty in detecting them at birth. They are flat, from 1 to 3 cm in greatest dimension, and typically well-circumscribed, with the lance-ovate shape from which the appellation ash-leaf spot is derived, and although hypopigmented, are not completely amelanotic, in contradistinction to vitiligo. They may not be noticed until the patient has acquired some degree of suntan. They are more easily visualized with the use of an ultraviolet light,[83] which causes an increase in their perceived lightness with respect to the surrounding skin.

The hypopigmented macules in tuberous sclerosis may appear unremarkable by histologic methods unless compared with surrounding skin. Unlike the case in piebaldism and vitiligo, normal numbers of melanocytes are present in the macules.[90] The melanocytes, however, contain decreased amounts of pigment, and this difference is accentuated by a decreased DOPA reaction.[83,90]

Ultrastructurally there is a decrease in the size, number, and degree of pigmentation of melanosomes in the macules,[83,90] which is reported to be distinguishable from the aggregation of melanosomes of normal size and pigmentation seen in nevus depigmentosis.[90]

Shagreen Patch. Shagreen patch is an anglicised name for a lesion described in French as "peau chagrine," meaning "skin like untanned leather." Such lesions are present on 70 to 80 percent of adult tuberous sclerosis patients,[84,86] but on only 21 percent of the children studied by Lagos and Gomez,[48] suggesting that most appear during childhood.

These lesions usually occur in the lumbar region, although they may be gluteal or on other aspects of the dorsal trunk.[86] Ventral examples are rare but have been reported.[47,84] The shagreen patch lesions are classically single, lateral, and several centimeters in greatest dimension, although none of these characteristics is always present. They are slightly raised and poorly circumscribed, with a mammillated, rough surface resembling pigskin. They are usually the color of the surrounding skin, although they may be slightly lighter or darker. They have a variable consistency, and seem to be separable from the subcutaneous tissue.

By light-microscopy, the dermal portion of the shagreen patch lesions resembles scleroderma.[84] There is usually a zone of unremarkable connective tissue separating the epidermis from increased, randomly arranged collagen in the deeper

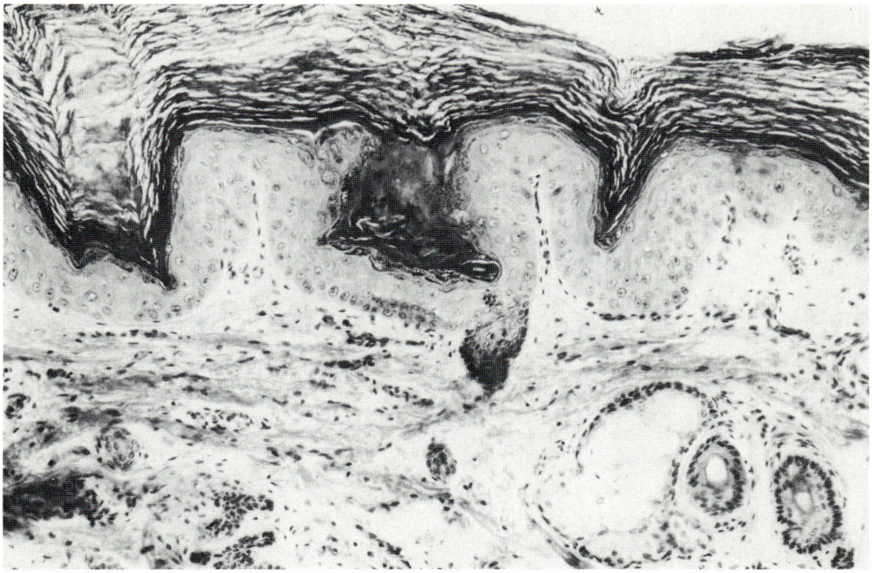

FIG. 13. Shagreen patch: Hyperplastic redundant epidermis overlies increased connective tissue. Rete ridges are absent, appendages are present. H&E. ×135.

dermis (Fig. 13); a variation has no normal upper dermis. Occasionally the collagen forms dense bands.[84] Elastic tissue is usually normal but may be increased or decreased.[91] No inflammation is present. A tendency to clustering of hair follicles has been described.[86] The overlying epidermis may be hyperplastic and hyperkeratotic (Fig. 13).

Ultrastructurally, collagen bundles in the lower dermis of shagreen patch lesions have been reported to be thicker than normal,[28] with fibers arranged in parallel bundles and having a 55 nm periodicity. Occasional abnormal collagen fibrils were present, 20 to 100 nm in thickness, with curling or twisted shapes. There was irregularity of the fibrillar margins, with the fibrils having whisk-like ends. Threadlike material was present. These findings differ from those reported in scleroderma by the same group,[92] in having the above abnormalities and not having a marked variation in thickness.

Neither the clinical appearance nor the histology of shagreen patch is distinguishable from that of connective tissue nevus.[47,93] Their presence in a child with seizures is therefore suggestive, but not diagnostic, of tuberous sclerosis.

Parungual Fibroma. Parungual fibromas appear during the second decade and are present in approximately 50 percent of all tuberous sclerosis patients. They have more capacity for continued growth and regrowth after excision than do other cutaneous lesions. It has been suggested that they may be stimulated by shoes,[86] since they are more common on the toes than the fingers, and predominate in females. The similarity between the frequency and apparent time of occurence of parungual fibroma and renal angiofibromas has been noted,[84] although no increased association of these lesions with each other has been demonstrated.

The parungual fibromas measure up to 1 cm in diameter[84] and are dull red or tan, moderately firm,[86] well-circumscribed nodules which usually protude above the surrounding tissue. No distinction is made between lesions next to the nail bed and those in it. The larger lesions may lead to nail dystrophy or cause pain.

Histologically, the parungual fibromas in tuberous sclerosis are fibromas or angiofibromas, with a proliferation of connective tissues similar to that of facial angiofibroma.[94] The proliferating cells may have a glial appearance. Occasionally the epithelium is acanthotic.[84]

Although they may be confused clinically with epithelial inclusion cysts, infantile digital fibromatosis, or verruca vulgaris, the histologic appearance of the parungual fibromas in tuberous sclerosis allows a differentiation to be made. These lesions are also virtually diagnostic of tuberous sclerosis.

Fibrous Plaques The forehead and scalp of tuberous sclerosis patients may have large, plaque-like pink or brown lesions.[95] These are of variable consistency and have a smooth, hairless surface. They are raised but appear to be subcutaneous[86] by palpation.

The incidence of these lesions is unclear. They have been stated to be common among severely affected,[84] and uncommon in older,[84] patients, although this finding is not widely reproduced. They are uncommonly noted in children,[47] but a case has been described in which a small red mark was noted on the scalp at birth and was unchanged until 9 years of age, when it started to grow and eventually produced a huge fibroma.[95] These lesions may be severely deforming; their successful removal has been reported.[95]

Histologically the fibrous plaques in tuberous sclerosis exhibit the same fibrous proliferation with stellate cells that is seen in facial angiofibroma,[84,86] without any vascular component. There may be entrapment of adnexae,[84] and older lesions have a tendency to formation of dense collagen bands.[88] The fibrous plaques are considered to be a variant of facial angiofibroma.[47,87,89]

Nonspecific Lesions. Café-au-lait spots and soft fibromas have been reported frequently in patients with tuberous sclerosis.[47,86,89] Although Nickel and Reed believe that the soft fibromas are more cellular than those in the normal population,[84] others see no histologic difference.[47] It has been shown that the incidence of cafe-au-lait spots does not exceed that of the general population.[47] Although it is possible that the occurence of cafe-au-lait spots and soft fibromas is one of the more subtle aspects of the generalized tissue dysplasia of tuberous sclerosis, it is also possible that they are incidental findings. Many other cutaneous lesions have been reported with this complex, but these are also probably incidental findings.

Kidneys

Two different renal lesions are highly associated with tuberous sclerosis: angiomyolipoma and epithelial cysts.

Angiomyolipoma. It has been estimated that 80 percent of patients with complete expression of tuberous sclerosis have renal angiomyolipoma,[44] with other estimates as low as 42 percent[96] and as high as 100 percent.[97] Conversely, approximately 50 percent of all renal angiomyolipomas occur in patients with tuberous sclerosis.[98] In Farrow's series[43] of 32 cases, the diagnosis of tuberous sclerosis was suspected in only 3 patients. However, upon follow-up, seven additional adult patients had extrarenal findings typical of tuberous sclerosis, and two patients without such extrarenal findings had children with classical tuberous sclerosis.

In most tuberous sclerosis patients, angiomyolipoma is totally asymptomatic. However, renal colic occasionally occurs, usually secondary to hemorrhage.[43,98,99] Renal failure due to replacement of renal tissue by an angiomyolipoma may occur.[100] The incidence of angiomyolipoma in patients with tuberous sclerosis increases with age.[47]

Angiograms reveal a whorled pattern[101] without arteriovenous shunting.[102] Multiple aneurysmal dilatations of the interlobar and interlobular arteries are also seen.[101,102]

Pathologically, the angiomyolipomas of tuberous sclerosis are most easily distinguished from those not associated with tuberous sclerosis by gross (Fig. 14) characteristics. Those in the former group tend to be multiple and larger, a finding which led Price[103] to state that they were more likely to be palpable in tuberous sclerosis patients. They range in size from microscopic collections of abnormal cells to huge masses which completely replace the kidney. They are circumscribed but not encapsulated, and may bulge from the renal surface. Their color varies from yellow to pink to gray depending upon their composition, and they may have a

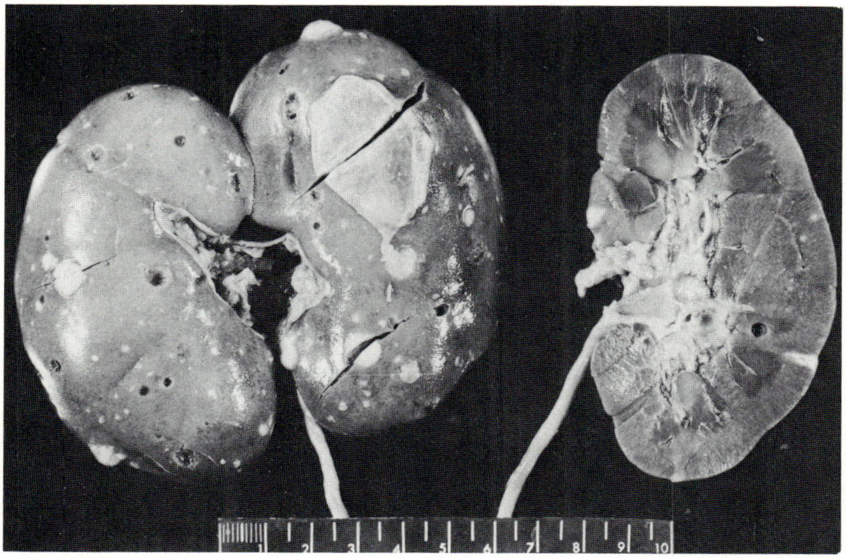

FIG. 14. Multiple circumscribed angiomyolipomas protrude from the surface of these kidneys. Multiple cysts are also apparent. The cut surface contains several white angiomyolipomas and a cyst.

lobulated appearance. These tumors may transgress the renal capsule and invade surrounding fat or invade the renal vein on rare occasions.[43,47]

Microscopically, there is a mixture of fat, spindled smooth muscle cells, and dysplastic vessels in the tumors (Fig. 15). Many fat cells are mature signet-ring forms (Fig. 15B). There are also scattered foamy cells which may be either

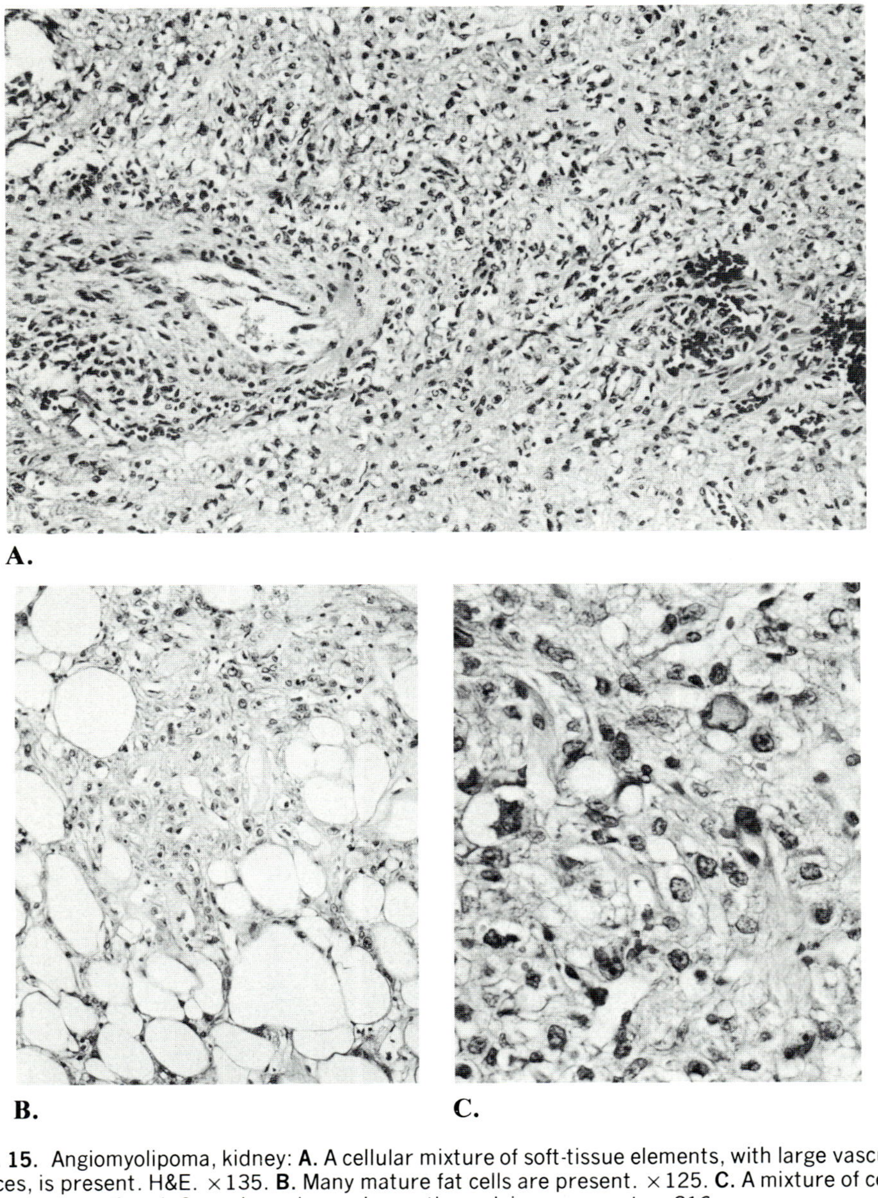

FIG. 15. Angiomyolipoma, kidney: **A.** A cellular mixture of soft-tissue elements, with large vascular spaces, is present. H&E. ×135. **B.** Many mature fat cells are present. ×125. **C.** A mixture of cells. Many are vacuolated. Some large hyperchromatic nuclei are present. ×316.

histiocytes or less mature fat cells; these cells may be multinucleated. The spindled cells are frequently dysplastic, with large immature nuclei and occasional mitoses (Fig. 15C).[47,103,104] There may be a large number of moderate- to large-size vessels with thick, eccentric walls. The elastic lamina of these vessels is usually incomplete both internally and externally. There is no encapsulation, and apparently trapped renal glomeruli and tubules are frequently present.

Many of the angiomyolipomas in tuberous sclerosis have been misdiagnosed as sarcomas.[103,104] This is probably due to three factors which were summarized by Price[103]: (1) The tumors are multiple; (2) the smooth muscle cells have a dysplastic appearance with nuclear hyperchromatism and mitoses; and (3) the tumors exhibit invasion of large vascular channels, which are probably tumorous vessels. The variation in composition of these tumors, with some having a single predominant cell type, may also lead to erroneous diagnoses of sarcoma. In any patient with multiple renal hamartomas, with or without atypicality, a search for other signs of tuberous sclerosis should be undertaken and a diagnosis of malignancy should be avoided.

In one electron microscopic report[26] the cells of angiomyolipoma were described as having an abundant, electron-lucent cytoplasm without filaments. They had many long cytoplasmic protrusions which ran adjacent to each other. No junctional apparatus or basement membrane was recognized. In another such report,[105] two types of cells were described, some with the characteristics of smooth muscle, including basement membranes, and some like fibroblasts.

Cysts. The second lesion in the kidneys of patients with tuberous sclerosis is a cystic malformation. This is probably less common than angiomyolipoma,[106] but its true incidence is unknown, since its significance has been recognized more recently. Many authors reporting on renal diseases in tuberous sclerosis have described cysts but considered them incidental,[107] and many have undoubtedly missed them or left them out of reports. In our series cysts were found in all eight cases of children with tuberous sclerosis from whom renal tissue was available. Many of these were microscopic, and two had pale lining cells rather than the usual eosinophilic cells.

Renal involvement with these cysts can consist of totally asymptomatic microscopic foci, or almost complete replacement of one or both kidneys by cystic spaces, with the usual consequences of cystic kidneys: hypertension and renal insufficiency. These two effects may be some of the earliest signs of tuberous sclerosis in patients who develop other stigmata later.[47,106,108]

Grossly, cystic spaces are present in the cortical region of the kidney, more commonly in the more superficial areas. Although they are poorly circumscribed, they tend to be clustered within a segmental area (Fig. 16), with multiple cysts adjoining each other and ending abruptly at normal renal parenchyma.

Microscopically, the cystic lesions are highly distinctive (Fig. 17).[106,109] They consist of dilated spaces which are lined by cells resembling tubular epithelium, with abundant eosinophilic cytoplasm and a small, round, benign appearing nucleus (Fig. 17 Bottom). Mitoses are not seen, nor is atypicality present. The cells may pile upon one another and protrude into the lumen of the cyst.[109] Occasionally there is the appearance of ciliation of the surface cells. The cysts are limited by an

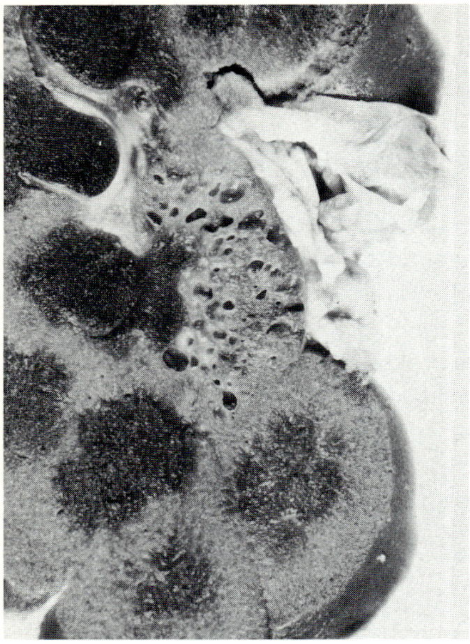

FIG. 16. A cluster of cysts in the cortex of a kidney.

unremarkable tubular wall. Occasionally, the cells lining the cysts do not have the typical enlarged eosinophilic appearance but are flattened and pale.

The piling up of eosinophilic, unflattened, epithelial cells is distinctly unusual in other renal cystic diseases. It may indicate that the cysts in tuberous sclerosis are not obstructive. The finding of these lesions in a renal biopsy is probably diagnostic of tuberous sclerosis, even in patients without other stigmata of the disease at the time of biopsy.[108,109]

Microdissection in a single case of tuberous sclerosis revealed thin-walled cysts in the kidney to be enlargements of Henle's loops and other cysts to arise in collecting tubules.[110] In routine microscopic sections, however, dilated Bowman's capsules are seen, with glomerular tufts, within cysts (Fig. 17 Top). It is therefore likely that the cysts can arise anywhere in the nephron.

Ultrastructurally the cells in the renal cysts are similar to tubular cells. They do not contain fibrils or dense bodies.

Various malformations, including dilatation of the renal pelvis, large kidneys, distorted calyces, double ureters, supernumerary kidneys, and a single kidney have been reported in association with tuberous sclerosis.[2] However, these associations are probably incidental.

Heart

There is only one strongly associated cardiac lesion in tuberous sclerosis. This is the tumor most frequently referred to as rhabdomyoma. The coincidence of tuberous sclerosis of the brain and rhabdomyoma of the heart has been apparent since von

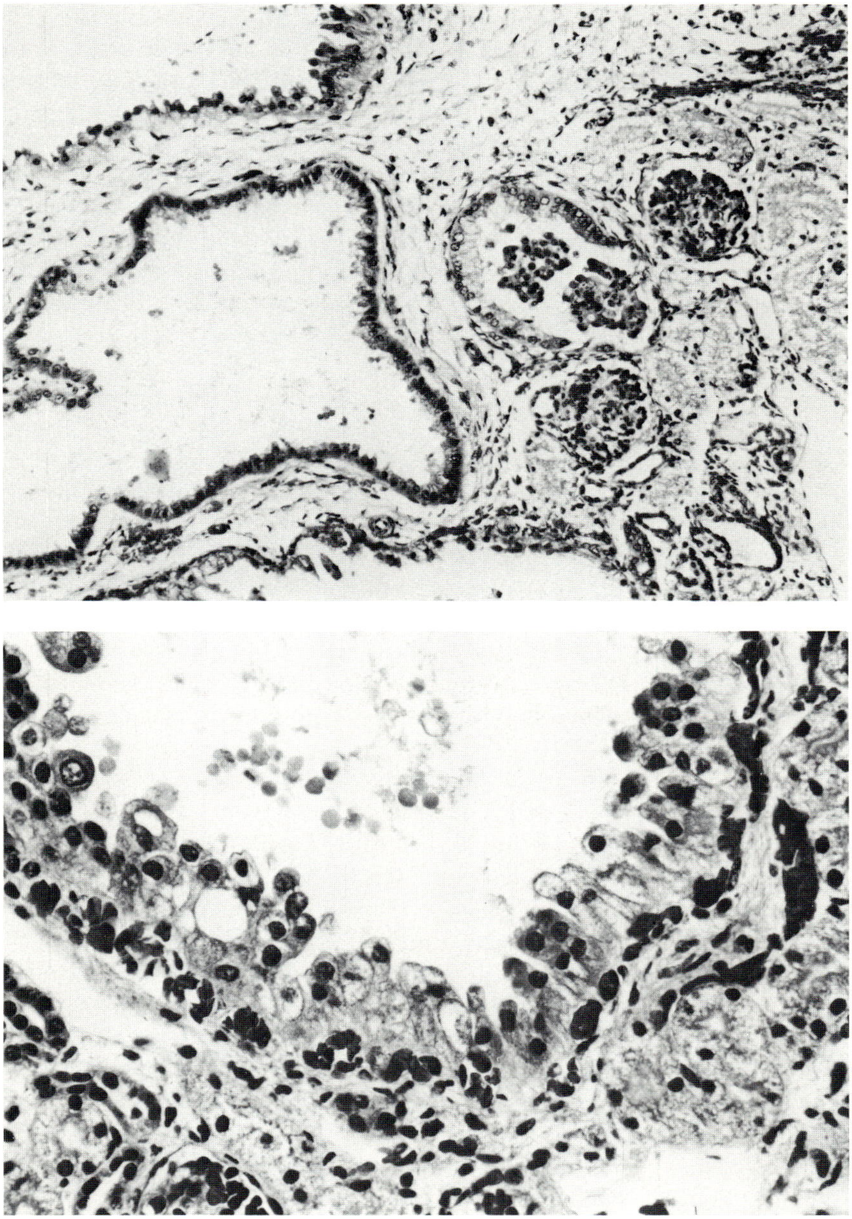

FIG. 17. Renal cysts: **Top.** Cysts of variable size are present. Glomeruli are included within them. Their lining is not flattened. They are separated by loose connective tissue. H&E. ×135. **Bottom.** The lining of this cyst is columnar. H&E. ×340.

Recklinghausen's original description of both.[1] It is conservatively estimated that approximately 30 percent of patients with tuberous sclerosis have rhabdomyomata, and that approximately 30 percent of patients with rhabdomyomata have tuberous sclerosis.[47] Other authors have suggested that the incidence of tuberous sclerosis in patients with rhabdomyomata is closer to 50 percent,[111-113] and have emphasized that many of the neonates who die of rhabdomyoma might have developed other stigmata of tuberous sclerosis had they lived longer.[113]

It is clear that patients with multiple rhabdomyomata have a much higher incidence of tuberous sclerosis than those with a single cardiac tumor.[112,114] Farber found that tuberous sclerosis was present in 24 of 28 reported cases of multiple rhabdomyomata where the head was mentioned, and in only 1 of 4 single rhabdomyomata.[115] Of our 10 cases of tuberous sclerosis in children, 7 had been autopsied, and 6 of these had rhabdomyomata; the other 3 are alive and have no cardiac problems, but small lesions cannot be excluded.

Clinically, cardiac involvement may be asymptomatic, a minor problem, or the only symptomatic aspect of the disease. Although the age range at diagnosis is reported to be from 6 months to 45 years,[116] most patients have circulatory difficulty during the first few days of life and most of these die shortly. In one series of 63 cases, 15 presented as newborns, 18 others at under 1 year, 9 at from 1 to 3 years, 12 at from 3 to 15 years, and only 7 at over 15 years.[112] In another series of 36 patients, 78 percent were under 1 year of age.[117]

The symptoms are those of any mass lesion, which can mimic those of many other cardiac lesions. Obstruction of blood flow by intracavitary tumor has produced symptoms resembling tricuspid,[116] pulmonary,[101] and subaortic stenosis.[116,118,119] Congestive heart failure may result from poor ventricular motion. Arrhythmias are common.[111,120-122]

In the past, the diagnosis of rhabdomyomata was frequently made only at autopsy.[115,122,123] However, the introduction of echocardiography has provided a good noninvasive technique of visualizing this lesion.[47,124] Angiography, although more invasive, has become the definitive diagnostic tool.[120,121] With the advent of premortem diagnosis, several patients have undergone operation, and a few successful removals of these tumors have been performed.[111,114,116,117,121,125] Shaker et al. believe that those patients in whom a diagnosis of rhabdomyoma can be made preoperatively—usually children with other stigmata of tuberous sclerosis—should have surgery only if obstructive symptoms occur.[116] This is based on the frequent occurrence of multiple tumors and their presumably very limited capacity for growth. Simcha et al.[120] have emphasized the need to treat childhood cardiac tumors surgically, a viewpoint supported by the inability to tell rhabdomyomata from other cardiac tumors, which have a greater capacity for growth. Fenoglio believes that patients who are symptomatic should be surgically treated even if multiple tumors are present, because the symptoms are probably due to only one tumor.[117]

The rhabdomyomata in tuberous sclerosis may be up to several centimeters in diameter.[112,115] They may occur anywhere in the heart, and can project from the epicardium or endocardium (Fig. 18). It has been noted that patients with tuberous sclerosis have more intramyocardial tumors than other patients with rhabdomyomata.[47,117] The tumors are well circumscribed but not encapsulated, lighter

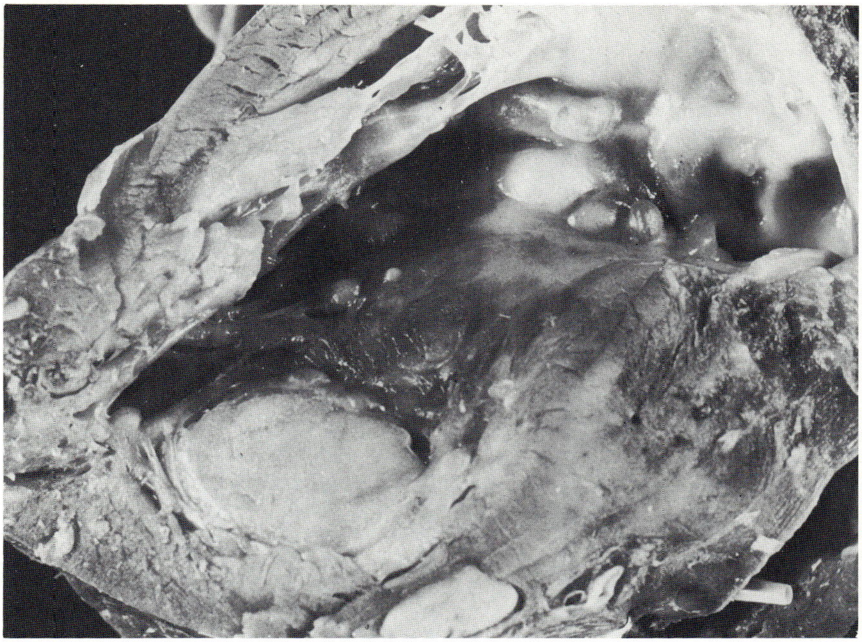

FIG. 18. Multiple well-circumscribed rhabdomyomas. Most are subendocardial but one appears to be intramyocardial.

than the surrounding myocardium, and firm, but not as firm as fibrous tissue. The cut surface may bulge slightly above the myocardium.

Histologically the tumors have a highly distinctive appearance. They are unencapsulated (Fig. 19); the tumor cells range in size from 80 to 200 μ[115] and are larger than surrounding myocardial cells. Tissue fixed in formalin or Zenker's fixative has large irregular or round intracytoplasmic spaces; these may be so numerous as to be separated only by thin eosinophilic trabeculae of residual cytoplasm. Moderate-sized blood vessels, a few lymphocytes, extramedullary hematopoiesis, and large cells with coarsely granular cytoplasm are present in varying amounts. Calcification is unusual but occurs.[111,117] Fibrosis is rare.

At higher powers it is apparent that there is a spectrum of changes, from enlarged cardiac muscle cells with granularity of the cytoplasm to those with a few peripheral vacuoles, culminating in a single, very large vacuole, with the nucleus and cytoplasm pushed peripherally and barely apparent or unseen (Fig. 20). At times, the nucleus is in the center of the cell, with wisps of cytoplasm proceeding towards the periphery, producing a classic "spider" cell (Fig. 20 Top).

The cytoplasm of the rhabdomyoma cells in tuberous sclerosis has striations visible on H & E (Fig. 20 Bottom) staining, but which are accentuated by PTAH. Mallory's trichrome yields red staining of the cytoplasm. There is no cytoplasmic metachromasia with toluidine blue. Mucicarmine and alcian blue stains are negative. Alkaline and acid phosphatase stains are reported to be negative; but

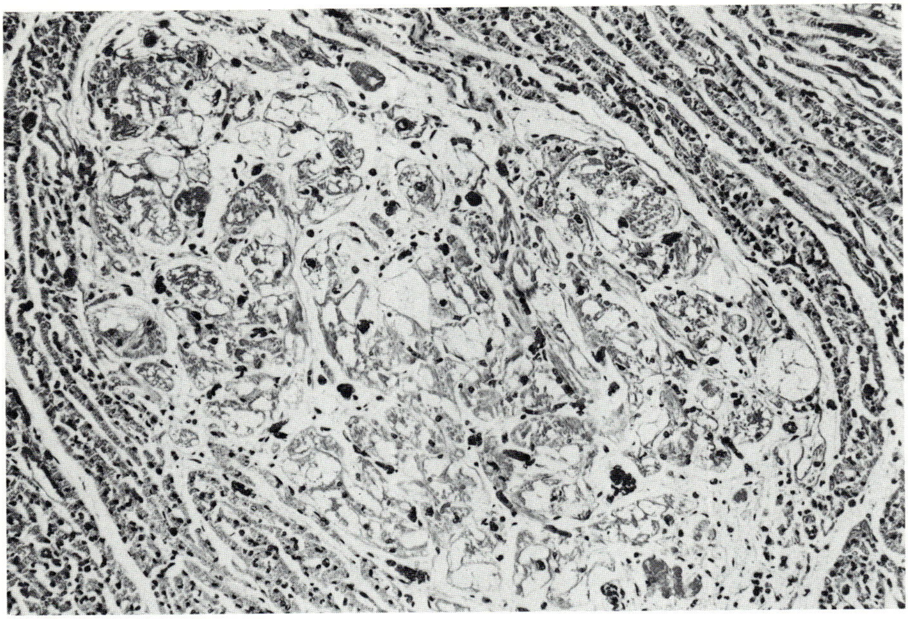

FIG. 19. Cardiac rhabdomyoma. This tumor is unencapsulated and composed of large cells with prominent vacuolization. H&E. ×135.

phosphorylase and debrancher enzymes are increased in involved cells.[111] Succinic dehydrogenase is decreased in relation to its concentration in surrounding myocardial cells.[111]

Alcohol-preserved tissue from rhabdomyomata stains strongly for glycogen. A few droplets of lipid may be visualized with lipid stains. The nuclei of the rhabdomyoma cells are usually single, but occasionally two or three are found within a cell. They are larger and have less dense hematoxylin staining than surrounding myocardial cell nuclei. A small nucleolus may be seen. Mitotic figures are very rare.

Ultrastructurally, the vacuoles are not delimited by membranes. They are either empty or contain glycogen granules, usually of the beta type.[117] The cytoplasm has scattered mitochondria, myofilaments and leptofibrils[117] (Fig. 21). Tubular mitochondrial cristae, lipid droplets,[125] and calcium may be seen.[117] Muscle fragments are variably well formed, with some cases having only Z bands and myosin filaments, while others have thick and thin filaments with Z, I, A, H, and M bands[125] (Fig. 21). No T tubules have been found. The nuclei are ovoid with peripheral chromatin.

The cells are bound by a membrane which contains long segments resembling intercalated discs, with desmosomes, zonulae adherens, large undifferentiated areas, and infrequent nexuses.[117] The intervening stroma contains scattered collagen, including some of the long-spacing variety.

The ultrastructure of cardiac rhabdomyoma has been compared with that of skeletal rhabdomyoma.[117,125] Although cardiac tumors were fixed immediately in

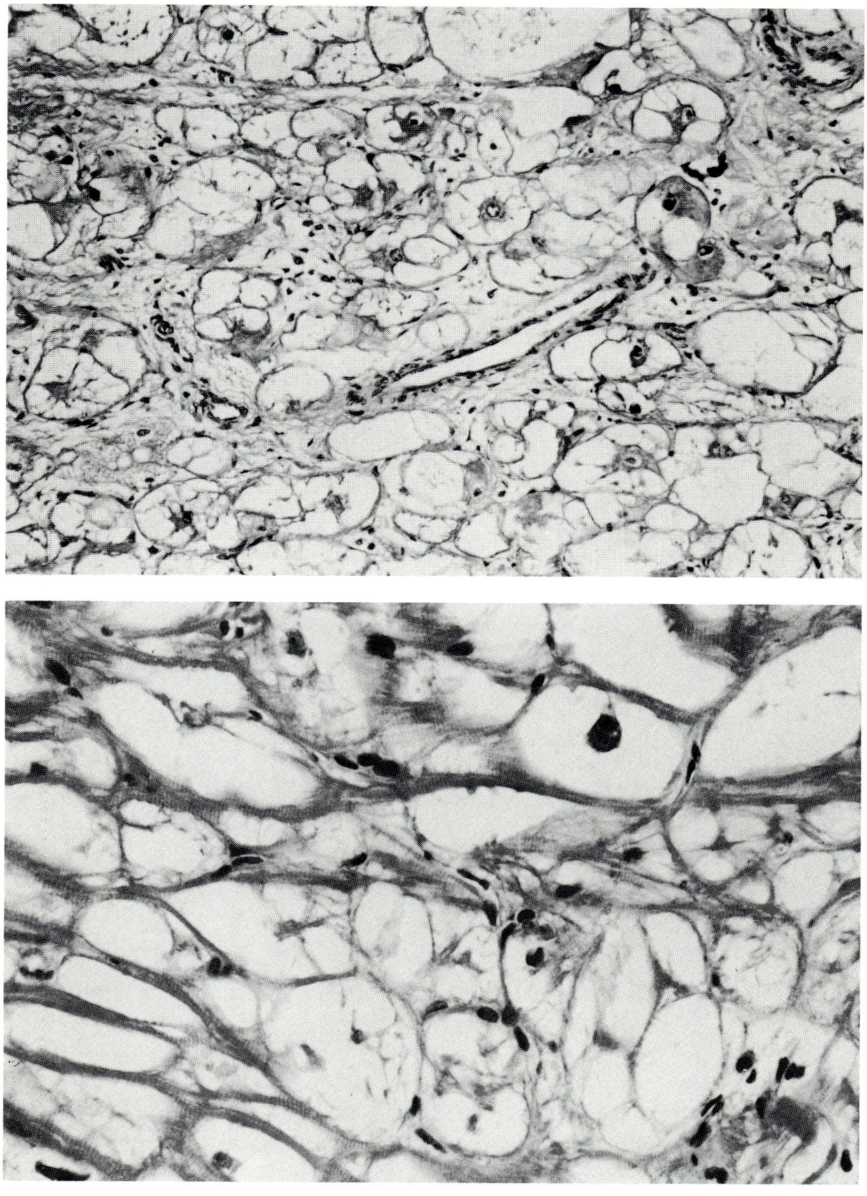

FIG. 20. Rhabdomyomas: **Top.** Only a small amount of interstitium and a few blood vessels separate the tumor cells. These cells have variable proportions of granular cytoplasm to vacuoles. Several "spider" cells are present. H&E. ×135. **Bottom.** Cross striations are evident in residual cytoplasm. H&E. ×340.

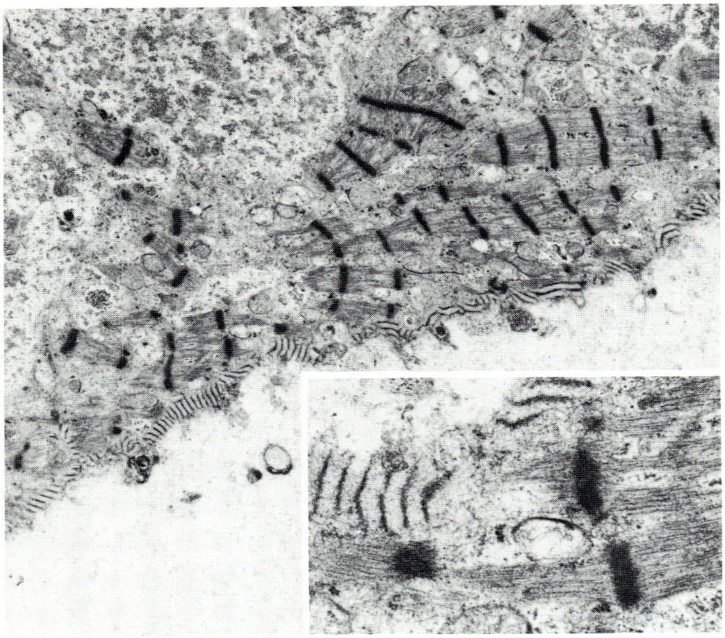

FIG. 21. Rhabdomyoma: Strands of unremarkable muscle are adjacent to leptofibrils and at the edge of a pool of glycogen. ×7,000. Inset: Higher-power view of muscle and leptofibrils. ×21,000.

glutaraldehyde and the skeletal tumor was fixed in formalin for 24 hours in one comparison,[125] there were some differences: The presence of leptofibrils was restricted to the cardiac tumors and hypertrophic Z bands were more apparent in the skeletal tumors. Fenoglio[117] has noted more glycogen and fewer contractile elements in the cardiac tumors. He stated that extracardiac rhabdomyoma cells never have specialized cell junctions. T tubules have been found in extracardiac rhabdomyomas.[126,127]

Normal Purkinje cells differ from myocardial cells in having no demonstrable T tubules or intercalated discs, although they do demonstrate all the components of intercalated discs.[127] Some specialized conducting cells and many atrial muscle cells lack T tubules.[117] Primitive myocardial cells have contractile elements at their periphery, with randomly located intercellular junctions. These similarities led Fenoglio et al. to hypothesize that cardiac rhabdomyoma cells arise aberrantly from primitive cardiac muscle cells before complete differentiation.[117]

Congenital rhabdomyomata in patients with tuberous sclerosis have little or no growth potential. Metastases have never been convincingly demonstrated, and patients treated without surgery have survived for long periods.[114,116] These facts, combined with the histologic appearance of poorly developed cardiac muscle cells in these tumors, have led to the currently accepted hypothesis that they are hamartomas[47,117,125] and not true neoplasms. These tumors probably represent a disordered maturation of clusters of myocardial cells, with no disturbance of organization beyond the cellular level.

Lungs

Pulmonary lesions in tuberous sclerosis were first described by Berg[128] and by Berg and Veglens.[53,130] Less than 50 cases have been reported, and it has been estimated that 1 percent or less of patients with tuberous sclerosis have pulmonary involvement.[131] However, similar pulmonary lesions are vanishingly rare in patients without tuberous sclerosis. The lesion has been designated "tuberous sclerosis of the lung,"[129,132] myomatosis, lymphangiomyoma,[133] and lymphangiomyomatosis.[134,135]

Clinically, patients with pulmonary lesions form a distinct subset of those with tuberous sclerosis. They are older, with an average age of onset of 34 years,[131] have considerably less mental deficiency,[80,99,131] frequently not having been diagnosed as having tuberous sclerosis or any other central nervous system disorder, and are almost all females.[2,47,99,131,134,135] There has been some debate about whether some of these patients have tuberous sclerosis or not,[133] but several who had very few manifestations of tuberous sclerosis have had severely affected children[80] or family members.[136]

These patients frequently present with dyspnea or pneumothorax. Respiratory insufficiency is severe and generally progressive.[80,129,131] The average survival from the age of diagnosis is 3 to 5 years.[80,131] Pneumothorax may be a recurrent and incapacitating problem. One feature that has been noted more frequently in patients who have lymphangiomyomatosis without the stigmata of tuberous sclerosis than in those with tuberous sclerosis is chylothorax.[133,137] However, some cases of tuberous sclerosis with chylothorax have been reported.[138]

The lungs of affected patients have a honeycomb[139,140] or reticular pattern[131] radiologically. Large cysts or pneumothoraces are occasionally visualized. It has been suggested that the radiologic findings of tuberous sclerosis in the brain, kidneys, skeletal system, and chest may be diagnostic in and of themselves.[140]

The gross appearance of affected lungs is striking. The normal lacy parenchymal pattern is replaced, usually diffusely, by a multitude of cysts varying from a few millimeters to several centimeters in size, "resembling a sponge." These cysts are usually empty, but may contain chylous[119] or serous[129] fluid. Their walls vary from paper thin to up to 0.5 cm in thickness, with the thicker areas containing multiple minute cysts.[129] Despite careful examination and the occasional confluence of cysts, their origin from the bronchial tree has been impossible to demonstrate.[129,131] The pleura is frequently thickened and may have scars indicative of old pneumothorax. The lungs are normal to moderately heavy at autopsy, weighing 400 to 800 gm.[107,135] The pulmonary vasculature, including the lymphatics, is usually unremarkable. There may be associated cor pulmonale or a chylous effusion.

Microscopically, the cysts are usually unlined, although occasionally they are cuboidal or, less frequently, they contain ciliated epithelium.[80,137] The tissue between the cysts seems to be the lesion, and consists of a proliferation of spindled, somewhat immature, smooth-muscle cells with interdigitating cleft-like lymphatic spaces (Fig. 22).[80,99,134] These cells are present throughout the lung parenchyma and prominent subpleurally. The mixture of smooth-muscle and endothelial cells has been confirmed ultrastructurally.[141] Fibrosis is not prominent.[135] There may be

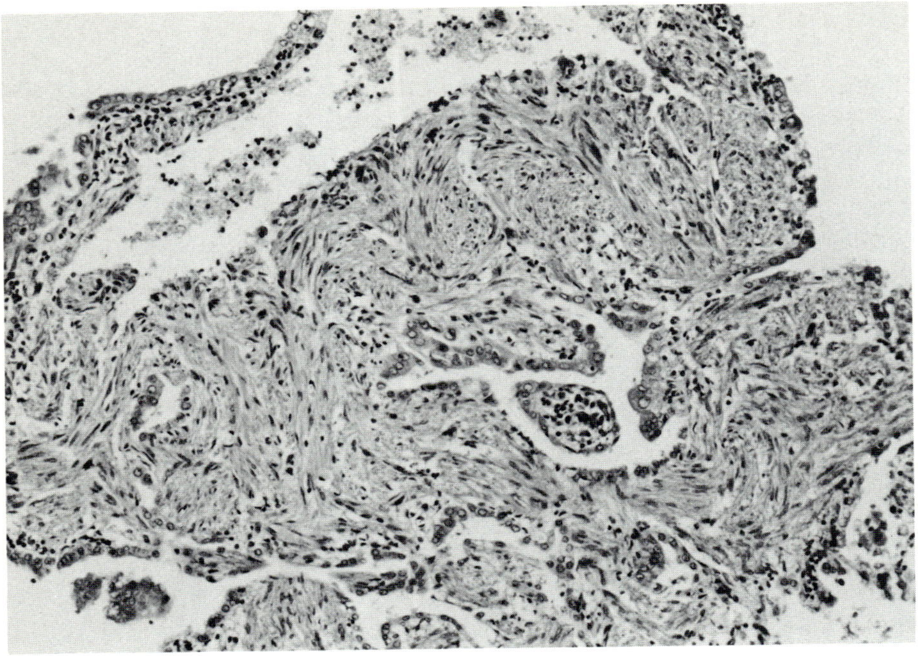

FIG. 22. A pulmonary lesion with bands of smooth muscle and vascular spaces separating alveoli. Material courtesy of Dr. Lynne Reid, Boston, Massachusetts. H&E. ×79.

multiple, enlarged firm white lymph nodes in the mediastinum,[142] containing a similar proliferation of smooth-muscle and endothelial cells. These cells are distributed more randomly throughout the mediastinum in patients with tuberous sclerosis than in those without the disease, with involvement of the thoracic duct more prevalent in the latter. This has been invoked as a possible explanation for the higher incidence of chylothorax among patients without tuberous sclerosis.[133]

The histologic appearance of muscular as opposed to fibrous proliferation is supported by the finding of pulmonary function changes which resemble those of emphysema rather than of diffuse interstitial fibrosis.[132,134,135]

Despite some arguments to the contrary,[143] the lesions found in lymphangiomyomatosis with and without tuberous sclerosis are considered indistinguishable from each other.[133-135,141]

Spleen

Hemangiomatous Hamartoma. Splenic abnormalities of two types have been reported in tuberous sclerosis.[13,24,25,114,129,144] The one usually considered most common is a hemangiomatous malformation, which has been reported in four patients.[24,25,47,144] Two of these patients were evaluated clinically for abdominal masses.[24,25] In one a loud abdominal bruit was present over the mass, and arteriography revealed a vascular lesion with arteriovenous shunting, filled entirely by the splenic artery.[24] The other two patients had no clinical findings referable to their splenic lesion. Despite the vascular nature of the splenic lesions, clinically significant hemorrhage has not been reported.

All of the spleens involved were over 350 gm and contained one or more discrete, deep red, multinodular masses 5 to 11 cm in diameter. On cross section the masses were well demarcated and occasionally had a partial fibrous capsule,[47] with an irregular consistency and a mixed red, yellow, and white surface. Microscopically they were composed of vascular elements in a distorted pattern, with no malpighian corpuscles. Markedly dilated sinusoids formed frequently thrombosed vascular lakes lined by a single layer of endothelial cells.

These vascular hamartomas bear a superficial resemblance to renal angiomyolipomas, but muscle and fat have not been demonstrated. The lesions reported have been large, and even small ones should not be easily missed. Therefore it is unlikely that splenic hemangiomatous hamartoma is a very common lesion in patients with tuberous sclerosis. However, the extreme rarity of such lesions in the general population suggests that they are related to tuberous sclerosis and should be considered a part of that complex rather than incidental findings.

Histiocytoid Cells. The second splenic lesion in tuberous sclerosis is much more subtle than the first, and has never been reported to have any clinical manifestations. It consists of foci of large, eosinophilic histiocytoid cells in the intersinusoidal portions of the red pulp. This lesion was first reported by Morales,[13] and in a recent review,[47] is stated to be unique, despite the report of an identical finding by Tsakraklides et al.[114] and by Östör.[22] We have demonstrated it in a retrospective search in three of five neonates with tuberous sclerosis,[145] making a total of six cases that have been found. All of the patients have been neonates.

Grossly, the involved spleens are unremarkable. By light-microscopy there are occasional clusters of abnormal cells in the red pulp; these are frequently perivascular. Although intrasinusoidal in Tsakraklides'[114] report, the location of the clusters was not consistent in our cases. They are unencapsulated and uncircumscribed, mingle with normal splenic cells, and do not compress or destroy surrounding tissue (Fig. 23). Morales reported collections 2 low-power fields in diameter.[13] The largest in our series was approximately 1 mm.

The histiocytoid cells range from 20 to 75 μ in diameter. They have a large, round, central nucleus with unremarkable chromatin and no nucleolus. Mitoses are not seen. Occasional binucleate cells are present. The cytoplasm is abundant, eosinophilic, and finely granular. The resemblance of these cells to the giant cells of central nervous system tubers is striking. There is no autofluorescence, birefringence, or Ziehl-Neelsen, naphthol-ASD, or Sudan IV[114] staining. The granularity of the cytoplasm is more apparent on PAS staining, which has marked diastase-resistant positivity. Best's carmine staining is positive.[13] Immunostaining for glial fibrillary acidic protein, frequently positive in the central nervous system lesions of tuberous sclerosis, was negative in the single case of a histiocytoid-cell lesion upon which it was perfomed.

The nucleus of the histiocytoid cells is ultrastructurally unremarkable. The

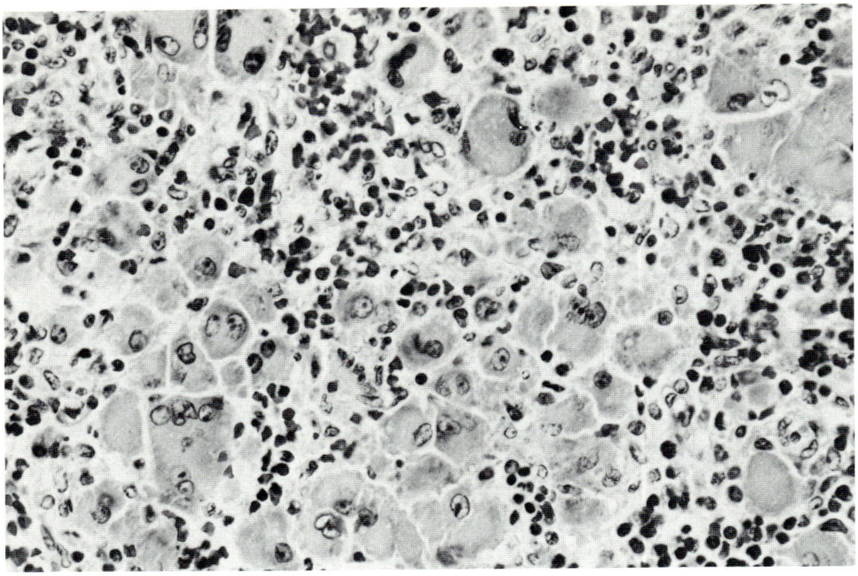

FIG. 23. Splenic histiocytoid cells. An uncircumscribed cluster of large cells with abundant eosinophilic cytoplasm is present. ×340.

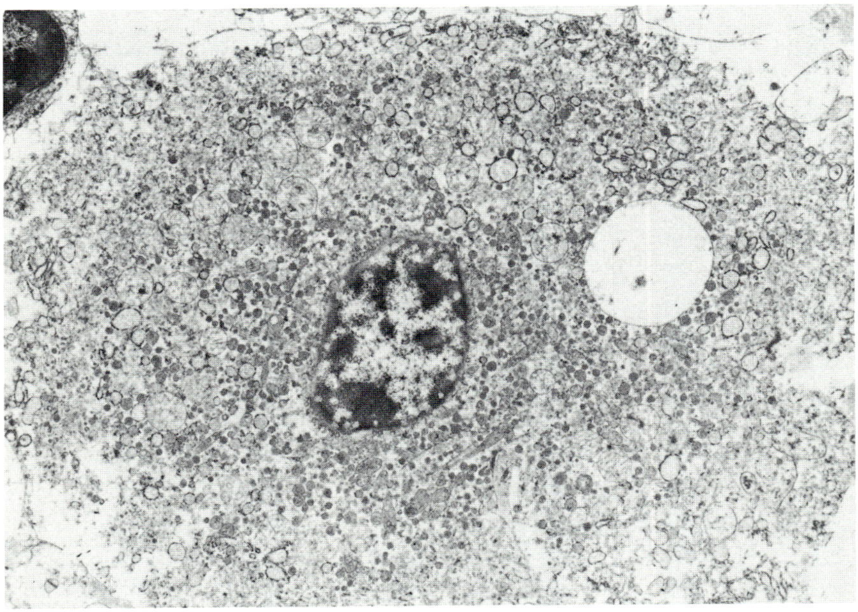

FIG. 24. Histiocytoid cell, spleen. There is prominent perinuclear accumulation of organelles resembling lysosomes. ×6,500.

cytoplasm is characterized by many 90 to 270 nm membrane-bound structures with an amorphous, moderately electron-dense interior (Fig. 24). These organelles frequently had internal membranous circles, and occasionally a more electron-dense core. The peripheral membrane of the organelles was trilaminar. The organelles were most frequently perinuclear. Unremarkable mitochondria and spheres of rough endoplasmic reticulum (RER) containing a small amount of lacy, moderately electron-dense material were present. No fibrils were found, but the tissue studied had been fixed in formalin, and its preservation was suboptimal. The cell membranes were poorly preserved but specialized junctions and processes were not seen.

The origin of the histiocytoid cells is unclear. They do not appear to be the same as the giant cells of the central nervous system. They were designated histiocytes by both Morales[13] and Tsakraklides,[114] and that is still the best designation. It is possible that the 90- to 270-nm organelles are aberrant lysosomes, and the possibility that they are related to the crystalline structures in central nervous system lesions in intriguing, but neither of these speculations is proven. The apparent limitation of the cells to neonates suggests that they are either transient or occur only in the most severely affected tuberous sclerosis patients.

Bone

Cranium. The most commonly described osseous changes in tuberous sclerosis are radiologically visible densities of the cranium. Although some authors believe many of these lesions to be calcified cerebral tubers,[146] Holt and Dickerson have demonstrated that a large fraction are intraosseous.[147,148]

Radiologic changes of the skull are visualized in from 40[148] to 60[63] percent of patients. They are usually finely calcified, poorly defined nodules of the inner table or diploe,[149] with a pagetoid appearance.[150] Thickening of the vault of the skull[56] and of the cranial sutures has also been noted.

Histologically, the nodular lesions are poorly circumscribed areas of hyperostosis[147] surrounded by fat in the marrow space. Haversian canals may be lacking.[89] Many are in close proximity to cerebral tubers,[147,150] and they are much more frequent in patients over the age of 10 years[147]—findings suggesting that most of the nodular lesions are secondary to irritation and pressure from adjacent tubers.

Digits. Cystic spaces in the phalanges and periosteal new bone formation in the metatarsals are also found in tuberous sclerosis[148,151-153]; the former is more common in the hands and the latter in the feet.[148] These lesions have been found in about half of the patients examined. They are unusual in small children, and their progression with time has been illustrated.[148] The rarefied areas are in the periphery of the bone. The lesions are poorly circumscribed and do not distort the bone.

The histologic appearance of these lesions has been described as focal bony resorption with osteoclastic activity in combination with abundant osteoid formation and few osteoblasts[151]; there was dense bone with poorly formed lamellae around fat and dense connective tissue.[151] These changes were considered indicative of old bony resorption and disordered replacement.

The histologic observations described above were obtained from a patient with marked parungual fibromas of all phalanges. The relation of one to the other is unclear. It is possible that they are both effects of local trauma on tissue with a disordered growth capacity.

Periosteal new bone formation in the digital lesions is wavy and irregular,[148] and many other bony changes have been described in tuberous sclerosis,[89,154] including a peculiar myxoid tumor followed by hyperostosis of the mandible.[155] However, the relation of these lesions to the tuberous sclerosis complex is unclear.

Liver

Hamartomas of the liver have been reported several times in tuberous sclerosis.[60,101,102,104,107,144] They are usually discovered at autopsy, but have also been demonstrated angiographically.[101,102] In one series they were demonstrated in five of eight patients upon whom celiac angiography was performed[101]; their incidence and time of occurrence are undocumented. The liver hamartomas are usually multiple,[101] soft, light brown nodules up to several centimeters in diameter. Microscopically, some are entirely composed of fat cells distributed among unremarkable hepatocytes.[104] One example of this type was seen in the seven livers that we examined (Fig. 25). Others occur within the portal regions and consist of a mixture of fat cells, capillaries, and spindled cells. The bile ducts may be dilated and distorted. Fibrosis may be prominent, and Landing[156] has suggested that this

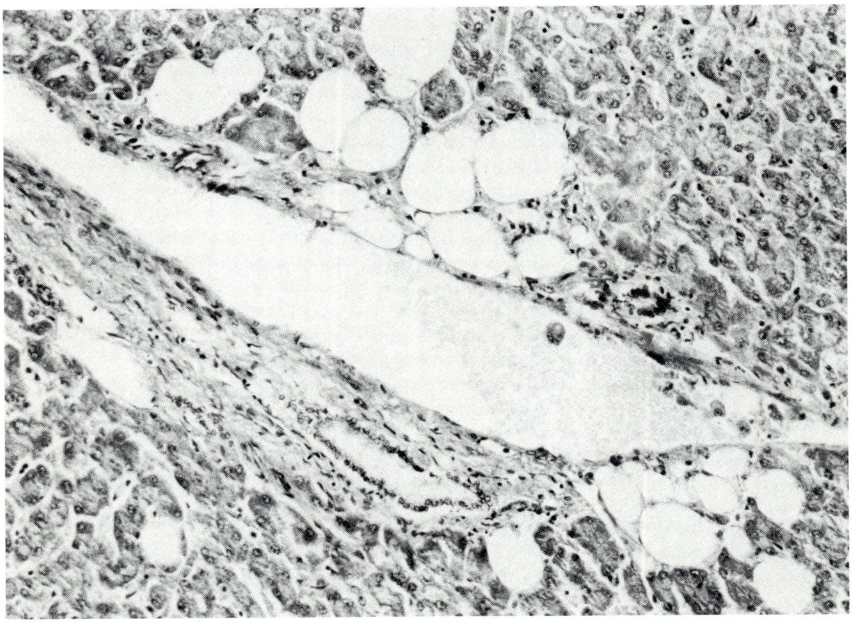

FIG. 25. Periportal adipocytes in the liver. H&E. ×135.

change merits the designation hepatic ductular "polycystic" disease in tuberous sclerosis. The bile-duct changes may well not be the main change in the liver, however, and we believe that retention of the more general designation hamartoma or dysplasia conveys the nature of the lesion more accurately.

Oral Cavity

Two types of lesion have been described in the oral cavity in tuberous sclerosis,[47] both in small numbers of patients and with no reliable data concerning the age at which they appear, their frequency, or whether they are increased in individuals with tuberous sclerosis as opposed to the normal population. Therefore, despite claims to the contrary,[157] these lesions cannot be considered a proven aspect of the tuberous sclerosis complex.

Gingival papillomas[158] or fibromas[86,159] have been reported several times; the tongue and palate have also had such lesions.[86,159] The lesions are usually the color of the surrounding mucosa, but may be grey, red, or yellow.[78] They are firm and nonpainful. Their histologic appearance has not been illustrated. It is most likely that they are fibrous overgrowths similar to the skin lesions, with which they were grouped by Butterworth,[86] and that any papillomatous aspect is secondary.

Small pits were reported on all tooth surfaces of six institutionalized patients with tuberous sclerosis;[157] no control population was studied. Teeth removed for "routine dental treatment" were examined and the roots of teeth from three of four patients had grossly visible enamel pearls. The pits, which were classified as "small pits," "indentations," or "craterlike structures" were studied by light- and scanning electron microscopy (SEM), and were found to consist of simple enamel defects that proceeded as far as the amelodentinal border and were surrounded by normal enamel.

Other Organs

Hamartomas of the mesentery, small intestine,[160] pancreas,[59,104] adrenal glands,[144] and thyroid[60,104] have been reported rarely in tuberous sclerosis. Lymph nodes may contain a proliferation of vascular and smooth-muscle cells, similar to that seen in the lungs.[161]

Diminution of the number of eosinophilic cells in the pituitary, and occasional diabetes insipidus have been reported.[53] This finding has not been systematically evaluated and is of unknown significance.

The lesions noted above can be grouped as mesenchymal and vascular tumors, as in the liver and lymph nodes, or adenomas. The mesenchymal hamartomas are probably a part of the tuberous sclerosis complex; the adenomas may not be.

One study found multiple endocrine and metabolic abnormalities in seven patients with tuberous sclerosis and concluded that such abnormalities were a part of the tuberous sclerosis complex.[162] No tissue was obtained, however.

CONCLUSION

It is apparent that the tuberous sclerosis complex includes far more than epilepsy, adenoma sebaceum, and mental retardation. This developmental disorder may be expressed in almost any tissue or combination of tissues, and has clinical manifestations ranging from minor changes diagnosable only by family study to profound mental disturbance and infant death.

Most of the lesions are hamartomas—abnormal proliferations of tissue indigenous to the involved organ. The cells involved in different organs differ from each other, allowing the dismissal of theories that a single cell line is involved in this disease. In many organs, particularly the brain and eyes, involved cells are very similar to embryonic, undifferentiated cells.

It is likely that tuberous sclerosis is a disease that affects all cells at a very early stage, as has been suggested many times before. As the affected individual matures, these abnormal cells differentiate in unusual directions and eventually manifest themselves as the multitude of lesions catalogued above.

ACKNOWLEDGMENTS

We gratefully acknowledge the secretarial assistance of Ms. Mary Jo Bush and Mrs. Cheryl Myerowitz.

REFERENCES

1. von Recklinghausen F: Ein Herz von einem Neugeborenen welches mehrere Theils nach aussen, Theils nach den Höhlen prominirende Tumoren (Myomen) trug. Verh Ges Geburtsch Monatschr Geburtsk 20:1–2, 1862
2. Bourneville DM: Contribution a l'étude de l'idiotie: Sclérose tubéreuse des circonvolutions cérébrales; idiotie et épilepsie hémiplégique. Arch Neurol (Paris) 1:81–91, 1880
3. Bourneville DM, Brissaud E: Contribution a l'étude de l'idiotie: Encéphalite ou sclérose tubéreuse des circonvolutions cérébrales. Arch Neurol (Paris) 1:397–412, 1881
4. Bourneville DM: Idiotie et épilepsié symptomatiques de sclérose tubéreuse ou hypertrophique. Arch Neurol (Paris) 10:29–39, 1900
5. Rayer PFO: Traite Theorique et Practique de Maladies de la Peau, ed 2. Paris, J.B. Balliére, 1835
6. Balzer F, Menetrier P: Etude sur un cas d'adénomes sébacés de la face et du cuir chevelu. Archiv Physiol Norm Pathol 6 (Série III): 564–576, 1885
7. Pringle JJ: A case of congenital adenoma sebaceum. Br J Dermatol 2:1–14, 1890
8. Perusini G: Über einen Fall von Sclerosa tuberosa hypertrophica. Monatsschr Psychiatr Neurol 17:69–255, 1905
9. Vogt H: Zur Diagnostik der tuberösen Sklerose. Z Erforsch Behandl Jugendl Schwachsinns 2:1–12, 1908
10. Campbell AW: Cerebral sclerosis. Brain 28:382–396, 1905
11. Marcus, cited by: Dalsgaard-Nielsen T, in: Tuberous sclerosis with unusual roentgen picture. Nord Med 10:1541–1548, 1935
12. Van der Hoeve J: Les phakomatoses de Bourneville, de Recklinghausen et de von Hippel-Lindau. J Belge Neurol Psychiatr 33:752–762, 1933

13. Morales JM: Congenital rhabdomyoma, tuberous sclerosis and splenic histiocytosis. Arch Pathol 71:485–493, 1961
14. Hirano A, Tuazon R, Zimmerman HM: Neurofibrillary changes, granulovacuolar bodies and argentophilic bodies observed in tuberous sclerosis. Acta Neuropathol (Berl) 11:257–261, 1968
15. Pellissier JF, Tripier MF, Berard-Badier M, Toga M: Étude ultrastructurale de la tumeur du noyau caudé dans un cas de sclérose tubéreuse de Bourneville. Arch Anat Pathol 20:277–284, 1977
16. Ribadeau-Dumas JL, Poirier J, Escourolle R: Étude ultrastructurale des lésions cérébrales de la sclérose tubéreuse de Bourneville. Acta Neuropathol (Berl) 25:259–270, 1973
17. Probst A, Ohnacker H: Sclérose tubéreuse de Bourneville chez un prématuré. Acta Neuropathol (Berl) 40:157–161, 1977
18. Poirier J, Escourolle R: Etude ultrastructurale d'une tumeur cérébrale dans un cas de sclérose tubéreuse de Bourneville. In: Proceedings, VI Congrès International de Neuropathologie. Paris, Masson, 1970, pp 992–993
19. Arseni C, Alexianu M, Horvat L, et al.: Fine structure of atypical cells in tuberous sclerosis. Acta Neuropathol (Berl) 21:185–193, 1972
20. de Chadarévian J, Hollenberg RD: Subependymal giant cell tumor of tuberose sclerosis: A light and ultrastructural study. J Neuropathol Exp Neurol 38:419–434, 1979
21. Barth PG, Stam FC, vd Harten JJ: Tuberous sclerosis and dysplasia of the corpus callosum: Case report of their combined occurence in a newborn. Acta Neuropathol (Berl) 42:63–64, 1978
22. Östör AG, Fortune DW: Tuberous sclerosis initially seen as hydrops fetalis: Report of a case and review of the literature. Arch Pathol Lab Med 102:34–39, 1978
23. Bender BL, Yunis EJ: The CNS pathology of tuberous sclerosis in children. Ultrast Pathol 1:287–299, 1980
24. Darden JW, Teeslink R, Parrish RA: Hamartoma of the spleen: A manifestation of tuberous sclerosis. Amer Surg 41:564–566, 1975
25. Van Heerden JA, Longo MF, Cardoza F, Farrow GM: The abdominal mass in the patient with tuberous sclerosis. Arch Surg 95:317–319, 1967
26. Mori M, Ikeda T, Onoe T: Blastic Schwann cells in renal tumor of tuberous sclerosis complex: An electron microscopic study. Acta Pathol Jpn 21:121–129, 1971
27. Bhawan J, Edelstein L: Angiofibromas in tuberous sclerosis: A light and electron microscopic study. J Cutan Pathol 4:300–307, 1977
28. Kobayasi T, Wolf- Jürgensen P, Danielsen L: Ultrastructure of shagreen patch. Acta Dermvenereol (Stockh) 58:275–278, 1973
29. Bielschowsky M: Über tuberose Sklerose and ihre Beziehungen zur Recklinghausenschen Krankheit. Z Gesamte Neurol Psychiat 26:133–155, 1914
30. Bielschowsky M: Zur Histopathologie und Pathogenese der tuberösen Sklerose. Z Psychol Neurol 30:167–200, 1923
31. Bolsi D: Contributo all'istogia patologica cerebrale della sclerosi tuberosa. Riv Patol Nerv Ment 33:656–680, 1928
32. Yakolev PI, Guthrie RH: Congenital ectodermoses (neurocutaneous syndromes) in epileptic patients. Arch Neurol Psychiatr 26:1145–1194, 1931
33. Van Bogaert L: Les dysplasies neuro-ectodermiques congenitales. Rev Neurol 63:353–398, 1935
34. Ferraro A, Doolittle GJ: Tuberous sclerosis (diffuse neurospongioblastosis) Psychiat Q 10:365–416, 1936
35. Moolten SE: Hamartial nature of the tuberous sclerosis complex and its bearing on the tumor problem. Arch Intern Med 69:589–623, 1942
36. Kissel P, Beurey J: Les géno-neuro-dermatoses. In: VIII Congrès Dermat et Syphil de Langue Française. Nancy, Vittel, 1953, pp 273–280

37. Inglis K: The relation of the renal lesions to the cerebral lesions in the tuberous sclerosis complex. Am J Pathol 30:739–755, 1954
38. Gunther M, Penrose LS: The genetics of epiloia. J Genet 31:413–430, 1935
39. Marshall D, Saul GB, Sachs E: Tuberous sclerosis: A report of 16 cases in two family trees revealing genetic dominance. N Engl J Med 261:1102–1105, 1959
40. Nevin NC, Pearce WG: Diagnostic and genetical aspects of tuberous sclerosis. J Med Genet 5:273–280, 1968
41. Singer K: Genetic aspects of tuberous sclerosis in a Chinese population. Am J Hum Genet 23:33–40, 1971
42. Stevenson AC, Fischer OD: Frequency of epiloia in Northern Ireland. Br J Prev Soc Med 10:134–135, 1956
43. Farrow GM, Harrison EG, Utz DC, Jones DR: Renal angiomyolipoma: A clinicopathologic study of 32 cases. Cancer 22:564–570, 1968
44. Critchley M, Earl CJC: Tuberous sclerosis and allied conditions. Brain 55:311–346, 1932
45. Kofman O, Hyland HH: Tuberous sclerosis in adults with normal intelligence. Arch Neurol Psychiatr 81:43–48, 1959
46. Duvoisin RC, Vinson WM: Tuberous sclerosis: Report of three cases without mental defect. JAMA 175:869–873, 1961
47. Gomez M: Tuberous Sclerosis. New York, Raven Press, 1979
48. Lagos JC, Gomez MR: Tuberous sclerosis: Reappraisal of a clinical entity. Mayo Clin Proc 42:26–49, 1967
49. Brun A: The subpial granular layer of the foetal cerebral cortex in congenital cortical malformations. Arch Pathol Microbiol Scand (Suppl 179), 1965
50. Borberg A: Clinical and genetic investigations into tuberous sclerosis and Recklinghausen's neurofibromatosis. Contribution to elucidation of interrelationship and eugenics of the syndromes. Acta Psychiatr Scand (Suppl 71):11–239, 1951
51. Velasco ME, Dahl D, Roessman U, Gambetti P: Immunohistochemical localization of glial fibrillary acidic protein in human glial neoplasms. Cancer 45:484–494, 1980
52. Hartdegen A: Ein Fall von multipler Verhärtung des Grosshirns nebst histologisch Eigenartigen harten Geschwulsten der Seitenventrikel (Glioma gangliocellulare) bei einem Neugeborenen. Arch Psychiatr Nervenkr 11:117–131, 1881
53. Rubinstein LJ: Tumors of the Central Nervous System, Washington DC, Armed Forces Institute of Pathology, 1970, p 302
54. Van der Hoeve J: Eye symptoms in tuberous sclerosis of the brain. Trans Ophthalmol Soc UK 40:329–334, 1920
55. Font R, Ferry AF: The phakomatoses. In Ferry AF (ed): Ocular and Adnexal Tumors. Int Ophthalmol Clin 12:1–50, 1972
56. Hall GS: The ocular manifestations of tuberous sclerosis. Q J Med 15:209–220, 1946
57. Nyboer JH, Robertson DM, Gomez MR: Retinal lesions in tuberous sclerosis. Arch Ophthalmol 94:1277–1280, 1976
58. Miles PW, Dixon JM: Tuberous sclerosis in three siblings. Arch Ophthalmol 41:473–480, 1949
59. Pagenstecher WJ: Tuberous sclerosis: Historical review and report of two cases. Am J Ophthalmol 39:663–676, 1955
60. Reed WB, Nickel WR, Campion G: Internal manifestations of tuberous sclerosis. Arch Dermatol 87:715–728, 1963
61. Grover WD, Harley RD: Early recognition of tuberous sclerosis by funduscopic examination. J Pediatr 75:991–995, 1969
62. Atkinson A, Sanders MD, Wong V: Vitreous haemorrhage in tuberous sclerosis. Br J Ophthalmol 57:773–779, 1973
63. Kranias G, Romano PE: Depigmented iris sector in tuberous sclerosis. Am J Ophthalmol 83:758–759, 1977
64. Harley RD, Grover WD: Tuberous sclerosis: Description and report of 12 cases. Ann Ophthalmol 1:477–481, 1970

65. Koch FLP, Walsh MN: Syndrome of tuberous sclerosis: Report of a case. Arch Ophthalmol 21:465–475, 1939
66. Walsh MN, Koch FLP, Brunsting HA: The syndrome of tuberous sclerosis, retinal tumors and adenoma sebaceum: Report of a case. Mayo Clin Proc 13:155–160, 1938
67. Lagos JC, Holman CB, Gomez MR: Tuberous sclerosis: Neuroroentgenologic observations. Am J Roentgenol 104:171–176, 1968
68. McLean JM: Glial tumors of the retina in relation to tuberous sclerosis. Am J Ophthalmol 41:428–432, 1956
69. Cleasby GW, Fung WE, Shekter WD: Astrocytoma of the retina: Report of two cases. Am J Ophthalmol 64:633–637, 1967
70. Gass JDM: Differential Diagnosis of Intraocular Tumors: A Stereoscopic Presentation. St. Louis, CV Mosby, 1974, p 371
71. Morris WE, La Piana FG: Spontaneous regression of bilateral multifocal retinoblastoma with preservation of normal visual acuity. Ann Ophthalmol 6:1192–1194, 1974
72. Reese AB: Relation of drusen of the optic nerve to tuberous sclerosis. Arch Ophthalmol 24:187–205, 1940
73. Messinger HC, Clarke BE: Retinal tumors in tuberous sclerosis. Review of the literature and report of a case with special attention to microscopic structure. Arch Ophthalmol 18:1–11, 1937
74. Wolter JR, Mertus JM: Exophytic retinal astrocytoma in tuberous sclerosis. J Pediatr Ophthalmol Strabismus 6:186–191, 1969
75. Barsky D, Wolter JR: The retinal lesions of tuberous sclerosis: An angiomatous hamartoma? J Pediatr Ophthalmol Strabismus 8:261–265, 1971
76. Van der Hoeve J: Augengeschwülste bei de tuberosen Hirnsklerose (Bourneville) und verwandten Krankheiten. Arch f Ophthalmol 111:1–16, 1923
77. Zolli C, Rodrigues MM, Shannon GM: Unusual eyelid involvement in tuberous sclerosis. J Pediatr Ophthalmol Strabismus 13:156–158, 1976
78. Luo TH: Conjunctival lesions in tuberous sclerosis. Am J Ophthalmol 23:1029–1034, 1940
79. Tridon P, Marchand P, Coffe P: Sclerose tubereuse de Bourneville et malformations oculaires. Rev Otoneuroophthalmol 49:43–46, 1977
80. Dawson J: Pulmonary tuberous sclerosis and its relation to other forms of the disease. Q J Med 23:113–145, 1954
81. Bundey S, Evans K: Tuberous sclerosis: A genetic study. J Neurol Neurosurg Psychiatry 32:591–603, 1969
82. Gold AP, Freeman JM: Depigmented nevi: The earliest sign of tuberous sclerosis. Pediatrics 35:1003–1005, 1965
83. Fitzpatrick TB, Szabo G, Hori Y, et al.: White leaf-shaped macules: Earliest visible sign of tuberous sclerosis. Arch Dermatol 98:1–6, 1968
84. Nickel WR, Reed WB: Tuberous sclerosis: Special reference to the microscopic alterations in the cutaneous hamartomas. Arch Dermatol 85:209–226, 1962
85. Kiun TP: A propos de deux cas de tumeurs de Koenen isolées. Bull Soc Franc Derm Syph 71:586–587, 1964
86. Butterworth T, Wilson M: Dermatologic aspects of tuberous sclerosis. Arch Derm Syph 43:1–41, 1941
87. Chao DH: Congenital neurocutaneous syndromes in childhood. J Pediatr 55:447–459, 1959
88. Ross AT, Dickerson WW: Tuberous sclerosis. Arch Neurol Psychiatry 50:233–257, 1943
89. Donegani G, Grattarola FR, Wildi E: Tuberous sclerosis: Bourneville disease. In Vinken PJ, Bruyn GW (eds): Handbook of Clinical Neurology: the Phakomatoses, Vol 14. New York, American Elsevier, 1972, pp 340–389
90. Jimbow K, Fitzpatrick TB, Szabo G, Hori Y: Congenital circumscribed hypo-

melanosis: A characterization based on electron microscopic study of tuberous sclerosis, nevus depigmentosis, and piebaldism. J Invest Dermatol 64:50–62, 1975
91. Rague CJ, Wood MG: Connective tissue nevus. Arch Dermatol 102:390–396, 1970
92. Kobayasi T, Asboe-Hansen G: Ultrastructure of generalized scleroderma. Acta Dermvenereol 52:81–93, 1972
93. Lever W, Shaumberg-Lever G: Histopathology of the Skin, ed 5. Philadelphia, JB Lippincott, 1975, p 575
94. Noon ZB, Williams OO: Tuberous sclerosis: Report of a case. Arch Derm Syph 50:96–98, 1944
95. Good CK, Garb J: Symmetric nevi of face, tuberous sclerosis, epilepsy, and fibromatous growth of scalp. Arch Derm Syph 47:197–206, 1943
96. Kissel P, Schmitt J: Les formes viscérales des phakomatoses. In Michaux, Feld (eds): Les Phakomatoses Cérébrales. Paris, SPEI, 1963, pp 221–253
97. Fischer W: Die Nierentumoren bei der tuberösen Hirnsklerose. Beitr Pathol Anat 50:235–282, 1911
98. McCullough D, Scott R, Seybold H: Renal angiomyolipoma (hamartoma): Review of the literature and report of 7 cases. J Urol 105:32–44, 1971
99. Murphy ES, Fuyü Y, Yasuda A, Sasabe S: The tuberous sclerosis complex: A study of a new case. Arch Pathol 65:166–173, 1958
100. Schnitzer B: Tuberous sclerosis complex: Report of a 62-year-old patient who died of renal involvement. Arch Pathol 76:626–632, 1963
101. Compton WR, Lester PD, Kyaw MM, Madsen JA: The abdominal angiographic spectrum of tuberous sclerosis. Am J Roentgenol 126:807–813, 1976
102. Viamonte M, Ravel R, Politano V, Bridges B: Angiographic findings in a patient with tuberous sclerosis. Am J Roetgenol 98:723–733, 1966
103. Price EB, Mostofi FK: Symptomatic angiomyolipoma of the kidney. Cancer 18:761–774, 1965
104. Perou ML, Gray PT: Mesenchymal hamartomas of the kidney. J Urol 83:240–261, 1960
105. Sun CN, White HJ, Bissada NK: Renal angiomyolipoma in a case of tuberous sclerosis, an electron microscopy study. Beitr Pathol 156:401–410, 1975
106. Bernstein J, Brough AJ, MacAdams AJ: The renal lesion in syndromes of multiple congenital malformations. In: Birth Defects: Original Article Series 10 (4):35–43, 1974
107. Chonko AM, Weiss SM, Stein JH, Ferris TF: Renal involvement in tuberous sclerosis. Am J Med 56:124–132, 1973
108. Wenzl JE, Lagos JC, Albers DD: Tuberous sclerosis presenting as polycystic kidneys and seizures in an infant. J Pediatr 77:673–676, 1970
109. Stapleton FB, Johnson D, Kaplan GW, Griswold W: The cystic renal lesions in tuberous sclerosis. J Pediatr 97:574–579, 1980
110. Osathanondh V, Potter EL: Pathogenesis of polycystic kidneys. Arch Pathol 77:459–516, 1964
111. Golding R, Reed G: Rhabdomyoma of the heart: Two unusual clinical presentations. N Engl J Med 276:957–959, 1967
112. Batchelor TM, Maun ME: Congenital glycogenic tumors of the heart. Arch Pathol 39:67–73, 1945
113. Kidder LA: Congenital glycogenic tumors of the heart. Arch Pathol 49:55–62, 1950
114. Tsakraklides V, Burke B, Mastri A, et al. Rhabdomyomas of heart: A report of four cases. Am J Dis Child 128:639–646, 1974
115. Farber S: Congenital rhabdomyoma of the heart. Am J Pathol 7:105–130, 1931
116. Shaher RM, Mintzer J, Farina M, et al. Clinical presentation of rhabdomyoma of the heart in infancy and childhood. Am J Cardiol 30:95–103, 1972
117. Fenoglio JJ, McAllister HA, Ferrans VJ: Cardiac rhabdomyoma: A clinicopathologic and electron microscopic study. Am J Cardiol 38:241–251, 1976

118. Shaher RM, Farina M, Alley R, et al.: Congenital subaortic stenosis in infancy caused by rhabdomyoma of the left ventricle. J Thorac Cardiovasc Surg 63:157–163, 1972
119. Kuehl KS, Perry LW, Chandra R, Scott LP III: Left ventricular rhabdomyoma: A rare cause of subaortic stenosis in the newborn infant. Pediatrics 46:464–468, 1970
120. Simcha A, Wells BG, Tynan MJ, Waterston DJ: Primary cardiac tumors in childhood. Arch Dis Child 46:508–514, 1971
121. Kayaba T, Hoshino S, Abe T, Honda K: Cardiac rhabdomyoma: Report of a case. Int Surg 46:88–93, 1966
122. Sussman W, Stasney J: Congenital glycogenic tumor of the heart. Am Heart J 40:312–315, 1950
123. Labate JS: Congenital rhabdomyoma of the heart: Report of a case. Am J Pathol 15:137–140, 1939
124. Farooki ZQ, Henry JC, Arciniegas E, Green FW: Ultrasonic pattern of ventricular rhabdomyoma in two infants. Am J Cardiol 34:842–844, 1974
125. Silverman JF, Kay S, Chang CH: Ultrastructural comparison between skeletal muscle and cardiac rhabdomyomas. Cancer 42:189–193, 1978
126. Cornog J, Gonatas NK: Ultrastructure of rhabdomyoma. J Ultrastruct Res 20:433–450, 1967
127. Rhodin JAG: Histology: A Text and Atlas. New York, Oxford University Press, 1974, p 240
128. Berg G: Spontan pneumothex vid fall au "Cystlunga": Sv lakaretidningen 52, 1938
129. Veglens G: Specific pulmonary alterations in tuberous sclerosis. Acta Pathol Microbiol Scand 18:317–330, 1941
130. Berg G, Vejlens G: Maladie kystique du poumon et sclérose tubéreuse du cerveau. Acta Paediatr 26:16–30, 1939
131. Dwyer JM, Hickie JB, Garvan J: Pulmonary tuberous sclerosis: Report of three patients and a review of the literature. QJ Med 40:115–125, 1971
132. Lie JT, Miller RD, Williams DE: Cystic disease of the lungs in tuberous sclerosis. Mayo Clin Proc 55:547–553, 1980
133. Jao J, Gilbert S, Messer R: Lymphoangiomyoma and tuberous sclerosis. Cancer 29:1188–1192, 1972
134. Silverstein EF, Ellis K, Wolff M, Jaretzki A III: Pulmonary lymphangiomyomatosis. Am J Roentgenol 120:832–850, 1974
135. Vadas G, Pare JA, Thurlbeck WM: Pulmonary and lymph node myomatosis. Can Med Assoc J 96:420–424, 1967
136. Malik SK, Pardee N, Martin CJ: Involvement of the lungs in tuberous sclerosis. Chest 58:538–540, 1970
137. Joliat G, Stalder H, Kapanci Y: Lymphangiomatosis: A clinicoanatomical entity. Cancer 31:455–461, 1973
138. Broughton RBK: Pulmonary tuberous sclerosis presenting with pleural effusion. Br Med J 1:477–478, 1970
139. Oswald N, Parkinson T: Honeycomb lungs. QJ Med 18:1–20, 1949
140. Teplick JG: Tuberous sclerosis: Extensive roentgen findings without the usual clinical picture. A case report. Radiology 93:53–55, 1969
141. Monteforte WJ, Kohnen PW: Angiomyolipomas in a case of lymphangiomyomatosis syndrome: Relationships to tuberous sclerosis. Cancer 34:317–321, 1974
142. Wolff M: Lymphangiomyoma: Clinicopathologic study and ultrastructural confirmation of its histogenesis. Cancer 31:988–1007, 1973
143. Stovin PGI, Lum LC, Flower CDR, et al. The lungs in lymphangiomatosis and in tuberous sclerosis. Thorax 30:497–509, 1975
144. Cares RM: The tuberous sclerosis complex. J Neuropathol Exp Neurol 17:247–254, 1958
145. Bender BL, Yunis EJ: Splenic involvement in tuberous sclerosis. Report of three cases. Virchows Arch [Pathol Anat] 391:363–369, 1981

146. Yakolev PI, Corwin W: A roentgenographic sign in cases of tuberous sclerosis of brain (multiple "brain stones"). Arch Neurol Psychiatry 40:1030–1037, 1939
147. Dickerson WW: Characteristic roentgenographic changes associated with tuberous sclerosis. Arch Neurol Psychiatry 53:199–204, 1945
148. Holt JF, Dickerson WW: The osseous lesions of tuberous sclerosis. Radiology 58:1–7, 1952
149. Ravault PP, Colomb D, Lejeune E, et al.: Sclérose tubéreuse de Bourneville à déterminations multiples, en particulier osseuses. Lyon Méd 93:815–822, 1961
150. Dalsgaard-Nielsen T: Tuberous sclerosis with unusual roentgen picture. Nord Med 10:1541–1548, 1935
151. Dickerson WW: Nature of certain osseous lesions in tuberous sclerosis. Arch Neurol Psychiatry 75:525–529, 1955
152. Ravault PP, Colomb D, Lejeune E, et al.: Les déterminations osseuses de le sclérose tubéreuse de Bourneville. Rev Rhum Mal Osteoartic 29:158–164, 1962
153. Gottlieb JS, Lavine GR: Tuberous sclerosis with unusual lesions of the bones. Arch Neurol Psychiatry 33:379–388, 1935
154. Paterson JH: Tuberous sclerosis with ? melorheostosis. Proc R Soc Med 45:228–229, 1952
155. Rushton MA: Some less common bone lesions affecting the jaws. Oral Surg 9:284–304, 1956
156. Landing BH, Wells TR, Claireaux AE: Morphometric analysis of liver lesions in cystic diseases of childhood. Hum Pathol 11:549–560, 1980
157. Hoff M, van Grunsven MF, Jongebloed WL, 's-Gravenmade EJ: Enamel defects associated with tuberous sclerosis: A clinical and scanning-electron-microscope study. Oral Surg 40:261–269, 1975
158. Papanayotou P, Vezirtzi E: Tuberous sclerosis with gingival lesions: Report of a case. Oral Surg 39:578–582, 1975
159. Gorlin RJ, Chaudhry AP, Kelln EE: Oral manifestations of the Fitzgerald-Gardner, Pringle-Bournevelle, Robin, adrenogenital, and Hurler-Pfaundler syndromes. Oral Surg 13:1233–1244, 1960
160. Engstrom N, Ljungquist A, Persson B, Wetterfors J: Tuberous sclerosis with a localized malformation in the ileum and excessive albumin loss into the lower gastrointestinal tract. Pediatrics 30:681–693, 1962
161. Berg G, Vejlens G: Cystic lungs of rare origin-tuberous sclerosis. Acta Radiol 36:425–436, 1941
162. Sareen CK, Ruvalcaba RHA, Scotvold MJ, et al.: Tuberous sclerosis: Clinical, endocrine, and metabolic studies. Am J Dis Child 123:34–39, 1972

VITAMIN D AND METABOLIC BONE DISEASE: A CLINICOPATHOLOGIC OVERVIEW

ARNOLD FELSENFELD AND FRANCISCO LLACH

A review of a major topic should provide a historical background against which our current knowledge can be put in perspective. The history of vitamin D and the vitamin D deficiency diseases is essential to the understanding of present knowledge of these two entities.

At the beginning of the twentieth century, rickets was a common disease whose etiology was not known. Thus, Professor Clemens Pirquet believed that rickets, like tuberculosis, was an infectious disease, affecting children made susceptible by inherited and nutritional factors. Lawson Dick published a book on the topic of rickets, and in the book, while attributing the etiology of rickets to some nutritional factor—probably protein deficiency—recommended treatments such as massage with skin friction.[1] In 1919, Mellanby published his work on the production and cause of experimental rickets, proving that dietary deficiencies could produce rickets in puppies.[2] The Medical Research Council studied rickets in postwar Vienna (1919 to 1922) and demonstrated that either cod liver oil or sunlight exposure would prevent its development or heal the condition if it already existed.[1] Also, Huldschinsky, in 1919, showed that ultraviolet irradiation of a solitary limb could cure rickets of the entire body, suggesting that the ultraviolet light might have been activating a substance capable of action at a distant site.[3]

In 1927, Parsons, in two separate papers, described the rickets of chronic renal disease and celiac disease.[4,5] Albright, in 1937, reported a nonnutritional rickets that failed to respond to the usual dosages of cod liver oil. Albright termed the disease "vitamin D resistant rickets."[6] During the 1930s, Fanconi and DeToni provided a description of a new form of renal rickets. They described patients who were not severely azotemic but had defects in urinary concentrating capacity, hydrogen ion secretion, and reabsorption of filtered substances such as glucose, phosphate, and

This work has been supported in part by a grant from the Veterans Administration Research Advisory Group.

amino acids.[7-9] With the advent of paper chromatography in 1944, the analysis of amino acids became possible, and allowed the entity known as cystinosis to be separated from other forms of renal tubular disease.[10]

As might be expected, the past three decades have produced a further expansion of knowledge of vitamin D and its deficiency states. New disease entities have been described and the elaboration of previously described diseases has been accomplished. In addition, new investigative techniques have provided details of the metabolic pathway of vitamin D. However, many unanswered questions remain with regard to vitamin D and its metabolism.

VITAMIN D METABOLITES

Vitamin D and its metabolites are sterol hormones that are major regulators of mineral metabolism in man and other species. The pathway for the metabolism of vitamin D includes the production of vitamin D_3 (cholecalciferol) from the activation of 7-dehydrocholesterol maximally concentrated in the malphigian layer of the skin. This activation is accomplished by exposure to ultraviolet light of wavelength 290 to 320 nm.[11] In addition, a comparable substrate, vitamin D_2 (ergocalciferol), can be ingested in the diet and absorbed in the small bowel. Although more than 80 percent of metabolized vitamin D exists in the form of vitamin D_3 (cholecalciferol) in man,[12] there appears to be little difference in activity between the cholecalciferol and ergocalciferol. However, this fact does not appear to be universal, since in birds and New-World primates, vitamin D_2 is less effective than vitamin D_3 in enhancing calcium absorption.[13]

The next principal step in the metabolism of vitamin D is the hepatic hydroxylation of the 25 position of the vitamin. This reaction occurs either in the microsomal fraction or the endoplasmic reticulum of hepatic cells.[14] Once the liver produces 25-hydroxy-vitamin D_3 (25-OHD_3), the hydroxylated compound is bound to an alpha globulin, molecular weight approximately 58,000, and is released into the circulation.[15]

Although it is not certain whether the level of 25-OHD_3 controls 25-hydroxylase activity, several known factors do contribute to the circulatory level of 25-OHD_3.[16,17] First, it is well known that marked seasonal variations in the level of 25-OHD_3 do exist; thus, plasma levels of 25-OHD_3 are highest during the summer and lowest in the winter months.[18] In addition, a geographic variability is known to exist for values of 25-OHD_3. For example, in the United States, most assays for 25-OHD_3 have yielded plasma concentrations ranging from 10 to 80 ng/ml; in the United Kingdom, the normal range is between 4 and 20 ng/ml. There is little doubt that climate and resultant sunlight exposure are major contributing factors to these variations in concentration.[19] Besides sunlight exposure, vitamin D fortification of such common staples as milk and bread may also have a role. The best natural sources of vitamin D are eggs, butter, cream, liver, and fish.[13]

Dietary vitamin D_2 is absorbed principally in the proximal small intestine. The absorption is facilitated by bile salts and the formation of chylomicrons. Hence, any disease process that either involves the small bowel mucosa or the production of bile salts can affect the quantity of vitamin D presented to the liver for 25-hydroxylation.[20] In addition to being affected by disease states, vitamin D_2 may be bound in the small bowel lumen by drugs such as cholestyramine, or by phytate contained in whole-grain cereals.[21]

Impaired 25-hydroxylase activity may occur in hepatocellular disease and affect the level of 25-OHD_3. Certain drugs, such as anti–convulsants, may alter the turnover or metabolism of 25-OHD_3.[22] Recent studies have demonstrated that 25-OHD_3 undergoes an enterohepatic circulation. After an intravenous injection of radioactive 25-OHD_3, approximately one-third of this radioactive substance is secreted into the duodenum within 24 hours, and 85 percent of this amount is reabsorbed by the ileum.[23] Hence, any process that affects the ileal resorptive capacity may theoretically alter 25-OHD_3 levels.

The second major step in the metabolism of vitamin D, 1-alpha hydroxylation, occurs in the mitochondria of the renal cortical cells.[24,25] The 1-alpha-hydroxylase activity is localized to the kidney cortex in every vertebrate class. In fish, reptiles, birds, and mammals, 1,25-$(OH)_2D_3$ is produced in the renal cortex. From such evidence, it would appear that 1,25$(OH)_2D_3$ production has been confined to the kidney since early in vertebrate evolution.[13]

The principal modulation of 1-alpha-hydroxylase activity appears to be by both parathyroid hormone (PTH) and phosphorus. Parathyroidectomy eliminates the response of 1-alpha-hydroxylase to hypocalcemia; however, the activity of the enzyme and the production of 1,25-$(OH)_2D_3$ can be restored by exogenous parathyroid hormone.[26,27] Similarly, 1-alpha-hydroxylase activity can be restored and increased in a parathyroidectomized animal by producing hypophosphatemia.[28,29] In addition to the currently well-recognized effects of parathyroid hormone and phosphorus, a variety of other hormones—growth hormone, prolactin, estrogen, and progesterone—appear to influence 1,25$(OH)_2D_3$ concentrations.[19] Whether these hormones act directly through 1-alpha-hydroxylase remains to be clarified. Nevertheless, increased circulating levels of 1,25-$(OH)_2D_3$ are present during such conditions as pregnancy, lactation, and the growth period.

Another major vitamin D metabolite is 24,25-dihydroxycholecalciferol (24,25-$(OH)_2D_3$). It has been demonstrated that 24,25-$(OH)_2D_3$ is produced in the kidney[30]; however, whether 24,25-$(OH)_2D_3$ is produced in extrarenal sites remains unclear.[31] Present evidence suggests that 24-hydroxylase activity is induced by the presence of 1,25-$(OH)_2D_3$. This results in the 24-hydroxylation of both 25-OHD_3 and 1,25-$(OH)_2D_3$.[32] The 24-hydroxylation of 1,25-$(OH)_2D_3$ results in 1,24,25-$(OH)_3D_3$, whose role at present is totally unknown.[33] Another vitamin D metabolite that should be mentioned for the sake of completeness is 25,26-dihydroxyvitamin D_3;[34] little information is available regarding its biologic significance.

Considerable debate has been directed to whether an increase in the levels of 1,25-$(OH)_2D_3$ results in a direct inhibition of parathyroid hormone (PTH) secretion. In vitro inhibition of PTH secretion by 1,25-$(OH)_2D_3$ has been demonstrated[35]; however, the results of in vivo experiments have provided conflicting results.[36,37] A recent series of experiments by Canterbury et al. have suggested that 24,25-$(OH)_2D_3$ may be directly responsible for the suppression of PTH secretion.[38,39] Further investigation into this issue may be forthcoming.

The estimated biologic half-lives of vitamin D, 25-OHD_3, 24,25-$(OH)_2D_3$, and 1,25-$(OH)_2D_3$ are 19 to 25 hours, 12 days, 15 to 40 days, and 12 hours, respectively. The accepted normal serum concentrations are: 25-OHD_3, 15 to 80 ng/ml (United States); 24,25-$(OH)_2D_3$, either 8 ng/ml (St. Louis) or 1.5 to 1.7 ng/ml (Great Britain); 1,25-$(OH)_2D_3$, 25 to 33 pg/ml (adults) and 49 to 66 pg/ml (adolescents).[13,19] It should be mentioned that the concentration of 1,25-$(OH)_2D_3$ in picograms is approximately 1/1,000 that of 25-OHD_3 and 24,25-$(OH)_2D_3$ in nanograms.

PHYSIOLOGIC ACTIONS

Vitamin D and its metabolites are integrally involved in calcium homeostasis and bone metabolism, and probably have a role in the maintenance of muscle strength.

Once radioactively labeled vitamin D compounds became available, in 1965, it was soon readily apparent that additional modifications of the parent compound were necessary to produce the resultant biologic activity. After a physiologic intravenous or oral dose of vitamin D_3, 9 and 16 hours, respectively, were required to achieve a target-organ response, and pharmacologic doses of vitamin D_3 failed to accelerate the time required for this target-organ response. It has subsequently been shown that 1,25-$(OH)_2D_3$ can augment intestinal calcium absorption 2 to 3 hours after its administration.[13,40]

Hydroxylation at the 25 position of vitamin D_3 occurs in the liver. The initial belief that 25-OHD_3 is an inactive metabolite on the pathway to the final agent of vitamin D activity—1,25-$(OH)_2D_3$—has been contradicted by several lines of evidence. First, there are data to the effect that in muscle, 25-OHD_3 may be the principal metabolite of vitamin D. Large quantities of 25-OHD_3 are found in muscle, and muscle has a high binding affinity for 25-OHD_3.[41,42] In such conditions as nutritional osteomalacia and anticonvulsant-induced osteomalacia, muscle weakness is a major finding.[43] In both conditions, 1,25-$(OH)_2D_3$ has been measured and found to be normal, while 25-OHD_3 values are markedly diminished.[44,45] Second, evidence has been presented that 25-OHD_3 may have a role, independent of 1,25-$(OH)_2D_3$, in the reabsorption of phosphate from the urine.[46] Third, evidence exists suggesting that 25-OHD_3 may have an important function in the mineralization of bone. Such evidence is derived from several sources. As already mentioned, levels of 1,25-$(OH)_2D_3$ have been recorded as normal in two forms of osteomalacia in which 25-OHD_3 levels are very low.[44,45] Bordier et al. have demonstrated that 25-OHD_3, given in cases of nutritional osteomalacia, restores normal mineralization, while 1,25-$(OH)_2D_3$ fails to correct the mineralization defect, despite normalizing the serum calcium.[47] However, it should be noted that a recent publication contradicted this result and suggested that the Bordier study failed to restore normal mineralization because the serum phosphorus was not adequately corrected.[48] Finally, it was shown in a group of anephric patients that mineralization abnormalities were not a frequent finding.[49] This group of patients would be expected to have undetectable levels of 1,25-$(OH)_2D_3$.

It was in the late 1960s and early 1970s that several groups of investigators demonstrated the existence of the dihydroxylated vitamin D metabolite, 1,25-

$(OH)_2D_3$, with the second hydroxylation occurring in the kidneys. 1,25-$(OH)_2D_3$ has proven to be faster and more potent in augmenting intestinal calcium absorption than 25-OHD_3. In addition, it has proven one hundred times as active as 25-OHD_3 in promoting bone calcium reabsorption in tissue culture.[50] Besides increasing intestinal calcium absorption, 1,25-$(OH)_2D_3$ increases intestinal phosphate absorption independent of calcium transport.

Like other sterol hormones, 1,25-$(OH)_2D_3$ appears to bind to nuclear receptors and modulate RNA synthesis;[51] the nuclear effects of 1,25-$(OH)_2D_3$ can be blocked by actinomycin D.[52] The question of how 1,25-$(OH)_2D_3$ increases intestinal calcium absorption remains unanswered. In the normal chick, 2 percent of the total protein content is calcium-binding protein (CaBP); in the vitamin D-deficient state, however, CaBP is absent.[19] After the administration of 1,25-$(OH)_2D_3$ to the vitamin D-deficient chick, there is a rapid appearance of CaBP. Nevertheless, the major concern in ascribing a specific role to CaBP is that the calcium transport decays at a faster rate than CaBP disappears.[53] Another protein of interest is calcium ATPase, but this protein appears more slowly than the increase in calcium absorption.[54]

Both in vitro and in vivo evidence exist that 1,25-$(OH)_2D_3$ is involved in bone resorption. The study by Raisz demonstrated that 1,25-$(OH)_2D_3$ was capable of greatly increasing calcium resorption in tissue culture.[50] The calcium resorption could be blocked by the prior use of actinomycin D. Studies in renal failure have shown skeletal resistance to the effects of parathyroid hormone.[99,106] This skeletal resistance could be partially but not completely corrected by the administration of 1,25-$(OH)_2D_3$.[55] Such studies suggest that 1,25-$(OH)_2D_3$ augments the capacity of parathyroid hormone to resorb bone.

Levels of 1,25-$(OH)_2D_3$ appear to be not as constant as initially believed. Levels above those previously considered normal have been found in children of less than 2 years, during the adolescent growth spurt, and during the third trimester of pregnancy.[19] In addition, increased levels have been reported in such conditions as primary hyperparathyroidism and acromegaly.[31,56] Low levels of 1,25-$(OH)_2D_3$ have been reported in hypoparathyroidism, tumor-induced osteomalacia, vitamin D-dependent rickets, and senile osteoporosis.[33,57,58] The exact governance of the modulation of 1,25-$(OH)_2D_3$ levels in physiologic conditions and pathologic states requires further elaboration.

Another dihydroxylated vitamin D metabolite, 24,25-$(OH)_2D_3$ is receiving increased attention. In normal humans, the minimum effective dose of this metabolite needed to augment intestinal calcium absorption is eight times that of 1,25-$(OH)_2D_3$ and one-tenth the dose of 25-OHD_3. Also, the maximal stimulation of intestinal calcium absorption is less for 24,25-$(OH)_2D_3$ than for 1,25-$(OH)_2D_3$.[59] However, an interesting and potentially important feature of 24,25-$(OH)_2D_3$ is that despite augmenting intestinal calcium absorption, it does not increase urinary calcium, as happens with both 25-OHD_3 and 1,25-$(OH)_2D_3$, suggesting that the calcium may be deposited in bone.[39,59,60] Further studies are needed to assess the importance of 24,25-$(OH)_2D_3$.

Other vitamin D metabolites, such as 1,24,25-$(OH)_3D_3$ and 25,26-$(OH)_2D_3$ exist, but knowledge regarding their function is limited, and even speculation on this is not warranted.

DISEASE STATES PROBABLY INVOLVING VITAMIN D

Parathyroid Disorders

Primary Hyperparathyroidism. As already stated, PTH acts as a stimulus for 1-alpha hydroxylation.[26,27] In addition, excess PTH produces hypophosphatemia, which is also a stimulus for 1,25-$(OH)_2D_3$ production.[28,29] Thus, in primary hyperparathyroidism, levels of 1,25-$(OH)_2D_3$ should be elevated, which would increase intestinal calcium absorption and bone resorption as the result of the combined action of PTH and 1,25-$(OH)_2D_3$.[19,33]

However, despite these theoretical considerations, clinical studies show two distinct groups of patients with primary hyperparathyroidism; those with extensive bone disease and those with renal calculi (stones). Peacock et al. have shown that stone-forming patients display increased intestinal calcium absorption compared to non-stone-formers.[61] A recent study by Broadus et al. has classified two subpopulations of hyperparathyroid patients: (1) those who exhibit hyperabsorption with the calcium tolerance test, plus hypercalciuria, marked elevations of 1,25-$(OH)_2D_3$ levels, and a high incidence of renal stones; (2) those with a normal level of 1,25-$(OH)_2D_3$ and a low incidence of stones.[56]

Thus, the initial clinical impression of two clinical groups of patients with primary hyperparathyroidism[62] seems to be supported by recent biochemical data. However, the question of why patients with comparable levels of immunoreactive PTH should manifest different clinical expressions remains to be answered.

It has been our experience, using 5-μ-thick, Goldner-stained, undecalcified preparations that bone involvement in primary hyperparathyroidism is less extensive than that seen in secondary hyperparathyroidism due to renal disease. Although increased bone resorption, endosteal fibrosis, and increased osteoblastic activity are frequently present in primary hyperparathyroidism, the involvement is generally localized to small areas. Thus, an increased resorptive surface and osteoclast count are observed in primary hyperparathyroidism, although these findings are sometimes recognized only when quantitative histomorphometric analysis is undertaken.[63,64]

The areas of resorptive activity in bone are easily recognized (Fig. 1) from the irregular, deeply scalloped margins produced by the active osteoclasts. There is an increased number of osteoclasts and, under the stimulation of parathyroid hormone, these cells may have multiple nuclei. Behind the cutting edge of the osteoclasts, in the resorption cavity, the osteoblasts can be appreciated; their primary function is osteoid deposition and the formation of new bone. The osteoblasts nearest to the osteoclasts are mononuclear, cuboidal cells, and the more distant these cells are from this interface, the more they progressively foreshorten.

When endosteal fibrosis is present, it is usually observed within the resorption cavity produced by the increased osteoclastic activity. With increased PTH stimulation, the endosteal fibrosis can extend into the marrow space.

Hypoparathyroidism. Hypoparathyroidism comprises a diverse group of disorders including: (1) primary hypoparathyroidism, most commonly idiopathic or surgically induced; (2) pseudohypoparathyroidism; and (3) pseudo-pseudohypo-

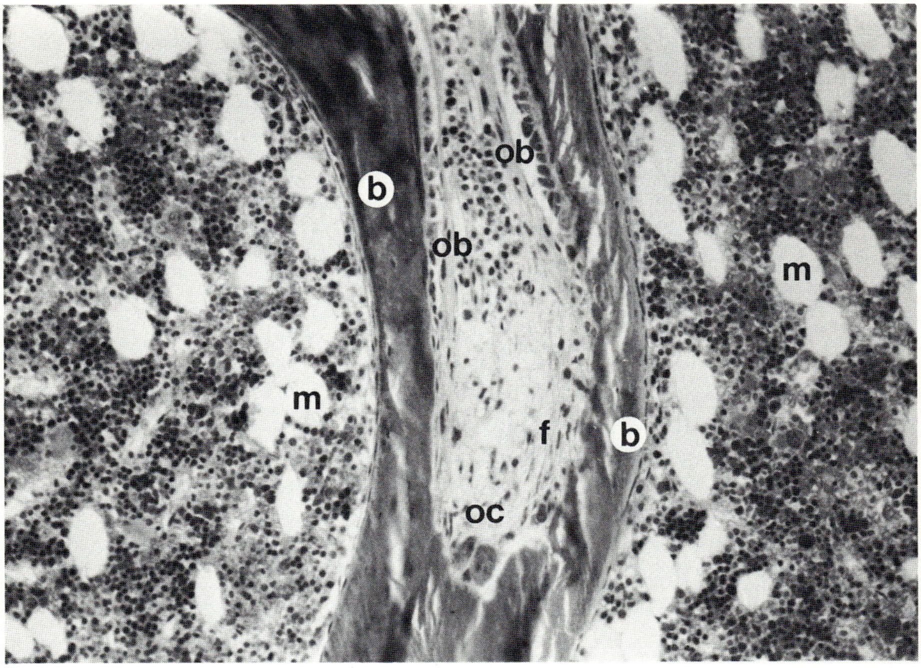

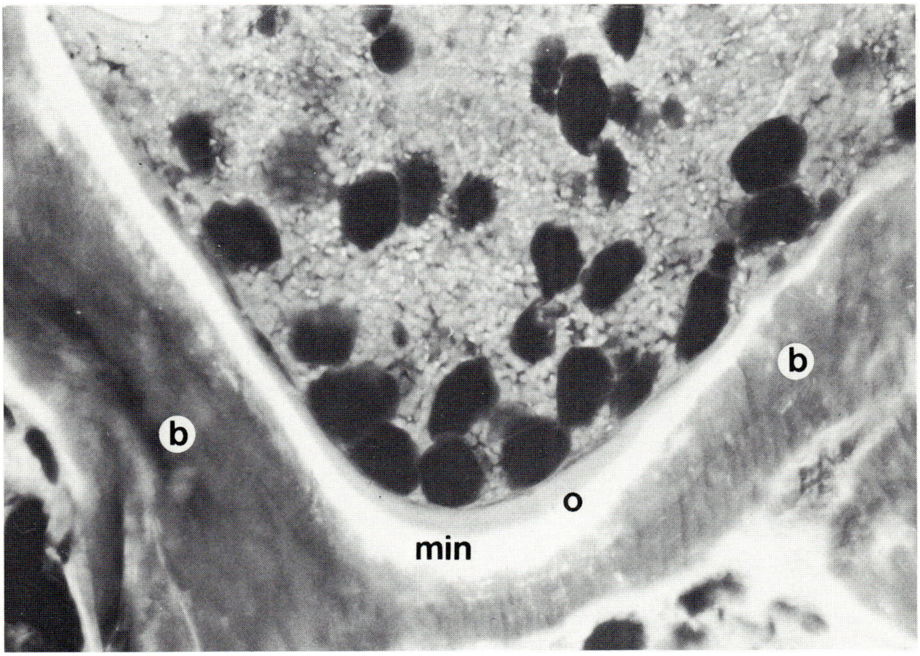

FIG. 1. Primary hyperparathyroidism. **Top.** A resorption cavity in a patient with primary hyperparathyroidism. Within the resorption cavity are osteoclasts (*oc*), endosteal fibrosis (*f*), and osteoblasts (*ob*). Normal marrow (*m*) is present along both lateral margins of trabecular bone (*b*). × 150. **Bottom.** In the same patient, a single tetracycline label indicates normal mineralization (*min*) at the interface of bone (*b*) and osteoid (*o*).

parathyroidism.[65,66] A better way to categorize these entities is a consideration of their pathogenesis: (1) decreased production of PTH; (2) physiologically inactive parathyroid hormone; and (3) target-organ resistance.

The basic defect in primary hypoparathyroidism is the failure to produce physiologic amounts of PTH. In this condition, levels of 1,25-$(OH)_2D_3$ are low as a consequence of PTH deficiency and hyperphosphatemia.[67] The latter results from decreased renal excretion of phosphate, caused by lack of PTH. One of the principal manifestations of primary hypoparathyroidism is marked hypocalcemia, which occurs because of: (1) failure of PTH and 1,25-$(OH)_2D_3$ to resorb calcium from bone; (2) defective renal tubular calcium reabsorption secondary to decreased PTH; and (3) deficient intestinal calcium absorption secondary to decreased levels of 1,25-$(OH)_2D_3$.[66]

Pseudohypoparathyroidism is an entity in which there is a defective response to PTH. At the kidney, there is a failure of PTH to elicit a response in terms of increased cyclic AMP excretion.[68] Initially, it was also believed that the hypocalcemia resulted from the failure of PTH to act on bone. However, the plasma concentration of 1,25$(OH)_2D_3$ in pseudohypoparathyroidism is low, so that both the hypocalcemia and the decreased calcemic response to PTH are corrected by vitamin D.[69] A normocalcemic variant of pseudohypoparathyroidism has been reported. In this entity, the levels of 1,25-$(OH)_2D_3$ and the calcemic response to parathyroid extract are normal, while there is a continued failure to generate a urinary cyclic AMP response.[70]

Pseudo-pseudohypoparathyroidism is diagnosed by normal or elevated PTH concentrations, the normal generation of urinary cyclic AMP, and the failure of PTH to produce a phosphaturic or calcemic response. Many patients with this condition have characteristic somatic features, including short stature, a round face, and shortening of the metacarpal and metatarsal bones.[65,66]

Rickets

Rickets is a mineralization defect involving both cartilage and bone. The earliest described and most common form was due to a lack of vitamin D intake. With adequate prophylaxis, initially by cod liver oil and subsequently by vitamin D supplementation of dairy products, classic rickets has become an infrequent occurrence. As mentioned previously, the prevention and treatment of classic rickets unmasked the existence of other causes of rickets.[1]

Vitamin-D-Dependent Rickets (VDDR). This entity is an inherited autosomal recessive form of rickets, refractory to physiologic doses of vitamin D. The signs and symptoms of rickets usually appear during the first year of life. In addition to the skeletal involvement, severe muscular weakness is characteristic. Intestinal malabsorption of calcium is a general finding in this entity.[3]

Children afflicted with VDDR universally fail to respond to physiologic doses (400 IU) of vitamin D; therapeutic responses have been attained using pharmacologic doses of the vitamin (50,000 IU). The pathogenesis of VDDR is ascribed to the lack of 1-alpha-hydroxylase, and the subsequent failure to form

$1,25\text{-}(OH)_2D_3$. Fraser et al. showed that small doses of $1,25\text{-}(OH)_2D_3$ (1 μg) were capable of healing.[71] Scriver et al. have reported that in six patients with VDDR, the levels of $1,25\text{-}(OH)_2D_3$ were low despite treatment with pharmacologic doses of vitamin D_2.[72]

A type-II VDDR has been reported, in which the presumed defect is postulated to be end-organ unresponsiveness to $1,25\text{-}(OH)_2D_3$. In this case report, hypocalcemia was present despite an increased level of $1,25\text{-}(OH)_2D_3$ and PTH.[73]

Vitamin D-Resistant Rickets (VDRR). VDRR is a familial disorder transmitted by an X-linked dominant gene. The clinical presentation is characterized by short stature and by varus and valgus knee deformities in children.[3] The biochemical hallmark of VDRR is severe hypophosphatemia. The presumed defect in the condition appears to alter the transepithelial transport of the phosphate anion in both the intestine and kidney.[74] Parathyroid hormone concentrations in VDRR have been reported by various authors to be both normal or increased.[75,76] Scriver et al. have reported low concentrations of $1,25\text{-}(OH)_2D_3$, while Haussler et al. have reported normal concentrations.[58,72] Theoretically, these results are not representative of what would be expected; since hypophosphatemia is a strong stimulus for the production of $1,25\text{-}(OH)_2D_3$, increased levels of $1,25\text{-}(OH)_2D_3$ should be present.

Osteomalacia

Osteomalacia is by definition a failure to mineralize bone. Although certain radiographic criteria are helpful in the diagnosis of the condition, the most accepted means of assessing bone mineralization is by the tetracycline labeling of a bone biopsy specimen.[77] The most frequent causes of osteomalacia are due to the lack of or the abnormal processing of vitamin D. These may include: (1) deficient intake of vitamin D and/or lack of sunlight exposure; (2) malabsorption of both ingested vitamin D and of $25\text{-}OHD_3$ during the enterohepatic cycle; (3) defective production or increased metabolism of $25\text{-}OHD_3$ secondary to hepatic disease, anticonvulsants, or nephrotic syndrome; and (4) defective production of $1,25\text{-}(OH)_2D_3$ secondary to a presumed inhibitor (tumor-induced), or to a decreased stimulus (hypoparathyroidism) for production of this metabolite.[21]

Nutritional Deficiency. Inadequate intake of vitamin D and the lack of sunlight exposure are infrequent causes of osteomalacia in Western society. A possible exception is the occurrence of osteomalacia in the elderly population. Approximately 10 to 30 percent of elderly patients with osteopenia will demonstrate evidence of defective mineralization that is responsive to treatment with vitamin D.[78,79] The presumed etiology of this last-named condition probably reflects a combination of decreased vitamin D intake and mild intestinal malabsorption, common in the geriatric population.

Gastrointestinal Disease. Malabsorption of vitamin D_3 and $25\text{-}OHD_3$ has been found in patients with adult celiac disease, pancreatic steatorrhea, blind loop syndrome, obstructive jaundice, and visceral scleroderma; low serum concentrations of

25-OHD_3 and osteomalacia have been described in these entities.[80] The presence of low levels of serum 25-OHD_3 and osteomalacia in patients after gastrectomy is not well understood; whether the etiology of these low levels of 25-OHD_3 is secondary to poor vitamin D intake or to malabsorption remains controversial.[81,82] Jejunoileal bypass has also been associated with decreased levels of 25-OHD_3,[83] presumably due to malabsorption of vitamin D. After bypass, hepatic dysfunction also may be a contributing factor in the genesis of osteomalacia.

Hepatic Disease. Controversy exists regarding the mechanism of decreased 25-OHD_3 levels in hepatic parenchymal disease. The question centers around whether decreased 25-OHD_3 levels are secondary to impaired vitamin D conversion because of a diseased liver, or result from malabsorption of vitamin D.[84] Whether parenchymal hepatic disorders result in detectable metabolic bone disease remains debatable, although documented rickets has been reported in neonatal hepatitis.[85]

Anticonvulsant-Induced Disease. Serum 25-OHD_3 levels have been reported to be low in children receiving chronic anticonvulsant therapy.[22] The low 25-OHD_3 concentration is believed to be secondary to induction of hepatic microsomal enzymes. However, despite the low level of 25-OHD_3, the plasma concentration of 1,25-$(OH)_2D_3$ in these patients is normal.[44] Treatment of the condition with vitamin D requires doses that exceed recommended physiologic doses, although a prompt response is attained with physiologic doses of 25-OHD_3.[21,86]

Rickets and osteomalacia are the metabolic bone diseases found in some children and adults receiving anticonvulsants. Healing can be attained with vitamin D, and prophylactic weekly administration of the vitamin may be indicated.[74]

Nephrotic Syndrome. This entity may induce osteomalacia as a consequence of increased loss of 25-OHD_3 in the urine; in the blood, this metabolite circulates bound to an alpha globulin with a molecular weight of about 58,000. In certain renal diseases characterized by increased glomerular permeability, there is leakage of 25-OHD_3 into the urine. In a recent study, Goldstein et al. demonstrated that levels of 25-OHD_3 were depressed in patients with the nephrotic syndrome, and that an inverse relationship was present between the level of 25-OHD_3 and the magnitude of proteinuria.[87] A subsequent study in six patients with the nephrotic syndrome and normal glomerular filtration rates (GFRs) revealed that all six patients had bone biopsy changes consistent with osteomalacia. In these six patients, the level of 25-OHD_3 was very low.[88]

Tumor-Induced Osteomalacia. Several case reports have described the coexistence of mesenchymal tumors and osteomalacia.[57,89] Characteristic biochemical abnormalities in these cases have included hypophosphatemia, phosphaturia, and hyperaminoaciduria. In a well-documented case, Drezner et al. found the level of 1,25-$(OH)_2D_3$ to be very low; after physiologic doses of 1,25-$(OH)_2D_3$ the biochemical abnormalities were corrected and the osteomalacia healed.[57] Resection of the tumor resulted in healing of the osteomalacia, normalization of 1,25-$(OH)_2D_3$ levels, and the restoration of all biochemical abnormalities. The proposed mechanism for the production of tumor-induced osteomalacia is that a tumor-secreted factor inhibits 1,25-$(OH)_2D_3$ synthesis. However, such a hypothesis still requires verification.

Bone Histology in Osteomalacia and Rickets. The histology of iliac crest bone is similar in rickets and osteomalacia. There is an increased amount of osteoid which results in an increase both in the amount of osteoid covering the trabecular surface and in the osteoid seam width. However, an excess of osteoid is not the sole diagnostic criterion for osteomalacia[77]; any metabolic disorder with accelerated bone turnover can produce both an increase in surface osteoid and osteoid seam width. Such is the case with hyperparathyroidism, hyperthyroidism, and Paget's disease.[77] In these disorders, as opposed to the case in osteomalacia, there is no mineralization defect and the excessive osteoid is secondary to increased osteoid deposition, which exceeds the capacity for mineralization.[90]

The primary criterion for diagnosing osteomalacia is the demonstration of defective mineralization. This is best accomplished by the use of a tetracycline label (Fig. 2). Because of certain physicochemical properties, tetracycline is localized at the interface of osteoid and bone only when active mineralization is occurring.[91] Therefore, unstained bone sections, when viewed under fluorescent light, will reveal a linear, yellow label (tetracycline hydrochloride) provided that a normal, active mineralization process is ongoing. With osteomalacia and rickets, the deposition of tetracycline is diminished and results in a decreased label.

Although tetracycline labeling is the most accurate tool in the assessment of bone mineralization, several other findings may be helpful in the diagnosis of osteomalacia. For instance, since other causes of excess osteoid are usually accompanied by an increase in osteoblastic and osteoclastic activity, it follows that the absence of any cellular activity is suggestive of osteomalacia. The outline of the margin between the osteoid and the bone may also be helpful. In the presence of active mineralization, the osteoid–bone interface is linear and smooth, and can become irregular and scalloped when mineralization is abnormal. Finally, when 40-μ unstained sections are viewed, the presence of a granular layer observed at the margin of the osteoid and the bone is indicative of active mineralizaton.[92] This layer is absent if mineralization is not proceeding normally.

Renal Disease

The metabolic bone disease associated with renal failure is complex and multifactorial. The interactions between serum calcium and phosphorus, PTH, vitamin D metabolites, collagen maturation, and uremic toxins are incompletely understood.[93-99] Bricker and colleagues suggest that the principal factor leading to hypocalcemia in early renal failure is phosphate retention.[100-102] As a consequence of phosphate retention, the serum ionized calcium falls, which results in increased PTH secretion; the increased PTH secretion restores the ionized calcium level and produces a phosphaturia lowering the serum phosphorus. To attain the normalization of serum phosphorus and ionized calcium requires an increased baseline secre-

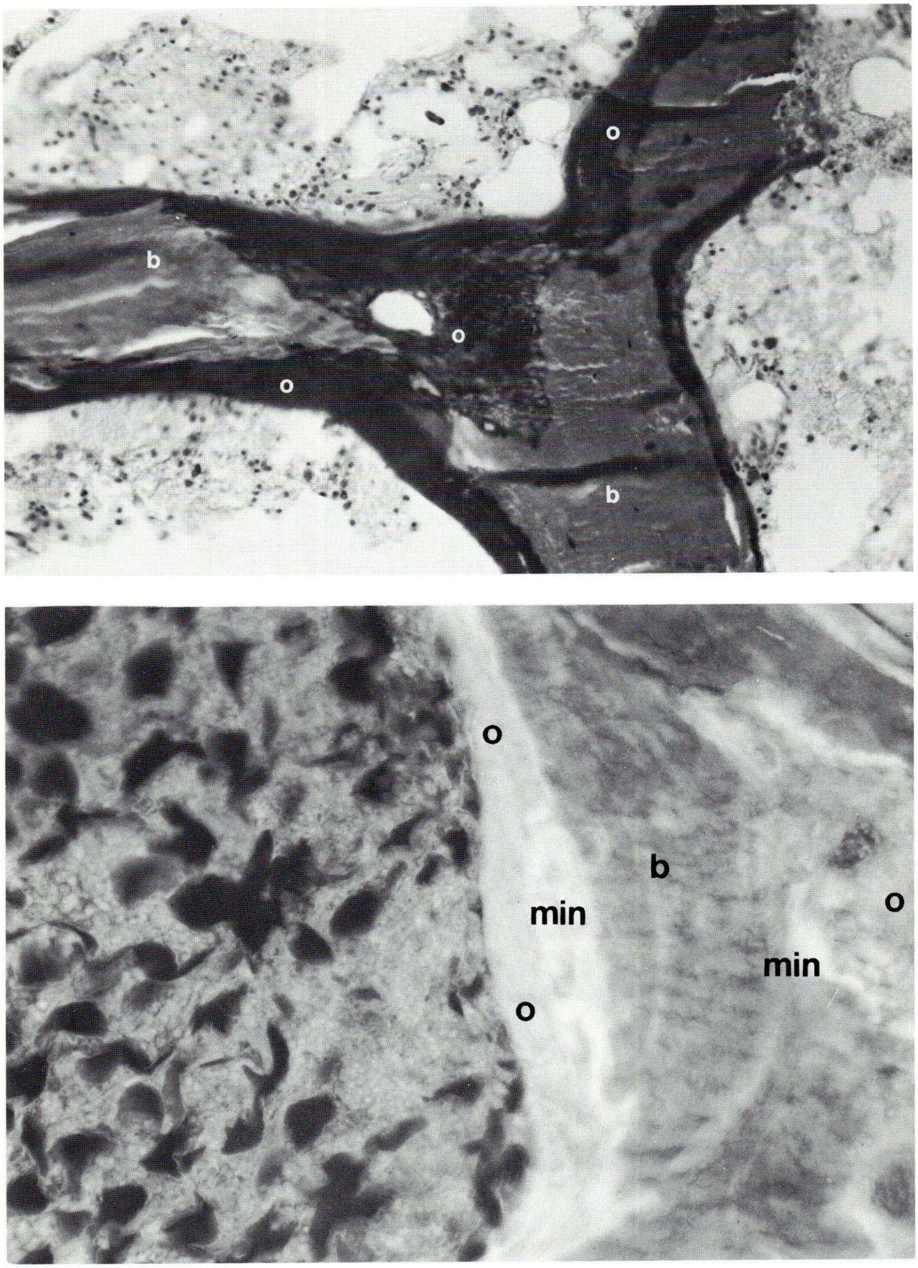

FIG. 2. Osteomalacia secondary to malabsorption. **Top.** A bone biopsy from a patient with osteomalacia secondary to malabsorption. The prominent features are the presence of osteoid (*o*) covering most of the trabecular bone (*b*) surface and the excessive width of the osteoid. ×150. **Bottom.** A single tetracycline label in the same patient demonstrates disordered and diminished mineralization (*min*) at the interface of bone (*b*) and osteoid (*o*). The uptake of the tetracycline occurs over only a small fraction of the osteoid–bone interface, and the deposition is disorganized. ×150.

tion of PTH. As renal function continues to deteriorate, increasing amounts of PTH are required to restore baseline values, and this process results in parathyroid gland hyperplasia. At a glomerular filtration rate of approximately 25 ml/min, PTH secretion is no longer capable of producing a phosphaturia sufficient to maintain a normal level of serum phosphorus, and thus hyperphosphatemia results.

Although the current belief is that phosphate retention is the initial factor leading to hypocalcemia and parathyroid gland hyperplasia in renal disease, contradictory evidence also exists. Many patients with early renal failure will exhibit mild hypophosphatemia, which suggests that phosphate accumulation may not be the main factor leading to hypocalcemia.[99,103]

Other major considerations in the genesis of the hypocalcemia concern the metabolism of vitamin D. As has been previously stated, the kidney is involved in the 1-alpha hydroxylation of 25-OHD_3 to form 1,25-$(OH)_2D_3$.[24] In addition, the majority, if not the total production of 24,25-$(OH)_2D_3$ occurs in the kidney.[30,31] The exact levels of 1,25-$(OH)_2D_3$ and 24,25-$(OH)_2D_3$ with changing renal function, and their complex interaction with PTH and phosphate metabolism have not really been fully evaluated. It is generally accepted that baseline levels of 1,25-$(OH)_2D_3$, and consequently calcium absorption from the gastrointestinal tract, remain normal until the glomerular filtration rate falls below 25 ml/min.[104,105]

A third factor leading to hypocalcemia in patients with renal failure is the presence of skeletal resistance to the calcemic actions of PTH.[55] Thus, when exogenous PTH extract was given to normal persons, dialysis patients, and stable kidney transplant recipients, the calcemic response was recorded. The ability to attain a normal calcemic response was markedly diminished in dialysis patients and mildly altered in the renal transplant recipients. Pretreatment of the dialysis patients with 1,25-$(OH)_2D_3$ partially restored the calcemic response.[106]

A probable exception to the aforementioned events concerns the renal tubular disorders. During the late 1920s and through the 1930s, Parsons (1927), DeToni (1933)[8], and Fanconi (1931 and 1936)[7,9] described rickets as a consequence of renal tubular disorders. Early in their course, the majority of patients with such disorders manifest only minimal alterations in the glomerular filtration rate, and yet demonstrate severe metabolic bone disease. The etiology of the bone disease may be multifactorial in origin, secondary to hypophosphatemia, hyperphosphaturia, acidosis, hypercalciuria, and altered metabolism of vitamin D. These patients, in general, demonstrate marked resistance to therapy with vitamin D, and doses of 50,000 to 250,000 IU of the vitamin have been employed in their treatment.

The spectrum of renal osteodystrophy in dialysis patients is quite diverse. There appear to be vast differences in renal osteodystrophy from country to country and within different geographic areas of a single country[107]. In addition to the metabolic abnormality created by the lack of excretory and metabolic functions of the kidney, environmental factors, such as aluminum contamination of the water, have been implicated in the causation of this condition.[108,109]

In mild and moderate renal failure, the predominant bone disease reflects the increased resorption characteristic of secondary hyperparathyroidism.[98,110] Considerably greater experience has been gathered in dialysis patients. The types of bone disease include: (1) osteitis fibrosa-increased resorption, and endosteal fibrosis; (2) mixed osteitis fibrosa and osteomalacia-increased resorption, minimal endosteal fibrosis, and evidence of mild mineralization deficits; and (3) osteomalacia, a marked mineralization deficit, abundant osteoid, and the virtual absence of osteoblastic and osteoclastic activity.

Bone Histology. The osteitis fibrosa observed in chronic renal failure is quite apparent when undecalcified, stained bone sections are reviewed. The characteristic findings include a marked increase of bone resorption, extensive osteoclastic and osteoblastic activity, and endosteal fibrosis. When quantitative bone histomorphometry is employed, the amount of endosteal fibrosis and active resorption (defined by the presence of osteoclasts at the bone interface), correlates with the plasma levels of carboxy-terminal PTH (Fig. 3). Osteoblastic activity is extensive and there is also a correlation between active resorption and osteoblastic activity (Fig. 4).

The numbers of osteoclasts are markedly increased in osteitis fibrosa and they are frequently multinucleated and large, many containing more than six nuclei. In addition to the extensively increased surface resorption, there frequently exist many

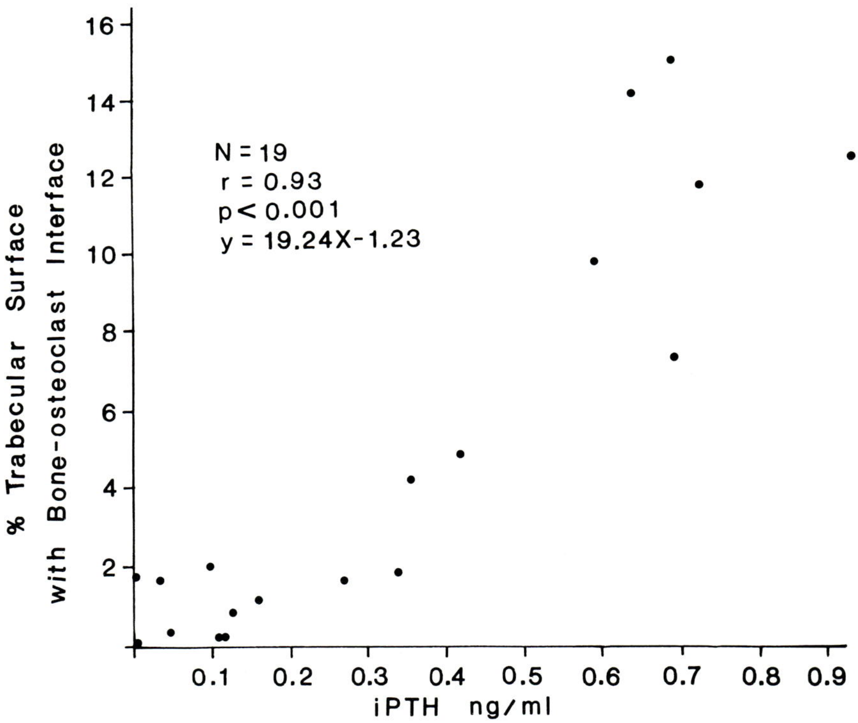

FIG. 3. Correlation of serum immunoreactive parathyroid hormone (iPTH) concentration with the proportion of bone–osteoclast interface on iliac bone biopsy. The upper limit for the C-terminal iPTH assay is < 0.1 ng/ml. The correlation with the iPTH and bone–osteoclast interface on iliac bone biopsy was performed in patients receiving chronic maintenance dialysis. Bone–osteoclast interface is defined as the fraction of trabecular surface covered by osteoclasts. Reprinted with permission from Felsenfeld: Calcif Tissue Int (in press)

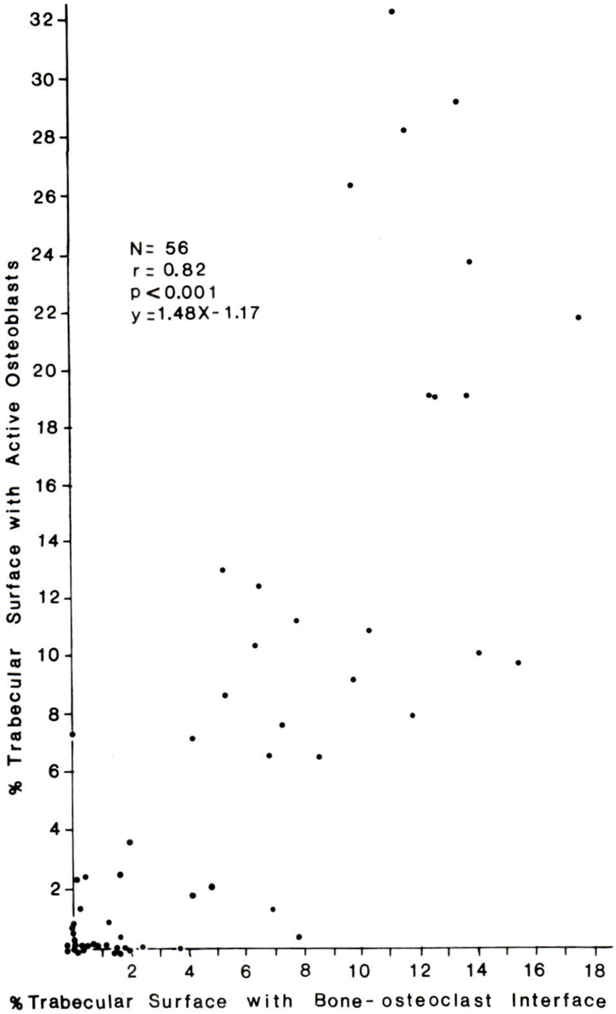

FIG. 4. Correlation of osteoblastic and osteoclastic activity noted in iliac bone biopsy specimen of patients with renal osteodystrophy. In renal osteodystrophy patients, the bone biopsy demonstrates a significant correlation between osteoblastic and osteoclastic activity, suggesting that the formative and resorptive processes may be coupled. Active osteoblasts are defined as cuboidal osteoblasts. The bone–osteoclast interface is the fraction of trabecular surface covered by osteoclasts. Reprinted with permission from Felsenfeld: Calcif Tissue Int (in press)

dissecting cavities in which the osteoclasts tunnel through the body of the trabecular bone (Fig. 5).

The presence of endosteal fibrosis is characteristic of osteitis fibrosa, and can be first appreciated in a resorption lacuna. With continued marrow stimulation, the endosteal fibrosis extends beyond the resorption cavities in a narrow band along the peritrabecular surface (Fig. 6). The next stage of extension is represented by bridging areas between trabecular spicules. Finally, fibrosis of large contiguous areas of marrow space may occur (Fig. 7).

Despite the presence of increased osteoid in chronic renal failure patients with osteitis fibrosa, mineralization, as assessed by tetracycline labeling, occurs with only minimal alteration. The osteoid, although abundant, contains many active osteoblasts (Fig. 8).

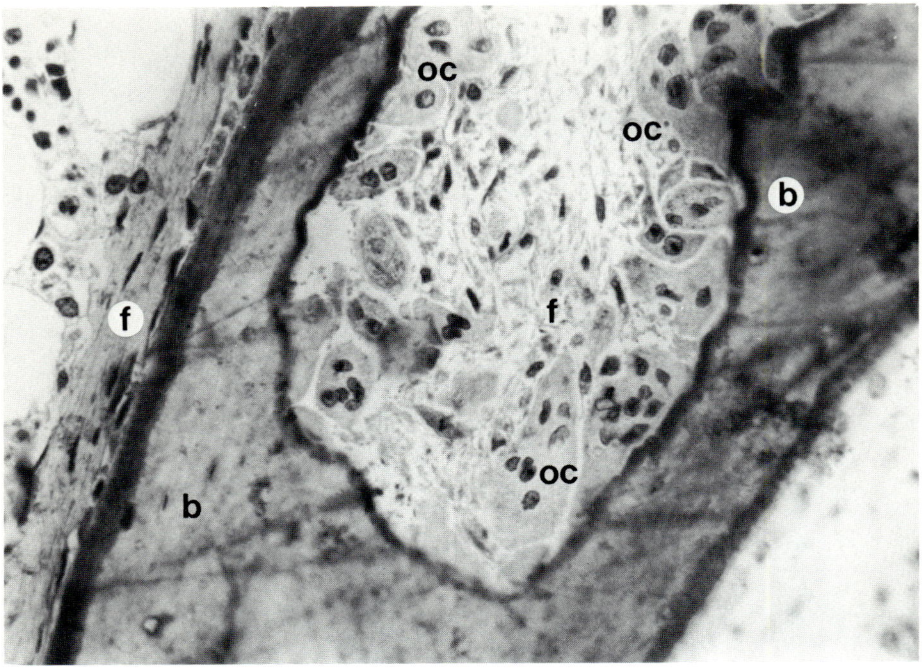

FIG. 5. Dissecting osteitis in a patient with chronic renal failure and osteitis fibrosa. The multinucleated osteoclasts (*oc*) have tunneled through trabecular bone (*b*). Other features to note are the presence of endosteal fibrosis (*f*) within the dissection cavity and along the lateral trabecular surface. × 375.

From our experience, it appears that with osteitis fibrosa, two subgroups exist. One subgroup will have osteosclerosis and increased bone volume; when viewed with polarized light, abundant deposits of woven bone will be seen, as opposed to the normal lamellar pattern (Fig. 9). The second subgroup will have osteopenia, increased osteoclastic and osteoblastic activity, and endosteal fibrosis. The pathogenetic factors involved in the development of osteosclerosis are not known.

The predominant bone disease found in chronic dialysis patients is osteitis fibrosa, in which bone resorption is excessive. There also exists a minority of patients who have a mixed osteitis fibrosa and osteomalacia. The extent of osteitis fibrosa (viz., endosteal fibrosis, resorptive and osteoblastic activity) is mild, and there is a concomitant mild-to-moderate mineralization defect, characteristic of osteomalacia. The third group of dialysis patients has pure osteomalacia, characterized by a severe mineralization defect and a reduced tetracycline label. The amount of osteoid is excessive and no osteoblastic activity is observed; the osteoid covers more than 75 percent of the trabecular surface, and the seam width is from 2 to 4 times normal. The bone–osteoid interface is irregular and deeply scalloped (Fig. 10). A characteristic feature is the absence of endosteal fibrosis. These patients with pure osteomalacia are characterized by a high incidence of spontaneous skeletal fractures, a significant myopathy, a normal to minimally elevated serum

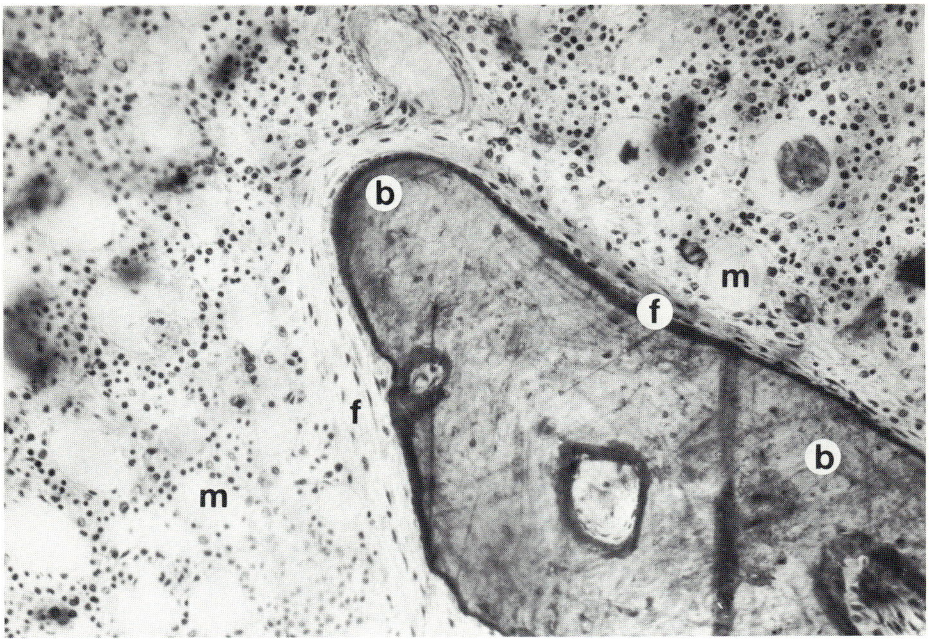

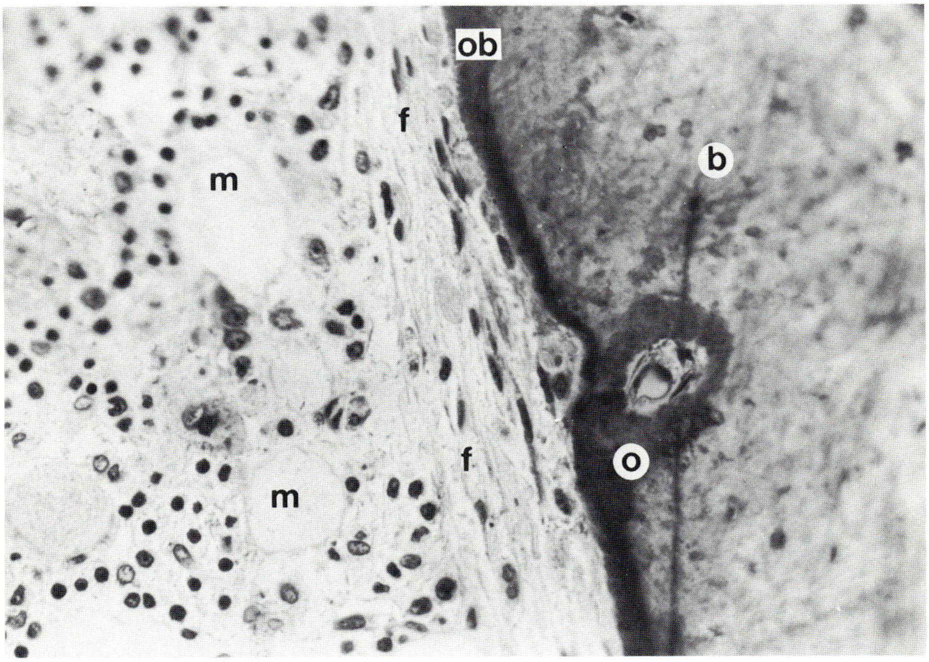

FIG. 6. Peritrabecular fibrosis in a chronic renal failure patient. **Top.** Endosteal fibrosis (*f*) is localized to an area adjacent to trabecular bone (*b*). The remainder of the marrow space (*m*) is normal. × 150. **Bottom.** The same area highlighted by increased magnification. The endosteal fibrosis (*f*) is adjacent to the trabecular bone (*b*) and the osteoid (*o*) with osteoblasts (*ob*). Normal marrow (*m*) is also present. × 375.

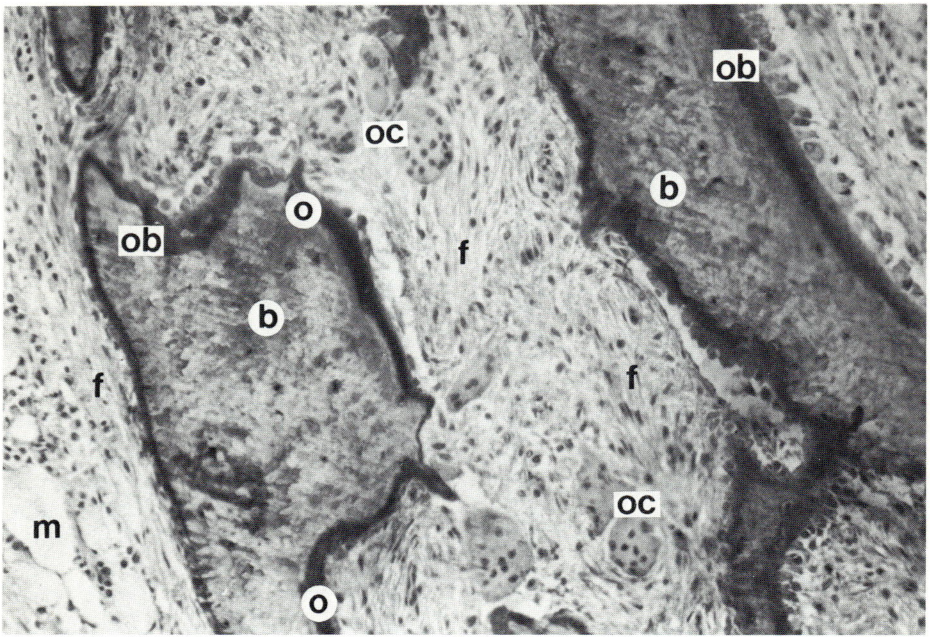

FIG. 7. Diffuse endosteal fibrosis of the marrow. Endosteal fibrosis (*f*) occupies large, contiguous areas of the marrow. Many giant multinucleated osteoclasts (*oc*) are visible. Osteoid (*o*) and osteoblastic osteoid (*ob*) cover much of the trabecular bone (*b*) surface. Normal marrow (*m*) is seen in one corner. × 150.

alkaline phosphatase, and normal PTH levels and serum calcium concentrations; however, they show a tendency to become hypercalcemic with vitamin D therapy.

The frequency of osteomalacia appears to have a marked geographic variation.[107] In addition, it has only been reported in patients receiving maintenance dialysis,[98,111] although we have seen a patient with osteomalacia prior to the initiation of chronic dialysis. Investigation for a pathogenetic agent has been centered upon possible exposure to an environmental toxin that might occur during dialysis. Epidemiologic evidence has implicated the presence of aluminum in water, since the incidence of this osteomalacic syndrome increases greatly in areas in which the aluminum content of the water is high.[108,109] Pretreatment of the water with reverse osmosis has decreased the incidence of the osteomalacic syndrome. Besides the epidemiologic evidence implicating aluminum, it has been shown that aluminum has a predilection for bone deposition.[112] However, whether the bone aluminum concentration plays a pathologic role or is an innocent bystander in the syndrome remains to be established. The etiology of these patients' low PTH concentrations and the predilection of the patients to develop hypercalcemia are unknown.

Treatment of renal osteodystrophy has proven difficult; during the 1970s it was hoped that treatment with 1,25-$(OH)_2D_3$ would result in healing of the condition.[113,114] However, from the initial studies until the present, it has been increas-

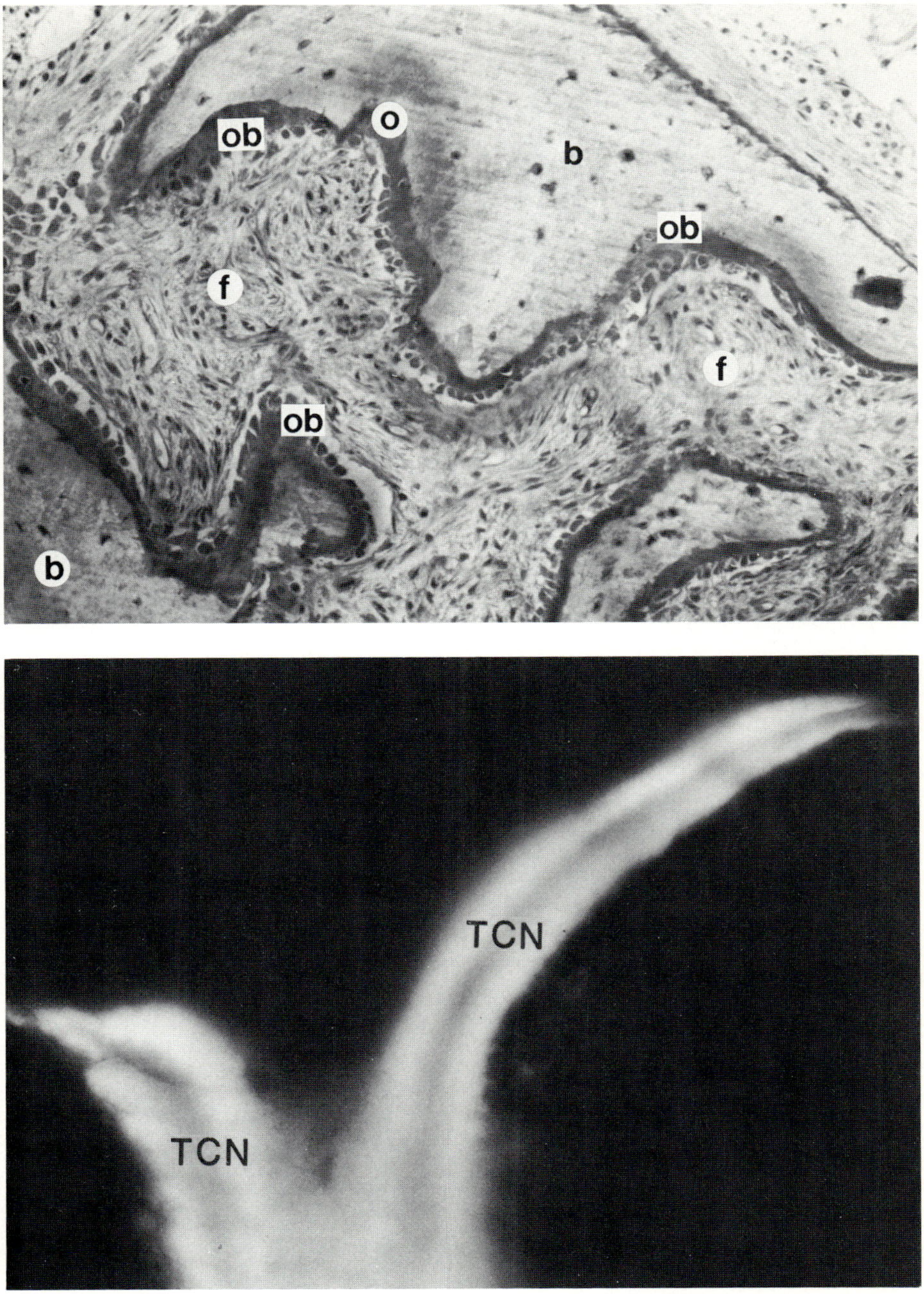

FIG. 8. Osteoblastic osteoid and bone mineralization in osteitis fibrosa. **Top.** Despite the presence of abundant osteoid (*o*) in osteitis fibrosa, the existence of many active osteoblasts (*ob*) suggests that mineralization is proceeding. Bone (*b*); endosteal fibrosis (*f*). × 150. **Bottom.** Mineralization in osteitis fibrosa, as assessed by a double tetracycline label (*TCN*), demonstrates both normal percent mineralization and bone appositional rate (the distance between labels divided by time). × 375.

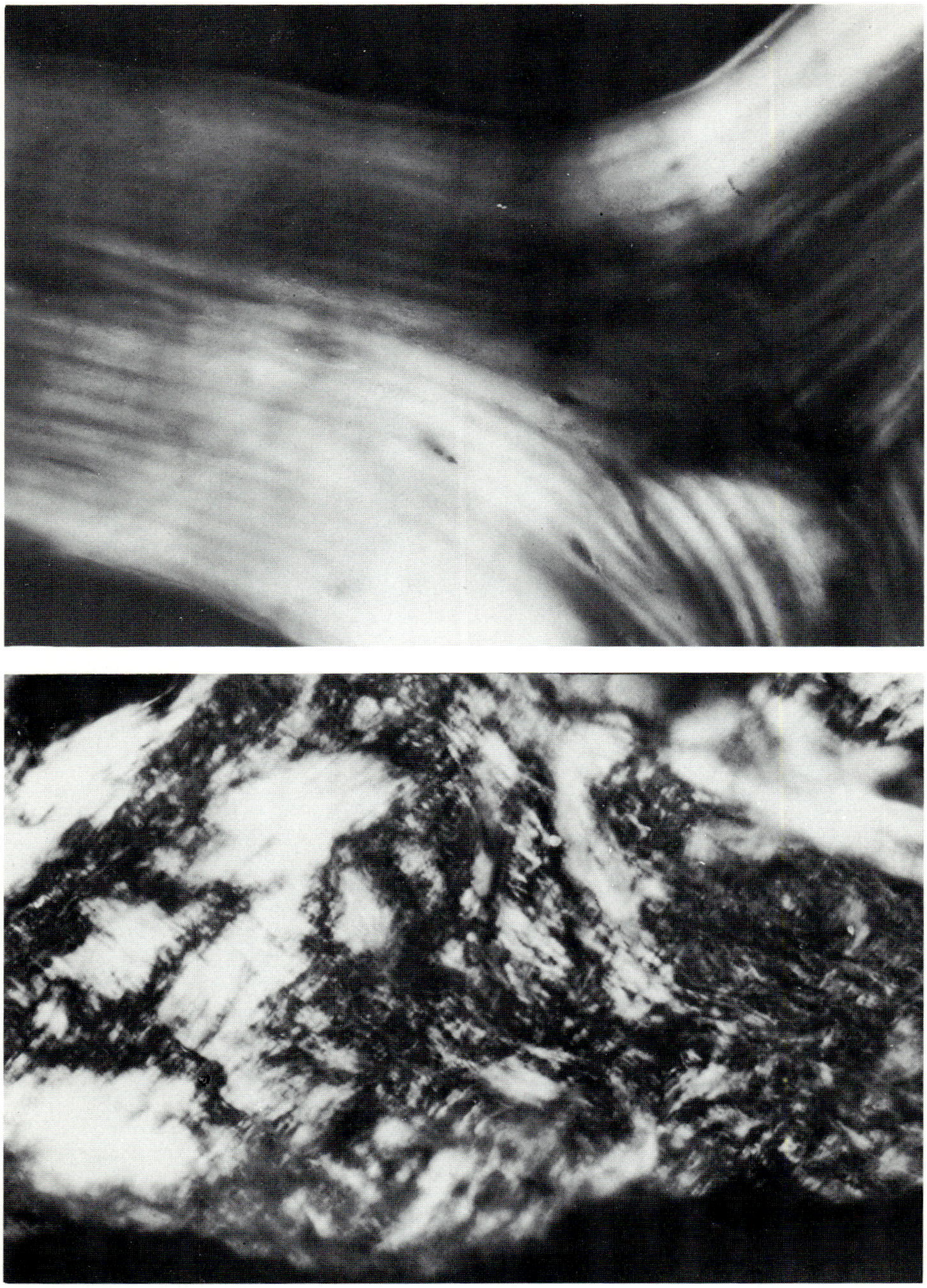

FIG. 9. Lamellar and woven bone. **Top.** Normal bone when viewed under polarized light possesses a lamellar pattern. × 150. **Bottom.** The bone of osteitis fibrosa when viewed with polarized light has a woven (disorganized) pattern. × 150.

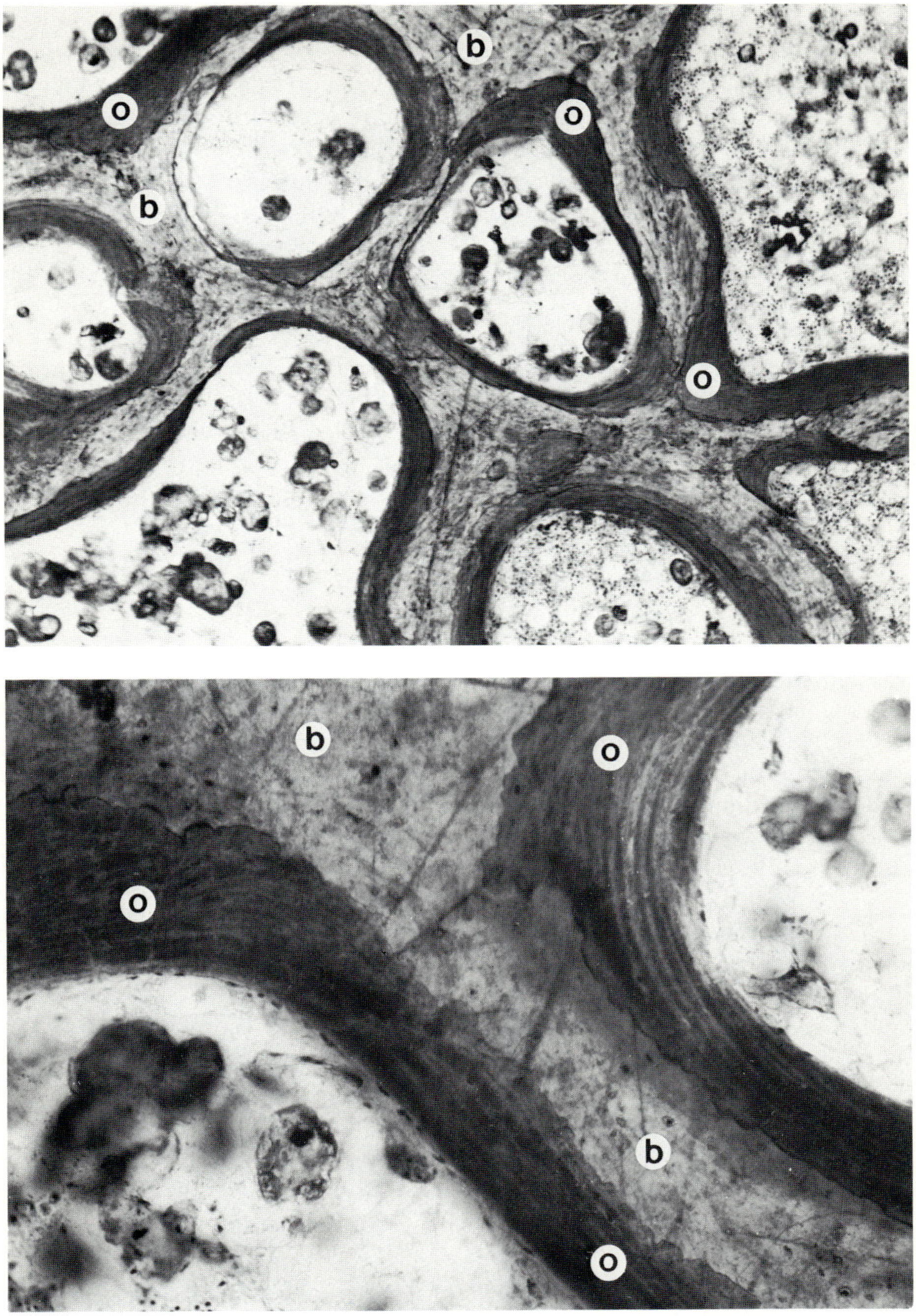

FIG. 10. The osteomalacia of renal failure. **Top.** Large irregular deposits of osteoid (*o*) cover almost the entire trabecular bone (*b*) surface. Additional features to be noted are the absence of osteoblasts, osteoclasts, and endosteal fibrosis. × 150. **Bottom.** An excessively wide, scalloped osteoid (*o*) seam covers the trabecular bone (*b*) surface. Note the irregularity of the bone–osteoid interface. This feature is commonly observed in the osteomalacia of renal failure. × 375.

ingly apparent that 1,25-$(OH)_2D_3$, although having a beneficial effect in the treatment of some forms of renal osteodystrophy, does not induce bone healing in the majority of patients.[115] Improved calcium balance, increased serum calcium levels, and lowered PTH concentrations[114,116,117] have occurred with the use of 1,25-$(OH)_2D_3$ and its analog 1-alpha-$(OH)D_3$. Despite the significant improvement in biochemical parameters, however, changes in bone histology have not been dramatic even after long-term therapy.[115,118] In addition, patients with severe osteitis fibrosa have developed severe hypercalcemia after treatment with 1,25-$(OH)_2D_3$.[115,119] Such a result has necessitated subjecting these patients to either a subtotal parathyroidectomy or a total parathyroidectomy with a forearm autograft.

The use of 1,25-$(OH)_2D_3$ or 1-alpha-$(OH)D_3$ in the osteomalacic syndrome has, for the most part, been disappointing. Hypercalcemia has developed with very low doses of 1,25-$(OH)_2D_3$, and the treatment has failed to produce any significant remission in the osteomalacia[111,115,120,121]; therapy has failed to prevent the relentless course of skeletal deterioration. Preliminary results from a recent study suggest that a combination of 24,25$(OH)_2D_3$ and 1,25-$(OH)_2D_3$ may be beneficial.[122]

Miscellaneous Bone Diseases

Heavy Metals. A number of heavy metals ingested as enviromental toxins have caused bone- and vitamin D-metabolism abnormalities. Exposure to cadmium has produced "itao-tai byo" (ouch-ouch disease) in Japan.[123] The name was derived from the painful and crippling osteomalacia. At least in vitro, small amounts of cadmium can completely inhibit the 1-alpha hydroxylation of 25-OHD_3.[124] A recent report by Rosen and colleagues implicated lead as the cause of decreased 1,25-$(OH)_2D_3$ levels in children with increased serum lead concentration.[125]

Corticosteroid Therapy. An important area of consideration is corticosteroid-induced osteopenia. The reported bone findings in this condition have demonstrated a greater loss of trabecular than of cortical bone, with decreased formation and increased resorption.[126] With regard to corticosteroid-induced osteopenia, intestinal calcium absorption appears to be inhibited, although the exact mechanism of causation of the condition remains to be elucidated. The current evidence suggests that secondary hyperparathyroidism occurs as a result of decreased intestinal calcium absorption. For the most part, 25-OHD_3 levels are normal in patients receiving less than the equivalent of 40 mg of prednisone per day.[127,128]

Osteoporosis. Integrating this common and crippling disorder into a discussion of vitamin D metabolites is quite preliminary. Obviously, a great deal of interest is centered both upon the development and the treatment of this devastating affliction. Reports measuring 1,25-$(OH)_2D_3$ levels in postmenopausal osteoporosis have produced conflicting results.[33] At present, the best assessment is that osteoporosis is probably not dependent upon a single deficiency.

ACKNOWLEDGMENTS

We would like to thank Dr. Samuel Wells for measurement of parathyroid hormone, Mrs. Jeanne Ray and Mr. Carl Haygood for technical assistance, and Mrs. Alvia M. Woodfork and Mrs. Carolyn Clay for preparation of the manuscript.

REFERENCES

1. Dent CE: Rickets and osteomalacia, nutritional and metabolic (1919–69). Proc R Soc Med 63:401–408, 1970
2. Mellanby E: An experimental investigation on rickets. Lancet 1:407–412, 1919
3. Dent CE: Vitamin D, rickets, and osteomalacia. In Avioli LV and Krane SM (eds): Metabolic bone disease, Vol I. New York, Academic Press, 1977, p 239
4. Parsons LG: Bone changes occurring in renal and coeliac infantilism, and their relationship to rickets; renal rickets. Arch Dis Child 2:1–25, 1927
5. Parsons LG: Bone changes occurring in renal and coeliac infantilism and their relationship to rickets; coeliac rickets. Arch Dis Child 2:198–215, 1927
6. Albright F, Butler AM, Bloomberg E: Rickets resistant to vitamin D therapy. Am Dis Child: 54:529–547, 1937
7. Fanconi G: Die nicht diabetischen Glykosurien und Hyperglykamien des alteren Kindes. Jahrbuch Fur Kinderheilkunde 133:257–300, 1931
8. De Toni G: Remarks on relations between renal rickets (renal dwarfism) and renal diabetes. Acta Paediatr (Uppsala) 16:479–484, 1933
9. Fanconi G: Der fruhinfantile nephotisch-glykosurische Zwergwuchs mit hypophosphatamischer Rachitis. Jahrbuch Fur Kinderheilkunde 147:299–338, 1936
10. Consden R, Gordon AH, Martin AJP: Qualitative analysis of proteins: A partition chromatographic method of using paper. Biochem J 38:224–232, 1944
11. Holick MF, Frommer J, McNeill S, et al.: Photometabolism of 7-dehydrocholesterol to previtamin D_3 in skin. Biochem Biophys Res Commun 76:107–114, 1977
12. Haddad JG, Hahn TJ: Natural and synthetic sources of circulating 25-hydroxyvitamin D in man. Nature 244:515–517, 1973
13. Coburn JW, Hartenbower DL, Norman AW: Metabolism and action of the hormone vitamin D—Its relation to diseases of calcium homeostasis. West J Med 121:22–44, 1974
14. Bhattacharyya MH, DeLuca HF: Subcellular location of the rat liver calciferol-25-hydroxylase. Arch Biochem Biophys 160:58–62, 1974
15. Haddad JG Jr, Walgate J: 25-hydroxyvitamin D transport in human plasma. Isolation and partial characterization of calcifidiol-binding protein. J Biol Chem 251:4803–4809, 1976
16. Tucker G, Gragnon R, Haussler M: Vitamin D_3-25-hydroxylase: Tissue occurrence and apparent lack of regulation. Arch Biochem Biophys 155:47, 1973
17. Bhattacharyya MH, DeLuca HF: The regulation of rat liver calciferol-25-hydroxylase. J Biol Chem 248:2969–2973, 1973
18. McLaughlin M, Ragatt PR, Fairney A, et al.: Seasonal variations in serum-25-hydroxycholecalciferol in healthy people. Lancet 1:536–538, 1974
19. Haussler MR, McCain TA: Basic and clinical concepts related to vitamin D metabolism and action. N Engl J Med 297:974–983, 1041–1050, 1977
20. Haddad JG Jr: Vitamin D economy in gastrointestinal disease. Ann Intern Med 87:629–630, 1977
21. Frame B, Parfitt AM: Osteomalacia: Current concepts. Ann Int Med 89:966–982, 1978
22. Hahn TJ, Hendin BA, Sharp CR, et al.: Effect of chronic anti-convulsant therapy on serum 25-hydroxycalciferol levels in adults. N Engl J Med 287:900–904, 1972

23. Arnaud SB, Goldsmith RS, Lambert PW, et al: 25-hydroxyvitamin D_3; evidence of an enterohepatic circulation in man. Proc Soc Exp Biol Med 149:570–572, 1975
24. Fraser DR, Kodicek E: Unique biosynthesis by kidney of a biologically active vitamin D metabolite. Nature 228:764–766, 1970
25. Gray R, Boyle I, DeLuca HF: Vitamin D metabolism: The role of kidney tissue. Science 172:1232–1234, 1971
26. DeLuca HF: The kidney as an endocrine organ for the production of 1,25-dihydroxyvitamin D_3, a calcium-mobilizing hormone. N Engl J Med 289:359–365, 1973
27. Henry HL, Midgett RJ, Norman AW: Regulation of 25-hydroxyvitamin D_3 1-hydroxylase in vivo. J Biol Chem 249:7584–7592, 1974
28. Tanaka Y, DeLuca HF: The control of 25-hydroxyvitamin D metabolism by inorganic phosphorus. Arch Biochem Biophys 154:566–574, 1973
29. Galante L, Colston KW, Evans IMA, et al.: The regulation of vitamin D metabolism. Nature 244:438–440, 1973
30. Knutson JC, DeLuca HF: 25-hydroxyvitamin D_3-24-hydroxylase. Subcellular location and properties. Biochemistry 13:1543–1548, 1974
31. Hay A: Complexities of vitamin D metabolism still increasing. Nature 278:509–510, 1979
32. Larkins RG, MacAuley SJ, MacIntyre I: Feedback control of vitamin D metabolism by nuclear action of 1,25-dihydroxyvitamin D_3 on the kidney. Nature 252:412–414, 1974
33. DeLuca HF: Vitamin D metabolism and function. Arch Intern Med 138:836–847, 1978
34. Avioli LV, Haddad JG: Vitamin D's more and more measured better and better. N Engl J Med 297:1006–1007, 1977
35. Chertow B, Baylink D, Wergedal J, et al.: Decrease in serum immunoreactive parathyroid hormone in rats and in parathyroid secretion in vitro by 1,25-dihydroxycholecalciferol. J Clin Invest 56:668–678, 1975
36. Llach F, Coburn JW, Brickman AS, et al.: Acute action of 1,25-dihydroxyvitamin D_3 in normal man: Effect on calcium and parathyroid status. J Clin Endocrinol Metab 44:1054–1060, 1977
37. Care AD, Bates RFL, Pickard DW, et al.: The effects of vitamin D metabolites and their analogues on the secretion of parathyroid hormone. Calcif Tiss Res 21:142–146, 1977
38. Canterbury JM, Lerman S, Claflin AJ, et al.: Inhibition of parathyroid hormone secretion by 25-hydroxycholecalciferol and 24,25-dihydroxycholecalciferol in the dog. J Clin Invest 61:1375–1383, 1978
39. Canterbury JM, Gavellas G, Bourgoignie JJ, et al.: Metabolic consequences of oral administration of 24,25-dihydroxycholecalciferol to uremic dogs. J Clin Invest 65:571–576, 1980
40. DeLuca HF: Vitamin D endocrinology. Ann Intern Med 85:367–377, 1976
41. Birge SJ, Haddad JG: 25-hydroxycholecalciferol stimulation of muscle metabolism. J Clin Invest 56:1100–1107, 1976
42. Rodman JS, Baker T: Changes in the kinetics of muscle contraction in vitamin D-depleted rats. Kidney Int 13:189–193, 1978
43. Schott GD, Wills MR: Muscle weakness in osteomalacia. Lancet 1:626–629, 1976
44. Jubiz W, Haussler MR, McCain TA, et al.: Plasma 1,25-dihydroxyvitamin D levels in patients receiving anticonvulsant drugs. J Clin Endocrinol Metab 44:617–621, 1977
45. Eastwood JB, de Wardener HE, Gray RW, et al.: Normal plasma $1,25(OH)_2D_3$ concentrations in nutritional osteomalacia. Lancet 1:1377–1380, 1979
46. Puschett JB, Moranz J, Kurnick WS: Evidence for a direct action of cholecalciferol and 25-hydroxycholecalciferol on the renal transport of phosphate, sodium, and calcium. J Clin Invest 51:373–385, 1972
47. Bordier P, Rasmussen H, Marie P, et al.: Vitamin D metabolites and bone mineralization in man. J Clin Endocrinol Metab 46:284–294, 1978
48. Nagant de Deuxchasnes C, Rombouts-Lindemans C, Huaux JP: Healing of vitamin

D-deficient osteomalacia by the administration of $1,25(OH)_2D_3$. In MacIntyre I and Szelke M (eds): Molecular Endocrinology. Amsterdam, North-Holland Biomedical Press, Elsevier, 1979
49. Bordier PJ, Tun Chot S, Eastwood JB, et al.: Lack of histological evidence of vitamin D abnormality in the bones of anephric patients. Clin Sci 44:33–41, 1973
50. Raisz LG, Trummel CL, Holick MF, et al.: 1,25-dihydroxycholecalciferol: a potent stimulator of bone resorption in tissue culture. Science 175:768–769, 1972
51. Brumbaugh PF, Haussler MR: 1α,25-dihydroxycholecalciferol receptors in intestine. I. Association of 1α,25-dihydroxycholecalciferol with intestinal mucosa chromatin. J Biol Chem 249:1251–1257, 1974
52. Corradino RA: 1,25-dihydroxycholecalciferol: Inhibition of action in organ-cultured intestine by actinomycin D and α-amanitin. Nature 243:41–42, 1973
53. Wasserman RH, Corradino RA, Fullmer CS, et al.: Some aspects of vitamin D action; calcium absorption and vitamin D-dependent calcium-binding protein. Vitam Horm 32:299–324, 1974
54. Norman AW, Henry H: 1,25-dihydroxycholecalciferol—A hormonally active form of vitamin D_3. Rec Prog Horm Res 30:431–473, 1974
55. Massry SG, Stein R, Garty J, et al.: Skeletal resistance to the calcemic action of parathyroid hormone in uremia: Role of $1,25(OH)_2D_3$. Kidney Int 9:467–474, 1976
56. Broadus AE, Horst RL, Lang R, et al.: The importance of circulating 1,25-dihydroxyvitamin D in the pathogenesis of hypercalciuria and renal stone formation in primary hyperparathyroidism. N Engl J Med: 302:421–426, 1980
57. Drezner MK, Feinglos MN: Osteomalacia due to 1α,25-dihydroxycholecalciferol deficiency: Association with a giant cell tumor of bone. J Clin Invest 60:1046–1053, 1977
58. Haussler MR, Baylink DJ, Hughes MR: The assay of 1α,25-dihydroxyvitamin D_3: Physiologic and pathologic modulation of circulating hormone levels. Clin Endocrinol 5:151S–165S, 1976
59. Brickman AS, Gerszik D, Norman AW, et al.: 24,25-dihydroxyvitamin D_3. A sterol with unique effects in normal man. Clin Res 26:411A, 1978
60. Kanis JA, Cundy T, Bartlett M, et al.: Is 24,25-dihydroxycholecalciferol a calcium-regulating hormone in man? Br Med J 1:1382–1386, 1978
61. Peacock M: Renal stone disease and bone disease in primary hyperparathyroidism and their relationship to the action of parathyroid hormone on calcium absorption. In Talmage RV, Owen M, Parsons JA (eds): Calcium regulating hormones: Proceedings of the Fifth Parathyroid Hormone Conference. Amsterdam, Excerpta Medica, 1975, pp 78–81
62. Lloyd HM: Primary hyperparathyroidism: An analysis of the role of the parathyroid tumor. Medicine 47:53–71, 1968
63. Bordier PJ, Arnaud C, Hawker C, et al.: Relationship between serum immunoreactive parathyroid hormone, osteoclastic and osteocyte bone resorptions and serum calcium in primary hyperparathyroidism and osteomalacia. In Frame B, Parfitt AM, Duncan H (eds): Clinical Aspects Metabolic Bone Disease: Proceedings of the International Symposium, 1972. International Congress Series No. 270. New York, Elsevier, 1973, pp 222–228
64. Meunier P, Vignon G, Bernard C, et al.: Quantitative bone histology as applied to the diagnosis of hyperparathyroid states. In Frame B, Parfitt AM, Duncan H (eds): Clinical Aspects Metabolic Bone Disease, Proceedings of the International Symposium, 1972 International Congress Series No 270. New York, Elsevier, 1973, pp 215–221
65. Schneider AB, Sherwood LM: Pathogenesis and management of hyperparathyroidism and other hypocalcemic disorders. Metabolism 24:871–898, 1975
66. Breslau NA, Pak CYC: Hypoparathyroidism. Metabolism 28:1261–1276, 1979
67. Hughes MR, Brumbaugh PF, Haussler MR, et al.: Regulation of serum 1α, 25-dihydroxyvitamin D_3 by calcium and phosphate in the rat. Science 190:578–580, 1975

68. Chase LR, Melson GL, Aubach GD: Pseudohypoparathyroidism. Defective excretion of 3′5′-AMP in response to parathyroid hormone. J Clin Invest 48:1833–1844, 1969
69. Drezner MK, Neelon FA, Haussler M, et al.: 1,25-dihydroxycholecalciferol deficiency: The probable cause of hypocalcemia and metabolic bone disease in pseudohypoparathyroidism. J Clin Endocrinol Metab 42:621–628, 1976
70. Drezner MK, Haussler MR: Normocalcemic pseudohypoparathyroidism: Association with normal vitamin D_3 metabolism. Am J Med 66:503–508, 1979
71. Fraser D, Kooh SW, Kind HP, et al.: Pathogenesis of hereditary vitamin D-dependent rickets: An inborn error of vitamin D metabolism involving defective conversion of 25-hydroxyvitamin D to 1α, 25-dihydroxyvitamin D. N Engl J Med 289:817–822, 1973
72. Scriver CR, Reade TM, DeLuca HF, et al.: Serum 1,25-dihydroxyvitamin D levels in normal subjects and in patients with hereditary rickets or bone disease. N Engl J Med 299:976–979, 1978
73. Brooks MH, Bell NH, Love L, et al.: Vitamin D-dependent rickets type II: Resistance of target organs to 1,25-dihydroxyvitamin D. N Engl J Med 298:996–999, 1978
74. Drezner MK, Harrelson JM: Newer knowledge of vitamin D and its metabolites in health and disease. Clin Orthop 139:206–231, 1979
75. Lewy J, Cabana E, Repetta H, et al.: Serum parathyroid hormone in hypophosphatemic vitamin D-resistant rickets. J Pediatr 81:294–300, 1972
76. Arnaud C, Glorieux F, Scriver C: Serum parathyroid hormone in X-linked hypophosphatemia. Science 173:845–847, 1971
77. Byers PD: The diagnostic value of bone biopsies. In Avioli LV and Krane SM (eds): Metabolic Bone Disease, Vol I. New York, Academic Press, 1977, p 215
78. Sorensen OH, Andersen RB, Christensen MS, et al.: Treatment of senile osteoporosis with 1α-hydroxyvitamin D_3. Clin Endocrinol (Suppl 7): 169S–175S, 1977
79. Avioli LV: Osteoporosis: Pathogenesis and therapy. In Avioli LV and Krane SM(eds): Metabolic Bone Disease, Vol I. New York, Academic Press 1977, p 336
80. Sitrin M, Meredith S, Rosenberg IH: Vitamin D deficiency and bone disease in gastrointestinal disorders. Arch Intern Med 138:886–888, 1978
81. Stamp TCB: Intestinal absorption of 25-hydroxycholecalciferol. Lancet 2:121–123, 1974
82. Gertner JM, Lilburn M, Domenech M: 25-hydroxycholecalciferol absorption in steatorrhea and post gastrectomy osteomalacia. Br Med J 1:1310–1312, 1977
83. Teitelbaum SL, Halverson JD, Bates BS: Abnormalities of circulatory 25-OH vitamin D after jejunal-ileal bypass for obesity. Ann Intern Med 86:289–293, 1977
84. Long RG, Shiver RD, Wills MR, et al.: Serum 25-hydroxyvitamin D in untreated parenchymal and cholestatic liver disease. Lancet 2: 650–652, 1976
85. Yu JS, Walker-Smith JA, Burnard ED: Rickets, a common complication of neonatal hepatitis. Med J Aust 1:790–792, 1971
86. Stamp T, Flanagan R, Richens A, et al.: Anticonvulsant osteomalacia. In Copp DH, Talmage RV (eds): Endocrinology of Calcium Metabolism. Amsterdam, Excerpta Medica, 1978, pp 16–22
87. Goldstein DA, Oda Y, Kurokawa K, et al.: Blood levels of 25-hydroxyvitamin D in nephrotic syndrome. Ann Intern Med 87:664–667, 1977
88. Malluche HH, Goldstein DA, Massry SG: Osteomalacia and hyperparathyroid bone disease in patients with nephrotic syndrome. J Clin Invest 63:494–500, 1979
89. Prader A, Ielig R, Uehlinger E, et al.: Rachitis infolge Knochentumors. Helv Paediatr Acta 14:554–565, 1959
90. Meunier P, Edouard C, Courpron P, et al.: Morphometric analysis of osteoid in iliac trabecular bone: Dynamic significance of the osteoid parameter. In Norman AW, Schaeffer K, Grigoleit HG, von Herrath D, and Ritz E (eds): Vitamin D and Problems Related to Uremic Bone Disease. Hawthorne, New York, Walter de Gruyter, 1975, pp 149–155
91. Milch RA, Rall DP, Tobic JE: Fluoresence of tetracycline antibiotics in bone. J Bone Joint Surg 40:897–910, 1958

92. Jowsey J: The Bone Biopsy. New York, Plenum, 1977
93. David DS: Calcium metabolism in renal failure. Am J Med 58:48–56, 1975
94. Slatopolsky E, Rutherford WE, Hruska K, et al.: How important is phosphate in the pathogenesis of renal osteodystrophy? Arch Intern Med 138:848–852, 1978
95. Brickman AS, Massry SG, Norman AW, et al.: On the mechanism and nature of the defect in intestinal absorption of calcium in uremia. Kidney Int (Suppl 2):S113–S117, 1975
96. Slatopolsky E, Hruska K, Rutherford WE: Current concepts of parathyroid hormone and vitamin D metabolism: Pertubations in chronic renal disease. Kidney Int (Suppl 2): S90–S96, 1975
97. Russell JE, Avioli LV: Effect of progressive end stage renal insufficiency on bone mineral-collagen maturation. Kidney Int (Suppl 2): S97–S101, 1975
98. Bordier PJ, Marie PJ, Arnaud CD: Evolution of renal osteodystrophy: Correlation of bone histomorphometry and serum mineral and immunoreactive parathyroid hormone values before and after treatment with calcium carbonate and 25-hydroxycholecalciferol. Kidney Int (Suppl 2): S102–S112, 1975
99. Llach F, Massry SG, Singer FR, et al.: Skeletal resistance to endogenous parathyroid hormone in patients with early renal failure: A possible cause for secondary hyperparathyroidism. J Clin Endocrinol Metab 41:339–345, 1975
100. Slatopolsky E, Caglar S, Pennell JP, et al.: On the pathogenesis of hyperparathyroidism in chronic experimental renal insufficiency in the dog. J Clin Invest 50:492–499, 1971
101. Slatopolsky E, Caglar L, Bradowska L, et al.: On the prevention of secondary hyperparathyroidism in experimental chronic renal disease using ''proportional reduction'' of dietary phosphorus intake. Kidney Int 2:147–151, 1972
102. Rutherford WE, Bordier P, Marie P, et al.: Phosphate control and 25-hydroxycholecalciferol administration in preventing experimental renal osteodystrophy in the dog. J Clin Invest 60:332–341, 1977
103. Coburn JW, Koppel MH, Brickman AS, et al.: Study of intestinal absorption of calcium in patients with renal failure. Kidney Int 3:264–272, 1973
104. Massry SG, Goldstein DA, Malluche HH: Current status of the use of $1,25(OH)_2D_3$ in the management of renal osteodystrophy. Kidney Int 18:409–418, 1980
105. Slatopolsky E, Gray R, Adams ND, et al.: Low serum levels of $1,25(OH)_2D_3$ are not responsible for the development of secondary hyperparathyroidism in early renal failure. Proceedings of the 11th Annual Meeting of the American Society of Nephrology 11:99A, 1978
106. Massry SG, Coburn JW, Lee DBN, et al.: Skeletal resistance to parathyroid hormone in renal failure. Studies in 105 human subjects. Ann Intern Med 78:357–364, 1973
107. Parkinson IS, Feest TG, Ward MK, et al.: Fracturing dialysis osteodystrophy and encephalopathy. An epidemiological study. Lancet 1:406–409, 1979
108. Ward MK, Feest TG, Ellis HA, et al.: Osteomalacic dialysis osteodystrophy; evidence for a water borne aetological agent, probably aluminum. Lancet 1:841–845, 1978
109. Platts MM, Goode CC, Hislop JS: Composition of the domestic water supply and the incidence of fractures and encephalopathy in patients on home dialysis. Br Med J 2:657–660, 1977
110. Malluche HH, Ritz E, Lange HP, et al.: Bone histology in incipient and advanced renal failure. Kidney Int 9:355–361, 1976
111. Ellis HA, Pierides AM, Feest TG, et al.: Histopathology of renal osteodystrophy with particular reference to the effect of 1α-hydroxy vitamin D_3 in patients treated by long-term dialysis. Clin Endocrinol (Suppl 7): 31S–38S, 1977
112. Alfrey AC, LeGendre GR, Kaehny WD: The dialysis encephalopathy syndrome. N Engl J Med 294:184–188, 1976
113. Brickman AS, Sherrard DJ, Jowsey J, et al.: 1,25-dihydroxycholecalciferol: Effect on skeletal lesions and plasma parathyroid hormone levels in uremic osteodystrophy. Arch Intern Med 134:883–888, 1974

114. Berl T, Berns AS, Huffer WE, et al.: 1,25 Dihychoxycholecalciferol effects in chronic dialysis. Ann Intern Med 88:774–780, 1978
115. Kanis JA, Cundy T, Earnshaw M, et al.: Treatment of renal bone disease with 1-α-hydroxylated derivatives of vitamin D_3. Q J Med 48:289–322, 1979
116. Brickman AS, Coburn JW, Massry SG, et al.: 1,25-dihydroxy vitamin D_3 in normal man and patients with renal failure. Ann Intern Med 80:161–168, 1974
117. Ahmed KY, Varghese Z, Wills MR, et al.: Long-term effects of small doses of 1,25-dihydroxycholecalciferol in renal osteodystrophy. Lancet 1:629–632, 1978
118. Sherrard DJ, Coburn JW, Brickman AS, et al.: Skeletal response to treatment with 1,25-dihydroxy vitamin D in renal failure. Contr Nephrol 18:92–97, 1980
119. Coburn JW: Renal osteodystrophy. Kidney Int 17:677–693, 1980
120. Coburn JW, Sherrard DJ, Brickman AS, et al.: A skeletal mineralizing defect in dialysis patients; a syndrome resembling osteomalacia but unrelated to vitamin D. Contr Nephrol 18:172–183, 1980
121. Prior JC, Cameron EC, Ballan HS, et al.: Experience with 1,25-dihydroxycholecalciferol therapy in patients undergoing hemodialysis with progressive vitamin D-treated osteodystrophy. Am J Med 67:583–589, 1979
122. Coburn JW, Wong EGC, Sherrard DJ, et al.: Use of 24,25-dihydroxy Vitamin D_3 in dialysis osteomalacia: Preliminary results. Clinical Research 28:532A, 1980
123. Friberg L, Piscator M, Nordberg GF, et al.: Cadmium in the Environment, ed 2. Cleveland, CRC Press, 1974
124. Gonick HC: Trace metals and the kidney. Mineral Electrolyte Metab 1:107–120, 1978
125. Rosen JF, Chesney RW, Hamstra A, et al.: Reduction in 1,25-dihydroxy vitamin D in children with increased lead absorption. N Engl J Med 302:1128–1131, 1980
126. Hahn TJ: Corticosteroid-induced osteopenia. Arch Intern Med 138:882–885, 1978
127. Hahn TJ, Halstead LR, Haddad JG Jr: Serum 25-hydroxy vitamin D concentration in patients receiving chronic corticosteroid therapy. J Lab Clin Med 90:399–404, 1977
128. Klein RG, Arnaud SB, Gallagher JJ, et al.: Intestinal calcium absorption in exogenous hypercortisolism. J Clin Invest 60:253–268, 1977

INDEX